Bioethics
a nursing perspective

third edition

To Olga and Bill, with thanks for your many years of friendship, and unwavering support of my work.

You should not decide until you have
heard what both have to say.

Aristophanes, *The Wasps*

Nobody is infallible; and for that reason many
different points of view are needed.

Mary Midgley, *Can't we make moral judgements?*

Bioethics
a nursing perspective

third edition

Megan-Jane Johnstone

RN, BA, PhD, FRCNA, FCN (NSW)
Professor of Nursing
Department of Nursing and Public Health
Faculty of Biomedical and Health Sciences and Nursing
RMIT University, Melbourne

SAUNDERS
An Imprint of Elsevier Science
Philadelphia London Toronto Montreal Sydney Tokyo

Saunders
is an imprint of Elsevier Science

Elsevier (Australia) Pty Limited
30–52 Smidmore Street, Marrickville, NSW 2204

This edition © 1999
by Elsevier (Australia) Pty Limited ACN 000 910 583
Reprinted 2000, 2002

First edition published 1989
Second edition published 1994

National Library of Australia Cataloguing-in-Publication Data

---

Johnstone, Megan-Jane 1955–
Bioethics: a nursing perspective

3rd ed
Includes index.
ISBN 0 7295 3403 0.

1. Nursing ethics. 2. Bioethics. 3. Medical ethics
I. Title.

174.2

Publishing Services Manager: Helena Klijn
Project managed, edited and indexed by Forsyth Editorial Services
Cover design by Maria Miranda
Typeset by Sun Photoset
Printed in Australia by Southwood Press Pty Limited

Contents

Preface

It is ten years since the first edition of this book was published, and it is no small measure of the importance of the topic that there presently exists a demand for this third revised edition. In 1989, when the first edition of this work was published, very little had been written on bioethics from a nursing perspective, and nursing ethics itself was largely invisible and poorly understood. This situation made it very difficult for nurses to have their concerns about ethical issues heard, let alone addressed, and many nurses suffered intolerably at both a personal and a professional level as a result.

At the time of its 1989 publication, *Bioethics: a nursing perspective* stood as the first text of its kind to be written from an Australasian perspective, and attempted to give 'visibility' to nursing concerns about ethical issues in health care and to remedy the palpable lack of understanding about nursing ethics that existed at the time. It also attempted to give nursing a much needed 'voice' in both the health professional and bioethics literature, and to 'defend' a nursing point of view. To this end, a key aim (and focus) of the first and second editions was to demonstrate that bioethics was a legitimate professional concern for nurses and one that warranted serious attention by all concerned. In this aim, the first two editions succeeded beyond all expectations.

Today, much has changed. Significantly, the 'defensive' position taken in the first two editions is no longer warranted, and has for the most part been abandoned in this third revised edition. Nursing ethics now enjoys recognition and respect as a legitimate and discrete field of inquiry and practice in its own right, and is no longer regarded (as it once was) as being merely adjunct to the ethical concerns of the medical profession and medical ethics. Nursing ethics is taught in all undergraduate nursing education programs around Australia, and increasing numbers of nurses are undertaking important research and scholarship in the area. This third revised edition reflects this change in attitude — not merely by the addition of new material, but by the removal and/or radical revision of large portions of the discussions advanced in the previous two editions.

Notable among the revisions and additions included in this third revised edition (and which distinguishes it from the previous two editions) are the new and/or expanded discussions on the following issues: the changing moral world and its implications for nurses (including the problems of moral pluralism, postmodern ethics, and the demise of traditional moral certainty in health care domains); the history and nature of mainstream bioethics and its relationship to nursing ethics; the nature and implications of nursing ethics (including a new and more substantive definition of what constitutes and distinguishes nursing ethics from other branches of ethics); theoretical perspectives informing ethical practice in nursing (including theories of moral justification, the revitalisation of other previously abandoned traditional perspectives on ethics such as virtue ethics and casuistry ethics; the role of emotion in moral decision-making; and the relationship between virtue theory and nursing as ethical practice); moral problems in nursing (including moral stress, moral distress and moral perplexity in nursing care contexts); patients' rights issues (including paternalism and informed consent; the right to be treated with respect); human rights and the mentally ill; ethical issues associated with the reporting of child abuse; ethical issues associated with matters of life and death (including abortion, euthanasia and assisted suicide, unassisted suicide and parasuicide, and 'Not For Treatment'

[NFT] decisions); and the promotion of ethical practice in nursing (including the formulation and enactment of meaningful standards of ethical nursing conduct, providing preventive and remedial nursing ethics education programs, ethical management and improving the moral culture of the organisations in which nurses work, supporting nursing research and scholarship, and taking political action aimed at achieving public policy and law reforms to facilitate the ethical practice of nursing). In making these revisions, it is hoped that nurses will be assisted further in their quest to gain knowledge and understanding about the ethical issues affecting their practice, to use this knowledge and understanding to challenge and change the status quo in health care contexts — particularly where this is not conducive to the welfare and wellbeing of patients — and thereby to *make a difference* to the moral world in which they live and work.

Acknowledgments

The writing and revision of this text would not have been possible without the stalwart support of several of my friends and colleagues. My deepest gratitude goes to my good friend and colleague, Olga Kanitsaki AM, of La Trobe University, who read large portions of the original manuscript as well as the revised manuscript for the third edition, and made many helpful suggestions. I am particularly indebted to Olga for sharing her views on the fundamental relationship between culture and ethics, and the important role that culture plays in shaping and mediating our ethical thinking and conduct. The final text is, however, entirely my own, as are any weaknesses, omissions or mistakes. My deep gratitude is also due to my good friend, Dr Bill McArthur, who has always supported me and taken a keen interest in my work. His unwavering encouragement and good advice over the years has, on many occasions, given me the courage to 'fight the battles' which this work represents. The dedication of this third edition to Olga and Bill stands as a small token of my appreciation for their support.

Special thanks and acknowledgment are also due to the many people (nurses, psychotherapists, patients/clients, students and others) whose generosity in sharing their experiences and views has, in many ways, made writing and revising this text possible. I especially want to thank Naomi Halpern, psychotherapist in private practice, for sharing her insights on the nature and aftermath of child abuse. This sharing has been influential in my writing and including in this edition the new chapter entitled 'Ethical issues associated with the reporting of child abuse', although the chapter as it stands is entirely my own work. And I wish to thank Ekura Emery for her helpful comments on the case discussed in this text involving a young Maori woman who gave birth prematurely to a 20-week-old fetus. Thanks are also due to my colleagues and friends Sue Harvey and Lois Kennedy (of the Austin & Repatriation Medical Centre in Melbourne) and Gay Edgecombe (Associate Professor at RMIT University in Melbourne) for their continuous encouragement, enthusiasm and unending belief in me during the arduous months of revising this third edition.

I also wish to acknowledge the Royal College of Nursing, Australia (RCNA) which has, over the past decade, provided me with many important opportunities to contribute to the advancement of nursing ethics in Australia. In several respects, the status of nursing ethics in Australia would not have improved had it not been for the foresight and professional support of the RCNA.

Finally, these acknowledgments would not be complete without thanks being given to Gina Brandwood and Helena Klijn, at Harcourt Brace & Company, and Forsyth Editorial Services for their contribution to the successful production of this text.

Chapter 1

The changing moral world and its implications for the nursing profession[1]

Introduction

Nurses live and work in a world that has become — and will remain — unequivocally pluralistic in nature and outlook. To put this another way, nurses now live and work in a world in which there is no one single reality, but many coexisting realities (multiple realities) among which they must choose (Anderson 1990).

The development of a pluralistic world view has had a significant impact on our moral ways of seeing, believing and acting. The more pluralistic our world has become, the more value systems there have been available to us and the more complex our ideas about what constitutes the moral life and how best to achieve it (Anderson 1990; Engelhardt 1996). Little wonder then, that in the 1990s, the world in which we live, and the contexts in which we work, have all become increasingly characterised by moral indiscernability, ambiguity, uncertainty, controversy and perplexity (Bauman 1993; Wildes 1993, 1994; Wear et al. 1994; Singer and Kuhse 1994; McCullough 1995; Kane 1994). For some, these difficulties have been compounded by what they refer to as the 'postmodern predicament' wherein, it is assumed, 'we no longer share any common grounds to which we might appeal for the adjudication of our differences' (Wear et al. 1994, p. 147; see also Engelhardt 1996). To add to this predicament, we continue to face moral problems in our day-to-day personal and professional lives, we continue to worry about whether the moral choices we make are 'correct', and continue to suffer the moral perplexity and distress that inevitably follows from 'not getting it right' or from being unable, for various reasons, to translate our moral reflections and judgments into action. Against this backdrop, at least two important questions can be raised: what are the implications of this scenario for the nursing profession? and how can nurses be prepared best to deal with them? In this and the following chapters of this book, attention will be given to addressing these questions.

---

1. An earlier version of this chapter was presented and published as the Inaugural Bennett Lecture: Moral Controversy and the Search for Solution: Some Critical Reflections for the Nursing Profession, Faculty of Nursing, RMIT University, 20th Year Anniversary Celebration Dinner, Melbourne, 7 September, 1995. It has been revised for publication in this text.

The demise of traditional moral certainty

There is increasing recognition that our moral standards are not absolute, but are 'ever-changing social creations' (adapted from Anderson 1990, p. x). As Anderson puts it:

> Morality ... is the product of hard-won wisdom, a way of being that expresses wherever a person happens to be along the (hopefully) never-ending path of understanding and reunderstanding life, constructing and reconstructing the rules of relationship between self and others.
>
> (Anderson 1990, p. 156)

He goes on to point out that many have come to accept 'morality, and moral discourse, as a living and central element in human existence', explaining:

> We see our interpersonal relationships as collaborative efforts in constructing values. We see education as, among other things, a training in the skills of moral reasoning — morality not merely handed down but learned and created and re-created out of experience. And when there is conflict about that, as there inevitably will be, we accept the conflict also as an arena for expressing and creating values ... Morals are not being handed down from the mountaintop on graven tablets; they are being created by people out of the challenges of the times. The morals of today are not the morals of yesterday, and they will not be the morals of tomorrow.
>
> (Anderson 1990, pp. 258–59)

This new understanding of morality as a 'constructed reality' has, among other things, provided an arena for 'expressing and creating [new] values' (Anderson 1990, p. 258). However, it has also seriously challenged our traditional certainty about moral matters. With this loss of certainty has also come a loss of confidence about our choices: while our choices and decisions might be 'right', they might also be 'wrong'. Thus, at the end of the day, we are left concerned about whether we — and others — have succeeded in 'getting it right' (Smith 1994).

The demise of our traditional moral certainties (if indeed such certainties ever existed) has witnessed not just the emergence of moral disagreement between people (this, in itself, is not problematic and has always existed), but the emergence of *radical* and *irreconcilable* moral disagreement (Boyle 1994; Milo 1986). This latter type of disagreement is very serious since, unlike 'ordinary' moral disagreement, people's viewpoints are so radically incompatible and so implacably opposing in nature, there is no hope whatsoever of achieving any acquiescence, compromise, agreement or reconciliation between the disputing parties. Further, in the absence of a once (classically) posited single 'universal' moral truth, and the moral certainty and associated confidence this once brought to the Western World's moral deliberations, there is no 'objective' measure against which radically competing views can be soundly adjudicated. The pessimistic outcome of this kind of scenario is that differing and competing opinions will remain polarised, with each of the disputing parties whose opinions are at issue insisting on the absolute 'truth' and 'rightness' of their own respective viewpoints.

The rise and manifestation of moral fanaticism

Regrettably, radical moral disagreements have not always been confined to the relatively safe boundaries of philosophical texts. In recent times, we have increasingly seen these disagreements spill out into the wider community, with strangers not only intruding in scandalous ways into the private lives and grief of innocent others, but committing extraordinary acts of violence against those whose viewpoints they do not share. For example, in 1993, Dr David Gunn, a medical practitioner engaged in abortion work at the Pensacola Women's Medical Services clinic in the Unites States, was fatally wounded by an anti-abortion demonstrator engaged in a pro-life protest outside of the clinic (Rohter 1993, p. 7). Described by authorities as the first slaying of its kind in the United States, the incident exemplified the increasing violence against abortion clinics and workers across the nation. In regard to the death of Dr Gunn, Rescue America (a pro-life group) was reported as commenting that 'while Gunn's death is unfortunate, it's also true that quite a number of babies' lives will be saved' (Rohter 1993, p. 3).

Just over a year later, again in the Unites States, a second doctor was killed outside an abortion clinic by a pro-life protester (Sharkey 1994, p. 3). At the time, a British commentator on anti-abortion protests in the United States was reported as saying that the slaying was 'the start of the new Pro-Life movement, the new activism' (Sharkey 1994, p. 3). This new 'pro-life activism' has involved bombing and arson attacks against clinics, and the murder and injury of health workers. It has been reported that 'one hundred per cent of the bombers, arsonists and now murderers are Christian fundamentalists' (Sharkey 1994, p. 4). The chances of these fundamentalists pursuing less violent forms of activism are considered to be slim.

The United States of America is not, of course, the only country troubled by the increasingly public and sometimes violent manifestations of radical moral disagreements about bioethical issues. Australia has encountered its own problems. For example, in 1995 the Brisbane *Courier-Mail* reported that a member of the group called Christians Speaking Out stated that 'it is a Christian's duty to stop abortionists by any means' (13 May, 1995). The member is also reported as condoning the killing of abortionists arguing that it was 'justifiable homicide' (*Courier-Mail* 13 May, 1995).

Perhaps one of the most poignant Australian examples of an aggressively intrusive if not violent manifestation of a radical moral disagreement, however, can be found in the much publicised Victorian case involving a severely disabled new born known under the legal pseudonym 'Baby M' (Kuhse 1992). The case became the subject of media attention and intense public debate when it was revealed that the local Right to Life association (a pro-life group) had become interested in the case, and had intruded in unwanted ways into the private lives and grief of the parents of the baby. In brief, the Right to Life had become privy to information that doctors at the baby's admitting hospital had decided to treat Baby M 'conservatively' and that, because of this, her chances of survival were remote. Upon learning this, the group tried unsuccessfully to gain access to the baby's parents to discuss 'other possible treatments for the child'. After visiting the hospital, and failing to achieve their objectives, members of the Right to Life reported the case to the police (Kuhse 1992). In the process of trying to access and lobby the parents to reconsider their decision about Baby M's treatment, the vice-president of Right to Life, Father Eugene Ahern, had gone to the parents' home in the middle of the night and slipped a letter under their door. Kuhse (1992) reports:

> In that letter, Father Ahern said that he was concerned that a deliberate decision had been made to allow Baby M to die, spoke of the guilt felt by parents who did not seek treatment for their spina bifida babies, and told

them that another couple had offered to care for the child, no matter how disabled she might be.

(Kuhse 1992, p. 236)

The actions of Right to Life members in this case were widely reported on by the media and, significantly, led to public outrage. Many onlookers viewed the Right to Life's actions as being unacceptably intrusive and even outrageous given that they occurred at a time when, to borrow from Kuhse (1992, p. 236), the parents of Baby M 'were suffering the anguish and grief that almost inevitably follows the birth of a severely disabled child'.

The lessons of moral fanaticism

Upon considering these and similar real-life case scenarios (and there are many of them [see, for example, Singer and Kuhse 1994; Macklin 1993]), it is perhaps understandable that we feel a certain degree of anxiety about the moral fanaticism — and the intolerable outcomes of this fanaticism — that have been exemplified. These cases are frightening insofar as they demonstrate the extent to which 'bioethics touches upon moral issues that men and women view with sharp disagreement' (Wildes 1994, p. 124), the propensity for these disagreements to spill over into acts of aggression and violence, and the disconcerting impotence of our ethical theories and practices to prevent these outcomes from occurring in the first place and/or supply remedies once they do occur. Another frightening aspect of this modern day moral fanaticism is that it appears to be on the increase, and no-one or thing seems to be able to stop it. The lessons that are inherent in these contemporary examples of radical moral disagreements are, then, important ones, and while we may choose to either accept or reject them, we cannot — and should not — ignore them. However, the question remains what, if anything, can we do about this state of affairs?

In search of solutions

It is understandable that when faced with the challenges posed by the moral problems of human life, people will want, need and search for answers to help guide them in their deliberations on what constitutes the morally right thing to do, and how best to do it (and, of importance to this discussion, nurses are no exception here). Further, as Wear (1991, p. 69) points out in the context of discussing the challenges posed by bioethics in clinical practice settings, 'it seems simply human to want simple answers and quick solutions to ... vexing and poignant problems'. Perhaps it is also 'simply human' to be tempted by 'Kentucky fried ethics' — or 'assembly line' ethics — and its promise of simple answers rapidly supplied (the moral principlism espoused by mainstream bioethics is an example here). The trouble is, however, that in our quest to find 'the answers', 'the solutions', 'the remedies', call them what you will, we have ended up with too many answers and not enough questions. Paradoxically, this has tended to compound rather than remedy the problems initially experienced, with people of differing moral persuasions being driven further apart rather than being brought closer together by their respective 'final solutions'.

In short, the multitude of 'final answers' discovered has served more to fragment and alienate the moral world, rather than bring it closer together as an orderly and harmonious whole striving toward a viable and peaceable future. At the end of the day we are well positioned to learn that, as Auschwitz and Hiroshima have long since warned, there are unimaginable dangers in embracing and trusting 'final solutions' (see Fasching 1993, p. 7). So, where do we go from here?

Toward a pluralistic vision of human life

Whether we wish to accept it or not, it cannot be ignored that human life has become 'multidimensional in a way it never was before' (Anderson 1990, p. 148). Furthermore, it is necessary to recognise that this multidimensionality and the multiple realities embedded in it are not going to go away. The important thing, however, is for people not to be frightened by this scenario. Rather than seeing the multidimensionality of human life (and the multiple realities that are constitutive of it) as positing a 'chaos of choices' from which one must flee (reactively) into the embrace of the prescriptive certainty and predictable orderliness of moral fundamentalism, it is important to view this situation as a creative opportunity for developing something new (Anderson 1990; Zohar 1991; Zohar and Marshall 1993). This, of course, will require us not just to think about new things, but to develop a whole new way of thinking.

In particular, we need to develop a whole new way of thinking about the moral world, our position(s) within it, and what it is we ought to be aiming to achieve. It will also involve learning to live with many points of view; that is, to adopt a pluralistic vision of human life (Zohar and Marshall 1993). If we do not do these things, and if we do not accommodate the 'multiplicities and diversities of our new experience', we will not actualise the multiple possibilities of a 'better' (moral) life (Zohar and Marshall 1993). Instead, it is almost certain that the world will become so hopelessly fragmented, and its constitutive multiple dimensionalities and realities so alienated, that we will not survive.

In the past, when confronted by the moral problems of life, it has been 'too easy to reach solutions that fail to do justice to the difficulty of the problem' (Nagel 1991, p. xi). Indeed, we do not have to look far to see that many of the answers gained and the solutions reached in contemporary bioethics have been found seriously deficient and woefully inadequate when applied to and in the concrete circumstances of life. What is required to help remedy this situation is a mind set that not only seeks to ask questions, but seeks to *call into question* 'things as they are' (Freire 1970, 1972). There also needs to be a recognition that when faced with morally perplexing issues:

- we 'need to think better and harder' about the issues in question (Boyle 1994);
- we need to remember that moral indiscernability, uncertainty, controversy and disagreement can and do have many causes, both practical and theoretical (McCullough 1995); and
- we need to accept that addressing moral problems in a sound and effective manner requires an appeal to a moral schema that recognises a *multiplicity of possible solutions* to a given problem, and that a moral schema which insists on there being just one single correct answer to a given moral problem may compound rather than remedy that problem.

In other words, what is required is a whole new approach to thinking about and responding to moral issues. One such approach (quantum morality) will be considered in Chapter 15 of this text (under the subheading 'Moral decision-making by institutional ethics committees').

Moral controversies and the responsibilities of the nursing profession

Like other domains, the health care domain is not immune from and cannot escape the social, cultural and political impact of the pendulous backlashing swings between the extremes of fragmentation on the one hand, and fundamentalism on the other, of which the present traditionalist and inerrantist (or literalist)[2] backlashes against postmodernism is an example (Anderson 1990, pp. 14–17; Friedman 1994, p. 39). Nor can it escape the radical moral disagreements that are inherent in the swinging polarisations of these positions. As professionals working in the health care domain it is, then, very clear that nurses like other health care professionals cannot escape the tensions that are being caused by the radically opposing and competing moral viewpoints that are presently pulling the health care arena and indeed the world apart. An important question to arise here is: how can the nursing profession best respond to this predicament?

There is, of course, no simple 'final answer' to this question. Nevertheless there is at least one crucial point that needs to be made, and it is this: it is vitally important that nurses learn to recognise the cyclical processes of social and cultural change, and realise that they themselves are participants in this change. Once realising this, they also need to learn that, as participants in these cyclical transformations, they are positioned and have a stringent moral responsibility to sensitively and artfully advocate for the mediation of the extreme and multiple positions they might (and very often do) find themselves caught between (see, for example, Bishop and Scudder 1987; Andersen 1990; Winslow and Winslow 1991). Where able, they also have a moral responsibility to facilitate this mediation by acting as mediators themselves. However, the additional point needs to be made that fulfilling these responsibilities requires much more than ordinary commonsense and intuition. As well, it requires a sophisticated 'moral competency' that involves nurses:

- being well informed about ethical issues in nursing;
- having moral knowledge; and
- having a complex range of learned skills and guided experience that will enhance their ability to act wisely and creatively as reflective moral agents when confronted with moral problems (Johnstone 1998).

Such skills include the ability: to 'read the world' — to not only question, but to call into question 'things as they are'; to anticipate moral problems and take the necessary action to prevent them from occurring in the first place (otherwise known as 'preventive ethics' [McCullough 1995]); to think critically and reflectively about emergent and emerging moral issues; to discern a range of possible solutions to moral problems identified; to communicate effectively with others; to respect, listen to, understand and be compassionate toward others; to be tolerant, flexible, creative and imaginative when dealing with and attempting to resolve moral problems; to act as a moral negotiator and mediator when

---

2. Inerrantism or literalism advances the doctrine 'of the literal truth of the Bible — one truth, one infallible and unerring truth' (Anderson 1990, pp. 15–17). Relativism, by this view, is seen as the enemy of truth and the enemy of society. In the United States of America the rise of inerrantism in some public and theological schools has seen teachers lose their jobs for teaching the relativity of truth (Anderson 1990, pp. 14–17).

confronted by competing moral viewpoints; to maintain one's own personal and professional integrity; and to engage in the 'concrete exercise of the ethical virtues' (Reichlin 1994, p. 99; see also McCullough 1995; Boyle 1994; Khushf 1994; McCullough and Jonsen 1991; Winslow and Winslow 1991; Forrow et al. 1991; Johnstone 1998).

The ramifications of these 'new' (postmodern) moral responsibilities for the nursing profession, and not least for nursing education and research, are obviously enormous. They are not, however, insurmountable. So long as the nursing profession can keep its collective mind even and not become unbalanced by the 'vertigo of relativity' (Anderson 1990, p. 38), can view the present moral crisis of the world as a *crucial stage* or '*turning point*' (which, incidentally, is the meaning of the word crisis) rather than as destructive chaos, and can approach the future with vision, informed knowledge and skill, it will be able to correctly anticipate the challenges ahead in its practice, and in its education and research programs. By achieving these things, nurses will be enabled and empowered to honour their long-held historical, cultural and moral commitment to promoting and protecting human welfare and wellbeing.

Conclusion

Deciding and acting morally in a conflicted world, dealing constructively with moral controversy, finding satisfactory solutions to moral disagreements and coping effectively with moral distress are all complex, perplexing and demanding tasks. Compounding the problems associated with their achievement is the additional problem of the demise of traditional moral certainty and a concomitant rise in moral fanaticism which has seen acts of violence committed in the name of morality. It is, among other things, this increase in violence associated with moral fanaticism that underscores the need to find tenable solutions to moral disagreements and the controversies that have emerged as a result of them; that is, before they are transformed into acts of violence.

The responsibilities ahead may seem overwhelming. It needs to be remembered, however, that the nursing profession has a remarkable history of succeeding against the odds, and of overcoming what at times have seemed like insurmountable obstacles to the realisation of its ultimate professional and moral goals of practice (see, for example, Johnstone 1994). Nurses can and should take courage from this history in these difficult times, and have confidence in their ability to participate morally in the world and, through this participation, transform it into something better. It is hoped that the discussion and views advanced in this text will provide an important starting point for nurses to begin and/or advance further their quest to acquire the moral knowledge, understanding, wisdom and skills that are necessary to enable them to 'make a difference', morally speaking, when making difficult moral choices — and acting on those choices — not just in the course of their professional work, but in their personal lives as well.

Chapter 2

'Be good women but do not bother with a Code of Ethics'

Introduction

The nursing profession worldwide has a rich and distinctive history of identifying and responding substantively to ethical issues in nursing and health care domains. Since the inception of modern nursing in the last century, nurses globally have taken seriously their moral responsibilities as health care practitioners; they have also taken seriously the issues which have emerged as a consequence of their attempts to fulfil these responsibilities effectively (Johnstone 1993; Winslow and Winslow 1991). As the nursing literature dating as far back as Florence Nightingale's (1970) foundational text *Notes on nursing* demonstrates, the early modern nursing profession was as much concerned with the ethical dimensions of promoting the wellbeing and welfare of people requiring and or receiving nursing and health care as it is today. Further evidence of this can be found in the impressive chronology of nursing literature published on the subject over the past century. As Jameton (1984, p. 36) observes, since 1900 'no decade has passed ... without publication of at least one basic text in nursing ethics' with one of the first discrete texts on nursing ethics being published as early as 1888. Notable among some of the earliest nursing ethics texts are: Luckes' (1888) *Hospital sisters and their duties*, Dock's (1900) *Short papers on nursing subjects*, Parson's (1916) *Nursing problems and obligations*, Hampton Robb's (1903) *Nursing ethics: for hospital and private use*, Aikens' (1916) *Studies in ethics for nurses* (revised five times and still available in 1943), Gladwin's (1930) *Ethics talks to nurses*, and Densford and Everett's (1947) *Ethics for modern nurses: professional adjustments*. The plethora of nursing journal articles and public addresses published on the subject at the turn of this century (see Birnbach and Lewenson 1991, pp. 197–240), and the now vast body of 'new' nursing ethics literature published over the past twenty years, expands this volume of distinctive nursing ethics literature even further.

While it is conceded that some of the earliest discourses on nursing ethics and its practice might seem quaint by today's standards, it is important to note that others remain remarkably insightful, forthright, and visionary as examples to be given in this and subsequent chapters will show. Either way, it is important to treat these works in a way that reflects adequately their historical and cultural locations, and which does not undermine either the importance or significance of their moral intent even where their contents may be judged as 'lacking' by today's standards (a retrospective judgment that could, of course, be made of many other fields besides nursing ethics).

Despite this rich and accessible modern history of nursing ethics, it has not always been easy for members of the nursing profession to have their practice, views and concerns taken seriously by others outside of the profession. Even today, despite the remarkable progress that has been made by the nursing profession in recent years, the moral significance of nursing practice and the nurse–patient relationship, and the moral concerns of nurses generally, continue in varying ways to be marginalised, invalidated and/or even ignored altogether. This, in turn, has made it exceedingly difficult for nurses to fulfil their moral responsibilities as health professionals. Sometimes, nurses who have had the courage to speak out and/or take a stand on important issues have found themselves being either ridiculed, derogated, reprimanded or, worse, dismissed from their jobs (Johnstone 1994, 1998). This is especially so in cases where what nurses have had to say questioned and called into question the status quo and the powerful interests that were invested in it.

An examination of the field of inquiry appropriately named 'nursing ethics' would not be complete without also examining some of the powerful processes external to the nursing profession that have been influential in obstructing the development of nursing ethics generally and the ethical practice of nurses in particular. In this and the following chapters, attention will be given to examining some of these processes and influences. Meanwhile, it remains the task of this chapter to briefly examine some specific examples involving the medical profession, the media, interdisciplinary bioethics forums, the legal system (including formally constituted commissions of inquiry) and the internationally reputed *Encyclopedia of bioethics*, and the extent to which they have contributed to the marginalisation of a nursing perspective on ethical issues in health care.

The marginalisation of nursing ethics

Influences of the medical profession

Historically, members of the medical profession have not always understood or been supportive of the idea that nurses have 'moral agency' and are independently responsible and accountable for their own moral actions when caring for patients. The medical profession has been even less supportive of the idea and has rejected outright any thought that nurses are capable of and indeed make independent moral judgments and decisions when caring for patients, believing instead that only members of the medical profession are capable of these things which, in their view, are not always readily distinguishable from simply 'good medical judgments and decisions' being made.

One of the earliest advocates of a code of ethics for nurses in America was advised by a physician: 'Be good women but do not bother with a Code of Ethics' (Dock 1900, p. 37). Significantly, nurse leaders of the day were not impressed by this and other seemingly benevolent 'advice' offered to them by their medical colleagues. One leading nurse of the day, Lavinia Dock, was particularly critical of the role that the learned medical men were playing in regard to teaching nurses 'ethics', pointing out that what they were teaching was 'etiquette', not ethics which, although important, was 'not to be mistaken for ethics' (Dock 1900, p. 38). Dock goes on to fume:

> But what do they teach us of ethics? Well, this — as yet the extremist that we have heard — the nurse's whole duty, loyalty, and obedience begins and

ends in subordination to the doctor. Beyond this there is no horizon and outside of this she has no reason for existing.

(Dock 1900, p. 41)

Condemning the yearly recurring nursing ethics talks by doctors as 'wearisome, perennial rubbish', Dock goes on to conclude that in order to be ethical and to be able to fulfil their moral responsibilities as professional women, nurses *needed to be free* — to have 'the same amount of independence as any other moral being' (Dock 1900, pp. 41, 49). Anything less, she argued, would be to risk the moral cowardice of subordination and the slavishness of blind obedience.

Despite writing from a North American context, Dock's views were nevertheless relevant to the Australian context. An examination of early Australian nursing journals (such as *Una* and the *Australasian Nurses Journal*) reveals, for example, that Australian nurses were subjected just as much to the 'wearisome, perennial rubbish' on so-called 'nursing ethics' as were their North American counterparts, and in some instances were subjected to the exact same writings since many of the early articles addressing nursing ethics and professional conduct were reprinted from established Canadian and American nursing journals (Johnstone 1993, p. 36). And, despite being written almost 100 years ago, Dock's views remain remarkably pertinent to the present day context as the following examples demonstrate.

In 1986, a class of registered nurses undertaking a postgraduate diploma course in health administration attended a lecture on ethical issues in professional functioning. The lecturer (a medical doctor) told his audience, some of whom were senior nurse administrators, that 'nurses [were] unable to understand the intellectual concept of ethical models'. His reasoning seemed to be that nurses were 'too simplistic and practical, not generally capable of the objective, abstract thought that is required for this type of [ethical] decision' (*Report of the Study of Professional Issues in Nursing* 1988, p. 165). The lecturer is also alleged to have discouraged those present from attending a session on ethical decision-making that was planned for a neurosurgical conference later that year.

The attitude of this lecturer is by no means unique nor outdated. Anecdotal evidence abounds worldwide on how nurses are continually told by doctors that nursing practice is devoid of any sort of moral complication, and that it is nonsense for nurses to assume that they have any independent moral responsibilities when caring for patients. The nursing ethics literature also offers persuasive evidence of this kind of dismissive attitude toward nurses. For example, Yarling and McElmurry (1986) cite an American case in which a physician, responding to a particular case scenario, objected strongly to the suggestion that nurses have a moral duty to disclose information to terminally ill patients who request it. Medical students present at the time were, however, unanimous in suggesting that the nurse in the scenario, contrary to the physician's views, had a duty to disclose the information requested and that the physician's order was 'unjustifiable' (Yarling and McElmurry 1986, pp. 65–6).

When one of the medical students asked the physician why he disagreed with their view, the physician replied that 'the nurse's relationship with the patient is different than the physician's. It does not require independent moral judgment by the nurse' (Yarling and McElmurry 1986, p. 66). Another example of this kind of attitude can be found among some English physicians who participated in a survey investigating physician opinion on the nurse's duty to tell the truth to questioning patients. Of the nineteen doctors surveyed, most believed that nurses should avoid giving patients precise information in response to queries about their (the patients') health problems (*Nursing Times*, 11 July 1990, p. 9). Significantly, three doctors asserted that 'nurses should lie to patients if they were put on the spot by a direct question' (*Nursing Times*, 11 July 1990, p. 9). Like their American colleagues referred to above, it would seem that these English physicians do not recognise — or at least are reluctant to recognise — the moral nature of the nurse–patient relationship, or to concede that nurses have any independent moral (or professional) responsibilities to their patients (Johnstone 1994).

More recently, at a medical seminar on 'Not For Resuscitation' (NFR) which was attended by over 200 hospital staff (including doctors, nurses and legal representatives), once again medicocentric views about the assumed 'moral incompetence' and 'lack of independent moral (and legal) responsibilities' of nurses were advanced. A leading speaker at the seminar, a consultant cardiac physician, made it very plain that he believed: nurses had 'nothing to worry about' in the case of NFR directives, NFR had 'nothing to do with ethics', 'ordering NFR was simply a case of "good medical practice"', 'patients did not need or want to be troubled by the NFR decisions being made in their case and would become unduly distressed if given an opportunity to consent to such decisions', 'nurses were misguided in their moral beliefs about NFR practices', 'nurses were not doctors, lacked medical knowledge, and thus had no authority to question good medical practice', and 'nurses were obliged to follow medical orders'. A criminal barrister of law, who had also been invited to speak at the seminar, endorsed the physician's views. He argued, incorrectly, that where a patient dies as the result of a NFR directive, nurses would not face 'any trouble' because the patient would be 'brain dead' and that nurses thus 'could not be held negligently responsible for killing the patient because the patient would already be dead'. He also argued incorrectly that 'the doctor was ultimately responsible for the actions of nurses' and that 'nurses were obliged to follow doctors' orders'. It was only when a nurse speaker present at the seminar (and who was initially denied a right of reply) challenged these views with considerable evidence to the contrary, that both speakers retracted their contentions. She further challenged that if NFR directives being given at the hospital were so medically and legally correct, then why were doctors still refusing to formally document their NFR directives in patients' case notes as they did all other medical directives? (The issue of NFR directives and the problems nurses continue to experience in relation to them will be considered further in Chapter 14 of this text.)

The perception that nurses are not required to make independent moral judgments and do not have any independent moral responsibilities is not as uncommon as some would like to believe. Clay (1987), for example, writes:

> Many assume that because it is the doctors who decide when to turn off the ventilator, the lawyers who pronounce on issues such as surrogacy, the scientists who play around with *in vitro* fertilisation, and the managers and politicians who decide where limited health resources are put, then the nurses have no separate responsibilities. And there is a supposedly sympathetic way of thinking that wants to keep nurses out of all this intellectual and moral agonising.
>
> (Clay 1987, pp. 39–40)

Regardless of their popularity among those who choose to hold them, these views — that nursing practice is devoid of moral complication, that it is nonsense for nurses to presume they have any independent moral responsibilities when caring for patients, and that nurses are not required to make independent moral judgments in the nurse–patient relationship — are quite misleading and incorrect. Examples are given in the following chapters to illustrate clearly that nurses are just as much 'responders who encounter the claims of others' (in this instance, patients) as are doctors and other allied health professionals, and are just as stringently bound by moral considerations when responding to these claims (Beauchamp and Childress 1989; Johnstone 1987, pp. 31–2). Arguments are also given to show conclusively that nurses have as much independent moral responsibility for their actions (and omissions) as they have independent legal responsibility, and are just as accountable for their practice morally as they are legally. It is the contention of this book that to dismiss the moral authority and competence of nurses is to seriously undermine their ability to fulfil their very real moral responsibilities to patients. This, in turn, places at unacceptable risk the welfare interests and wellbeing of patients who may, in some circumstances, be dependent on nurses to advocate their welfare interests. Nurses must be accorded the recognition and legitimated authority necessary to enable them to fulfil their many and complex responsibilities as professionals bound by agreed standards of care. It is important for members of the medical profession to realise that nurses do have independent moral responsibilities (and, it should be added, legal responsibilities) when caring for patients and, indeed, can be (and have been) held independently accountable for their actions (Johnstone 1994, 1998). It is neither reasonable nor fair to expect nurses to ignore or violate their demonstrable responsibilities to patients and to practise below an acceptable standard of care.

It is acknowledged that many positive changes in attitude have occurred in recent years and that there does exist a much greater appreciation by many members of the medical profession of the kinds of moral burdens that nurses carry. There is also growing anecdotal evidence of a genuine willingness by members of both the medical and nursing professions to work together when needing to address difficult ethical issues in the workplace with demonstrable positive outcomes. However, it is also evident that there still exists considerable room for improvement. Perhaps an important starting point for securing this improvement is understanding that, contrary to what one general medical practitioner contends, nurses are not seeking to 'take clinical decisions away from the medical staff' (Rudd 1992, p. 15). Rather, nurses are trying to genuinely facilitate the realisation of morally just outcomes for patients for whose care they share responsibility.

The media

Members of the medical profession are not alone in their view that nurses have no independent moral concerns regarding ethical issues in health care. The media (with some notable exceptions involving sympathetic radio commentators and journalists) has also been extremely influential in marginalising and even obstructing a nursing perspective on important ethical issues in health care. In several respects, the nursing profession today is just as much at the mercy of unscrupulous lay editors as it was in the late 1800s and early 1900s. From the 1800s, the press succeeded in obstructing the professional development of nursing for almost thirty years until, in 1923, the International Council of Nurses (ICN) established an international nursing journal (the *International Nursing Review*), to be controlled by nurses and to reflect nursing opinion and nursing issues (Bridges 1968, p. 10). At the 1923 ICN Executive Committee meeting, at which the proposal to establish an international nursing journal was originally discussed, one of the delegates gave a solemn warning that reports in the lay press were a 'very serious peril to personal and professional liberty' (Bridges 1968, p. 10). Her warning is as pertinent today as it was in 1923.

An important example of the 'peril to nursing ethics' posed by the lay press can be found in a rough analysis of newspaper articles appearing in a major Melbourne newspaper during a ten-week period in 1988. Between 14 March 1988 and 20 May 1988, *The Age* featured over 38 main articles, 37 'Letters to the Editor', and over 52 'Access Age' comments on bioethical issues — mostly in relation to the Right to Die with Dignity movement and the Victorian State Government's then controversial Medical Treatment Bill (since proclaimed as the *Medical Treatment Act 1988*). These articles, letters and comments featured the views of doctors, lawyers, philosophers, theologians, sociologists — even groups such as the Right to Life movement — and, not least, the public at large (Johnstone 1988b, p. 8).

Superficially, it appears that the media in this instance made a stringent effort to present a balanced view on the issues under discussion. On closer inspection, however, it is clear that quite the reverse is true. For example, of the 127 or so items published, none (with the exception of a short 52-word 'Access Age' comment) seriously attempts to represent the views of nurses; yet nurses comprise the largest single body of health providers in the health care system. The term 'nurse' has generally been used (particularly by television media) in relation to the 'emotional' aspect of the moral dilemma or problem being discussed rather than the intellectual or 'rational' aspect. In some instances, the term 'nurse' has been loosely used in relation to the 'team' that is caring for a given patient — with acknowledgment being given more as a token gesture than as a serious recognition of the troubling dilemmas that nurses face in professional health care practice. In the 52-word comment that did appear, the author referred to an AIDS update article that had been recently printed in *The Age* and criticised the article for its 'glaring omission' of the contribution made by nurses in caring for AIDS patients (Mathews 1988, p. 12).

Editorial bias can also be found in individual newspaper reports and articles. For example, in an interesting newspaper article by Michael Pirrie (1987, p. 11), headed 'A disabled baby's right to live', the nursing perspective on the ethical issues under discussion was once again ignored. An analysis of the key terms used in this article is revealing: for example, the terms 'doctor', 'medical profession' and 'medical staff' are collectively mentioned at least fourteen times; the terms 'parents', 'family members', 'grandparents' and 'mother' are collectively mentioned at least eleven times; the terms 'medical treatment', 'treatment', 'medical care', 'medical practice', 'medical decisions' and 'medical technology' are collectively mentioned at least nine times; and the terms 'lawyers', 'judges' and 'the courts' are collectively mentioned at least three times. The term 'nurse', surprisingly, is mentioned only once, and the term 'nursing care' is not mentioned at all. The omission is extraordinary, given that nurses are involved twenty-four hours a day in caring for severely disabled newborns, and are inevitably concerned with the many moral problems that arise in this area.

In the same article, the views of five medical doctors, two judges, one other legal source, one philosopher and one sociologist are quoted. No parents or nurses are quoted.

The article also reported on a recommendation to set up a state advisory committee:

to set broad guidelines for those involved in caring for deformed babies, as well as to review difficult cases to be certain that the interests of the infant, as well as parents and medical staff, are given proper weight.

(Pirrie 1987, p. 11)

On the basis of this newspaper report, readers might well assume that nurses have no moral interests at stake in dilemmatic situations involving the care and treatment of disabled newborns, let alone an active care role. Such thinking would be quite mistaken. In these and similar situations nurses do have significant moral interests at stake — interests that are just as deserving of protection as are the interests of babies, parents and medical staff (Johnstone 1988c).

In fairness to *The Age*, it has reported on papers given by nurses at nursing ethics conferences, although not without constraint. A comprehensive report written by Ingrid Svendsen (1987) on two papers presented at a nursing ethics conference held at Monash University entitled 'The role of the nurse: doctors' handmaiden, patients' advocate or what?' was relegated to page 21 of the paper. Almost a year later, a well written and accurate report by Peter Schumpeter (1988) on a controversial paper on Not For Resuscitation directives presented at another nursing ethics conference was printed in *The Age*, but in the first edition only, and again on page 21. It is significant that the first edition generally goes to country areas only; copies are not generally kept on file. Only copies of the second or later editions are kept, which effectively means that the report has been lost to history. Another report, written by Philip McIntosh (1988), one of *The Age's* medical reporters, featured a very controversial paper presented by a nurse at the second South-East Asian Regional Nurses Conference at Dallas Brooks Hall on 12 May 1988. Interestingly, the report was not published in *The Age*, as might be expected, but in the *Australian Dr Weekly* — complete with a major front-page headline and photograph!

Significantly, the past decade has seen little change in media attitudes and biases against representing a substantive nursing perspective on important and controversial bioethical issues. An instructive example of this can be found in the media coverage given to a survey conducted by Kuhse and Singer (1992) exploring nurses' attitudes and practices in regard to euthanasia. In an unusual and extraordinary act of attentiveness, both the electronic and print media reported widely on the survey results, which were published initially in the *Australian Nurses Journal*. What made this particular instance of media attention so unusual is that, in the past, the media have demonstrated a great antipathy towards reporting on issues of specific concern and importance to the nursing profession. Even now, it is most unusual for the media to report on an article published in the *Australian Nurses Journal* and, what is more, to give it front-page headlines (see, for example, Magazanik 1992a, p. 1). Why then were nurses around the state not 'jumping for joy' at this unprecedented media attention?

The short answer is that, as in the past, the media fell far short of representing a realistic or complete nursing perspective on the issue being debated, and, as in the past, ended up marginalising rather than according authority to a nursing point of view. Further, at the time, many nurses felt that, whatever else the media debate was being motivated by, it was not a genuine concern for exploring and making public the many problems nurses have to deal with when caring for people who might otherwise be considered candidates for euthanasia. They even believed that the nursing profession was being exploited to further the ends of the pro-euthanasia lobby. Some nurses also regarded the media coverage of the survey as being grossly irresponsible on account of its failure to take into consideration public perceptions of, and the realities of, the role of nurses in pain assessment and management. What is not widely known is that the media coverage given to the euthanasia survey caused some patients considerable anxiety about whether or not to trust their nurses, and even, in some instances, resulted in patients refusing responsibly prescribed and needed narcotic analgesia which would otherwise have been administered by their attending nurses. This, in turn, caused the nurses involved to suffer considerable and unnecessary distress. Other nurses were just plain angry, and responded by arguing that the original survey, which involved the views of just 943 nurses (just over 1 per cent of nurses holding practising certificates in Victoria), was not representative of the 82 280 nurses who held practising certificates in Victoria, and therefore could not be relied on (see, for example, Cotterhill 1992, p. 4; Millership 1992, p. 4; Monkivitch 1992, p. 12; Muirden et al. 1992, p. 12; O'Connor 1992, p. 4).

In several respects, the nurses' anger and concerns were justified. Consider the following: on 2 March 1992, *The Age* carried the front-page headline: 'Nurses back euthanasia, survey finds' (Magazanik 1992a, p. 1); on the same day, the *Herald-Sun* carried the more provocative headline 'NURSES ADMIT DEATH ROLE' (p. 3). The next day, 3 March, the *Herald-Sun* carried another provocative headline: 'Nurses death aid "no shock"' (Gartland 1992, p. 5); *The Age*, meanwhile, carried the more subdued headline: 'Nurses in call for euthanasia inquiry' (Bock 1992, p. 6). On 4 March 1992, *The Age* carried another article headed 'When death is part of the quality of life', in which the views of four experienced nurses were reported in an informative and thought-provoking manner (Magazanik 1992b, p. 3). As the days passed, however, the nursing voice and perspective paled into insignificance as others with 'more authority' added their voices to the growing media debate on the nature of euthanasia, the circumstances in which it should or should not be permitted, and the need for the law to reflect community opinion on the matter. Significantly, most of these others (doctors, lawyers, politicians, philosophers, clergymen, and members of the Right to Life movement) all failed to place their comments in the context of nursing care, and, more specifically, failed to identify and address the very real problem of the unfair burden that nurses often have to carry when caring for people who are living lives characterised by intolerable suffering, or who are dying, or both (*The Age* 5 March 1992, p. 13; Magazanik 1992c, 1992d, 1992e; Tighe 1992, p. 10; Syme 1992, p. 10; Briggs and McDonald 1992, p. 12; Skene 1992).

A good example of the extent to which the plight of nurses was overlooked in the media coverage of the survey can be found in the reported comments of Loane Skene, who was at that time the principal research officer of the now disbanded Victorian Law Reform Commission. Commenting on the need for law reform with regard to euthanasia and severely disabled newborns, Skene is reported to have said that 'doctors justifiably felt uncertain about their legal position when treating critically ill babies', and that:

> there are lots of cases where doctors are required to do something that contravenes the letter of the law and there is a real risk that doctors might be charged with criminal offences for making those decisions.
>
> (Reported by Magazanik 1992e, p. 5)

Although nurses also harbour uncertainties about their legal position when caring for critically ill babies (and, it should be added, adults), and although there are many instances in which nurses are required (often by doctors) to do something that 'contravenes the letter of the law' (unconsented 'Not For

Resuscitation' [NFR] directives being a case in point), no mention was made of this in the media reports covering Skene's comments. Further, although nurses are intimately involved in the care and treatment of sick babies, no nurse was quoted in the report; the views of a director of neonatology, the health minister, the president of the Victorian branch of the Australian Medical Association (AMA), and the president of the Right to Life movement were, however, all quoted (Magazanik 1992e, p. 5). The initial media reports on the euthanasia issue began with nurses, but it was as though suddenly nurses no longer existed.

More recently, the opportunity to represent a substantive nursing view on an important ethical issue in health care was again missed. Over the past two years, following the passage and subsequent overturning of the Northern Territory of Australia's *Rights of the Terminally Ill Act (1995)*, there has been intense public debate about the issue of the legalisation of euthanasia and the so-called 'right to die'. Despite the obvious importance of the euthanasia question for the nursing profession, media reports on the issue (too numerous to list here) consistently failed to represent the views of informed nurses even though nurses stand to be implicated in and significantly affected by any public policy or legislative changes relating to end-of-life practices such as euthanasia and assisted suicide. (The issues of euthanasia and assisted suicide will be discussed in greater depth in Chapter 12 of this text.) Despite the fact that nurses are at the forefront of providing care to people at the end stages of life, during which euthanasia might be considered as an option, the views and concerns of nurses were not adequately represented (see also Johnstone et al. 1996, p. 120).

In 1998 there was one notable exception to this demonstrable media bias against representing a nursing perspective, significantly, in relation to the abortion issue. This 'shift' in attitude occurred during a period of intense media publicity that was given to a Western Australian case of two doctors who were charged, in February 1998, with the criminal act of 'attempting to procure an abortion' (O'Brien and Price 1998a, p. 5). Predictably, both the print and electronic media (the citations of which are too numerous to list here) gave ample publicity nationally to the plight of these doctors, to the Australian Medical Association (AMA) advising doctors in Western Australia to refuse performing abortions, and to the Western Australian Government 'clearing doctors to perform abortions after women injure themselves in attempts at termination' (Ewing 1998a, 1998b; O'Brien and Price 1998a, 1998b). Within a week of the initial media reports covering the case of the two Perth doctors, it was reported nationally that the Australian Nursing Federation (ANF), on legal advice, was advising nurses in Western Australia that they, like the two doctors, also risked criminal prosecution if they directly or indirectly engaged in the termination of pregnancies (O'Brien 1998a, p. 3; see also Reeves 1998, p. 11). Interestingly, the legal advice received by the ANF contradicted earlier advice received from the Health Department that 'nurses who assist in terminations might be fulfilling their contract of employment' (Reeves 1998, p. 11). The involvement of nurses was mentioned again in at least two other reports published in a newspaper that has national distribution (O'Brien 1998b, 1998c). While this media coverage gave some visibility to the concerns and involvement of nurses, however, it stopped short of providing a comprehensive account of the situation of nurses. For example, in a national newspaper report given the bold headline 'Stop abortions or face charges, nurses told' (O'Brien 1998a, p. 3), only two out of the sixteen paragraphs of the report dealt with nursing concerns. (The issue of abortion and the moral problems faced by nurses will be considered in detail in Chapter 11 of this text.)

An important implication of nurses not being represented accurately or fairly, or being given a low media profile in bioethical debates, is, arguably, that it makes it easier for those in positions of power — and even for the community at large — to ignore the enormous moral burdens that nurses often face in health care domains. It may make it easier for those outside nursing to maintain and enforce the expectation that nurses will not question the morally troubling reality around them, nor speak out against any injustices and moral violations they witness. It may also make it easier to maintain the traditional image of nurses as merely 'good women' who do not — and thus should not — have a code of ethics, much less a substantive moral position on ethical issues in health care.

Interdisciplinary ethics seminars and conferences

Until relatively recently, a nursing perspective was largely ignored by the organisers of 'interdisciplinary' bioethics conferences. If it was included, it was usually scheduled in an insignificant slot on the program. For example, at a 1987 conference on AIDS run by the Monash University Centre for Human Bioethics, the nurse speakers were programmed last, making it very difficult for them to make any sort of impact at the end of a very demanding day (Centre for Human Bioethics 1986).

The Centre for Human Bioethics 1988 conference on institutional ethics committees also did not provide for a substantive nursing perspective to be given, despite the obvious interest that the nursing profession had at the time in the setting up and functioning of institutional ethics committees. A nurse did appear on the program, but her role amounted to nothing more than closing the conference. The Centre for Human Bioethics, however, has been instrumental in assisting nurses to explore the issue of bioethics in relation to nursing practice. In 1987 for example, the centre organised one of the first serious conferences in Victoria on ethical issues in nursing: 'The role of the nurse: doctors' handmaiden, patients' advocate, or what?' (Centre for Human Bioethics 1987a).

Another example of the extent to which the nursing perspective has been neglected in interdisciplinary bioethics conferences can be found in the program of the inaugural meeting of the Australian Summer School of Medicine, Science and Humanities (December 1988). The school chose as its theme 'Current topics in medical ethics', and focused on such topics as Not For Resuscitation directives, AIDS, clinical trials, and transplant surgery. (Why the notion of medical ethics rather than bioethics was used is a question worth considering.) Of the twenty or so panellists scheduled to participate in the school's inaugural program, only three were women and only two were nurses, both males. At least twelve were male medical doctors. In light of these statistics, it is clear that the representation of doctors and nurses on the program was unbalanced. The faculty itself included a human rights commissioner, a professor of law and two doctors.

Although considerable progress has been made in regard to this issue, and nurses are now featuring more equitably on interdisciplinary bioethics seminar and conference programs in Australia, the views of philosophers, lawyers and doctors of medicine still tend to dominate, and still tend to be regarded as more authoritative than the views of nurses. Adding to this, there is now a new and unforseen problem emerging, namely, for these ethics forums to be used as a platform by some for denigrating the nursing profession and for presenting misrepresentative, misleading and potentially damaging accounts of where nurses are situated in relation to certain ethical issues. An example of this can be found in the case of a conference that was held in Melbourne, Australia, in 1995. During this conference a distinguished bioethicist, who was an invited speaker at the conference, began her presentation with the following unwarranted attack on nurses: 'It is time you nurses got out of your ghetto mentality. Look at you — all nurses. Where are the doctors in the audience?'. She then proceeded to attack and denigrate nurses for not taking a leadership role in calling for the legalisation of euthanasia notwithstanding the fact that this issue was at the time — and remains — controversial both within and outside of the nursing profession (for further details of this incident, see Johnstone et al. 1996, p. 118). In another more recent incident, a bioethicist speaking at an interdisciplinary ethics seminar similarly launched an unwarranted stinging attack on nurses; this time, for allegedly being 'silent' on bioethical issues. It was, however, evident to nurses present in the audience that this commentator had little knowledge and understanding of how proactive nurses had in fact been in addressing ethical issues not only in the nursing literature but in their places of work. In response to this critic, one of the nurses present made reference to the now vast body of ethics literature authored by nurses and pointed out: 'Nurses have not been silent. It is just that others — like you — have not listened ...' (seminar participant, personal communication).

It remains to be said that, despite the many obstacles confronting them, members of the nursing profession have been extremely resourceful in addressing ethical issues and in responding effectively to the unwarranted criticisms of others outside of the profession. Nursing ethics workshops, seminars and conferences are organised regularly across Australia as well as overseas, and have been influential in assisting the nursing profession grapple with the many ethical issues that confront it. A good portion of the material presented in this text has been informed by the responses of nurses attending such workshops, seminars and conferences.

The courts

The courts have also been influential in the marginalisation and invalidation of nursing ethics through being unsupportive of nurses in their attempts to provide morally responsible and accountable nursing care to patients. Notable legal cases, both in Australia and overseas, have made it plain that nurses are bound to follow the lawful and reasonable orders of a superior on the one hand, and yet paradoxically are also bound to be independently accountable on the other (Johnstone 1994; Sanders 1988). The courts have continued to find in favour of employer hospitals who have dismissed nurses for conscientiously refusing to participate in morally controversial medical procedures. In at least two cases, legal proceedings resulted in the authority of the nursing profession's formally adopted code of ethics being rejected (Johnstone 1988a, 1994). On matters relating to morally responsible nursing practice, evidence suggests that the courts are not only frequently unsympathetic; they have even been a major factor in ensuring that the moral authority of nurses and the agreed ethical standards of the nursing profession have not achieved either the legal, social or cultural legitimation they deserve (Johnstone 1994, 1998).

The respect, or lack of it, paid by courts of law to nurses who have taken a strong moral stand on a matter involving their own individual nursing practice is an area worthy of some consideration. One compelling example of how unsympathetic the courts can be to nurses who have been caught up in a morally troubling situation is the case of *Warthen v Toms River Community Memorial Hospital* (1985).

This case involved a registered nurse who was dismissed from her employing hospital of eleven years for refusing to dialyse a terminally ill bilateral amputee patient. Warthen's refusal in this instance was based on what she cited as '"moral, medical and philosophical objections" to performing this procedure on the patient because the patient was terminally ill and ... the procedure was causing the patient additional complications' (*Warthen's case* 1985, p. 205).

Warthen had apparently dialysed the patient on two previous occasions. In both instances, however, the dialysis procedure had to be stopped because the patient suffered severe internal bleeding and cardiac arrest (*Warthen's case* 1985, p. 230). It was the complications of severe internal bleeding and cardiac arrest that she was referring to in her refusal. Her dismissal came when she refused to dialyse the patient for a third time.

Believing she had been wrongfully and unfairly dismissed, Warthen took her case to the Supreme Court, where she argued in her defence that the Code for Nurses of the American Nurses' Association (ANA) justified her refusal, since it essentially permitted nurses to refuse to participate in procedures to which they were personally opposed (Blum 1984, p. 50; *Warthen's case* 1985, p. 229).

The court did not find in her favour, however, and she lost her case. In making its final decision, the court made clear its position on a number of key points, three of which are relevant to this discussion:

1. An employee should not have the right to prevent his or her employer from pursuing its business because the employee perceives that a particular business decision violates the employee's personal morals, as distinguished from the recognised code of ethics of the employee's profession ... (p. 233).

2. [In support of the hospital's defence] it would be a virtual impossibility to administer a hospital if each nurse or member of the administration staff refused to carry out his or her duties based upon a personal private belief concerning the right to live ... (p. 234).

3. The position asserted by the plaintiff serves only the individual and the nurses' profession while leaving the public to wonder when and whether they will receive nursing care ... (p. 234).

(Warthen's case 1985)

There can be small doubt, given these comments, that the court had little regard for the nurse's conscientious objection to the tasks she was being compelled to perform. And there can also be little doubt that the court, in dismissing altogether the ANA Code for Nurses as an authoritative statement of public policy, had poor regard for the nursing profession's position on conscientious objection generally (Johnstone 1994, pp. 251–67, 1988a).

Two years later, another American court demonstrated a dismissive attitude toward the agreed ethical standards of nursing. This case involved a registered nurse by the name of Francis Free who unsuccessfully appealed a decision by her employer to dismiss her after she had refused to evict a seriously ill bedridden patient (*Free v Holy Cross Hospital*, 1987). Free's refusal was based on grounds that to evict the patient would have been:

in violation of her ethical duty as a registered nurse not to engage in dishonourable, unethical, or unprofessional conduct of a character likely to harm the public as mandated by the *Illinois Nursing Act*.

(Free's case 1987, p. 1190)

The patient in question had been arrested for possession of a hand gun. Meanwhile, an order had been given for her to be transferred to another hospital. The police officer guarding the patient pointed out, however, that because of certain outstanding matters, the other hospital would probably not accept the patient and it was likely that she would be returned to Holy Cross Hospital. Free communicated this information to the hospital's chief of security who responded by telling her that the patient was to be removed from the hospital 'even if removal required forcibly putting the patient in a wheelchair and leaving her in the park' which was across the road from the hospital (*Free's case* 1987, p. 1189). Although Free disagreed with removing the patient, she gave the necessary instructions for the patient's transfer to the other hospital.

As part of the process of dealing with this situation, Free contacted the vice-president of her employing hospital to discuss the matter with him. It is reported that the vice-president 'became agitated, shouted and used profanity in telling Free that it was he who had given the order to remove the patient' (*Free's case* 1987, p. 1189). After this incident, Free contacted the patient's physician who stated that 'he opposed the transfer' and instructed Free 'not to touch the patient but to document his order that the patient should remain at the hospital' (*Free's case* 1987, p. 1189). After checking the patient and 'calming her down', Free received a telephone call 'ordering her to report to the office of the vice-president'. When she arrived at the vice-president's office Free was advised 'that her conduct was insubordinate and that her employment was immediately terminated' (*Free's case* 1987, p. 1189). Significantly, in the unfair dismissal court case that followed, Free's actions were characterised by the court 'as being of a personal as opposed to a professional nature and therefore as falling outside the scope of the *Illinois Nursing Act*' (Johnstone 1994, p. 256).

This dismissive attitude towards nursing ethics has also been experienced in an Australian context. An example of this can be found in the Victorian industrial relations case *In re the alleged unfair dismissal of Ms K Howden by the City of Whittlesea* (1990). This case involved a maternal and child health nurse (MCHN) who was dismissed from her place of employment for 'professional misconduct' after it was alleged she had maliciously breached confidentiality while dealing with a case of suspected child (sexual) abuse. (It should be noted that the MCHN was later cleared of the misconduct charges against her, and an order given that she should be reinstated to her former position [for further details of the case see Johnstone 1994, pp. 259–61]). Of significance to this discussion is that, in reaching his decision about the case, the deputy president of the Industrial Relations Commission was particularly critical of the International Council of Nurses (1973) *Code for Nurses* which the MCHN cited in defence of her actions. In response to the MCHN's defence and referring to the code's statement that 'the Nurse holds in confidence personal information and uses judgment in sharing this information', the deputy president concluded, controversially, that although 'well-meaning', the code's statement was 'so imprecise as to be of limited value in circumstances like those which concerned [the MCHN]'(*Howden's case* 1990). He then instructed the nurse's employer, the City of Whittlesea, that it:

> would be wise to become involved in the development of [precise and clear-cut] guidelines. Otherwise the city leaves the field to an imprecise code of nursing ethics, to standards of a professional peer group with whom the city may disagree.
>
> (*Howden's case* 1990, p. 29)

The influential role that the courts have played in marginalising and invalidating professional nursing ethics is an important issue in its own right and one which unfortunately is beyond the scope of this present work to advance. Since I have considered this issue at length elsewhere (Johnstone 1994, pp. 252–67), I shall venture nothing more on the subject here suffice to say that we would be hard-pressed to find comparable examples of the agreed ethical standards of other professions, for example medicine and law, being treated in such a dismissive way.

A National Commission of Inquiry

Other legal processes, besides law courts, have also played an influential role in the marginalisation and invalidation of professional nursing ethics. An important example of this can be found in the case of the 1987 New Zealand national inquiry into what has become popularly referred to as the 'unfortunate experiment' at the National Women's Hospital. The details of this inquiry and the 'unfortunate experiment' in question are well documented in the *Report of the Cervical Cancer Inquiry* (prepared by the Committee of Inquiry into Allegations Concerning the Treatment of Cervical Cancer at National Women's Hospital and into Other Related Matters 1988), and in Sandra Coney's book *The unfortunate experiment* (1988). Nevertheless, there are aspects of this inquiry that are highly pertinent to our discussion here, and that are therefore worth considering at length.

The 'unfortunate experiment' began in 1958, under the direction of four National Women's Hospital doctors — one of whom, Dr Herbert Green, had once been described as 'one of the 25 outstanding physicians in the world' (Johns 1988, p. 9). The experiment, involving 948 women, sought to examine the invasive potential of carcinoma *in situ* (CIS) of the cervix. The experiment reached the public's attention when, in 1987, *Metro* magazine published an article by Sandra Coney and Phillida Bunkle in which allegations were made that not only had women with CIS been used as unconsenting subjects in a medical experiment, but also that, as a result of being a part of this experiment, some of these women had not had their condition adequately treated (claims which were to be fully vindicated by the inquiry's findings).

Initially, according to Coney, the article caused 'virtually no reaction', and both she and her co-author feared that the 'unfortunate experiment' had once again 'dropped into a hole' (Coney 1988, p. 71). The media would not take up the issue. One radio reporter stated that legal advice had been received to the effect 'if it was anything to do with doctors to keep away from it', while another newspaper reporter was told by the editor that it was 'too dangerous' (Coney 1988, p. 71). On top of this, as Coney wrote:

> No women's groups commented. Civil liberty groups were silent. Some individuals in the Cancer Society were supportive, but the society's executive contained a large number of doctors and they weren't sure they wanted to get involved. There was no one to quote.
>
> (Coney 1988, p. 72)

As a result of the efforts of some individual newspaper journalists and radio commentators, the information gradually filtered through to the public arena, and on 5 June 1987 the then Prime Minister of New Zealand, David Lange, announced that there would be a 'very rapid inquiry' (Coney 1988, p. 74). This 'rapid inquiry' was eventually to see the documentation of over two million sheets of evidence (*New Zealand Herald* 1988b).

As the inquiry got under way, the magnitude of what had happened began to be realised. It was not long before the public came to fully appreciate the extent to which the hospital and, more particularly, the doctors involved, had failed the women who had been unwitting participants in the 'unfortunate experiment' (*Report of the Cervical Cancer Inquiry* 1988, pp. 101, 210). The public also came to appreciate that not only had these women suffered unnecessarily but, in some cases, had also died unnecessarily, as was made evident by the inquiry's findings.

The 948 women used in the 'unfortunate experiment' had been divided into two groups. Those in group one (817 women) received treatment, while those in group two (131 women) received only 'limited' or no treatment. The outcome was that those in group two developed invasive carcinoma at the rate of 22 per cent, compared with only 1.5 per cent in group one, and had a mortality rate of 6 per cent, 5.5 per cent higher than that of group one (*Report of the Cervical Cancer Inquiry* 1988, p. 57; Coney 1988, pp. 14–15). Media reports also claimed that some women experienced as many as sixty hospital admissions and over fifty vaginal examinations — but received no treatment. As *a New Zealand Herald* article (1987a) reports, the women 'got more and more diagnoses but not always treatment, or treatment was left too late'.

As the inquiry progressed, the media began to reveal the disturbing details of other morally questionable medical practices that had been allowed to continue, unchecked, over the past twenty or so years. The *Waikato Times* (1987a), for example, revealed that '... the decision whether a patient received surgery or deep X-ray treatment in addition to radium was decided by the random process of tossing a coin'.

Two months later, the *New Zealand Herald* (1987b, p. 14) revealed that over 2200 newborn baby girls had been subjected to vaginal swabs at the National Women's Hospital without parental consent. It was also alleged that over 200 fetal cervixes were collected from stillborn baby girls for histological studies — again without parental consent. One researcher is reported to have said that the samples were collected with 'a minimum of fuss and a maximum of discretion, but not with the knowledge of the mothers' (*New Zealand Herald* 1987e). It was also alleged that there was never any intention to get parental consent.

In the Report of the Cervical Cancer Inquiry it was later confirmed that not only had these babies been subjected to vaginal swabbing but that the swabbing had been done in vain. Judge Cartwright, the commissioner of the inquiry, explained that Dr Green, the chief researcher, had:

> lost interest in this trial after 200 babies had had smears taken. Unfortunately this decision not to continue the trial was not communicated to the nursing staff and the trial continued until smears had been taken from 2244 newborn babies.
>
> ... there was no system in place that ensured that the trial stopped ... an effective system for monitoring research and ensuring that unnecessary procedures are not conducted, should have been in place. If this had been so, then more than 2000 babies would not have been subjected to a useless and possibly damaging procedure.
>
> (Report of the Cervical Cancer Inquiry 1988, p. 141[1])

---

1. Quotations from this report are reprinted by permission of the Government Printing Office, Wellington, New Zealand.

Most of the swabs were taken from newborn babies of Maori and Pacific Island women, as well as from unmarried mothers — in short, women who were least likely to be able to stand up for themselves (Coney 1988, p. 217). One nurse witness made the further claim that the 'babies of private patients were not swabbed', but that claim was contradicted by another witness (Coney 1988, p. 213).

Nurses, it seems, were actively involved in performing the swabbing. It is alleged that if mothers asked questions about the 'test', nurses would 'explain the test ... and reassure them' (Coney 1988, p. 213). Interestingly, none of the nurses involved gave evidence publicly, making it very difficult for the issue of informed consent to research to be discussed in full (Coney 1988, p. 213). Furthermore, one medical witness, Professor Dennis Bonham, allegedly attempted to discredit the evidence of a nurse witness on the overall matter by commenting that 'the remarks were out of character for the nurse concerned' (*New Zealand Herald* 1988a).

In the same inquiry, it was revealed that groups of medical students had been performing, and were still performing, vaginal examinations on anaesthetised women without consent. The National Women's Hospital was also alleged to have been allowing anaesthetised and unconsenting women to have intrauterine devices (IUDs) inserted and withdrawn, first by the duty surgeon as a demonstration, and then by attending postgraduate course doctors seeking educational experience (*Report of the Cervical Cancer Inquiry* 1988, pp. 190–1; Coney 1988, pp. 207–8). These examinations (also exposed in Australia at about the same time) were alleged to have been performed for over twenty years. Medical professors sought to justify this 'penetration without consent' (or 'rape' or 'indecent assault', as it is referred to in some circles) by arguing that 'in a teaching hospital the patients' rights had to be balanced against the need to teach' (*Waikato Times* 1987b). Other medical authorities claimed that women gave 'implied consent' to pelvic examination by medical students simply by attending a teaching hospital (Roberts 1987). At the inquiry, however, the practice was defended on the grounds that 'to teach a student with a conscious patient will create tensions for the patient, hence the decision to examine under anaesthetic' (*Report of the Cervical Cancer Inquiry* 1988, p. 191).

Two pressing questions arise from this inquiry. First, why had vaginal examinations — not to mention insertion and withdrawal of IUDs — been performed on *unconsenting* anaesthetised women for more than twenty years without any public protest by representative bodies of the nursing profession? Second, are we to understand that attending theatre nurses had no knowledge of these practices or, if they did, that they failed to see them as morally objectionable and thus did not pass the information on to their professional representatives (Johnstone 1987, p. 19)?

The report on the inquiry offers interesting answers to these questions. In response to the first question, representatives of the nursing profession apparently tried to have the practices condemned and stopped. The commissioner's findings on this matter are quoted here at length:

> Teaching examination techniques on anaesthetised patients without their consent is not a new issue at National Women's Hospital. In 1978 the Nurses Society of New Zealand made representation to the Auckland Hospital Board condemning the practice. Their allegations concerned teaching sessions involving the insertion and removal of intra uterine contraceptive devices on patients under general anaesthetic for other

purposes, without patient consent or knowledge. According to their evidence, no public comment was made by the Hospital Board as a result of the representations. The Nurses Society, however, published the matter and a newspaper article commented on the issue. Although a television interview was taped, it was never transmitted, apparently because of adverse reactions from a member of the Postgraduate [Medical] School.

(Report of the Cervical Cancer Inquiry 1988, p. 191)

In answering the first question, the commissioner's findings also partly answered the second question. In order for the Nurses Society of New Zealand to make its claim, it must have had reliable information, which presumably came from theatre nurses who were troubled by the practices they had been witnessing. Nevertheless, it is possible that there were instances in which it was genuinely difficult for theatre nurses to have a full grasp of the situation; for example, citing the evidence (given anonymously) of one theatre charge nurse, the commissioner explained:

unconscious patients were examined vaginally by up to four students. She [the nurse] *was not told whether the vaginal examination was part of that patient's treatment or not.* Her concern centred on the possible discomfort the woman might experience later, and her anxiety that the patient's permission had not been sought. When she voiced her concerns, they were dismissed by her supervisor.

(Report of the Cervical Cancer Inquiry 1988, p. 191, emphasis added)

Nurses also apparently tried to take positive action in relation to other morally questionable practices. Coney showed, for example, that nurses had 'tried for eight months to find out from the Ethical Committee why they were expected to send pancreases from aborted fetuses for research, "to no avail". Finally, they simply stopped supplying the fetuses because they could not get anything in writing' (Coney 1988, p. 141).

That nurses were expected to collect and send fetal material to the hospital laboratory for research should come as no surprise. It is not uncommon for hospitals to regard aborted fetuses as 'hospital property' and thus as items to be treated as the hospital (or rather, its doctors) see fit. Aborted fetal tissue is often sent 'routinely' to the hospital laboratory for 'analysis'.

At one point during the inquiry, the commissioner noted that she had 'a big gap in her information'. This, she is reported to have said, was because 'she had not heard from any nurses'. The commissioner then proceeded to criticise nurses for having been 'less than brave in coming forward to give evidence at the inquiry' (*New Zealand Herald* 1987d).

One nurse who gave evidence at the inquiry reportedly responded to this criticism by alleging that the medical superintendent of the National Women's Hospital, Dr Collison, had sent out a memo to the effect that:

nurses currently employed by National Women's Hospital are advised not to go forward to the hearing, and it is in their hospital's best interests and their own interests that they do not take part in the hearing.

(*New Zealand Herald* 1987c)

The media went on to report that Dr Collison had denied these allegations, stating that the only memo she recalled sending out was one that 'reminded staff ... that it was an offence [under the Hospital Act concerning confidentiality of patient information] to disclose to anyone information concerning the condition or medical history of any patient' (*New Zealand Herald* 1987c).

Coney stated that the memo advised staff that, if they wished to give information at the inquiry, they should see Collison. One obvious implication of this directive was that any staff members presenting themselves to Collison would, of course, be identified. Collison, however, refused to accept that her memo 'had acted as a disincentive' (Coney 1988, p. 224).

The New Zealand Nurses' Association had quite a different view on the matter from Collison, however. Coney wrote:

> The Nurses' Association said it had heard from several members that Collison's memo was 'interpreted as an instruction not to cooperate with the inquiry'. Two had given confidential interviews anonymously because of a very clearly expressed perception that their jobs would be in jeopardy or any future prospects for study hampered if they came out in the open.
>
> (Coney 1988, p. 224)

It was later revealed that the special authority given by the minister of health providing for the release of information to the inquiry had not been communicated to staff (Coney 1988, p. 224).

The outcome of the Cervical Cancer Inquiry in regard to the New Zealand nursing profession was not encouraging. Early nursing commentary on the whole affair was at the time less than satisfactory and not entirely optimistic. The New Zealand Nurses' Association, for example, was clearly relieved that nurses were not implicated in any substantial way in the practices exposed. The then professional officer of the New Zealand Nurses' Association, Joy Bickley, commented:

> Minimal discussion of nurses in the report implies they played only a peripheral part in the matters investigated at the inquiry. But in general, Cartwright says the nursing staff at National Women's were 'highly praised' for the caring attitude to the women they looked after.
>
> (Bickley 1988, p. 15)

Bickley, however, goes on to correctly criticise the report's grave reservations about the ability of nurses to defend patients' rights and the commissioner's comment that:

> Nurses, who most appropriately should be the advocates for the patient, feel sufficiently intimidated by the medical staff (who do not hire and fire them) that even today they fail or refuse to confront openly the issues arising from the 1988 trial.
>
> (Bickley 1988, p. 15)

In some respects, the commissioner's criticisms were well founded. In other respects, however, her findings reflected the malaise and inadequacy of a system that does not provide for the experiences and views of nurses to be made visible. Her report contained 'only a partial analysis of nurses' role in the inquiry and in health care' and, as Bickley (1988) put it, encouraged the 'side-lining of nursing'. Of particular concern was the report's recommendations which stopped far short of recognising the role and responsibilities of nurses in the whole matter. As Bickley (1993) explains in a later work:

> There was no explicit role identified for nurses in Judge Cartwright's recommendations regarding peer review, informed consent and research.

Auckland University was urged to improve the teaching of ethical principles but there was no acknowledgment that nursing schools included ethical principles in their teaching. There was no direction, for example, that nursing students could possibly be made more courageous by being helped to understand what their ethical obligations to clients should be. The NZNA [New Zealand Nurses' Association] Patients' Code of Rights and Responsibilities was first published in 1978 and the Code of Ethics in 1988. The Cartwright Report did not point to these documents as a contribution to greater nursing accountability in the future. It was recommended that half of ethics committees should consist of lay members but nurses were not identified as appropriate members of those committees.

(Bickley 1993, p. 126)

Bickley suggests that these omissions are possibly indicative of nursing being seen as being merely 'an ancillary to the medical profession' (1993, p. 126). There is, however, another explanation: had the nurses been found independently responsible for their part in the 'unfortunate experiment' and had they been found accountable for their actions, in effect this would have legitimated the moral authority of nurses to question medical practice; that is, on grounds other than clinical medical knowledge (historically recognised as being the only grounds upon which medicine could be legitimately challenged, and something which nurses are not seen as genuinely having). Regrettably, by overlooking the responsibility of nurses in the whole affair, and by failing to acknowledge or deal with the constraining effects that doctors and hospital administrators obviously had on the ability of nurses to act morally, the commission of inquiry in essence preserved the status quo, rather than challenged it. In so doing it not only also preserved the hegemonic power of the medical profession in health care, but reinforced the notion that nurses should be 'good women' (vessels of 'caring attitudes') and 'not have a code of ethics' prescribing independent moral responsibility and accountability.

The aftermath of the 'unfortunate experiment' and the inquiry into it is one of 'unfinished business' (Coney 1993). Among other things, there thus remains considerable scope to argue that unless nurses' continued lack of legitimated authority to match their responsibilities is addressed, unless the institutional constraints upon nurses' ability to be moral is confronted, and unless the issue of hegemonic power relations within health care institutions is addressed, the danger of there being recurrence of other 'unfortunate experiments' — not to mention medical malpractice and negligence — will remain high. Nurses may well have been 'less than brave in coming forward to give evidence at the inquiry'. It is a matter of deep regret that the commission failed, in this instance, to challenge the status quo in a way that would have accorded the legitimated authority nurses need in order to be able to fulfil their moral responsibilities to patients.

As a point of interest, Dr Herbert Green, the chief researcher of the cervical cancer project, ultimately evaded charges of disgraceful conduct relating to his project on grounds that he was ' "unfit mentally and physically" to face charges' (*Sun Herald* 17 June 1990, p. 168). However, Professor Bonham, who was head of the committee which approved the original project, and was also head of the department of obstetrics and gynaecology at the time the project was being carried out, is reported to have been found guilty by the New Zealand Medical Council of a 'total of six misconduct charges, including four of disgraceful conduct' (*Waikato Times* 15 October 1990, p. 3; see also Coney 1990, pp. 201–45).

The Nazi era

The complicity of nurses in morally questionable medical acts and the sidelining of nurses by important inquiries into medical malpractice and criminal behaviour is not unique. An instructive historical example can be found by examining some notable events that occurred during the Nazi era in Germany during the 1930s and 1940s.

Nazi Germany witnessed the shameful involvement of doctors, nurses, psychiatrists, dentists and pharmacologists in Hitler's euthanasia, or 'medicalised killing', programs (Aly and Roth 1984; Lifton 1986; Proctor 1988; Lagnado and Dekel 1991; Steppe 1991, 1992; Caplan 1992). Nazi doctors quickly emerged as the guardians of what Lifton called the 'Nazi biomedical vision, which saw the mass murder of millions in the name of "healing" the racially "diseased" body of the German nation' (Lifton 1986).

Nazi doctors were primarily responsible for the administration of lethal injections to 'patients'. However, as the German nurse historian Hilde Steppe (1991) has pointed out, it is very clear that 'nurses followed orders and were [likewise] involved in all phases of the systematic annihilation of masses of people' (p. 29). In his remarkable book, *The Nazi doctors: a study of the psychology of evil*, Lifton (1986) suggests that nurses played a fundamental part in determining the necessary drug dosages for 'putting to sleep' those patients whose names had been placed on 'special lists' (p. 101). In instances where patients were not cooperative, nurses would 'reassure' them by explaining that the prescribed injections were simply for 'the treatment of their lung disease' or whatever other 'disease' they may have had (Lifton 1986, p. 101).

Where nurses were involved, they were generally ordered by attending Nazi doctors to administer lethal drug regimes:

> the chief doctor was expected to give orders to the head male nurse to kill male patients, and the head female nurse to do the same to female patients ... the orders were passed along by the head male and female nurses to the ward nurses, who carried them out.
>
> (Lifton 1986, pp. 100–1)

Steppe explains that, once the choice of patients to be killed had been made, their names were noted by the nurse in charge, and the patients:

> were brought to a room which was especially set aside for the purpose and were then killed with medication or an injection of air. The killing was to a large extent carried out by the nursing personnel.
>
> (Steppe 1991, p. 31)

Aly and Roth (1984) and Caplan (1992) also cite examples of nurse involvement in Nazi atrocities.

There is evidence to suggest that, if a doctor felt uneasy and could not perform a certain murderous act, the difficulty could be solved by ordering a nurse to administer a prescribed 'treatment'. In one case, when a doctor refused to send a pregnant woman to a gas chamber, the problem was 'resolved' by ordering a nurse to give the woman a lethal injection (Lifton 1986, pp. 64, 100).

Nurses were also both directly and indirectly involved in the killing of children. For example, midwives were required to report the births of disabled newborns to attending Nazi physicians (Aly and Roth 1984, p. 156). Consequently, many of the disabled newborns were marked for death or experimental research that invariably led to death (Lifton 1986, p. 52). As well, nurses working in select departments or institutions (euphemistically referred to as 'children's specialty departments' or 'therapeutic convalescent institutions') were involved · in administering legally prescribed 'therapeutic regimes' to 'subnormal' or 'excitable' children who were 'completely idiotic [and who] could not be kept quiet with the normal dose of sedatives' (Lifton 1986, p. 54). These 'therapeutic regimes' included large and accumulatively lethal doses of luminal, followed by a morphine-scopolamine preparation. When children receiving these drugs eventually died, the cause of death was listed as 'a more or less ordinary disease such as pneumonia' (Lifton 1986, p. 55).

It is also now known that nurses played a fundamental role in preparing patients for death, and in some instances were especially chosen to be present in the death chambers. Their work consisted of helping to carry a patient's personal belongings to the gas chamber, helping patients to undress, accompanying them and generally helping them to calm down; some nurses even stayed to observe the actual gassing process (Steppe 1991, pp. 30–1). Commenting on the role of nurses working in psychiatric institutes, Steppe describes their involvement in the killing programs as follows:

> They packed up the personal belongings of the patient, gave identification numbers to the objects and to the patient, they accompanied the transport to an intermediate location or to the death site. They rode back to their workplace in the empty buses, and later said in court proceedings that they had given no thought to the question of what happened with their patients.
>
> (Steppe 1991, p. 29)

Some, however, gave considerable thought to what happened to their patients. In 1941, for instance, nurses were among those who celebrated the cremation of a ten-thousandth patient at a psychiatric hospital in Hadamar (Proctor 1992, p. 36).

It should be noted that not all nurses were willing accomplices to the workings of the Nazi biomedical machine; many acted under threat of death or imprisonment, or both (Steppe 1991, p. 35). Others courageously risked their lives to help patients escape from the institutions in which they were held. In one report a nurse blatantly refused to take part in the killings because she 'felt herself becoming "hysterical" from the mental strain' (Lifton 1986, p. 57). One nurse also cared for Jewish patients when they could not get needed medical or hospital treatment (Steppe 1991, p. 35). This included working secretly at night in a Jewish hospital at which she had been forbidden to work.

In another report, it is claimed that Catholic nurses refusing to participate in sterilisation procedures lost their jobs. Interestingly, these dissenting Catholic nurses were replaced by non-Catholic Brown Sisters who belonged to the Nazi Order of Nurses. Koonz (1987) explains:

> These women with a crash course on Nazi doctrine and eugenics as well as basic nursing skills, took the jobs of registered nurses who had received a minimum of four years of formal education. The 'brown sisters' received lower pay than nurses and, perhaps more importantly, they brought Nazi beliefs to their clients.
>
> (Koonz 1987, p. 284)

An example of how strong these Brown Sisters' Nazi beliefs were can be found in the oath they swore on the completion of their training:

> I solemnly swear that I will be steadfastly faithful and obedient to Adolf Hitler, my Fuhrer. I promise to fulfil my duties, wherever I may be designated to work, faithfully and conscientiously as a national socialist nurse in the service of the national community, so help me God.
>
> (Archives Koblenz N S 37/1039, cited in Steppe 1991, p. 24)

As a point of interest, it appears that no nurse involved in the Nazi atrocities was later barred from practising as a nurse (Steppe 1991, p. 18). Further, of those nurses who appeared in court to account for their Nazi activities, most were eventually acquitted, or, if found guilty, were released from prison after only a short time.

Curiously, formal literature on the subject (including publicly available literature on the Nuremberg trials) makes very little mention, if any, of nurses' participation in Nazi biomedical atrocities. Popular nursing history texts are also conspicuously silent on the subject. Moreover, neither the International Council of Nurses, the International Red Cross, the United Nations Information Centre, the United States National Archives nor the Melbourne Jewish Holocaust Centre has been able to provide useful information on either the involvement of nurses in Nazi biomedical practices or the postwar prosecution of nurses that might have taken place. There is an alleged incident where a registered nurse repeatedly used a bed sheet to bind together the legs of a woman in the advanced stages of labour. Both the woman and her unborn child suffered enormously as a result of this single and barbaric act. Unfortunately, there appears to be no formal documentation of this incident, or any others like it. This failure to document the involvement of nurses in Nazi war crimes, together with the failure of postwar legal proceedings to apportion any blame to the nurses who complied with the medicalised killing programs, is not without troubling consequence. Among other things, it has deprived the nursing profession globally of an important historical lesson on the conditions and circumstances under which nurses might either misrepresent or abandon the ethical ideals of their profession, and be coerced into unscrupulous or evil behaviour by others (including and perhaps especially the state). It has also served to reinforce cultural-stereotypical notions of nursing being merely ancillary to medicine, of nurses responsibilities being only vicarious to those of doctors, of nurses being subordinate to doctors and hence 'obliged' (professionally, legally and morally) to 'obey' their orders, and of nurses generally lacking the competence necessary to question medical practice. As in the case of the 'unfortunate experiment' (discussed above on pp. 22–7 of this chapter), by failing to hold offending nurses accountable and responsible for their actions in the ill-treatment of people victimised and terrorised by the Nazi medicalised killing programs, postwar legal proceedings have lost an important opportunity to legitimate the moral authority of nurses to question unscrupulous medical practice and to take the necessary action in accordance with their authoritative judgments to stop such practice when identified. Instead, their has been a powerful reinforcement of the notion of nurses being merely 'good women' (read, obedient servants to doctors) who 'should not bother with a Code of Ethics'. Nevertheless, this should not preclude nurses from learning from the important historical lessons that the Nazi nurse question poses; as Hilde Steppe so succinctly puts it:

> We must never forget that nursing never takes place in a value free, neutral space but is always a socially significant force. This means we cannot simply observe what is taking place around us, but must also take a stand, take our responsibilities actively.
>
> (Steppe 1991, p. 36)

'Taking our responsibilities actively', in this instance, could begin by nurses identifying and comprehending the conditions that made it possible for their sister members of a 'caring' profession to engage in and support the kinds of atrocities they did. (See also Wikler and Barondess 1993; Caplan 1992.)

The *Encyclopedia of bioethics*

The *Encyclopedia of bioethics* (edited by Warren T. Reich) is an internationally reputed and leading bioethics reference text. The first edition of this work was published just over two decades ago in 1978, and stands as the first encyclopedia in the field. Developed with the support of the Kennedy Institute of Ethics at Georgetown University, Washington DC, the complete unabridged volumes of the encyclopedia gave the world at that time (and since) possibly one of the most comprehensive and valuable literature resources in contemporary moral philosophy.

Of significance to this discussion is that, in the introductory statements of the first edition, the encyclopedia claimed to have provided coverage of a broad range of issues in bioethics from an interdisciplinary, intercultural and international perspective. Despite this claim, it was evident that the encyclopedia had failed to do justice to the moral experiences of nurses and to a nursing perspective on bioethics generally. A critical review of the encyclopedia revealed that it contained a number of omissions and biases that minimised and disadvantaged nursing's position both within it (the text) and the field of bioethics it was advancing. In sum, nursing ethics was minimised, marginalised and to some extent invalidated in and by this impressive work.

In 1995, a new and substantively revised edition of the *Encyclopedia of bioethics* was released. This new edition has corrected many of the omissions and biases contained in the first edition, the details of which will be given shortly. Given the importance of the first edition, however, and its significance to the history and politics of nursing ethics and nursing ethics inquiry, an examination of its earlier omissions and biases is warranted.

As already stated, the first edition of the *Encyclopedia of bioethics* claimed to advance an impressive interdisciplinary, intercultural and international approach to the new field of bioethics. Nevertheless, despite its comprehensiveness and outstanding list of contributors, this early edition of the encyclopedia failed to do justice to a nursing perspective on bioethics. Examples of omissions and inadequacies can be found in the encyclopedia's preface, list of editorial advisory board members, list of contributors, index to contents and appendix of ethical codes.

The preface states that several editors from a number of scholarly journals served both as advisory and critical reviewers of the encyclopedia project. Included are editors of scientific, theological, philosophical, psychological, medical, ethical and medical ethics journals. No nurse editors and no nursing journals are mentioned.

Of the sixty members of the editorial advisory board, most of the disciplines converging on bioethics are represented, but no professors of nursing or lecturers in nursing are mentioned. Of these sixty members, only six are women.

The list of contributors rates a little better, but yields no grounds for optimism. Of the 285 contributors, only about 15 per cent are female. The 285 include, in substantial numbers, professors and associate professors of philosophy, religion and moral theology, medicine, surgery, psychiatry and law, as well as professors and associate professors of ethics, medical ethics, history of medicine, law and medicine, biology, behavioural studies and psychology, dentistry, sociology, humanities and English, economics, social demography, political science, oriental studies, anthropology and zoology. Numerous directors of organisations, research fellows and lecturers are also listed. Of these only one appears to be a nurse — Teresa Stanley, who is described as a Kennedy Nursing Faculty Fellow in Bioethics, Director, Division of Nursing, Incarnate Word College, San Antonio, Texas. Stanley wrote the only article devoted specifically to nursing. Nursing is mentioned specifically in only one other article, which appears last in the encyclopedia, entitled 'Women as health professionals'. This article, a historical account of women health professionals, is co-authored by two Harvard University associate professors of psychiatry.

The encyclopedia's editors claim that 'all manuscripts were thoroughly reviewed for appropriateness of scope, accuracy of content, and clarity of style'. In terms of scope and accuracy, a few points need to be considered in relation to Stanley's article.

Stanley (1978, p. 1138) points out that nurses in the United States began seriously to question ethical issues in nursing as early as 1900. One of the great pioneers of nursing ethics at that time was Isabel Hampton Robb who, in 1903, wrote *Nursing ethics for hospital and private use* — one of the first texts of its kind. By the 1930s and 1940s, ethics courses were a strong component in nursing curricula. Special courses in ethics were eventually deleted from nursing curricula, however. This did not go unnoticed by the 1976 Commission on the Teaching of Bioethics in the United States, which reported that 'ethics as an integral part of nursing education has been seriously overlooked' (Stanley 1978, p. 1138).

Stanley raises the issues of nursing education, the need for theory and knowledge-based practice, the moral significance of nursing, the special responsibility of the nursing profession to the community at large, and popular ethical concerns in nursing practice (including conflict in the nurse–doctor relationship, conscientious objection to abortion, informed consent, truth telling, nurse participation in ethics committees and the ethical responsibilities of nurse researchers). Nevertheless, she cannot be expected to do justice to the issues she raises in the mere nine pages of her article. The space cannot compare with the overwhelming volume of other views given in the total of 1813 pages allocated for articles in the encyclopedia. Moreover, Stanley does not give an 'intercultural and international' perspective on the development of ethical concerns in nursing. Her article is presented entirely from a United States perspective and gives the misleading impression that this perspective accurately reflects the position of nursing worldwide.

Stanley omits the information that the International Council of Nurses (ICN) established an Ethics of Nursing Committee in 1933 to study and to collect data to formulate an international view on the ethical problems being encountered by nurse practitioners. The activities of this committee were delayed, partly because of World War II (Kelly 1985, p. 207). Nevertheless, it eventually formulated a code of conduct which was formally adopted in 1953, at a Grand Council meeting held in Brazil. A major revision of the 1965 version of this code was prompted rather forcefully by a group of Canadian student nurses who objected strongly to the statements in the code supporting 'nursing subservience to medicine' (Bergman 1973, p. 140). Their objections were formally presented to the ICN as well as to their national association representatives. The offending clause was eventually deleted. The ICN's current code of conduct is the legacy of these nursing students' initiative and foresight.

Stanley omits some other historical information. She states, for example, that 'there was no formal code of ethics to guide nursing practice in the early stages of the profession' (Stanley 1978, p. 1138). It is not clear whether this statement refers to universal or United States practice, but either way it is incorrect. In 1893, United States nurses had the Nightingale pledge, written by Lystra E. Gretter, superintendent of the school at Harper Hospital in Detroit (Kelly 1985, p. 44). This pledge had (and has) an ethical orientation, just like any other similar pledge, not least the celebrated Hippocratic Oath. Nursing codes or standards of care go back much further than this, however. There is evidence of formal standards of care existing in ancient India as early as 1000 BC (Smith and Lew 1968, p. 2). The author of this set of standards was the physician Charaka, who insisted, among other things, that those who care for the sick must be:

> of good behaviour, distinguished for purity; possessed of cleverness and skill; imbued with kindness; skilled in every service a patient may require; competent to cook food; skilled in bathing and washing the patient; rubbing and massaging the limb/s; lifting and assisting him [sic] to walk about; well skilled in the art of making beds; ready, patient and skilful in waiting upon one who is ailing and never unwilling to do anything that is ordered.
>
> (Smith and Lew 1968, p. 2)

It is evident that Charaka is not directing physicians in this instance, but those who care for the sick, notably, by modern-day interpretations, nurses.

The early Christian deaconesses and matrons (1–500 AD), the precursors of nursing as we know it today, conducted their activities in caring for the sick in strict accord with the moral demands of their religion. The early Christian 'golden rules' of 'do unto others' and 'love thy neighbour' that they rigorously observed prevail to this day — even in the more rationalistic and secular moralities. (Consider, for example, Kant's famous 'categorical imperative', which holds that people should only act on those principles that would be good for everybody to follow; and more recently the increasing attention being given to the sentiments of love and care as moral principles of conduct.) The deaconesses endeavoured to practise strictly the Corporal Works of Mercy (the formalisation of which stood as a kind of code) and to care and provide compassionately for those who were suffering. These Corporal Works of Mercy obligated the deaconesses:

- to feed the hungry;
- to give water to the thirsty;
- to clothe the naked;
- to visit the imprisoned;
- to shelter the homeless;
- to care for the sick;
- to bury the dead.

(Dolan et al. 1983, p. 45)

It might be objected here that this statement of the Corporal Works of Mercy is not an ethical code as such. However, if analysed from the perspective of a care-based ethic, as opposed to an ethic based on rational moral principles, the Corporal Works of Mercy are clearly as much an embodiment of a moral (prescriptive) code of conduct as is any other code specifying prescriptive rules of conduct.

The deaconesses and matrons successfully established the principles of selfless devotion and self-sacrificing and altruistic commitment to caring for the sick — principles that still have some influence today. There is also evidence that early Roman women caring for the sick were formally expected to have 'literacy, anatomic understanding, a sense of patient responsibility, and ethical concerns, particularly about confidentiality' (Nadelson and Notman 1978, p. 1713).

The most surprising omission in the Stanley article is Florence Nightingale's contribution to nursing ethics. As Olga Kanitsaki (AM of La Trobe University) has observed, in many respects Nightingale was the first modern nurse ethicist (personal communication). Benefiting from a liberal arts education, Nightingale firmly believed that nurse leaders 'must be just and candid, looking at both sides, not moved by entreaties or by likes and dislikes but only by justice and always being reasonable' (cited in Barritt 1973, p. 18). Nightingale also urged nurses to be chaste, sober, honest, truthful, trustworthy, discreet, kind, benevolent, duty bound, and respectful of patient autonomy (Kelly 1985, p. 34). Nightingale emphasised that nursing had a moral influence (Barritt 1973, p. 29), and her writings and work all reflect the resolve and commitment she had to transforming nursing into a moral profession — one that was fully accountable to the community and that was able to prevent human beings from suffering unnecessarily.

Nightingale has often been blamed for having established the principle of 'blind obedience to physicians' and thus for establishing nursing as a docile and subservient profession — seen by some as the source of many of our modern-day professional and moral problems. However, in many respects this blame is unfair. Although she had a profound respect for 'the rules' and for the 'principle of obedience', she was very aware that rules could be restrictive, that regulations 'were usually made by men who were incapable of devising suitable regulations for women', and that nurses required an 'obedience of intelligence, not obedience of slavery' (Barritt 1973, pp. 18–19, 34; Johnstone 1994, p. 55). Nightingale believed that devotion and obedience might well be fine qualities in a porter and 'might even do for a horse' (Woodham-Smith 1964, p. 262). They would not do for a nurse, however, and would render her little more than a servant and, thereby, a professional failure (Nightingale 1970, p. 75). She also firmly believed that nursing education and nursing practice should be controlled by nurses, and rejected the authority of doctors and hospital administrators over these domains. Her deeds and her writings stand as testimony that she most certainly did not believe that nurses should be 'blind obedient slaves'.

Stanley's article makes an important contribution to the encyclopedia's consideration of a nursing perspective on bioethics. However, the encyclopedia's shortcomings in presenting a full nursing perspective on bioethics are very apparent.

A brief analysis of the encyclopedia's index is also revealing. Subject titles beginning with the terms 'nurse' and 'nursing' have a total of five listings, with an additional twenty-six subheadings. Of these only two pertain to ethics — the subheadings 'nursing ethics for hospital and private use (Robb)' and 'ethics committees and', both of which refer to Stanley's article. This compares very poorly with the subject titles beginning with the terms 'medical', 'medicine' and 'physician', which receive approximately fifty listings, with an additional 314 subheadings. Within the subheadings, forty feature ethical considerations ranging from the history of medical ethics to medical codes of conduct. Unlike the nursing listings, these listings offer a cross-cultural, historical and international perspective, and include views from the Arab nations, Eastern and Western European countries, Latin America, North America, China and Japan. Both ancient and modern views are given. Stanley's account of nursing pales into insignificance next to this impressive profile of medicine. Also of significance is the fact that the subtitles feature the physician–nurse relationship, but do not include the nurse–physician relationship. Strike action by physicians is cited, but not strike action by nurses.

There is one further comment to be made, and this pertains to the encyclopedia's appendix entitled 'Codes and statements related to medical ethics' (pp. 1731–1815), in which the ICN 1973 Code for Nurses and the American Nurses' Association 1976 Code for Nurses are reprinted. The inclusion of these codes is commendable. Nevertheless, a number of observations remain to be made. First, it is philosophically and professionally questionable that all codes included in this appendix (including non-nursing and non-medical codes such as those of the American Chiropractic Association, and those of osteopathic, pharmacological, psychiatric, psychological and dental associations) are subsumed under 'medical ethics', rather than held to be codes in their own right. It is conceptually questionable to treat medical ethics as synonymous with bioethics, health care ethics or nursing ethics. The table of contents to this appendix introduces the codes as 'Codes of the health-care professions' (p. 1723), which is more accurate and appropriate, and gives each of the four sections an appropriate heading.

A second feature of this appendix is that over fourteen medical codes are included, together with another six related to the ethics of medical research. This total of twenty codes (which includes, among others, the ancient codes of Greece, India, Syria and Persia, and the modern codes of the USA, the USSR [now Russia] and the World Medical Association) completely overpowers nursing's almost imperceptible two codes. The inherent bias here speaks for itself. The medical codes are certainly worthy of inclusion, but the appendix is the poorer for not including some of nursing's older codes, not to mention other international nursing codes (see, for example, Sawyer 1989; Viens 1989).

The 1995 revised edition of the *Encyclopedia of bioethics* contains a number of improvements on the first edition, many of which were motivated and informed by the critical reviews authored by nurses (including, I am told, my own substantive and controversial critique which first appeared in the 1989 edition of this text). Notable among the improvements are:

- the inclusion of three North American nursing scholars (Mila Aroskar, Anne Davis and Sara Fry) as members of the Editorial Advisory Board;
- the inclusion of four internationally reputed nursing scholars (Mila Aroskar, Anne Bishop, Anne Davis and Sara Fry) on the List of Contributors (all of whom, however, are North American);
- an acknowledgment in the *Preface* to the work of the importance of 'including all voices, new and old, in as even-handed a way as possible' (p. xiii);
- the inclusion in the encyclopedia's *Introduction* of substantive references to nursing, including the extremely important and significant acknowledgment that the (past) 'medicalization of bioethics has tended to minimise the ethics of nursing and other health professionals' (p. xxii);

- the inclusion of entries in the index that refer specifically to *nursing ethics* including, but not limited to, the following issues: 'bioethics education, care perspective, civil disobedience, clinical ethics committees, confidentiality, conscience, death penalty stance, dying patients, history and emphasis [of nursing ethics], information disclosure, moral relations, philosophical issues and theory, professional code, strike action and whistleblowing'; and, not least,
- better recognition of and reference to various nursing position statements on ethical issues and codes of ethics.

It is acknowledged that these improvements are substantial and that, in a work like the *Encyclopedia of bioethics*, it is inevitable that some biases will still slip through. In the case of the 1995 revised edition of the *Encyclopedia of bioethics*, at least two key biases are apparent; these are the work's medicocentricity, and its North American ethnocentricity. For example, whereas approximately 107 pages of the encyclopedia are devoted to discussing the history of medical ethics, less than one page is given to discussing the history of nursing ethics which, controversially, is situated within the section on medical ethics. And whereas the history of medical ethics is considered from an impressive international perspective, the history of nursing ethics is considered from a North American perspective only and cites only North American authors. The history of nursing ethics in other countries is not examined even though information on this topic could have been readily located (see, for example, Johnstone 1993). To cite another example of ethnocentric bias, a discussion on the topic of bioethics education in nursing provides a relatively comprehensive overview of nursing ethics education in the United States together with supporting references by North American writers. Also considered in this discussion is an overview of nursing ethics education in other countries outside of the United States of America (for example, the United Kingdom, Canada, Finland, Norway, Sweden, Hungary, Latin America, Australia, New Zealand, China and Japan). Significantly, while references to North American authors are included in the bibliography, references to the leading works on nursing ethics written by authors from the other countries mentioned have been omitted (see, for example, the foundational British works by: Thompson et al. 1983; Rumbold 1986; Tschudin 1986; Hunt 1994; and the Australian works by Johnstone 1989, 1994).

A medicocentric and ethnocentric bias is also found in the appendix where various codes of ethics, oaths and ethical directives have been reproduced. As with the first edition of the encyclopedia, nursing codes, oaths and directives remain poorly represented in comparison to the medical codes, oaths and directives which have been included. Furthermore, whereas the respective codes of ethics of the American Nurses' Association and the Canadian Nurses' Association have been included, the ethical codes and directives adopted by other countries have not.

Having made these criticisms it nevertheless remains to be said that nursing ethics is now much better represented in the *Encyclopedia of bioethics*, and that this is an exciting and welcome development in the bioethics literature. The revisions in favour of a nursing perspective also underscore the importance of nurses speaking out against their constructed silence and marginalisation in important fields, and demonstrate that, among other things, through the strategic use of informed critique it is possible to challenge and change the status quo.

Conclusion

The examples and case scenarios discussed so far are by no means exhaustive. Nevertheless they are sufficient to illustrate how members of the medical profession, the media, the legal system and others have been influential in contributing to the minimisation, marginalisation and invalidation of the moral experiences of nurses and of ethical issues in nursing generally. It is important to note, however, that despite an historical lack of understanding and support of nursing ethics from those outside of the nursing profession, nursing ethics has nevertheless developed as a distinctive disciplinary field of inquiry in its own right. This is evidenced, among other things, by:

- the proliferation of nursing research and scholarship in the area (including the establishment of an international journal of nursing ethics);
- the inclusion of nursing ethics subjects as core subjects in the curriculums of both undergraduate and postgraduate nursing courses;
- the organisation of workshops, seminars, conferences and short courses on nursing ethics;
- the establishment of nursing ethics special interests groups (an example of which can be found in the Ethics Society of the Royal College of Nursing, Australia);
- the establishment of distinctive nursing ethics committees or forums in the institutions and organisation where nurses work (Zink and Titus 1994; Heitman and Robinson 1997; Johnstone 1997);
- the increasing representation of nurses on generic institutional ethics committees; and, not least,
- by the increasing numbers of nurses who are engaging in the political act of calling themselves 'nurse ethicists' (as opposed, for instance, to calling themselves bioethicists or medical ethicists or health care ethicists) and, in this capacity, who are beginning to be very influential in terms of contributing to public debate and public policy development on ethical issues relevant to the profession and practice of nursing and indeed to health care generally.

In the chapters to follow, attention will be given to examining some of the key ethical issues facing nurses at this time and which can be addressed, in beneficial ways, through using a nursing ethics framework. Before examining these issues, however, it is necessary first to gain some understanding of the theoretical underpinnings that have influenced nursing ethics inquiry. It is to guiding such an understanding that the next five chapters will now turn.

Chapter 3

Ethics, bioethics and nursing ethics: some working definitions

Introduction

In his celebrated work *Contemporary moral philosophy*, G.J. Warnock warned that:

> When we talk about 'morals' we do not all know what we mean; what moral problems, moral principles, moral judgments are is not a matter so clear that it can be passed over as simple datum. We must discover when we would say, and when we would not, that an issue is a moral issue, and why: and if, as is more than likely, disagreements should come to light even at this stage, we could at least discriminate and investigate what reasonably tenable alternative positions there may be.
>
> (Warnock 1967, p. 75)

The terms 'ethics', 'morality', 'rights', 'duties', 'obligations', 'moral principles', 'moral rules', 'morally right', 'morally wrong', 'moral theory', to name some, are all commonly used in ethics discourse. Nurses, like others, may use some of these terms when discussing life events and situations which are perceived as having a moral dimension. Whether nurses use these terms correctly, however, is another matter. For example, there is a popular tendency by nurses (including some nurse authors) to draw a firm but erroneous distinction between ethics and morality (see, for example, Kelly 1985; Leininger 1991; Thompson et al. 1994). Many see 'morality' as involving more a personal or private set of values, in contrast with 'ethics', which is seen as involving a more formalised, public and universal set of values. Another common error (see also Fagin 1975) is to regard the terms 'rights' and 'responsibilities' or 'duties' as being synonymous, and thus able to be used interchangeably. An example of this is found in the International Council of Nurses (ICN) position statement on the 'rights and duties of nurses', adopted at the ICN's Council of National Representatives meeting in Brazil in June 1983: 'Nurses have a *right* to practise within the code of ethics and nursing legislation' (Keireini 1983, p. 4, emphasis added). When we later examine the nature of rights and duties, it will become clear that the term 'right' in this example should, in fact, read 'duty'. Not surprisingly, the incorrect use of fundamental ethical terms and concepts has led to a certain degree of confusion in nursing ethics discourse. This is particularly evident in literature discussing the supposed role of the nurse as a patient's advocate. It has also caused confusion about and misunderstanding of a nursing perspective on bioethics generally; the language and grammar of ethics has, however, probably been misunderstood as much by doctors, lawyers, the media, theologians and other members of the community as by nurses. One unfortunate consequence of this distortion in communication has been (and in many respects continues to be) an inability of people in health care domains to achieve tolerable and peaceable solutions to many moral problems plaguing both them and the health care arena as a whole.

The need to understand clearly the moral language and grammar used in moral discourse is made explicit by the contemporary English philosopher, Richard Hare:

> in a world in which the problems of conduct become every day more complex and tormenting, there is a great need for an understanding of the language in which these problems are posed and answered. For confusion about our moral language leads, not merely to theoretical muddles, but to needless practical perplexities.

(Hare 1964, pp. 1–2)

These words are as relevant and as important for nurses as they are for the community of academic philosophers for whom Hare wrote. Nursing is just as vulnerable to the 'theoretical muddles' and 'needless practical perplexities' that flow from a confusion about moral language as are other disciplines engaged in the project of ethics. It is to clearing up some of the confusion surrounding the selection, interpretation, and use of moral language, and the concepts they import, that this chapter now turns.

Understanding moral language

The need for a common moral language

In order to be able to discuss ethics, bioethics and nursing ethics in a meaningful way, it is important, first, to share a common and working knowledge and understanding of these (and other) fundamental ethical terms. Unless nurses use the same moral language and grammar as others, little hope remains for either agreement or disagreement being reached on what is considered a competing moral view (i.e. a genuine difference of moral opinion), much less on what is considered a morally right or wrong course of action. For example, if two dissenting parties do not share a common conception of what nursing ethics is, then they cannot meaningfully debate whether or not it ought to be recognised as a distinctive and legitimate field of inquiry and practice in its own right. Similarly, for example, if two dissenting parties do not share a common conception about human rights and what these entail, they cannot even begin to debate the conditions under which a violation of human rights might be morally wrong or morally permissible. If those engaged in ethical, bioethical and nursing ethical debate do not use a common moral language, then they risk spending a lifetime arguing fruitlessly at cross-purposes and engaging in endless human misunderstanding. In this respect the philosophical adage that 'there must be agreement before there can be disagreement' is by no means trivial.

A second ingredient critical to any meaningful discussion on ethics, bioethics or nursing ethics is the use of clearly articulated, substantiated and mutually agreed upon *definitions* of ethical terms and concepts. This is necessary for at least two reasons. First, ethical definitions have an important role to play in evaluating moral disagreements and in commenting on how these might be best resolved. Second, ethical definitions are themselves 'ethically "loaded" with moral presuppositions, and therefore ... may need to be backed up by appeal to moral principles and an examination of specific instances' (Walton 1980, p. 16).

Consider, for example, the philosophical notion of 'person', which in mainstream Western moral philosophy relies very heavily on rational criteria and, to some extent, sentience (i.e. the capacity to feel and to experience sensations). The philosophical definition of 'person' (usually distinguished from the notion of 'human being') has an important bearing on deciding the moral permissibility of, for example, abortion, fetal tissue transplants, or the use of live-born anencephalic babies or brain-dead human beings as organ donors. In this instance, a philosophically defined notion of 'person' (together with its ethical 'loading') could make all the difference in the world between, say, a doctor being deemed, in the case of organ transplantation, to have 'committed murder' as opposed to having merely 'harvested organs', a notion that itself is designed to sound value neutral. In the same way, a mother could be deemed to have 'committed infanticide' as opposed to having merely 'got rid of the unwanted products of conception' in the case of abortion. A philosophical definition of 'person' could also determine which medical procedures nurses could be morally and reasonably expected to assist with — for example, organ transplants, abortions and experimental research procedures.

The important lesson to be learned here is that unless ethical definitions are scrupulously formulated, given and revised, moral language will be in danger of corrupting and/or distorting sound and purposeful bioethical debate, rather than contributing reliably and constructively to it. Poorly or inappropriately defined ethical terms and concepts can also seriously impinge upon and limit the moral imagination, and not least the moral options and choices that might otherwise be apprehended, contemplated and chosen in the face of moral adversity (Johnstone 1988). The notion of 'quality of life' is a good example. Many writers on bioethics assume that when a life ceases to be 'independent' it has diminished worth. In such instances, euthanasia might be considered a right and proper course of action to take. Here the ethically loaded notion of 'dependence' imparts a sense of permissibility of the euthanasia option and limits any thought of, say, pursuing a rehabilitation option. It also overrides any thought of the possibility that for some people 'dependence' may be quite irrelevant to the notion of a worthwhile life. Kanitsaki (1989, 1993, 1994), for example, has shown that in some traditional cultural groups, familial and friendly relationships are characteristically *collective and interdependent*, and thus any thought of *individual independence* is quite irrelevant to the assessment of 'a life worth living'.

The limiting effects of language on the moral imagination will be demonstrated more thoroughly as the discussions in this book are advanced. It remains the task here, meanwhile, to identify and provide brief working definitions of some key terms commonly used in discussions on bioethical issues: 'ethics'/'morality', 'bioethics', and 'nursing ethics'.

What is ethics?

It is appropriate to begin the task of defining commonly used ethical terms and concepts by first examining the terms 'ethics' and 'morality' themselves. Contrary to popular nursing opinion, there is no philosophically significant difference between the terms 'ethics' and 'morality' (Ladd 1978, p. 400; Beauchamp and Childress 1994, p. 5). If a distinction is to be drawn between these two terms it is one that is based on etymological grounds, with 'ethics' coming from the ancient Greek *ethikos* (originally meaning 'pertaining to custom or habit'), and 'morality' coming from the Latin *moralitas* (also originally meaning 'custom' or 'habit'). This means, of course, that it is not incorrect to use the terms interchangeably, as many philosophers in fact do, and as is done here. With respect to deciding which terms should be used in ethical discourse (i.e. whether to use the term 'ethics' or the term 'morality'), this is very much a matter of personal preference rather than of rigorous philosophical debate. Of course, contemporary definitions of the terms ethics and morality are far more sophisticated than those given earlier of 'custom' or 'habit' as will soon be shown.

Meanwhile, it remains the task here to clarify what this thing is that we call 'ethics'.

Ethics, popularly used as a generic term for referring to 'various ways of understanding and examining the moral life' (Beauchamp and Childress 1994, p. 4), can be traced back to the influential works of the Ancient Greek philosophers Socrates (born 469BC), Plato (born 428BC) and Aristotle (born 384BC). The works of these ancient Greek philosophers were especially influential in seeing ethics firmly established as a branch of philosophical inquiry which sought dispassionate and 'rational' clarification and justification of the basic assumptions and beliefs that people hold about what is to be considered morally acceptable and morally unacceptable behaviour. Ethics thus evolved as a mode of philosophical inquiry (known as moral philosophy) that asked people to question why they considered a particular act right or wrong, what the reasons (justifications) were for their judgments, and whether their judgments were correct. This view of ethics remains an influential one and, although the subject of increasing controversy over recent years, retains considerable currency in the mainstream ethics literature. Today, ethics is generally regarded as being a critically reflective activity fundamentally concerned with a systematic examination of the moral life and 'is designed to illuminate what we ought to do by asking us to consider and reconsider our ordinary actions, judgments and justifications' (Beauchamp and Childress 1983, p. xii).

It is important to clarify that ethics has three distinct 'sub-fields', namely: *descriptive ethics*, *metaethics* and *normative ethics*. *Descriptive ethics* is the sub-domain of moral philosophy that is concerned with describing the variant moral values and beliefs (that is, values and beliefs concerning what constitutes 'right' and 'wrong'/'good' and 'bad' conduct) that different people hold across and within different cultures and sub-cultural groups. *Metaethics*, in contrast, is the sub-domain of moral philosophy that is concerned with the nature, logical form and language of morality. *Normative ethics*, in turn, is the sub-domain of moral philosophy that is concerned with establishing a standard of correctness by the prescription of certain rules and principles. Unlike descriptive ethics and metaethics, normative ethics is evaluative and prescriptive (hortatory) in nature. In the case of the latter, ethics inquiry is not so much concerned with how the world is, but with how it *ought* to be. In other words, it is not concerned with merely *describing* the world (although, of course, a description of the world is necessary as a starting point for an evaluative inquiry), but rather in *prescribing* how it should be and providing *sound justification* for this prescription. Just what is to count as a 'sound justification', however, is an open question and one that will be considered in the following chapter. In this text, all three sub-fields are drawn upon in varying degrees to advance knowledge and understanding of ethical issues in nursing.

What is bioethics?

In order to gain some understanding of the nature and implications of bioethics (a form of moral philosophy) to and in nursing, it would be helpful to first consider briefly the origins and historical use of the term 'bioethics' which, in several respects, has emerged as a synonym for health care ethics.

Bioethics can be defined as 'the systematic study of the moral dimensions — including moral vision, decisions, conduct and policies — of the life sciences and health care, employing a variety of ethical methodologies in an interdisciplinary setting' (Reich 1995a, p. xxi). The term 'bioethics' (from the Greek *bios* meaning 'life', and *ethikos, ithiki* meaning 'ethics') is a neologism which first found its way into public usage in 1970–71 in the United States of America (Reich 1994). Although originally the subject of only cautious acceptance by a few influential North American academics, the new term quickly 'symbolised and influenced the rise and shaping of the field itself' (Reich 1994, p. 320). Significantly, within three years of its emergence, the new term was accepted and used widely at a public level (Reich 1994, p. 328). Interestingly, it is believed that the term 'bioethics' caught on because it was 'simple' and because it was amenable to exploitation by the media which had placed a great premium 'on having a simple term that could readily be used for public consumption' (Reich 1994, p. 331). It is worth noting that initially the term 'bioethics' was used in two different ways reflecting both the concerns and ambitions of two respective academics who, it is suggested, quite possibly created the word independently of each other. The first (and later marginalised) sense in which the word was used had an 'environmental and evolutionary significance' (Reich 1994, p. 320). Specifically, it was intended to advocate attention to 'the problem of survival: the questionable survival of the human species and the even more questionable survival of nations and cultures' (Potter 1971 — cited by Reich 1994, p. 321). In short, it advocated long-range environmental concerns (Reich 1995b, p. 20). Reich (1994) explains that the key objective in creating this term was:

> to identify and promote an optimum changing environment, and an optimum human adaptation within that environment, so as to sustain and improve the civilised world.
>
> (Reich 1994, pp. 321–2)

The other competing sense in which the word 'bioethics' was used referred more narrowly to the ethics of medicine and biomedical research. The primary focus of this approach was:

1. the rights and duties of patients and health care professionals;
2. the rights and duties of research subjects and researchers;
3. the formulation of public policy guidelines for clinical care and biomedical research (Reich 1995b, p. 20).

Significantly, it was this latter sense which 'came to dominate the emerging field of bioethics in academic circles and in the mind of the public' — and which remains dominant today (Reich 1994, p. 320). There are a number of complex reasons for this, not least, the climate at the time which saw the rise of the civil rights movement (including women's rights and the legal right to abortion which helped to keep bioethical issues 'before the public' as it were). Given the significant shift in social and moral values that was occurring at the time, however, it is perhaps not surprising that this essentially medicocentric sense of bioethics prevailed (Jonsen 1993; Singer 1994). For instance, it is now almost certain that the ideas behind the development of the field of bioethics in its medicocentric sense had been simmering for almost a decade before the field was eventually named (Jonsen 1993, S3). Notable among the events inspiring the development of the field were: the dialysis events of the early 1960s, the publication in 1966 of Henry Beecher's legendary and confronting article on the unethical design and conduct of twenty-two medical research projects, the heart transplant movement, and later the now famous 1975 Karen Ann Quinlan case (Jonsen 1993; see also Singer 1994; McNeill 1993; Pappworth 1967; Beecher 1966).

Today, the dominant concerns of mainstream Western bioethics are still essentially medicocentric, with the most sustained attention (and, it should be added, the most institutional support) being given to examining the ethical and legal dimensions of such 'exotic' issues as: abortion, euthanasia, organ transplantation (and the associated issue of brain-death criteria), reproductive technology (for example, in vitro fertilisation (IVF), genetic engineering, and so forth), ethics committees, informed consent, confidentiality, the economic rationalisation of health care (and the relatively new associated issue of 'medical futility'), and research ethics (particularly in regard to randomised clinical trials and experimental surgery). Not only has mainstream bioethics come to refer to and represent these issues, but, rightly or wrongly, has given legitimacy to them — through the power of naming — as *the* most pressing bioethical concerns of contemporary health care in the Western World.

It is alleged that Potter (one of the authors of the term, bioethics) was himself very frustrated with this narrow conception of bioethics and is reported as responding that 'my own view of bioethics calls for a much broader vision' (Reich 1995b, p. 20). Indeed, Potter feared (prophetically as it turned out) that 'the Georgetown approach would simply reaffirm medical professional inclination to think of issues in terms of therapy versus prevention' (Reich 1995b, pp. 20–1). Whereas Potter viewed bioethics as a 'new discipline' (of science *and* philosophy) emphasising a search for wisdom, the Georgetown group saw bioethics as an old discipline (applied ethics) to resolve concrete moral problems; that is, 'ordinary ethics applied in the bio-realm' (Reich 1995b, p. 21; see also Clouser 1978).

It has been claimed that 'bioethics is a native-grown American product' reflecting distinctively American concerns and offering distinctively American solutions and resolutions to the bioethical problems identified (Jonsen 1993, S3–4). Whatever the merits of this claim, there is little doubt that bioethics in its medicocentric sense has become an international movement. This movement (propelled along by a variety of processes) has witnessed a number of spectacular achievements, not least: the development of an awesome international body of literature on the subject of bioethics (including the powerfully legitimating publication in 1978 of the internationally reputed *Encyclopedia of bioethics*, discussed in Chapter 2 of this text; and the international dissemination of a more recent innovation, namely, the CD-ROM 'Bioethics Line'), the global establishment of research centres devoted specifically to investigating ethical issues in health care and related matters, the emergence of a new profession of hospital ethicists/consultant ethicists, the establishment of prestigious university chairs in applied ethics, the rise of a commercially viable and even lucrative bioethics education industry, and, not least, the stimulation of public and political debate on 'life and death' matters in health care which, in many instances, has had a positive effect on influencing long overdue social policy and law reform in regard to these matters. At the time of writing this chapter, there is a sense that these developments are still gathering momentum and have not yet reached a plateau. However, whether this momentum is travelling in the right direction — or, more correctly, *directions* — remains an open question.

The medicocentric sense of the term 'bioethics' has indeed dominated intellectual and political thought over the past two or three decades. Nevertheless, there are signs that this dominance is being called into question, if not beginning to weaken (see, in particular, the *Introduction to the Encyclopedia of bioethics* [Reich, 1995a]). At present, there is considerable room to speculate that in the not too distant future the term 'bioethics' might once again hold an environmental and evolutionary significance, and be more reflective of the interests and concerns of entities who, in the past, have been marginalised in and by mainstream bioethics discourse. An important objective of this text is to challenge the minimisation and marginalisation of nurses and nursing ethics in mainstream bioethics discourse.

What is nursing ethics?

In Chapter 2 of this text it was asserted that the nursing profession has its own rich and distinctive history of professional (nursing) ethics. Despite this history, the idea that nursing ethics is a distinctive field in its own right has not been without controversy. For instance, it has been suggested by some authors, incorrectly in my view, that nursing ethics is merely 'a subcategory of medical ethics' (see, for example, Veatch 1985; Veatch and Fry 1987), or, at the very least, should not to be treated 'in contradistinction to medical ethics or bioethics' (Melia 1994). While it could be contended, controversially, that nursing ethics is a subcategory of bioethics (and thus, borrowing from Reich [1995b, p. 30], could be called 'nursing bioethics'), it is demonstrably not the case that nursing ethics is a subcategory of medical ethics as hopefully the discussion below will now show.

In clarifying what nursing ethics is, it is important to first understand that 'medicine', 'nursing' and 'health' are quite distinct concepts, as are the notions and practices of 'medical care', 'nursing care' and 'health care'. To hold 'medicine' as being paradigmatic of 'health' or 'health care' (or, for that matter, of 'nursing' and 'nursing care') is, as Kleinman (1980, p. 37) correctly points out, 'ethnocentric and reductionistic', or, to borrow from Barnard (1988), 'medicocentric'. 'Health' involves a holistic concept of wellbeing; this is in contrast with traditional medicocentric notions of health being merely the 'absence of disease' or as something that can only be measured physiologically (Eberst 1984; Boddy 1985; Newman 1986; Nordenfelt 1987; Mordacci and Sobel 1998). Health care, in turn, can be — and is — provided by a range of people, not just members of the medical profession. Many people do not seek professional medical care; often they seek and receive help for their health problems from other people (Chrisman 1981; Waring 1988; Rowland 1988; Abel and Nelson 1990). These 'other people' include other health care professionals such as nurses, physiotherapists, osteopaths, chiropractors, psychotherapists, and 'alternative health therapists' such as herbalists, masseurs, aromatherapists, and so on. They also include lay carers such as parents, relatives, siblings, friends, partners and spouses, with women often sharing a disproportionate burden of care in lay caring contexts (Sax 1984; Abel and Nelson 1990; see also Toy 1998). While it is acknowledged that medical care is a form of health care, it can be seen that not all health care is medical care. Furthermore, while nursing care is obviously a form of health care, it is not a form of medical care. It also needs to be clarified that, while nursing care and medical care can and do overlap in some areas, this should not be taken to mean that nursing *ipso facto* is dependent on medicine, or that nursing knowledge does not exist independently of medical knowledge; similarly, neither should an overlap in medical and nursing care be taken as implying that nursing ethics is at best only vicarious to or a subcategory of medical ethics.

The generic use of the term 'medical' when referring to health and nursing care is misleading, and serves to promote the hegemony of the medical profession in these areas. Similarly in the case of the term 'medical' being used in reference to what might be broadly described as 'health care ethics'. The terms 'bioethics', 'biomedical ethics', 'health care ethics' and 'medical ethics' do not refer to one and the same thing. It has already been shown in the discussion on bioethics (pp. 43–5), that while bioethics tends to be medicocentric, it is not medical ethics *per se*. At best, medical ethics (taken here as ethics from the distinctive role differentiated perspective of medical practice) is a subcategory of bioethics, a form of moral philosophy. It is conceptually incorrect and misleading then to treat medical ethics as being synonymous with health care ethics or bioethics. It is also conceptually incorrect and misleading to treat nursing ethics as a subcategory of medical ethics given the quite distinct realms of inquiry, practice and theoretical perspectives to which these respective fields relate. If nursing ethics is to be regarded as a subcategory of anything (and it is far from clear that it is), it is more likely to be that of bioethics in much the same way that medical ethics is. This, however, begs the question of what is nursing ethics?

Nursing ethics can be defined broadly as the examination of all kinds of ethical and bioethical issues from *the perspective of nursing theory and practice* which, in turn, rest on the agreed core concepts of nursing, namely: person, culture, care, health, healing, environment, and nursing itself (or, more to the point, its *telos*; that is, its end good) — all of which have been comprehensively articulated in the nursing literature (too vast to list here). In this regard, then, contrary to popular belief, nursing ethics is not synonymous with (and indeed is much greater than) an ethic of care, although an ethic of care has an important place in the overall moral scheme of nursing and nursing ethics (a point that will be explored further in Chapter 5, 'A feminist perspective on ethics and bioethics'). Unlike other approaches to ethics, nursing ethics recognises the 'distinctive voices' that are nurses, and emphasises the importance of collecting and recording nursing narratives and 'stories from the field' (Parker 1990; Bishop and Scudder 1990; Benner 1991, 1994; Hodge 1993). Collecting and collating stories from the field are regarded as important since issues invariably emerge from these stories that extend far beyond the 'paramount' issues otherwise espoused by mainstream bioethics. Analyses of these stories tend to reveal not only a range of issues that are nurses' 'own', as it were, but a whole different configuration of language, concepts and metaphors for expressing them (examples of which will be given in Chapter 7 of this text on identifying and resolving moral problems). As well, these stories often reveal issues otherwise overlooked or marginalised by mainstream bioethics discourse. Given this, nursing ethics can also be described as *methodologically and substantively, inquiry from the point of view of nurses' experiences*, with nurses' experiences being taken as a more reliable starting point than other mainstream ethics discourses (texts, practices and processes) from which to advance a substantive and meaningful nursing ethics discourse.

Like other approaches to ethics, however, nursing ethics recognises the importance of providing practical guidance on how to decide and act morally. Drawing on a variety of ethical theoretical considerations (a kind of 'coherentist' approach; see Beauchamp and Childress 1994, p. 20), nursing ethics at its most basic could thus also be described as a practice discipline which aims to provide guidance to nurses on how to decide and act morally in the contexts in which they work.

The project of nursing ethics has been and remains multifarious in nature and approach. Among other things, it involves nurses engaging in 'a positive project of constructing and developing alternative models, methods, procedures [and] discourses' of nursing and health care ethics that are more responsive to the lived realities and experiences of nurses and the people for whose care they share responsibility (adapted from Gross 1986, p. 195). In completing this positive project, nursing ethics has had — and continues to have — the consequence of decentring mainstream (medicocentric) bioethics in the hierarchy of moral discourses and allowing other 'weaker' (read, minimised, marginalised, and repressed) discourses (for example, those of nurses and patients) to emerge and be heard. In this respect, nursing ethics is also intensely political — although, it should be added, no more political than other emergent role differentiated ethics, medical ethics being a case in point.

As in the case of moral philosophy, nursing ethics inquiry can be pursued by focusing on one or all of the following:

- *descriptive nursing ethics* (describing the variant moral values and beliefs that nurses hold and the various moral practices in which nurses engage across and within different cultures);
- *meta(nursing) ethics* (undertaking a critical examination of the nature, logical form and language of ethics in nursing); and
- *normative nursing ethics* (establishing standards of correctness and prescribing the rules of conduct with which nurses are expected to comply).

(Johnstone 1998, pp. 39–69)

In response to critics of nursing ethics, distinctive nursing ethics is not only necessary, but inevitable. It is necessary because 'a profession without its own distinctive moral convictions has nothing to profess' and will be left vulnerable to the corrupting influences of whatever forces are most powerful (be they religious, legal, social, political or other in nature) (Churchill 1989, p. 30). Furthermore, as Churchill (1989, p. 31) writes, 'Professionals without an ethic are merely technicians, who know how to perform work, but who have no capacity to say why their work has any larger meaning'. Without meaning, there is little or no motivation to perform 'well' (see also Johnstone 1998, pp. 74–6).

In regard to the inevitability of nursing ethics, as Churchill (1989, p. 31) points out, the 'practice of a profession makes those who exercise it privy to a set of experiences that those who do not practice lack'. By this view, those who practise nursing are privy to a set of experiences (moral experiences included) that others who do not practise nursing lack. So long as nurses qua nurses interact with and enter into professional caring relationships with other people, they will not be able to avoid or sidestep the 'distinctively nursing' experience of deciding and acting morally while in these relationships. It is in this respect, then, that nursing ethics can be said to be *inevitable*.

In summary, so long as nurses continue to work and practise in a professional capacity in these contexts, and practise in accordance with the agreed ethical standards of the profession, their professional ethics will be practised 'distinctively' (see Johnstone 1998). In this regard, it makes little sense to assert that 'nursing ethics has no right to an independent existence' (Melia 1994, p. 8). Nursing ethics already exists in its own right, and this existence is no less warranted than any other ethical perspective.

What ethics is not

Now that we have come some way in discovering what ethics (and its counterparts bioethics and nursing ethics) is, it would be useful to give some attention to what ethics is not. For instance, ethics is not 'legal' law (i.e. as distinct from moral law), a code of conduct or ethics, hospital etiquette, hospital policy, public opinion, or following the orders of a superior. Failing to distinguish ethics from these things could result in harmful consequences to people in health care domains.

Legal law

Ethics and legal law overlap in significant ways, but they are nevertheless quite distinct from one another. This distinction becomes particularly clear in instances where what the law may require in a given situation, ethics might equally reject, and vice versa. Consider, for example, the issue of active voluntary euthanasia and the plight of patients suffering intractable and intolerable pain who request euthanasia as a 'treatment' option. Current Australian legal law prohibits voluntary active euthanasia (Lanham 1993). As the law stands, it is quite clear that any nurse or doctor who administers a lethal injection to a patient with the sole intention of bringing about that patient's death would probably be charged with murder. The fact that such an act was demonstrably in accordance with the patient's rational wishes would not be a legitimate defence. Regardless of the benevolence and voluntariness of an act of euthanasia, it would still be deemed by law as illegal, and thereby *legally wrong*. This legal wrongness, however, is in no way synonymous with moral wrongness. Consider the following.

Secular moral law (the essence of which is discussed in greater detail in Chapter 4) essentially requires that people be respected as self-determining choosers, and further that the considered preferences of persons be maximised. This requirement holds even in instances where a person's individual preferences might be considered mistaken or foolish by others. Moral law also requires that otherwise avoidable harm (such as the needless suffering of intractable and intolerable pain) should be prevented where this can be done without sacrificing other important moral interests. Returning to our euthanasia example, it soon becomes clear that an application of moral law (or, more particularly, moral principles) in this instance would probably permit the administration of a lethal injection to a suffering patient who has autonomously requested it. Not only would moral law permit such an act; it would most likely demand it to be done. Given the benevolence and voluntariness of the act, it would be deemed as having accorded with moral law and thereby as being *morally right*.

Other compelling examples illuminating the difference between law and morality can be found by considering the laws enforced during wartime (such as those upheld by the Nazi regime), and the laws used to enforce apartheid (such as those upheld in early North America, and, until recently, in South Africa). The legal laws of the Nazis and of the apartheid-supporting regimes, although iniquitous, still stand as constituting valid *legal* law (Hart 1958). We would presumably want to resist condoning the *morality* of these laws, however.

Law and ethics are quite separate action-guiding systems, and care must be taken to distinguish between them. Making this distinction may not only help to prevent moral errors, but may also enforce moral and intellectual honesty about the undesirability of morally iniquitous law (Hart 1958). Further, if we do not make this distinction we will not have an independent value system from which to judge the moral acceptability or unacceptability of valid legal law. For instance, if morality were not distinct from legal law, we could not judge certain laws (e.g. Nazi laws) to be morally iniquitous.

The question remains, however, of how the distinction between law and ethics can be made, and, equally important, what the essential differences are between a legal decision and a moral/ethical decision, and, indeed, a clinical decision.[1]

A very traditional view of law is that it is the command or order of a sovereign (for example, a government) backed by a threat or sanction (for example, punishment) (Hart 1961). For instance, governments in the Western World have formulated laws which command their citizens to pay taxes; if the citizens in question fail to pay their taxes, they can expect to be punished in some way, such as by being fined or even sent to prison. The mere fact that they have not complied with the command — in essence, have broken the law — would probably be deemed sufficient justification for a sanction or punishment to be directed against them. Although this view of law does not capture its more political nature (see, for example, Kairys 1982; Thornton 1990; Fineman and Thomadsen 1991; Johnstone 1994b), it is nevertheless sufficient for the purposes of this discussion in regard to distinguishing between law and ethics.

Accepting the above view of law, there is a fundamental sense in which the concept 'legal decision' as it is used colloquially by nurses probably refers to a type of decision that is made on the basis of what is required or prohibited by law — together with a desire to avoid a legal sanction or punishment for non-compliance. In this respect, the notion 'legal decision' is probably more aptly described as a 'legally defensive' decision. Consider the following example. A nurse who regards voluntary euthanasia as morally justified in cases of intolerable and intractable suffering may nevertheless decline a patient's considered request for assistance to die in order to avoid any risk of receiving the penalty that would almost certainly be applied for murder should her actions be discovered. In this instance, the nurse's decision not to comply with the patient's request could be described as a 'legal decision' rather than a moral or clinical decision, and also as being 'legally defensive'. This is because her decision was influenced predominantly by considering the legal consequences of complying with the patient's request, rather than the moral or clinical consequences of doing so.

The question remains, however, of how a legal decision differs from an ethical decision. As is discussed more fully in the following chapter, ethics can be defined as a system of overriding rules and principles which function by specifying that certain behaviours are either required, prohibited or permitted. These principles are chosen autonomously on the basis of critical reflection, and are backed by autonomous moral reason (generally recognised in moral philosophy as the central organising principle of morality) and/or by feelings of guilt, shame, moral

---

1. The following discussion of these distinctions is drawn from Johnstone 1994a.

remorse and the like which operate as kinds of moral sanctions. For example, we may choose autonomously to follow a moral principle which demands truth telling; if we fail to tell the truth in a given situation, we may then reason the act to be wrong and/or experience feelings of guilt, shame or moral remorse accordingly. Unlike what happens in instances involving a breach of legal law, however, we are not generally 'punished' for lying — for example, by being fined or sent to prison — unless, of course, our lying entails an outright act of perjury in a court of law.

Accepting this view of ethics, it is probably correct to say that the concept 'ethical decision', as it is used colloquially in health care contexts, refers to a type of decision which is guided by certain prescriptive and proscriptive moral principles of conduct or other moral considerations (rather than by punitive legal laws) and a desire to achieve a given moral end. Thus, a doctor or a nurse tempted to tell a lie to either a colleague or a patient may choose instead to tell the truth in order to achieve some predicted overriding moral benefit and thereby also preserve her or his integrity as a morally autonomous person (as distinct from, say, a law-abiding citizen).

In light of these basic views on law and ethics, what is the essential nature of nursing and medicine in this decision-making schema? Primarily, nursing and medicine involve the skilful practice and application of tested principles of applied science and care to prevent, diagnose, alleviate or cure disease, illness and sickness and restore a person's health and sense of wellbeing. The practices of nursing and medicine are backed by legal and professional sanctions. For example, doctors and nurses can be found financially liable for negligence, and can be deregistered for professional misconduct, or even for civil misconduct unbefitting a professional person (see, for example, Pyne 1981; Johnstone 1998).

To say of a decision that it is a 'nursing decision' or a 'medical decision' in this context, however, is probably to say little more than that it has been made by a nurse or a doctor respectively, and is based on an established body of knowledge and 'reasonable' professional opinion on how this knowledge should or should not be applied in a clinical situation. For example, a doctor may venture the 'reasonable' medical opinion that if a certain life-saving treatment is stopped the patient will surely die. Or a nurse may venture the 'reasonable' nursing opinion that if a certain nursing care is not given the patient will suffer a particular type of harm. It must be understood here, however, that neither of the clinical opinions expressed in these instances is tantamount to expressing a valid moral judgment. For example, to say that a patient 'will die' if a certain drug or other treatment (for example, surgery) is given or withheld says nothing about the moral permissibility or imperatives of giving or withholding the drug or other treatment in question. The morality of a given clinical act is not implicit in the act itself; this is something which can be determined only by independent moral analysis.

Given these rough comparisons, it can be seen that legal, ethical and clinical decisions can be readily distinguished from one another. What is also obvious is the enormous potential for the respective demands of each of these three types of decisions to come into conflict. For example, a medical decision not to resuscitate a patient in the event of a cardiac arrest (on the grounds that the patient's condition is 'medically hopeless') may be supported by an established body of medical opinion, but nevertheless be deemed morally unsound or even illegal, or both. For instance, the patient's autonomous wishes may not have been established before the medical decision was made, or the patient's legally valid consent may not have been obtained to withhold cardiopulmonary resuscitation (CPR) in the event of a cardiac arrest. Or, to take another example, a medical decision to continue treating a patient may accord with a 'reasonable body of medical opinion', be legal (as in cases where patients have been deemed rationally incompetent under a mental health act), yet be quite unethical if the patient has expressly stated a wish not to be treated, and if this expressed wish, contrary to popular medical opinion, is not 'irrational' (as happened in the John McEwan case, cited in Chapter 8). We can also imagine cases where a medical decision to cease treatment accords with moral principles but may nevertheless invite legal censure — as in the case of withholding unduly burdensome life-prolonging treatment from severely disabled newborns or severely brain-injured adults.

Although there is potential for conflict between ethical, legal and clinical decisions, it is not the case that these are always on a direct collision course; indeed, they may even be in full harmony with each other, as examples given later in this text show.

In drawing comparisons between legal, ethical and clinical decisions, there remains another crucial point to be observed: that it is conceptually incorrect to regard nursing or medical decisions per se as synonymous with either legal or moral decisions. This is not to say that we cannot meaningfully speak of nursing or medical decisions as being legally or morally correct or incorrect, as the case may be. On the contrary, it merely makes the point that, in asserting the legal or moral status of a given clinical (nursing or medical) decision, a judgment *independent* of the generally accepted scientific or indeed conventional standards of nursing or medicine must be made. In the case of ethics, the moral status of a clinical decision requires independent *philosophical/moral* analysis and judgment based on relevant moral considerations (e.g. moral rules and principles); and in the case of law, the legal status of a clinical decision requires an independent *legal* analysis and judgment based on relevant legal considerations (e.g. legal rules and principles).

Codes of ethics

A code may be defined as a conventionalised set of rules or expectations devised for a select purpose. A code of professional ethics by this view could be described as (a document explicating) a conventionalised set of moral rules and/or expectations devised for the purposes of guiding ethical professional conduct. It is important to understand, however, that codes of ethics are not ethics per se since they are not fully developed *systematic theories* of ethics. Nevertheless, codes of ethics tend to reflect a rich set of moral values that have been explicated through a process of extensive consultation, debate, refinement, evaluation and review by practitioners over a period of time, and thus are well situated to function as meaningful action guides (Johnstone 1998, pp. 7–15).

It is important to state at the outset that codes of ethics can be either *prescriptive* or *aspirational* in nature. In the case of *prescriptive codes*, provisions are 'duty-directed, stating specific duties of members' (Skene 1996, p. 111). In contrast, *aspirational codes* are 'virtue-directed, stating desirable aims while acknowledging that in some circumstances conduct short of the ideal may be justified' (Skene 1996, p. 111). Either way, codes of ethics have as their principal concern directing:

> what professionals ought or ought not to do, how they ought to comport themselves, what they, or the profession as a whole, ought to aim at ...
> (Lichtenberg 1996, p. 14)

Codes of ethics are not, however, without difficulties — a point noted almost 100 years ago by the distinguished North American nurse leader and scholar, Lavinia Dock.

In a little-known but important essay entitled 'Ethics — or a code of ethics?', Dock challenged:

> What, exactly, could a Code of Ethics be? ... What are ethics and can they be codified? Do we aim at ethical exclusiveness and shall our ethical development be bounded or limited by a code? 'Code' suggests statutes, infringements, penalties, antagonisms. If we have the ethics, we will not need a code. The code is to regulate those who have no ethics, and in proportion as ethical principles are made a part of our natures and lives, our codes and restrictions will shrivel away and die the death of inanition.
>
> (Dock 1900, p. 37)

Dock goes on to explain that she is not advocating the total rejection of rules and regulations of professional conduct — to the contrary, particularly since such rules and regulations, as given in a code, could serve as helpful mechanisms 'to prop up the steps of those who are young in self-government or feeble in self-control' (p. 38). Rather, the issue was not to call codes of rules and regulations *ethics*, since, as she argued persuasively, there was a real risk that:

> If we call them ethics we may perhaps come to believe that they are all there is of ethics, and presently be worshipping the code rather than the thing, so unreasoning a reverence is there in our souls for statutes, fines, and punishments; so exaggerated a notion of the potency of drafted laws; so strong a tendency to make rules the end and aim of life rather than simply conveniences, changeable contrivances.
>
> (Dock 1900, p. 38)

Although written almost a century ago, Dock's visionary words are applicable today. Nurses globally would be well advised to be cautious in their use of formally stated and adopted codes of ethics, and to be especially vigilant not to fall prey to 'worshipping the code' at the expense of *being* ethical — and not to fall into the trap of treating the prescriptions and proscriptions of a code as absolute, and as ends in themselves, rather than as prima facie guides to ethical professional conduct.

It has long been recognised that a professional code of ethics is an important hallmark of a profession (Goldman 1980; Bayles 1981; Johnstone 1986). Whether professional codes as such have succeeded in fulfilling their intended purpose of 'formulating the norms of professional ethics' (Bayles 1981, p. 25) and guiding ethical professional conduct is, however, another matter. Some have argued that codes of ethics have failed to ensure this; instead, codes of ethics have served to protect the interests of the professional group espousing them, rather than the interests of the client groups whom the professionals are supposed to be serving (Kultgen 1982, pp. 53–69; Beauchamp and Childress 1994, pp. 6–8).

Despite the demonstrable shortcomings of professional codes of ethics, it is evident that many professional codes of ethics (such as those included as appendixes to this text) have been written with the noble intention of guiding ethically just professional practice. What needs to be understood, however, is that even the most scrupulously formulated and well-intended professional code of ethics is not without its limitations and, in the final analysis, may do little to either guide moral deliberation or ensure the realisation of morally just outcomes in morally problematic situations. In the case of the nursing profession, neither will following a code of ethics necessarily protect nurses when they are called upon to defend their actions, say, in a court or disciplinary hearing (see Johnstone 1994b, pp. 251–67; 1998).

In the noted North American law case of *Warthen v Toms River Community Memorial Hospital* (1985), for example, the court dismissed altogether the ANA Code for Nurses as an authoritative statement of public policy. And, in an Australian case involving the alleged unfair dismissal of a registered nurse involved in a case of suspected child sexual abuse (referred to earlier in Chapter 2 of this text), the deputy president of the Industrial Relations Commission of Victoria criticised and rejected the authority of the ICN (1973) *Code for Nurses*, which was referred to in defence of the nurse's actions in this area. It will be recalled that, the deputy president of the Commission criticised the ICN Code as being 'imprecise' and lacking the ability to provide 'clear guidance' in matters requiring fine discretionary professional judgment. He also pointed out that the 'code in its terms cannot stand alone' and must be considered in relation to the guidance which is also offered by the law (*In re alleged unfair dismissal of Ms K Howden by the City of Whittlesea* 1990). The fact that the ICN Code is widely accepted by professional nursing organisations around the world had little bearing on the deputy president's views in this case.

The legal status of the acclaimed *Code of Professional Practice* of the United Kingdom Central Council for Nursing, Midwifery and Health Visiting (1984) is also uncertain, its authority having been rejected by at least one court since its adoption in the early 1980s (Rea 1987, p. 534).

One question which arises here is that, if codes of ethics are problematic, and have only limited legal (and, it should be added, moral) authority, should nurses adopt them? The short answer to this question is yes. One justification for this is that, despite their limitations, codes of ethics have an important role to play in the broader schema of professional nursing ethics insofar as they can provide a public statement on the kinds of moral standards and values that patients and the broader community can expect nurses to uphold, and against which nurses can be held publicly accountable. Second, they can also inform those contemplating entering the profession of the kinds of values and standards which they will be expected to uphold, and which, if not upheld, could result in some sort of professional censure. For example, the ICN *Code for Nurses* makes explicit that a nurse's 'primary responsibility is to those people who require nursing care', and that, in providing care, the nurse will promote 'an environment in which the values, customs and spiritual beliefs of the individual are respected'. If people contemplating entering the profession of nursing are informed of these prescriptions, and do not agree with them, they will be in a better position to make an informed choice about whether or not to enter the profession.

Another justification is that codes of ethics can help with the cultivation of moral character (Johnstone 1998, pp. 7–15). They can do this by 'increasing the probability that people will behave in some ways rather than others' — specifically that they will behave in 'the right way' and, equally important, 'for the right reasons' (Lichtenberg 1996, p. 15). As already stated, although codes of ethics do not constitute systematic ethics per se (at best, they comprise only a list of rules that have been derived from systematic ethical thought), they nevertheless provide people with a reason to think and act ethically, not least by reminding them 'of the moral point of the sorts of activities they are involved in *as* members of the particular profession or group' (Coady 1996, p. 286). On this point, Lichtenberg (1996) contends:

> A code of ethics can increase the probability that people will think about it [what one is doing] — can make it more difficult to engage in self-deceptive practices — by explicitly describing behaviour that is undesirable or unacceptable.
>
> (Lichtenberg 1996, p. 18)

Crucial to the cultivation of moral character, is self-conscious moral reflection. And, as Freckelton (1996, p. 130) suggests controversially, codes of ethics 'are a means to this end'. He states:

> They [codes of ethics] have the potential to articulate the characteristics and ideals of a profession and to facilitate consciousness of and discourse about ethical issues. Through the process of moral deliberation thereby engendered, they may operate as the catalysts for ethical conduct both by heightening awareness of ethical priorities and by providing guidance from experienced professionals for the resolution of ethical conundra encountered at a practical level by practitioners ... By articulating the parameters of a profession and of acceptable professional conduct by its practitioners, a code defines what a profession is and is not, as well as the limits of proper conduct.
>
> (Freckelton 1996, p. 130)

Self-conscious moral reflection and discourses about ethical issues are facilitated by codes of ethics in at least one other important way, namely, by what Fullinwider (1996, p. 83) describes as supplying a vocabulary (which can be used for the purposes of stimulating 'moral self-understanding') and helping to '*create* a community of users'. To put this another way, by articulating a given set of ethical values, a code of ethics makes ethics discourse possible within a given professional group (community); it provides a (common) moral language, which can be used meaningfully by subscribers to a given code, to identify and discuss matters of moral importance and to advance the task of professional ethics generally in their milieu.

The point remains, however, as already argued, that codes of ethics have only prima facie moral authority (that is, they may be overridden by other, stronger moral considerations), and hence can only guide, not mandate, moral conduct in particular situations. Further, as Seedhouse (1988, p. 65) points out, it is important to understand that a code cannot inform a nurse which principles to follow in a given situation, how to interpret chosen principles, how to choose between conflicting principles, or 'how to decide when it is most ethical to disregard the rules and deliberate instead as a unique and independent individual' as is sometimes required. Accepting this, and as the examples given in the following chapters show, it can be seen that no code of professional nursing ethics should be regarded as an authoritative statement of universal action guides. Rather, it should be regarded only as a statement of prima facie rules which may be helpful in guiding moral decision-making in nursing care contexts, but which can be justly overridden by other, stronger moral considerations.

Hospital or professional etiquette

Nothing could be more different from ethics than etiquette. Although both seek to guide behaviour and conduct, they do so in quite different ways and for quite different purposes. Ethics, for example, speaks to morally significant rights and wrongs, with behaviour being guided by critically reflective moral thought and the application of sound moral values which seek to maximise the moral interests of all people equally. Etiquette, by contrast, speaks more to maintaining style and decorum, with behaviour being guided by the unreflective and arbitrary dictates of custom and convention. In application, etiquette paves the way for coordinated, consistent, predictable and, where possible, aesthetically pleasant practice and conduct, and serves only the interests of particular persons in particular circumstances (May 1983). As with legal law, what etiquette might demand in one situation, systematic ethics might reject, and vice versa.

The extent to which the notions of ethics and etiquette are confused in health care settings is well illustrated by the following cases — all of which, in varying degrees, emphasise the reluctance by health professionals (including nurses) to advise patients to seek a second medical opinion, in the mistaken belief that doing so would constitute a serious breach of ethics.

The first case (personal communication) involves a middle-aged woman suffering moderately severe retrosternal chest pain and shortness of breath who presented to the accident and emergency department of a large city hospital. The nursing staff admitted the woman into a cubicle equipped to deal with 'cardiac emergencies' and proceeded to perform an electrocardiograph (ECG). The ECG showed a number of cardiac arrhythmias, all of which were suggestive of an acute cardiac condition warranting immediate specialised medical and nursing care. Upon further questioning, it was revealed that the woman was also suffering a mild pain in her left arm (a pain she had 'never had before'), which is characteristic of cardiac disease. The pain improved, however, while she rested in the casualty department. Her past medical history indicated no known heart disease or any previous incidence of chest pain. This was the first time she had ever experienced such symptoms — symptoms which were indicative of significant underlying cardiac disease.

A junior first-year medical resident examined the woman and decided she should be admitted immediately into the coronary care unit for further cardiac monitoring and tests. As required by the hospital's admission policy, he contacted the registrar 'on call' to have his diagnosis confirmed and to arrange the woman's admission formally. Upon examining the patient, however, the registrar declined to admit her, since there were no 'cardiac beds' available in the hospital and he was not convinced that the ECG findings indicated a life-threatening cardiac condition. He discharged the woman, advising her to see her own general practitioner the following morning. He gave her a medical note and a prescription for an oral cardiac anti-arrhythmic agent.

The nursing staff were very concerned, as was the first-year medical resident. All felt the patient should have been seen by another doctor for a 'second opinion', but could not decide whether to advise the woman to go immediately to another hospital. After some twenty minutes of deliberation, the attending nursing supervisor concluded it would be 'unethical' to advise the patient to go to another hospital for a second examination. The nursing staff and junior doctor involved agreed. The patient walked out of the door and was not informed that it would be in her interests to seek a second medical opinion. At this hospital, it was not 'standard practice' to advise patients to seek second medical opinions.

What was at issue here, however, was breaching hospital *etiquette*. Advising the woman to seek a second medical opinion, in this case, would not have been unethical; indeed, there is considerable scope to suggest that offering such advice was morally obligatory in this case.

The second case is taken from Wendy Carlton's '*In our professional opinion ...*': *the primacy of clinical judgment over moral choice* (1978), and concerns an 11-year-old girl with Down's syndrome who was two months past menarche. The girl was admitted to hospital for a cardiac catheterisation in order to assess whether she could withstand the stresses of a hysterectomy (and a general anaesthetic); the hysterectomy had been recommended as a contraceptive measure. When a third-year medical student sought an explanation for why the girl was being admitted for such an elaborate procedure (it was evident to him that an oral contraceptive would have been quite sufficient to deal with the problem), a senior doctor admitted, 'it's a long drive on a short punt' (Carlton 1978, p. 33). When asked whether the girl's parents had been informed of the risks of the procedure, the attending doctor replied 'that he had minimised the risk rather than refusing to do the procedure, because "it turns people off, and they go elsewhere to get it done" ' (Carlton 1978, p. 33). Another doctor, however, was strongly against the idea of the girl having the hysterectomy. He argued that 'a tubal ligation at sixteen was a real possibility, but not a hysterectomy at eleven' (Carlton 1978, p. 33). Many involved in the case felt that the proposed procedures (i.e. the cardiac catheterisation and the hysterectomy) were unnecessary. Although the suggestion was made to contact the doctor who would be doing the cardiac catheterisation, 'the call was never made': '[No-one] was willing to incur the probable wrath of Dr Fine [the attending physician], who would resist any criticism of his clinical judgment. The proposed phone call would be a violation of *professional etiquette*' (Carlton 1978, p. 34, emphasis added).

The last case to be considered here concerns a woman who was advised by her surgeon to have a radical mastectomy for breast cancer (Johnstone 1987a). A domiciliary nurse involved in the care of this woman advised her to seek a second medical opinion, explaining that not all breast cancers warranted radical surgery, and that some conditions could be successfully treated by more conservative methods. Despite the fact that the woman's condition was indeed treatable by conservative methods (which the surgeon later admitted), the nurse was severely castigated by the surgeon in question — and by some of her nursing colleagues — and was criticised for being 'unethical'. The surgeon's response was: 'Yes, Mrs X would benefit from conservative treatment, but ...' (the 'but' implying he was a *surgeon* and was unable to offer a *medical* alternative). The patient did have a radical mastectomy. It is very clear that, contrary to popular criticism, and given a sound ethical analysis of this case, the nurse in question acted in a morally just way. Rather than breaching the demands of ethics, she had merely breached professional etiquette.

Etiquette obviously has its place in the professional and health care arena; it is not without limits, however. Unfortunately, as Blackburn (1984, p. 189) points out, people do 'often care more about etiquette, or reputation, or selfish advantage, than they do about morality'. The lesson to be learned here is that acting in accord with hospital or professional etiquette might sometimes be tantamount to acting unethically or immorally — or, in some instances, even illegally. It is, therefore, important that nurses learn to distinguish between the demands of etiquette and those of ethics.

Hospital or institutional policy

Hospital policy or institutional policy is often appealed to in order to legitimise a worker's actions and, in some cases, to settle a conflict of opinion about what course of action should be taken in a particular situation. In this respect, institutional or hospital policy plays an important practical role — it helps to coordinate 'the running of the system' and to make institutional practices consistent and predictable; nevertheless, it also paves the way for uncompromising control. Like legal law and etiquette, institutional policy can be morally iniquitous and in application can seriously conflict with the demands of ethics. The following case (taken from the author's personal observations) is a good example of how institutional policy can be at serious odds with ethics.

A 20-year-old woman in advanced premature labour was admitted to the casualty department of a city hospital. She was of a traditional Maori background, married, and the pregnancy had been planned. This was her third premature labour. On the two previous occasions she had spontaneously aborted at around twenty weeks' gestation. Her current pregnancy was also of approximately twenty weeks' gestation.

The obstetrics registrar was notified, but failed to appear before the young woman delivered her fully formed male fetus. The fetus was active upon delivery and was noted by nursing staff to have breathed, emitting a faint but audible high-pitched 'rasp' as it did so. In accordance with 'standard hospital procedure' the fetus was placed in a stainless steel kidney dish, taken immediately away from the mother's view, and placed, covered with a bed pan sheet, in the sluice room to die. The mother and her family, however, wanted to have 'the baby' near, not only to see it but more importantly to perform *karakia* (a kind of incantation or prayer), as stringently required by ancient Maori custom.[2]

Maori enrolled nurses working in the casualty department were greatly distressed by what was happening. As the mother and her family (one of whom was a *Tohunga* [priest]) were pleading to have the fetus returned, one of the Maori enrolled nurses went to the fetus in the sluice room 'to be with it, so that it would not die without knowing love'. Crying softly, she also admitted to a registered nurse involved in the case that she was going to offer a prayer 'for the child as he goes on his way ...'.

The doctor had, meanwhile, arrived in the department and examined the mother. He explained to her and her family that the fetus could not be released to them because 'tests had to be done on it'. He later explained to protesting nursing staff that fetuses delivered at the hospital were generally regarded as 'hospital property' and that it was 'hospital policy to send all aborted fetuses to the laboratory for analysis'. He also explained that the present case was particularly

---

2. The Oxford scholar Makereti (otherwise known as Maggie Papakura), the first Maori scholar to publish a comprehensive ethnographic account of Maori life, offers an illuminating explanation of this custom. In her celebrated work *The Old-Time Maori*, first published in 1938, she wrote (pp. 121–2):

> A case of premature birth seldom happened in the old days, and when it did, was supposed to be caused by the mother's breaking the laws of tapu [taboo]. A *Tohunga* [priest] then had to perform a *karakia Takutaku* over the woman to send away the *wairua* [spirit] of the unformed child, which was supposed to fly about in space — or it might enter a *mokomoko* [lizard] — and do harm to living people. A wairua of this kind, having never been properly formed, would never know any feelings of affection or love, and so would only try to do harm ... to living men, women and children ...

complicated because the fetus was of twenty weeks' gestation, and had breathed. It was therefore, technically speaking, a 'live birth', and thus an autopsy would have to be performed. This, he further claimed, was a legal requirement. Whether in fact this was correct was not known by those present at the time; informal sources have since indicated that autopsies cannot be performed without consent, and it is likely that the parents' claim to the fetus could have been legally upheld. Most of the registered nurses present nevertheless accepted the doctor's explanation and resigned themselves to 'hospital policy'.

One registered nurse, however, pressed the matter further and explained to the doctor that the 'hospital policy' in this instance was quite inappropriate given the situation at hand, and that to uphold the policy so rigidly stood to violate the Maori family's rights and interests. At the same time, the fetus had meanwhile been mistakenly submerged in the liquid preservative formalin and taken by a hospital orderly to the laboratory.

Fortunately, the doctor was sympathetic and sought to resolve the difficulties he perceived he would have with the hospital authorities by registering the fetus as being of less than twenty weeks' gestation, and as not having breathed. Nevertheless, the fetus was not retrieved from the laboratory for another twenty-four hours, by which time, sadly, considerable damage had already been done. The most the family and the *Tohunga* could now do was to try and appease the *wairua* (spirit) through *karakia*, and to try and persuade it to travel without taking harm with it. The mother's single room was turned into a *marae* (meeting place) setting, and a *tangi* (funeral) commenced. This was an act of sheer desperation, and in part an attempt to explain to the *wairua* why the violation and act of cruelty had occurred. It was also to grieve for what they had lost, and what would be lost to them forever.

Upholding hospital policy in this case resulted in an unacceptable level of human suffering — suffering which could have been avoided by a more critically reflective approach to the situation. Had those present been more aware of their moral obligations to respect the wishes of the mother and her family, a morally tolerable outcome could have been achieved. Fortunately, as a result of this particular incident, the hospital policy was revised, making it much easier for Maori mothers to claim their aborted fetuses.

This case demonstrates a situation where ethics is quite distinct from institutional policy, and where a review of ethical considerations may prompt reform of policy. It also shows how respect for hospital policy is not sufficient to ensure the realisation of morally desirable or morally tolerable outcomes.

Public opinion or the view of the majority

Ethics is not merely a matter of public opinion. If ethics were merely a matter of public opinion or majority view, all we would have to do is conduct an opinion poll on a given practice or procedure; its results would suffice to confirm whether the practice or procedure in question was morally right or wrong. Polling would quickly reduce moral testing to a crude 'might is right' formula — which goes against all the tenets of moral philosophy and the requirements of sound moral reasoning and justification (noting here that while public opinion might stand as a *good reason* for adopting a particular point of view on something, it nevertheless fails to provide a *sound justification* for doing so).

If ethics was determined by mere public opinion, our moral standards would be rendered unacceptably and intolerably fickle. Consider the following examples.

In 1987, a Saulwick poll published in *The Age* indicated that an overwhelming majority of Australians (66 per cent) 'approved of abortion in some circumstances' (Stephens 1987, p. 5). In April 1989, 300 000 people demonstrated their public support of legal abortion by marching on Capitol Hill in Washington, United States (Wainer 1989, p. 4). If ethics were merely a matter of public opinion, in these instances we would clearly be committed to accepting the permissibility of abortion. If public opinion were to change, we would likewise be committed to accepting the impermissibility of abortion. A public opinion view of ethics, in this instance, could change a judgment on the rightness or wrongness of abortion from one day to the next.

To take another example, in 1988 Kuhse and Singer published the results of their research project surveying medical opinion on active voluntary euthanasia. Their findings indicated that 'a clear majority of those who responded to the questionnaire support active voluntary euthanasia and that many doctors have provided active help in dying' (Kuhse and Singer 1988, p. 623). More recently, a New South Wales survey of 475 nurses found that 80 per cent of respondents favoured the legalisation of euthanasia in some circumstances (With AAP 1998, p. 9). If the majority view were to reign as the overriding moral view in this instance, doctors and nurses would be committed to support and practise active voluntary euthanasia until such time as the majority view changed.

A public opinion or majority view of ethics is open to serious objection. On a philosophical level, it violates a formal and necessary requirement for sound moral judgments, notably the requirement for *internal consistency* (Kuhse 1987, p. 25). Its findings are capricious, and thus morally unreliable. As well as this, on a more pragmatic level, there is the distasteful possibility that public opinion might be mistaken or wrong or misguided — particularly where public opinion has been manipulated by pressure groups or minorities (Brandt 1959, p. 59), or by the media, as occurred in the much publicised Chamberlain murder case in Australia, or by collective denial, as has occurred in cases of domestic and child abuse (Herman 1992). There is also, of course, the risk of opinion polls being fraudulent. As one woman wrote in a letter to the editor of *The Age*:

> If I felt strongly enough about the issue at hand [television phone-in polls] I could have spent the evening by my phone and, with the simple touch of one button, registered votes almost continuously without anyone being any the wiser to my hundreds and possibly thousands of votes ...

> ... Unfortunately many people never question the validity of opinion polls and instead take them at face value. I suspect that many think they represent general opinion, otherwise why conduct them.
>
> (Romanin 1988, p. 12)

It is not being denied here that public opinion is an important and relevant consideration that warrants some attention when deciding ethical issues. On the contrary, public opinion which reliably indicates a certain view on a given matter might well be a useful tool in guiding beneficial social policy and law reforms. However, public opinion is not infallible in matters of morality and mere *common acceptance* does not imply validity (Brandt 1959, p. 57). The moral rightness or wrongness of an act can be decided only by sound critical reflection, not merely by public opinion or 'collective desire' or 'collective preference'.

Following the orders of a superior

Contemporary bioethics relies heavily on the notion of autonomy, and in particular on persons autonomously and freely choosing the moral values and principles they are going to commit themselves to, and are going to rely upon for guiding their moral actions and decisions. By this account, it can be seen that following the moral commands or authority of another is quite incompatible with the notion of autonomous moral thinking and acting. Moreover, it paves the way for the abdication of moral responsibility and accountability. Superiors have superiors, and these superiors have still more superiors. A hierarchical system of authority may mean in practice that, because everyone is accountable for a given action, it is difficult or impossible to decide who is to be held ultimately accountable (Barry 1982, p. 13).

A classic example of this occurred at Waikato Hospital, New Zealand, in 1982. The incident in question involved a 28-year-old woman who died after being given an incorrectly prescribed dose of morphine. At the coronial inquiry into her death, it was revealed that the charge nurse who administered the 50-milligram intramuscular dose of morphine did so on the insistence of the prescribing 'doctor' (who was in fact a final-year medical student from Australia). The prescribing 'doctor' in turn insisted that she 'did not prescribe the morphine, but simply passed on [the covering registrar's] prescription for the nurse to administer' (*Waikato Times* 1984b, p. 3). The medical registrar, in turn, claimed that he had worked from eight in the morning on Saturday to midday Sunday, and had only had four hours' sleep during that time — implying that 'the system' was to blame. The medical consultant under whom the registrar was working meanwhile stated that 'if he was asked' he would not regard the duties of the medical student as being 'those of a house surgeon' (the New Zealand term for medical resident) — implying that his registrar was ultimately responsible (*Waikato Times* 1984a, p. 1). The medical superintendent, in turn, stated that the registrar 'should have been in charge of prescribing narcotics' (*Waikato Times* 1984a, p. 1), while the Waikato Hospital Board suggested that 'no one person be blamed for the overdose' (*Waikato Times* 1984b, p. 3).

The coroner concluded that it would be quite 'unfair, unkind and not based on the evidence' to blame the medical student who prescribed the morphine for the woman's death. On the basis of the coroner's overall findings, the police did not press charges.

Admittedly this case emphasises more the issues of legal responsibility and accountability than those of moral responsibility. Legal and moral responsibility and accountability, however, travel a common path, as made evident by the much noted *Bormann defence*, named after Martin Bormann, third deputy under the Nazi regime of World War II, who argued in defence of his involvement in wartime atrocities that he was 'just following orders' (Barry 1982, p. 13). This kind of defence is a convenient 'moral cop-out' for those who have no sense of moral accountability, or a poorly developed sense, and who ordinarily try to justify their behaviour as Bormann did: 'I was told to do it'; 'I was expected to do it'; 'I was just doing my job'; 'That's how things operate around here'; and so forth (Barry 1982, p. 13).

The outcome of the 1945–46 Nuremberg trials made it abundantly clear that a plea of following the orders of one's superiors was not to hold as a legitimate defence in the eyes of the law. Such a precedent had already been well established for nurses as early as 1929, however, with the successful prosecution in the

Philippines of a newly graduated nurse by the name of Lorenza Somera, who was found guilty of manslaughter, sentenced to a year in prison, and fined 1000 pesos because she had followed a physician's incorrect drug order (Grennan 1930). In court it was proved that the physician had ordered the drug, that Somera had verified it, and that the physician had administered the injection. But, as Winslow (1984) writes, 'the physician was acquitted and Somera found guilty because she failed to *question* the orders'. The case stunned nurses around the world. A campaign of protest was organised, and Somera was given a conditional pardon before serving a day of her sentence.

In an institutional setting, it is very easy to rationalise moral 'unaccountability':

> So many people, even institutions, can get involved at so many levels that moral buck-passing can become the order of the day. The blind pursuit of prestige and profits also blurs moral accountability. And most important, the intense pressure to keep one job and to secure promotions can be used to justify almost anything. The point is that working within an organisation provides easy excuses for abdicating personal moral accountability for decisions and actions.
>
> (Barry 1982, p. 13)

One way of avoiding this abdication is to draw a firm distinction between ethics and following the orders of a superior, and to recognise that moral demands are always the overriding consideration, irrespective of a superior's orders. (This point is explored further in Chapter 15 when conscientious objection is discussed.)

The task of ethics, bioethics and nursing ethics

In considering what ethics is, and what it is not, it is also important to have some understanding of exactly what ethics, in its broadest sense, is attempting to achieve; in short, what is the task of ethics and to what extent do bioethics and nursing ethics respectively contribute to this task?

In identifying and exploring the task of ethics, it is necessary to give a brief historical overview of the development of Western moral thinking. The task of ethics has been the subject of rigorous philosophical debate for almost 2500 years. In the Platonic dialogues, for example, we are told that the ultimate task of morality is to find out 'how best to live' or, in other words, how to lead 'the good life' and enjoy supreme wellbeing (Allen 1966, pp. 57–255). For the British philosopher Thomas Hobbes (1588–1679), the task of morality is a little different: notably, to find a device that will ensure mutual agreement and cooperation among each of society's members. It was Hobbes' view that, without such a device, the prospects of human survival would at best be slim (Hobbes 1968, p. 205).

Hobbes' concerns were echoed almost a century later by the Scottish philosopher David Hume (1711–76), who insisted, among other things, that morality was a subject of supreme interest since its decisions had the very peace of society firmly at stake (Hume 1888, p. 455). Like Hobbes, Hume recognised that the human mind was more than capable of courting the undesirable qualities of 'avarice, ambition, cruelty [and] selfishness'; and, like Hobbes, he recognised that society's hope for peace depended very much on the formulation of certain rules of conduct (Hume 1888, pp. 494–6). These rules of conduct need to be developed and enforced precisely because people fail to pursue the public interest 'naturally, and with a hearty affection' (Hume 1888, p. 496).

The influential German philosopher, Immanuel Kant (1724–1804) took a slightly different view from his predecessors. Unlike Hobbes and Hume, he saw the task of ethics (or rather, moral philosophy) as being 'to seek out and establish the supreme principle of morality' (Kant 1972, p. 57). Like those before him, Kant recognised that persons were vulnerable to being 'affected ... by so many inclinations and lacked the power to conduct their life in accordance with practical reason'. Kant went on to argue that as long as the 'ultimate norm for correct moral judgment' is lacking, morals themselves will be vulnerable to corruption (Kant 1972, p. 55).

Kant's overall investigation succeeded in providing a supreme, although not uncontroversial, principle of morality for guiding human actions. Upholding the tenets of *ethical rationalism* (now regarded as a controversial thesis), this principle took the form of a *categorical imperative* which essentially commands that rational autonomous choosers should 'act only on that maxim through which you can at the same time will that it should become universal law' (Kant 1972, p. 84). His final analysis made clear that the influences of self-interest and/or of individual 'feelings, impulses and inclinations' could have no place in a schema of sound morality (Kant 1972, p. 84). If 'rational agents' are to act morally, they must act in strict accordance with the dictates of 'rational moral law'.

The moral law was seen by Kant as providing ultimate, overriding principles of conduct and ones which all rational agents ought to respect. He was optimistic that if all rational persons lived absolutely by the moral law then they could hope to live in a world (or rather 'a kingdom', as he called it) where rational agents would be respected as ends in themselves and not as the mere means to the ends of others (Kant 1972, p. 96).

The influential views of Plato, Hobbes, Hume and Kant concerning the task of ethics continue to have force in modern moral philosophy. For example, the Australian philosopher John Mackie (born in Sydney in 1917) argues that so-called 'limited sympathies' exist as a profound threat to what might otherwise be regarded as the 'good life' (Mackie 1977, p. 108).[3] Mackie echoes the view that if an all-enduring and decent (harmonious) life is to be secured, the problem of limited sympathies needs to be counteracted. The only way this can be done is by finding something which will coordinate and marry together individual and differing choices of action. In other words, what is needed is a device which could act as a kind of 'invisible chain' keeping together many sorts of 'useful agreements' (Mackie 1977, pp. 116, 118).

The solution for Mackie lies squarely at the feet of morality, which he interprets as:

> a system of a particular sort of constraints on conduct — ones whose central task is to protect the interests of persons other than the agent and present themselves to an agent as checks on his [sic] natural inclinations or spontaneous tendencies to act.
>
> (Mackie 1977, p. 106)

Mackie argues further that a morality applied appropriately is a morality which will help to facilitate the realisation of the overall wellbeing of people. In order for morality to work in this way, however, it must have at its core the vital component 'humane disposition' (Mackie 1977, p. 194). A humane disposition in

---

3. Quotations from J.L. Mackie (1977), *Ethics: inventing right and wrong*, Penguin Books, Harmondsworth, Middlesex, are reproduced by permission of Penguin Books Ltd.

this instance is that which 'naturally manifests itself in hostility to and disgust at cruelty, and in sympathy with pain and suffering whenever they occur' (p. 194). People who are of humane disposition, suggests Mackie, 'cannot be callous and indifferent, let alone actively cruel either toward permanently defective human beings or toward non-human animals' (p. 194).

The English philosopher Richard Hare also views the task of ethics in terms of imposing stringent requirements on persons to act in morally just ways. On this, Hare argues that:

> Morality compels us to accommodate ourselves to the preferences of others, and this has the effect that when we are thinking morally and doing it rationally we shall all prefer the same moral prescriptions about matters which affect other people ...
>
> (Hare 1981, p. 228)

Hare ultimately advocates morality as a form of compelling 'rational universal prescriptivism', and concludes (in somewhat Kantian terms) that 'moral reason leaves us with our freedom, but constrains us to respect the freedom of others, and to combine with them in exercising it' (Hare 1981, p. 228).

The notion that the task of ethics is to supply a system of ultimate, overriding principles of conduct is also supported by the contemporary American philosopher Stephen Ross (1972, p. 283), who argues that the goal of morality is 'to reach a common set of moral ideals which everyone can follow' or, rather, to 'seek principles of conduct which everyone can live by'. According to Ross, moral principles are needed to regulate our moral decisions and to help settle competing alternatives. Moral principles remind us of our overriding duties to others and of the merits of morally principled action. Principles of morality also lend people 'tools' which can be used to deal appropriately and effectively with moral crises and dilemmas in both everyday and special (e.g. professional) worlds. They remind us that, without secure, ultimate and overriding rules of conduct, people may find it all too easy to abdicate their moral responsibilities and to commit atrocities (the My Lai massacre during the Vietnam War is a poignant example of how unclear and unstable rules of conduct can contribute significantly to the realisation of atrocious human behaviour [see in particular Peers 1979, p. 33; Bilton and Sim 1992; Kelman and Hamilton 1989]).

More recently, the contemporary American philosophers John Rawls, Tom Beauchamp and James Childress, David Gauthier, and H. Tristram Engelhardt Jr have described the task of modern moral philosophy in similar terms again. Rawls (1971) for example, sees the task of ethics as to validate the conception of morality 'as a set of rational, impartial constraints on the pursuit of individual interest', and to adjudicate cases in which there are conflicts of interest. Beauchamp and Childress, on the other hand, suggest that the task of ethics is to supply an 'ideal code consisting of a set of rules that guide the members of a society to maximise intrinsic value' (1983, p. 40). Gauthier (1986, p. 6), describes the task of ethics as that of developing a way of ordering interests. Engelhardt (1986, pp. 67–9), meanwhile sees the task of ethics as searching for common grounds to bind consenting individuals in a peaceable community — in short, to achieve peaceable bonds among persons without brute force. He also sees the task of ethics as being that which:

> aspires to provide a logic for a pluralism of beliefs, a common view of a good life that can transcend particular communities, professions, legal

jurisdictions, and religions, but whose grounds for authenticity are immanent to the secular world.

(Engelhardt 1986, p. 26)

Both bioethics and nursing ethics share the task of ethics.

Conclusion

Advancing ethics, bioethics and nursing ethics inquiry and practice requires at least a rudimentary knowledge and understanding of the definitions and meanings of such terms as 'ethics', 'bioethics' and 'nursing ethics'. In this chapter, working definitions of these notions have been provided (the definitions of other commonly used moral terms such as 'rights', 'duties' and 'obligations' will be given later in Chapter 4 of this text). In providing these working definitions, attention has also been given to demonstrating what ethics (bioethics and nursing ethics) *is not*. For example, ethics, bioethics and nursing ethics are not: legal law, codes of ethics, hospital or professional etiquette, hospital or institutional policy, public opinion or the view of the majority, or following the orders of a superior.

A brief examination has also been made of the task of ethics, namely, to find a way to motivate moral behaviour, to settle disagreements and controversies between people, and to generally bind people together in a peaceable community. Both bioethics and nursing ethics share in this task, acknowledging, however, that such a task has been and remains a complex and complicated one. To help understand the complexity of this task and how it might be achieved, it is necessary to first gain some understanding of the theoretical underpinnings of Western ethics generally and, concomitantly, bioethics and nursing ethics which are derivatives of it. It is to examining these theoretical underpinnings and their influences on the development of contemporary bioethics and nursing ethics that the next three chapters will now turn.

Chapter 4

Theoretical perspectives informing ethical conduct

Introduction

Deciding and acting morally (ethical practice), or, more simply, 'being ethical' never occurs in a theoretical vacuum; more than this, it actually requires a certain level of moral theorising on the part of moral agents — nurses being no exception in this regard. Here, three key questions can be raised: what is moral/ethical theory? what is its relationship to ethical practice? and what kinds of moral theories ought we to appeal to inform and guide our ethical practice in both our personal and professional lives? In this and the following three chapters an attempt will be made to answer these questions.

Moral theory and its relationship to ethical practice

Theory (from late Latin *theoria*, from Greek, meaning literally: *a sight, to gaze upon, to speculate*) is generally taken to mean abstract knowledge or reasoning. In the case of ethics, theory can be taken to mean one or all of the following: '(1) abstract reflection and argument, (2) systematic reflection and argument, and (3) an integrated body of principles that are coherent and well developed' (Beauchamp and Childress 1994, p. 44). Despite its 'abstract' nature (or, to put this another way, its lacking in material substance), theory is not passive. It can and does have a profound influence on the way in which we perceive, make meaning of, give order to, understand, and act in the world. More succinctly, theory and theorising (speculation) helps us to 'make sense' of our experiences as human beings.

As in everyday life, theory has an important role to play in assisting us to give meaning and order to our everyday *moral* experiences. Theory, or more accurately moral/ethical theory, does this by helping us to describe the moral world, devise meaningful moral standards and prescribe moral ideals, distinguish ethical issues from other sorts of issues, and to provide a systematic justification of the actual practice of morality. When well-developed, a moral/ethical theory 'provides a framework within which agents can reflect on the acceptability of actions and can evaluate moral judgments and character' (Beauchamp and Childress 1994, p. 44). It should be added, however, that 'good' ethical practice also provides a 'framework' for evaluating and reflecting on what constitutes a 'well-developed ethical theory'. In several respects, therefore, the relationship between moral theory and ethical practice is symbiotic; just as ethical practice cannot be evaluated independently of its theoretical underpinnings, neither can moral theory be evaluated independently of moral experience (including that of applying both ordinary and formal moral theories).

Ethical experience (practice) may, however, provide more than a evaluative framework for guiding theoretical reflections; in several respects it provides a — if not *the* — substantive methodological starting point for moral theory (both 'ordinary' and 'formal'). Moreno (1995, p. 113), for example, defending what he calls 'ethical naturalism', persuasively argues that 'moral values emerge from *actual human experience* and are not superimposed on it by some transcendental reality (Plato's Forms are the classic example)' (emphasis added). Clouser (1995, p. 235), takes a similar position. He states:

> Ordinary moral experience is our starting point. After all, morality cannot be *invented*. 'Look, here's my idea for a new morality ... those with the most education get to say what happens to anyone with less education ...!' We must begin with the moral system that is actually used by thoughtful people in making decisions and judgments about what to do in particular cases. Ordinary morality is generally expressed in what can be regarded as moral rules — e.g. don't cheat, don't kill, don't lie — and moral ideals — e.g. relieve pain, promote freedom, help the needy. If one were just initiating a study of morality as it is practiced, these rules and ideals would constitute the demarcations of the moral realm; they are the earmarks of morality at work; they are the phenomena on which the study would focus.
>
> (Clouser 1995, p. 228, emphasis original)

As we will go on to see, however, these views are just some among many that might be appealed to for providing an explanation of the origins of our moral values and beliefs and the moral schemas that are ultimately derivative of them.

Traditional and non-traditional theoretical perspectives

Western moral philosophy has given rise to many different and sometimes competing theoretical perspectives or 'viewpoints' on the nature and justification of moral conduct. These perspectives include 'modernist' and, more recently, 'postmodernist' views on ethics. Having some knowledge and understanding of these different perspectives is crucial not just to enhancing our understanding of the complex nature of moral problems and the controversy and perplexity to which they so often give rise, but to enhancing our abilities to devise satisfactory solutions to the moral problems we encounter in our everyday lives. While it is beyond the scope of this book to give an in-depth account of the vast array of ethical theories that have been and remain influential in Western moral philosophical thought, it is nevertheless possible to give a cursory overview of some of the key ethical theories here. Before doing so, however, some commentary is warranted on the nature and distinction between *modernist* and *postmodernist* ethics.

Modernist ethics

Modernist views on ethics rest on the presumption that morality is concrete, absolute, universal and 'available to all through rational reflection' (Engelhardt 1996, p. 3). This view has deep roots in Western history dating back to ancient Greece, and has been profoundly influenced by Judaeo–Christian religious values and beliefs through the ages. For instance, during the many centuries before modernity, ethics was 'almost totally identified with the moral theology of the Church' (Klostermaier 1998, p. 35). It was not until after the Enlightenment that 'reason was to take over what so far had been the realm of faith — and to improve upon it' (Klostermaier 1998, p. 35; Engelhardt 1996, p. 4). Whether in fact reason did improve the 'realm of faith' *apropos* ethics remains an open question, however, and one that will be considered more fully in the following chapters of this text.

Although a modernist approach to ethics has been — and continues to be — successfully challenged, it is nevertheless evident that it remains a powerful and dominant influence on contemporary moral thought and one which, it should be added, is extremely difficult to avoid. Modernist ethical theories such as *deontology* and *teleology* (to be discussed shortly in this chapter) still have currency, are still extremely influential, and continue to dominate mainstream discourses on ethics — including the views advanced in this text. The popular appeal to (and of) the modernist theoretical perspectives of (1) ethical principlism, and (2) moral rights theory (both of which will be considered later in this chapter), stands as an important example here. For instance, in the case of ethical principlism, autonomy discourse is so powerful that it is extremely difficult to challenge it. So successful has been the promotion of autonomy (and, drawing on moral rights theory, the assumed sovereign rights of individuals to exercise self-determining choices), that the imperatives of these theoretical perspectives (for example, as in the case of euthanasia/assisted suicide) have come to seem 'so self-evident to all "right thinking people" that to question them seems almost perverse' (Moody 1992, p. 50). Significantly, those who do question them risk being publicly ridiculed and dismissed by opponents as ill-informed and 'illogical', or worse as being 'insulting' to self-determining persons (see, for example, the reported comments in the Senate Legal and Constitutional Legislation Committee 1997 at pp. 71, 176).

Modernist views that hold morality to be concrete, absolute, universal, and 'available to all through rational reflection' are, however, being slowly overturned. There is increasing recognition that morality is not concrete, absolute, and universal, but changing and relative, and available through a variety of 'ways of knowing' (not just rational reflection) including the non-rational faculties of intuition and the emotions. Furthermore, rather than there being just *one warranted moral reality* (a legacy of, and analogous to, Christian monotheism), there are *many warranted moral realities* (analogous to polytheism), and these realities can be apprehended not by one rationality, but by many *rationalities* (Engelhardt 1996, p. 5), or more precisely many *subjectivities*. In short, contrary to modernist assertions, ethics is 'multiperspectival and multicultural' (or pluralistic) in its vision and, as such, is open to a diversity of interpretation and understanding (Engelhardt 1996, p. 11; Bauman 1993; Anderson 1990; Walzer 1987). This latter 'different' perspective is what can be roughly referred to as a 'postmodernist' view of ethics — referred to previously in Chapter 1 of this text, and now to be discussed briefly under the separate subheading to follow.

Postmodernist ethics

At its most basic, postmodernist ethics could be described as that which aims at:

> a possibly comprehensive inventory of moral problems which men and women living in a postmodern world face and struggle to resolve — new problems unknown to past generations or unnoticed by them, as well as new forms which old problems, thoroughly vetted in the past, have now taken.

> (Bauman 1993, p. 1)

Contrary to modernist concerns and criticisms, a postmodern perspective on ethics is not necessarily about abandoning or rejecting modern moral concerns. Rather, it is about rejecting what Bauman (1993) describes as 'the typically modern ways' of going about moral problems, advocating instead *new ways* of moral responsiveness. As Bauman reminds us:

> The great issues of ethics — like human rights, social justice, balance between peaceful co-operation and personal self-assertion, synchronisation of individual conduct and collective welfare — have lost nothing of their topicality. They only need to be seen and dealt with in a novel way.

> (Bauman 1993, p. 4)

Postmodern ethics or, more appropriately, a 'postmodern perspective' on ethics is increasingly being seen as offering 'new' or 'novel' ways of dealing effectively with contemporary moral problems. This new perspective is taken by Bauman (1993, p. 3) to mean 'above all the tearing off of the mask of illusions; the recognition of certain pretences as false and certain objectives as neither attainable nor, for that matter, desirable'. (Examples of certain 'masks of illusion' and 'false pretences' that have operated in mainstream moral philosophy and bioethics, and which are in need of being 'torn off', will be considered in the following chapters addressing feminist ethics and transcultural ethics.) In several respects, this book contributes to the project of the 'new' postmodern perspective on ethics, although it is acknowledged that this contribution is not without contradiction. For instance, this present work carries the paradoxical distinction of being both modernist and postmodernist in nature. It is modernist in that, in advancing its discussion, it draws extensively on modernist ethics discourse; it is postmodernist in that it advances and makes visible a perspective (a nursing perspective) that has previously been marginalised and rendered invisible in the hierarchy of contemporary moral discourses, and, in making visible this perspective, challenges the hegemony of other dominant discourses; for example, those of medical ethics and mainstream bioethics. This apparent contradiction, however, is not serious. One reason for this is that the linkages between modernist and postmodernist ethics are, in several respects, inevitable given the profound ways in which modernist values are so deeply embedded in and permeate our everyday language; the ways in which 'the cage of language' influences our patterns of thought and perception; and the ways in which our thinking, in turn, influences our behaviour. Second, although paradox imports ambiguity, ambiguity also carries with it an opportunity to create new meaning (Pylkkanen 1989). This is perhaps one of the most important promises of postmodern ethics: to enable the creation of new moral meanings in a world in which morality has otherwise lost its *meaning* (taken here as including *significance, purpose, intention [telos]*, and *value* [adapted from Bohm 1989; see also Johnstone 1998, p. 74]).

Whether people choose to accept or reject a postmodern perspective on ethics, one thing is clear: they cannot ignore it. As Engelhardt (1996, p. 3) reminds us: 'Moral diversity is real. It is real in fact and in principle. Bioethics and health care policy have yet to take this diversity seriously'. It is hoped that this text will offer a beginning step forward toward taking seriously the moral diversity that is so characteristic not just of health care domains, but the world.

Moral theory and justification

Before moving on to consider some of the more dominant traditional theoretical perspectives advanced by mainstream Western moral philosophy, some brief commentary is required on the issue that ethical theory is popularly considered as having a role regarding 'justifying' our moral decisions and actions.

Moral conflict and disagreement occurs frequently in health care contexts. This is not surprising given the profound 'value ladeness' of the health care practices that occur in health care domains. Indeed, it is inevitable that so long as we interact with other human beings, we will be faced with having to make choices to which morality is relevant (Hinman 1994, p. 1). It is equally inevitable that, given the complexity of the values that operate in health care domains, sometimes the choices we make will be 'problematic' insofar as they may express moral values, beliefs and evaluations which are not shared by others or which others do not agree with.

When experiencing situations involving moral disagreement and conflict, it is tempting to rely on our own ordinary moral apparatus and personal preferences to sustain the point of view we are advocating. Sometimes, however, our own 'ordinary moral apparatus' and personal preferences may not be reliable or worthy action guides because, as Kopelman (1995, p. 117) warns us, these can result from 'prejudice, self-interest or ignorance'. In light of this, we need to look elsewhere to strengthen the warranties of (in short, to justify) our moral choices and actions. Traditional moral theory is popularly regarded in modernist moral philosophy as the definitive source from which such warranties (justifications) can be reliably sought.

In modernist moral philosophy, it is not sufficient to merely *ascribe* moral values or judgments to things (for example, 'abortion is wrong', 'euthanasia is right'). There is also an onus of justification on the part of moral decision-makers; that is, to justify the basis upon which they have judged something to be 'right' and 'wrong'. This position, of course, begs the question of what is to count as a warranted model of moral justification?

Justifying a moral decision or action involves providing the *strongest moral reasons* behind them. According to Beauchamp and Childress (1994, p. 13), 'the reasons that we finally accept, express the conditions under which we believe some course of action is morally justified'. This account is not, however, free of difficulties. As Beauchamp and Childress (1994, p. 13) go on to point out, 'Not all reasons are good reasons, and not all good reasons are sufficient for justification'. For example, a majority public opinion supporting the legalisation of euthanasia may constitute a *good reason* for decriminalising euthanasia yet stop short of providing a *sufficient* reason for doing so (for example, other 'good and sufficient' reasons might be put forward demonstrating why public opinion is not relevant or adequate to justifying legalised euthanasia, for instance: majority opinion tells us only that a certain class of people hold a point of view, not whether that point of view is morally right [euthanasia could still be morally wrong despite a majority view to the contrary]; public opinion is notoriously fickle and hence unreliable as a moral action guide — what is deemed 'right' by the majority today, could equally be deemed 'wrong' tomorrow violating the standards of consistency and coherency otherwise expected in the case of sound moral decision-making). Decision-makers thus need to not only provide 'strong reasons' for their decisions and actions, but to also distinguish:

> a reason's *relevance* to a moral judgment from its final *adequacy* for that judgment, and also to distinguish an *attempted* justification from a *successful* justification.
>
> (Beauchamp and Childress 1994, p. 13, emphasis original)

Here, *relevance* (from the Latin *relevàre* to lighten, to relieve) can be measured by the extent to which the reason (belief) has *direct bearing* on and makes a *material difference* to the evaluation made as part of the process aimed at making moral judgments and choices/decisions. *Adequacy* (from the Lain *adaequare* to equalise, from *ad-to* + *aequus* Equal) can, in turn, be measured by the extent to which it fulfils a need or requirement (in this instance to provide sufficient grounds for belief or action) without being outstanding or abundant. An *attempt* is simply to 'make an effort'; to *succeed* is 'to accomplish'.

The notion of moral justification is not, however, without difficulties. One reason for this is that there exist a number of different accounts of what constitutes a plausible model of moral justification, and even of how a given or 'agreed' model of justification might be interpreted and applied (Kopelman 1995; Beauchamp and Childress 1994; Bauman 1993; Dancy 1993; Nielsen 1989). Some even suggest, controversially, that there can be no adequate model of justification since there is always room to question the grounds that are put forward as 'good reasons' supporting a particular act or judgment (see, for example, Hughes 1995; Johnston 1989).

The problem of moral justification has long been recognised as a crucial one in moral philosophy. As Kai Nielsen (1989) reflects:

> In ordinary non-philosophical moments, we sometimes wonder how (if at all) a deeply felt moral conviction can be justified. And, in our philosophical moments, we sometimes wonder if *any* moral judgments *ever* are *in principle* justified. Surely, we can find all sorts of reasons for taking one course of action rather than another. We find reasons readily enough for the appraisal we make of types of action and attitudes. We frequently make judgments about the moral code of our own culture as well as those of other cultures. But how do we decide if the reasons we offer for these appraisals are good reasons? And, what is the *ground* for our decision that some reasons are good reasons and others are not? When (if at all) can we say that these grounds are sufficient for our moral decisions?
>
> (Nielsen 1989, p. 53, emphasis original)

Beauchamp and Childress (1994, p. 14) suggest three possible answers to these questions, namely, that we can appeal to either: (1) moral rules, principles and theories; (2) lived experience and individuated personal judgments; or (3) a synthesis of both these (theoretical and experiential) approaches.

Moral rules, principles and theories

One way of justifying moral decisions and actions is by appealing to moral rules, principles and theories. By this view, an action is regarded as being morally justified:

> if it is in accordance with the relevant moral rules, where these rules have been derived from a set of adequate moral principles.
>
> (Solomon 1978, p. 410)

Underpinning this view is the generalised and widely accepted (modernist philosophical) assumption that moral rules are derived from (and justified by) sound moral principles, which in turn are derived from (and justified by) ethical theory. Particular judgments, in turn, are deemed to be justified if it can be shown that they accord with relevant moral rules and principles. This account can be portrayed diagrammatically as shown in Figure 4.1.

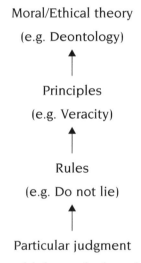

Moral/Ethical theory

(e.g. Deontology)

Principles

(e.g. Veracity)

Rules

(e.g. Do not lie)

Particular judgment

(e.g. Mr X ought to be told the truth about his medical diagnosis)

Figure 4.1 Moral justification and direction of appeal

(adapted from Beauchamp, T. and Childress, J. [1994], *Principles of biomedical ethics*, 4th edn, Oxford University Press, New York. p. 15)

Meanwhile, if the ethics of an action are called into question, attention will shift to one or all of the following: (1) the justification of the rules appealed to; (2) the adequacy of the moral principles from which the rules have been derived; and/or (3) the choice of the ethical theory applied (Solomon 1978, p. 410; Beauchamp and Childress 1994, p. 15). The justification provided, however, may still become unhinged on account of there being many competing ethical theories which moral agents might choose to justify their decisions and action. The point being that when chosen, different ethical theories commit their proponents 'to different norms and different solutions to problems' which, in turn, can cause further disagreements and controversies requiring still more justified responses (Beauchamp and Childress 1994, p. 15).

Lived experience and individuated personal judgments

Another way of justifying moral decisions and actions is by appealing to lived moral experience and individuated personal moral judgments. This approach takes lived experience rather than ethical theory as the source of moral justification. In contradiction to the tenets of modernist moral philosophy, this approach recognises that a society's moral views:

> are not justified by an ahistorical examination of the logic of moral discourse or by some theory of rationality, but rather by embedded moral traditions and a set of procedures that permit new developments.
>
> (Beauchamp and Childress 1994, p. 18)

It also recognises that ethics is culturally and socially constructed, that moral values and beliefs are informed and shaped by 'new experiences and innovations in the patterns of collective life' (Beauchamp and Childress 1994, p. 18), and that our moral standards are not absolute but, as previously mentioned in Chapter 1 of this text, are ever-changing social realities created and recreated by people out of their experiences and challenges of the times (Anderson 1990, pp. 258–59). By this view, an act would be morally justified if it accords with the moral standards and ideals that 'good thinking' people consent to on the basis of their collective experience.

Theory and experience

A third way of justifying moral decisions and actions can be found by appealing to a *combination* of moral rules, principles, ethical theory *and* the lived moral experiences of people. This approach assumes that justification is 'a matter of the mutual support of many considerations, of everything fitting together into one coherent view' (Rawls 1971, p. 21; Beauchamp and Childress 1994, p. 23). It also assumes the existence of a dialectic between theory and practice, and that experience has a crucial role to play in testing, corroborating, validating and revising our theories. For example, as Beauchamp and Childress explain:

> If a theory yields conclusions at odds with our considered judgments — for example, if it allows children but not adults to be used without consent as subjects of biomedical research — we have reason to be suspicious of the theory and to modify it or seek an alternative theory.
>
> (Beauchamp and Childress 1994, p. 23)

The justification of justification

It should be noted that none of the above three accounts of justification theory is free of difficulty. In the case of the theoretical model, a failure to provide an adequate account of selected moral rules, principles or theories could result in the absurd situation of an infinite regress of justification — that is, 'a justification of a justification of a justification' — with no final justification being achieved (Solomon 1978, p. 411; Beauchamp and Childress 1994, p. 17). Second, an appeal to given moral rules, principle and theories risks oversimplifying the otherwise complex process of moral judgment and decision-making, and the complex moral reasoning, evaluation and justification that is constitutive of this process. Third, following rules and principles can also render the moral decision-making process 'rigid, legalistic, and insensitive to the nuances of particular cases'

(Solomon 1978, p. 411). A fourth problem involves the following paradox: by demanding compliance with moral rules, the processes of autonomous and independent moral decision-making is undermined, and with it the ability of people to make choices where it really matters (Bauman 1993, pp. 132, 183). This situation is paradoxical because, by demanding compliance with 'agreed' rules, moral agents are rendered *rule followers*, not *rule makers* (Bauman 1993, p. 182). This, in turn, risks silencing and paralysing moral impulse — the very ingredient of personalised moral responsibility (Bauman 1993, p. 12).

The experiential approach is also problematic. Among other things it has little to say about 'the common circumstance in which conflicting judgments are reached in particular cases by equally well-informed and dispassionate moral agents' (Beauchamp and Childress 1994, p. 19). Further, it seems unable to provide a justification for the general moral standards that 'experience' suggests ought to be used to justify given moral decisions and actions. Finally, it leaves unanswered what we should do in the case of 'new experiences' *viz.* where our past experiences and otherwise generally agreed moral standards (based on past experience) are not adequate to the task of guiding our deliberations, and providing the 'good and sufficient reasons' we need to justify our actions in these new situations. The combined theory and experiential model of justification suffers from the problems of *both* the theoretical and experiential models of justification just outlined above.

An overview of key traditional ethical theories

Having briefly examined the different models of moral justification, it now remains the task of this chapter to explore some of the key ethical theories which have traditionally been appealed to in order to justify moral decisions and actions in given contexts. In particular, attention will focus on briefly examining: deontological ethics, teleological ethics (also known as consequentialism), ethical principlism, and moral (human) rights theory. Upon examining these key (and dominant) mainstream ethical theories, attention will then focus on providing a short examination of some emergent contemporary dissatisfaction with these mainstream theoretical perspectives, and the revival of other traditional theories — such as virtue ethics and casuistry ethics — as alternative perspectives, especially for and in the health care professions.

Deontological theories of ethics

'Deontology' comes from the Greek *deon*, meaning 'duty', and *logos*, meaning 'discourse'. As an ethical theory, deontology takes 'duty' to be the basis of morality and holds roughly that some acts are obligatory regardless of their consequences. A number of important views derive from deontological ethics, including the theological, rationalistic, emotivist and intuitionist views, and the view offered by social contract theory. All these views raise interesting ethical questions for nurses.

Theological ethics

Classic deontological theory has its origins in religious ethics, and relies heavily on the idea of 'divine command'. It emphasises the moral imperative of obeying God because 'he [sic] knows what is best for us, and what is best for us is to obey him [sic]' (MacIntyre 1966, p. 111). To disobey God would be to become estranged from God, and to risk denying ourselves the fruits of heaven. The ideal life is one marked by 'obedience to the will of God', regardless of one's own individual plans and desires.

For classic deontologists, it is God's command that determines whether something is to be regarded as morally right and good, and God's forbidding that determines whether it is to be considered wrong and bad. If God commands 'thou shalt not kill', 'thou shalt not steal', 'thou shalt love thy father and mother as thyself', and the like, then conduct that upholds or accords with these commands is both right and justified 'because and only because it is commanded by God' (Frankena 1973, p. 28).

This view is convenient, because it readily supplies concrete answers to otherwise complex problems. It is nevertheless problematic on a number of counts. First, it presumes the existence of God. The atheist (someone who has no sustained belief in the existence of God) would view God's supposed commands as having no content — as being 'fictitious' — and therefore totally lacking in terms of supplying compelling reasons for behaving in a 'divinely ordained' way. Atheist nurses working in a religious hospital (say, a Catholic or Jewish hospital) may find little if any consolation in any religious dogma put forward to justify certain moral–medical decisions made in the clinical setting. This also applies to atheist patients who might be admitted into a religious hospital for care.

A second problem here concerns the ethical limitations on God's omnipotence (Mackie 1962). If God is all-powerful, it follows that God has the capacity to create evil. This has important implications for the argument (generally raised in criticisms of a theological view of ethics) that, if God commands certain unjust and cruel acts, it follows that believers are committed to viewing such acts as morally right, good and obligatory. Believers might object, however, that, since God is all good, God is incapable of being cruel and would never command evil acts. While this is an interesting objection, it does little to rescue the thesis of God's being omnipotent. What is left seems to be the incompatible and logically contradictory thesis that God is both omnipotent (all-powerful and able to bring about all things — including evil) and not omnipotent (not all-powerful, and unable to bring about all things — especially evil) at the same time. A further, related, concern is raised by Socrates in Plato's Euthyphro: 'Is that which is holy loved by the gods because it is holy, or is it holy because it is loved by the gods?' (Allen 1966, p. 67). This famous Socratic dialogue questions the possibility of there being a superior reality that exists even above God. If such a reality does exist, God's Supreme Beingness together with his supposed omnipotence and omnipresence are immediately thrown into serious question.

A third difficulty with the theological perspective is the problem of how mere mortals could possibly know whether God's commands are right or wrong (Frankena 1973, p. 29). This gives rise to one of two possibilities — either morality is totally arbitrary (we act morally simply because God commands us to), or it is intrinsically self-interested (we act morally simply to avoid God's wrath) — both of which stand to condemn a systematic and critically reflective morality and all that it stands for.

A more practical difficulty relates to the problem of how to reconcile differing theological views and interpretations of God's commands. For example, how is the Catholic view on the sanctity of life (which would, among other things, probably condone the administration of a blood transfusion in a medically urgent and possibly life-saving situation) to be reconciled with the Jehovah's Witness view on the sanctity of God's commands (which are held to include a prohibition against the administration of a blood transfusion in the same situation)? Again, how is the Christian Science view on the sanctity of faith (which would be likely to prohibit the use of material cures such as drugs) to be reconciled with the Jewish view (Musgrave 1987, pp. 183, 186) on the sanctity of life (which would be likely to condone the use of life-saving drugs)?

These questions belong properly to theological discourse, and cannot be considered here. Nevertheless, they raise some important questions for nurses (see the following examples).

1. To what extent are nurses morally bound to conduct their practice in a way that respects the religious beliefs of others, particularly when doing so might result in foreseeable and otherwise preventable harmful consequences to patients (for example, as in the case of a Jehovah's Witness patient dying prematurely and 'unnecessarily' because of refusing a life-saving blood transfusion)?
2. Is it reasonable to expect nurses to respect the religious beliefs of others when doing so would result in them (the nurses) violating their own sincerely held moral beliefs and values? Can such an expectation be justified?
3. Can nurses validly claim conscientious objection when asked to assist with medical procedures to which they are opposed on the basis of religious beliefs (for example, abortion)? If so, what conditions need to be met before such a conscientious objection can be supported?

These and related questions will be explored further in the following chapters.

Rationalism

The theological or Judaeo–Christian view of deontology has been significantly modified under the influence of the famous German philosopher, Immanuel Kant (1724–1804). Kant's views to this day are a major influence on the development of Western moral thinking.

For Kant, the supreme principle of morality is 'reason', whose ultimate end is 'good will'. Reason is free (autonomous) to formulate moral law and to determine just what is to count as being an overriding moral duty. Kant held duty to be that which is done for its own sake — for its own intrinsic moral worth — and 'not for the results it attains or seeks to attain' (Kant 1972, p. 20). Just what is to count as one's duty is determined by appealing to some formal (reasoned) principle or 'maxim'. In choosing such a maxim, however, we must take care not to choose something which serves merely to uphold our own individual interests or to satisfy our own unruly desires. Indeed, Kant went on to assert that it is precisely because of our human weaknesses (especially our inclinations towards satisfying our own desires and interests) that the maxim we adopt must have the characteristics of being a universally valid 'law' — that is, something which 'commands or compels obedience' (Kant 1972, p. 21), and which is binding on all persons equally.

Kant's solution to the problem of establishing a universally valid law comes in his formulation of what he called the 'categorical imperative', which states: 'Act only on that maxim through which you can at the same time will that it should become universal law' (Kant 1972, p. 29). What this maxim or formal principle essentially demands is that we should only act in accord with a given principle or set of principles if we can, at the same time, reasonably will that it should become binding on all others throughout space and time. For example, if we are to adopt, and act, in accord with a principle that, let's say, permits our lying to others, then we are committed to accepting that all others are permitted to lie to us in return. If, in adopting this principle, however, we do not accept that others should be permitted to lie to us, then we are prohibited from adopting it, since, in adopting or acting on the maxim in question, we 'cannot at the same time will that it should become universal law' (Kant 1972, p. 29). As a point of interest, there are striking similarities between the demands of Kant's 'categorical imperative' and those of the Christian command to 'do unto others as we would have done unto ourselves', loosely referred to in moral philosophy as the 'golden rule'.

In summary, Kant believed that moral considerations are always overriding ones. Thus, in situations where a number of considerations are competing (for instance, between practical, economic, political, emotional, moral and cultural considerations), it is always the moral considerations which should 'win out', so to speak. For example, if a nurse is in the position of having to decide whether to risk losing his or her job (a practical consideration) by exposing the unethical conduct of a superior (a moral consideration), it is the moral consideration which is, according to Kant's view, the weightier of the two; the nurse, by this analysis, should expose the superior. Whether losing one's job is a purely practical consideration devoid of any moral content, however, is another matter.

As well as holding that moral considerations should always override non-moral considerations, Kant maintained that moral imperatives (as based on universal moral law) are by their very nature unconditional, absolute and inescapable. This means that moral imperatives, or duties in this instance, are both overriding and binding regardless of their consequences. Therefore we, as rational autonomous moral choosers, cannot escape the demands which a moral imperative may place upon us; the bottom line, given a Kantian deontology, is that we are absolutely required and therefore compelled to fulfil our moral duties. By this view, morally decent persons are those who fulfil their duties and who are not distracted by self-interested or practical considerations; morally indecent persons, on the other hand, are those who shirk or abandon their moral duties — probably in favour of other considerations such as the pursuit of material self-interest and pleasure.

Moral considerations and moral duties will be explored more fully as we go on to discuss the bioethical issues specific to grassroots nursing practice. In particular, two important questions will be considered.

1. Does a nurse always have a duty to care for a patient who has been assigned to her or his care in instances where other non-moral considerations have an important bearing on the situation at hand?
2. Can superiors, all things considered, decently order or compel a nurse to perform a task or an act which would otherwise stand to violate that nurse's reasoned or critical moral judgment?

Emotivism

For the emotivist, a moral statement is nothing more than an expression of emotion or an expression of attitude for or against things (Harmon 1977, p. 30; McNaughton 1988, pp. 24–7). Moral statements, by this view, can never be meaningfully judged as either true or false. At best they can only be deemed appropriate or inappropriate, genuine or fraudulent, justified or unjustified, rational or irrational, and the like (Frankena 1973, p. 107; Flew 1979, p. 104).

One of philosophy's most powerful advocates of emotivism was the Scottish philosopher David Hume (1711–76), who maintained, among other things, that 'reason is, and ought only to be, the slave of the passions and can never pretend to any other office than to serve and obey them' (Hume 1888, p. 415).

Hume utterly rejected reason or science as having ultimate moral authority, arguing that these things are nothing more than the 'comparing of ideas and the discovery of their relations' (Hume 1888, p. 466). He regarded reason as 'utterly impotent' (p. 457) in moral domains and said that it is 'perfectly inert, and can never either prevent or produce any action or affection' (p. 458). The only power reason has, in Hume's conceptual framework, is to shape beliefs — and, even then, beliefs cannot be relied upon to move one to action, unless they are relevant to the satisfaction of some passion, desire or need (Harmon 1977, p. 5).

The question remains, how does Hume's ontology capture the making of moral judgments? In essence, Hume's morality is something to be 'properly felt' rather than 'rationally judged', with goods and evils being known simply by particular sensations of pleasure and pain (Hume 1888, p. 470). He argued:

> Nothing can be more real, or concern us more, than our own sentiments of pleasure and uneasiness; and if these be favourable to virtue, and unfavourable to vice, no more can be requisite to the regulation of our conduct and behaviour.
>
> (Hume 1888, p. 469)

In summary, the Humean account of morality sees the sensations of pleasure as distinguishing that which is virtuous, and the sensations of pain or uneasiness as distinguishing that which is vicious. If something appears either virtuous or vicious, there is no reason to doubt that appearance — the sentiment just 'stands on its own', so to speak. In this respect, to quote the famous Humean quip, ' 'Tis not contrary to reason to prefer the destruction of the whole world to the scratching of my finger' (Hume 1888, p. 416).

One of philosophy's most sophisticated exponents of emotivism is the twentieth-century United States philosopher Charles Stevenson (born 1908). Stevenson argued that all moral statements are essentially an attempt to persuade others to share one's own attitudes about the rightness or wrongness of certain acts. He explained that to call something 'good' is to create an influence; that is, to try and influence the other person to have a 'pro-attitude' towards it. For instance, if we were to say to someone 'use of brain-dead babies as organ donors is always morally wrong or bad', we would not only be expressing our own dislike of and hostility towards this practice, but would also be trying to make the listener share that dislike and hostility. Likewise, if we were to say to a person something along the lines of 'euthanasia in medically hopeless cases is good', we would not only be expressing our own preference and support for euthanasia, but would also be trying to make the listener share that attitude.

Stevenson thought that the persuasive effect of ethical terms, insofar as their ability to direct attitudes is concerned, derives from what he called 'a characteristic and subtle kind of emotive meaning':

> The emotive meaning of a word is the power that the word acquires, on account of its history in emotional situations, to evoke or directly express attitudes, as distinct from describing or designating them.
>
> (Stevenson 1944, p. 33)

The lesson here (contrary to the rationalist thesis) is that 'ethical terms cannot be taken as fully comparable to scientific ones' (Stevenson 1944, p. 36); we must pay careful attention to the emotive meanings of the terms we use, and must distinguish their evaluative function from their descriptive function.

Emotivism has been heavily criticised on a number of counts. In particular it has been criticised for its exclusion of rationality from moral arguments and for its failure to distinguish serious moral arguments from irrational or non-rational propaganda. Stevenson's views are particularly vulnerable to the objection that not all moral statements are instances of trying to persuade others to share one's personal point of view. For example, we may talk with someone who already shares our views and wish merely to reach a private decision. Harmon (1977, pp. 39–40) offers the more scathing criticism that emotivism is trivial and is not much different from simple commonsense. The role of feelings in moral thinking will be raised again in Chapter 5 in the discussion on feminist moral theory.

Intuitionism

Like other moral theories, intuitionism has a long and respectable history, predating even Plato. Simply put, the thesis of moral intuitionism holds that moral principles and moral judgments are known to be true simply by intuition. For example, if a moral intuitionist were asked to justify why he or she judged abortion to be wrong, the reply would probably be: 'I just know it is', with the truth of this judgment taken as being more or less self-evident and thus not requiring any form of rational justification. Like emotivism, intuitionism totally rejects reason as having ultimate moral authority (Frankena 1973, pp. 102–5), and claims intuition as being the 'prime avenue to truth' (Goldberg 1983, p. 17).

The question remains, how does intuitionism actually determine the moral rightness or wrongness of a particular act? The short answer is that it determines the intrinsic good or bad nature of a given act, which in turn derives from the properties of that act — whether they are intrinsically good or bad. For example, an intuitionist might claim that the wilful act of leaving an innocent road-accident victim to die needlessly has the self-evident property of wrongness, whereas the thoughtful act of assisting and resuscitating an innocent road-accident victim and thereby preventing a needless and untimely death has the self-evident property of goodness.

The process of knowing by intuition the rightness or wrongness of an action goes something like this: first, properties making the act in question right or wrong must be determined. These properties in turn are classified as being either 'prima-facie right' (i.e. the 'rightness' of the properties may be overridden by stronger moral properties) or 'wrong, all things considered' (i.e. in light of other morally significant considerations, and when these considerations have been weighed up against each other, the act is wrong) (Baier 1978a, p. 415). For example, resuscitating an innocent road-accident victim may be regarded as 'prima-facie right' where other stronger moral considerations do not impinge (for example, the rescuer may risk her or his own life in the attempt to resuscitate or save the victim); whereas leaving the innocent accident victim to die needlessly might be regarded as 'wrong all things considered' (for example, when the rescuer is regarded as well qualified to instigate life-saving measures, and would be likely to succeed in the attempt, but is in too much of a hurry to stop, having promised to meet friends for a social dinner).

The second step involves determining the relative weight of given properties and deciding which imposes the more stringent of duties on a person to act. Once it has been decided which of the duties in question is the more stringent, the 'final duty', or 'duty, all things considered', can be established (Baier 1978a, p. 415). For example, once it is determined that the duty to save an innocent road accident victim's life is more stringent than the duty to fulfil one's promise to friends to share a social meal with them, so too is it established that saving the life of the innocent road accident victim is the 'final duty' or 'duty, all things considered'. How do we know this is our final duty, it might be asked? The answer: we 'just know', it is 'self-evident', and that is all there is to say on the matter.

Moral intuitionism is considered by many philosophers to be implausible. They have severely criticised intuitionism on the grounds that it is misleading; that it fails to answer important moral questions; that it is unable to define and analyse the properties to which ethical terms refer; that it lacks objectivity; that it fails to provide a theory of moral motivation (i.e. what motivates people to do morally good acts); that it fails to provide a convincing theory of moral justification; and, more seriously, that it cannot be relied upon to resolve moral conflict (Warnock 1967; Frankena 1973; Rawls 1971; Swanton 1987; Baier 1978a).

While these criticisms are serious, they should not be taken as implying that intuition has no role to play in moral or other forms of decision-making. Such a conclusion would be at odds with recent scientific and scholarly research demonstrating the nature of intuition and its practical importance to and in a range of activities characteristic of human living (see, for example, Davis-Floyd and Arvidson 1997). Furthermore, it is important to note that not all moral philosophers agree that intuition has no place in our moral schemas. For example, in his book *Moral Thinking: its levels, method and point*, Richard Hare (1981) concedes the role of intuition in moral thinking.

Although Hare completely rejects intuition as the basis of moral thinking, and rejects its independent ability to resolve moral conflict, he nevertheless accepts that 'the intuitive level of moral thinking certainly exists and is (humanly speaking) an essential part of the whole structure' (Hare 1981, p. 210).

Hare basically argues that neither intuition nor reason is adequate on its own to deal effectively with moral problems. A sounder or more complete approach to moral thinking, he suggests, would be to admit a kind of 'collaborative relationship' between these two faculties and to cease viewing them as being necessary opponents:

> Let us be clear, first of all, that critical and intuitive moral thinking are not rival procedures, as much of the dispute between utilitarians and intuitionists seem to suppose. They are elements in a common structure, each with its parts to play.
>
> (Hare 1981, p. 44)

Admittedly, Hare views intuition in somewhat rationalistic terms. He regards intuition essentially as being comprised of prima-facie moral principles which have been selected by critical thinking or reason (Hare 1981, pp. 49–50). This might lead intuitionists to be somewhat suspicious of his account of moral thinking. However, it should not detract from the worth of Hare's thesis or the significant contribution it can make to the development of a more progressive and flexible moral theory.

Psychologists also stress the importance of intuition in our everyday practical and working lives, and the need to enhance it if we are to make better rational decisions. Goldberg (1983, p. 33) argues that intuition is very much a part of reason, and in fact plays a crucial role in aiding the reasoning process itself.

Intuition does this by feeding and stimulating rational thought and then by evaluating its products. If a reason or a thought does not 'feel' right, the reasoner or thinker simply switches tracks. Goldberg even makes the radical suggestion that 'reason is merely slow intuition' (p. 37), and that intuition has a particularly important role to play when dealing with problems which are too complex to be solved by rational analysis (p. 23). Goldberg's thesis, again, is not incompatible with Hare's views, but his prescriptions are more fruitful. What is needed, concludes Goldberg, is:

> a balance and a recognition of the intricate, mutually enhancing relationship between intuition and rationality. We need not just more intuition but better intuition. We need not only to trust it but to make it more trustworthy. And at the same time we need sharp, discriminating rationality.
>
> (Goldberg 1983, p. 28)

Regardless of the classic modernist objections raised against intuition, it has its place both in our moral thinking and in our everyday lives (see also Vaughan 1979; Davis-Floyd and Arvidson 1997). (It also has an important place in nursing ethics, as is discussed in Chapter 7.) As Urmson (1975, p. 119) correctly points out, intuition is needed to weigh up the 'plurality of primary moral reasons for action', something which, in his view, is no cause for either surprise or distress. Why is this? The answer is that the need for an intuitive weighing up of a plurality of moral reasons is 'not an irrational anomaly but our ordinary predicament with regard to reasons in most fields' (Urmson 1975, p. 119).

Social contract theory

A social contract view of ethics holds actions to be right or wrong on the basis of whether they conform to or violate the terms of the social contract between the individual and the state. Early social contract theorists argued that the individual should form an agreement with the state (or given ruling power) to surrender freely certain liberties in return for the advantages of an orderly, beneficial and well-governed society. Remnants of this early contractarian approach can be found even today in many aspects of social living. For example, by observing the road rules, we surrender certain personal liberties in the hope of receiving safe road-driving conditions in return. If people did not agree to follow the road laws governing which side of the road to drive on, acceptable rates of speed, behaviour at intersections, safe blood alcohol limits and so on, chaos and death would result (and do result, as the nation's appalling road toll each year makes evident).

Remnants of early contractarianism can also be found in the social contract view of professionalism, which argues, roughly, that if society wishes to receive well-organised and skilful professional services, it must be prepared to relinquish a certain degree of autonomy and grant professionals special privileges of autonomy and power in return. In exchange for these privileges, professionals perform certain tasks and carry out certain duties that would not be expected of them were they acting as 'ordinary' persons (Newton 1981). By surrendering a portion of its liberty and autonomy, society can look forward in return to its interests being served by these all-powerful and autonomous professionals. If its interests are not served, and the professionals in question do not deliver the organised and skilful services they promised to deliver (as in the case of strike action), they may be deemed to have violated the terms of their 'social contract' and thus may be justly censured (for example, by being deregistered, charged with legal negligence, fined and so forth).

Whatever the nature of the social contract, what emerges is the classic position that the surrendering individuals become bound by the political and social contracts into which they enter, and can be justly censured for breaching their terms and conditions. Here the contract forms the very basis of obligation and determines the standard by which right and wrong actions, justice and injustice, are to be measured (Hobbes 1968; Locke 1947; Hume 1947; Rousseau 1947).

Recent contract theory, however, takes quite a different view from this classical position. It holds, for example, that right and wrong actions, justice and injustice, are determined by the 'cooperative maximisation of good'. This maximisation of good is achieved by all rational people choosing impartially (i.e. from behind a strictly hypothetical and decontextualised 'veil of ignorance') to adopt universal moral principles and to apply these in a way that ensures that no other person is unfairly disadvantaged. Individual interests are secured not by political or social bargaining (as in the case of classical contractarianism), but by a procedural principle of justice whose judgments seek to provide 'the most appropriate moral basis for a democratic society' (Rawls 1971, p. viii). Rawls, an influential proponent of contemporary social contract theory, explains that the contract, which 'implies a certain level of abstraction', emphasises social cooperation and ensures the distribution of advantages only to those who do their share' (Rawls 1971, p. 16). The principle of justice works meanwhile to regulate further agreements between cooperating individuals (Rawls 1971, p. 11). Although it is beyond the scope of this text to consider Rawls' thesis in detail, and the many criticisms raised against it, some important questions raised by his notion of choosing from a hypothetical and decontextualised position are touched upon in Chapters 5 and 6.

Applying deontological theory

Deontological theory can be applied to justify moral decisions either by the separate evaluation of a given act (act-deontology) or by an appeal to general rules (rule-deontology).

Act-deontology requires agents to make separate evaluations on their own when making moral decisions, rather than appealing to a general system of rules. This approach emphasises the individual situation as being the ultimate guide on how to respond, and accepts that 'circumstances alter cases' (Fletcher 1966, p. 29). In the words of the Christian ethicist Dietrich Bonhoeffer (executed for his part in an assassination attempt on Hitler):

> The question of good is posed and is decided in the midst of each definite, yet unconcluded, unique and transient situation of our lives, in the midst of our living relationships with men [sic], things, institutions and powers, in other words in the midst of our human existence.
>
> (cited in Fletcher 1966, p. 33)

It can be seen that an act-deontological approach could, if taken to its extreme, commit one to conclusions which would not ordinarily be accepted. For example, act-deontology could even permit murder, as Bonhoeffer's own actions against Hitler demonstrate.

Act-deontology requires the agent to make an extremely thorough and accurate assessment of the situation before making a decision. The rightness of the decision, in the final analysis, depends very much on the correctness of the facts gathered in that situation, and the correct interpretation of those facts. Apart from the facts of the situation, act-deontology offers no other guiding criteria or principles in moral decision-making (Frankena 1973, p. 23). This approach is sometimes referred to as 'situation ethics' (Fletcher 1966).

Rule-deontology, by contrast, requires agents to mediate their decisions by appealing to a system of general rules. This approach takes absolutely no account of the situation at hand; the general rules are to be followed regardless of the facts at hand. For example, if agents subscribe to rule-deontology and thereby accept the general rule 'always tell the truth', they would be compelled to tell the truth even in situations where a harmful consequence would follow from the truth-telling act (Frankena 1973, p. 17). Critics argue that rule-deontology, like act-deontology, could commit one to conclusions which ordinarily would not be accepted. The rule-deontologist's seeming over-reliance on rules has been criticised by modern philosophers as unmitigated 'superstitious rule worship' (Smart and Williams 1973, p. 6).

Teleological theories of ethics

Teleological ethics (from the Greek *telos*, meaning 'end', and *logos*, meaning 'word') refers to a group of ethical theories which differ from and compete with deontological ethics. In essence, teleology denies everything that deontology asserts — or at least almost everything. By this view, and in contrast with deontological ethics, actions are judged good or bad, right or wrong, on the basis of the consequences they produce. Disputes in teleological ethics generally centre on issues such as: What is to be regarded as a moral good? Whose good should be promoted? What kinds of guidance can a moral theory provide for persons deliberating about what should be done in a given situation (Baier 1978b, p. 417)?

Responses to the question 'what is good?' have ranged from the achievement of mere happiness and the satisfaction of desires (monistic goods), through to the acquisition of knowledge for its own sake, freedom, dignity, and so on (pluralistic goods). The good life quickly translates into a life characterised by monistic and/ or pluralistic goods — whichever is thought to hold.

Of equal importance has been the philosophical debate surrounding the questions 'whose good should be promoted?' or 'whose good should count?' This debate has raised four possibilities: ethical egoism, ethical elitism, ethical parochialism, and ethical universalism (Baier 1978b; Frankena 1973).

Ethical egoism holds that people should do only that which will promote their own greatest good (Frankena 1973, p. 15). If, for example, going out to dinner with friends is perceived as being a greater good than stopping at the scene of an accident to render life-saving measures to an unknown accident victim, the ethical egoist would probably decide to drive past the accident and continue on to the restaurant.

Ethical elitism, on the other hand, holds that only the good of the elite should be maximised. By this view, the interests of those who are 'less gifted' should be set aside in favour of those who have a better chance of achieving 'perfection' or excellence (Baier 1978b). A good example of this is the distribution of more resources to the elite or 'hard' sciences such as medicine, than to the 'less sophisticated' or 'softer' sciences such as nursing.

Ethical parochialism, by contrast, serves only the good of an individual's appropriate 'in-group'. The 'in-group' may be, for example, the individual's relevant profession, or else the family, circle of friends, class, gender, religion, political party, social club, or cultural group. Some professional codes of conduct are examples of 'ethical parochialism', particularly where these stand to serve more the interests of the professional group than the interests of those whom the professional group is supposed to be serving (e.g. the community at large and the individuals comprising it).

Ethical universalism, the fourth possibility, essentially demands that the good of all humankind must be given equal consideration, and that human interests should all be treated equally. Ethical universalism is generally regarded as being more acceptable than the limited approaches of ethical egoism, ethical elitism and ethical parochialism, since its outcomes are generally seen to be more just and more defensible. Utilitarianism is popularly regarded as one of the more compelling theories of ethical universalism, in that it promotes the 'greatest good for the greatest number' (Frankena 1973, p. 15). Before considering this theory, however, one or two comments should be made about a teleological account of moral duties.

Moral duties

A moral duty is an action which a person is bound, for moral reasons, to perform. From a teleological perspective, duties generally derive from the consideration of some predicted moral consequence that ought to be furthered or upheld. It might be argued, for instance, that one has a stringent moral duty to prevent otherwise avoidable harmful consequences from occurring where this can be done without sacrificing other important moral interests (Singer 1979a). Given this teleological maxim, if a person's action stands to prevent a particular harmful consequence from occurring, that person is duty-bound to perform that action, provided other important moral interests are not sacrificed in the process. An off-duty nurse, for example, could be said to be duty-bound to render life-saving care at the scene of a road accident, regardless of any inconvenience this might cause since mere inconvenience is not generally regarded as a morally significant consideration. If the life of the nurse were put at risk, however, the moral duty to render assistance would not be so clear-cut.

Duties are primarily concerned with avoiding intolerable results; they are thought to provide the basic requirements that may be universally demanded in an effort to achieve a 'tolerable basis of social life' (Urmson 1969, p. 73). They also work 'to secure reliability, a state of affairs in which people can reasonably expect others to behave in some ways and not in others' (Williams 1985, p. 187). If a duty fails to avoid an intolerable result, there is room for questioning whether in fact it was a duty in the first place (Urmson, 1969). It might also be argued that if a duty can be overridden (for example, where there appears to be a conflict of duties) it is not a duty at all; we have merely mistakenly thought that it was (Hare 1981, p. 26). On the other hand, it might be replied that just because a duty can be overridden this does not mean 'it was not a duty in the first place' but only that it was a 'prima-facie duty'. There is nothing philosophically wrong in holding that duties can be prima facie in nature (Ross 1930, p. 19).

Moral obligations

The notion of moral duty is related to the notion of moral 'obligation' (a notion that also finds usage in deontological moral discourse). The language of obligations is very similar to the language of duties, and typically involves expressions like: 'You have an obligation to ...', 'I have an obligation to ...', 'We have an obligation to ...', 'They have an obligation to ...', and so on. Although many philosophers treat the terms 'duties' and 'obligations' synonymously, an important and useful distinction can be drawn between them, which rests on the differing moral strengths each notion has, rather than on a difference in their essential moral nature. Duties are regarded as having a stronger force than obligations, or, to put this another way, duties are more morally compelling than are obligations. Dworkin (1977, pp. 48–9), an influential exponent of this distinction, gives the example that it is one thing to say a person has an obligation to give to a charity, but it is quite another to say that person has a duty to do so. While it would be 'good' if someone made a charitable donation, it would be erroneous to suggest a moral compulsion to do so. To a limited extent, Dworkin's thesis helps to alleviate the tension created by the problem of supposed conflicting duties.

The concept of obligation and its distinctiveness from duty has interesting and important implications for nurses, particularly in relation to the issue of following a doctor's or a superior's orders. For instance, it may well be that nurses have an obligation to follow a doctor's or a superior's orders, but it is far from clear that they always have a duty to do so, either morally or legally. In fact, if a doctor's or a superior's orders are 'dubious', a nurse has both a legal and a moral duty to question such orders. In some cases, the nurse may even have a duty to refuse to follow a given order when such an order is 'unreasonable', 'unlawful' or 'likely to cause otherwise avoidable harm'.

Classical utilitarianism

As mentioned earlier, utilitarianism is thought to be the more generally persuasive of the teleological theories on the grounds of its ethical universalism. Utilitarianism involves a principle which concerns itself more with the general welfare of people than the particular welfare of individuals. In other words, utilitarianism views the world not in terms of certain individual rights which people may or may not have, but in terms of people's collective and overall interests.

A broad view of utilitarianism is persuasive in that it promotes a universal point of view; that is, that one person's interests cannot count as being superior to the interests of another just because they are personal interests (Singer 1979b, p. 12). For example, I cannot claim that my interests count more than your interests just because they are my interests.

Modern utilitarianism was founded by the English philosopher Jeremy Bentham (1748–1832). Bentham's utility thesis holds that actions should be judged right or wrong on the basis of whether they tend to promote pleasure (and happiness) and diminish pain (and unhappiness) and, more specifically, whether they tend to maximise the balance of good over bad (Bentham 1962, p. 34).

Bentham held the principle of utility to apply equally to the private actions of individuals and to the public actions of government, and he took great pains to elaborate the principle's relevance to legal, political, educational and social institutions. One troubling aspect of his thesis, however, is that it is thoroughly tainted with ethical egoism. Bentham insisted, for example, that the key to maximising the community's interests is to maximise the individual's interests. He essentially saw the community as a 'fictitious body', and community interests as nothing more than 'the sum interests of the several members who comprise it' (Bentham 1962, p. 35).

The influence of the British philosopher John Stuart Mill (1806–73), who was the son of the Scottish philosopher James Mill (1773–1836), saw a major modification of Bentham's thesis. Mill was much more specific in his treatment of what he called the 'greatest happiness principle', and was quite adamant that the ultimate standard of utility is not the individual's 'own greatest happiness, but the greatest amount of happiness altogether' (1962b, p. 262).

Mill stressed that utilitarianism was quite distinct from mere ethical egoism (i.e. the promotion of one's own pleasure and happiness only), and in fact argued that in some instances individuals might even have a duty to sacrifice their own greatest good for the good of others (1962b, p. 268). He also advanced the notion that people should be striving to act cooperatively with one another and 'proposing to themselves a collective, not an individual interest as the aim ... of their action' (Mill 1962b, p. 285). Once people form a collective interest, suggested Mill, they are more inclined to view the interests of others as their own.

Although Mill essentially embraced a more cooperative and collective view of morality, he nevertheless upheld the notions of the sovereignty of the individual, individual independence and freedom of choice (1962a, p. 135). He generally considered rational persons as the best judges of their own best interests and entitled to make mistakes. However, he did recognise that in some instances a person's liberty of action may be justly interfered with. The first instance is where a given individual is incapable of exercising an informed choice, as in the case of children or other persons who lack the 'maturity of their faculties' (1962a, p. 135). The second instance is when an individual's conduct stands to hurt others or stands to 'affect prejudicially the interests of others', in which case both society and the law would have a prima-facie case for interfering with a person's liberty of action, and possibly even for punishing that person (1962a, pp. 136, 205).

For Mill, the principle of utility is the ultimate source of moral obligation. Utility can and should be used to decide between competing demands: its application may be difficult, argued Mill (1962b, p. 277), but it is better than no principle at all.

The works of Bentham and Mill sought to simplify ethics by providing one universally applicable principle by which all moral judgments should be made. Utility proved to be such a principle. As well as having philosophical appeal, the principle had the attraction of being democratic, and secular; that is, it could be upheld independently of any prevailing religious dogma or moral theology. Despite its appeal, however, classical utilitarianism has sustained heavy criticism on several grounds, some of which are:

- the difficulties likely to be encountered in reliably predicting the consequences of given actions;
- the time-consuming nature of utilitarian calculations and analyses;
- the risk of making mistakes in predicting and calculating the moral worth of outcomes;
- difficulties likely to be encountered in accurately trying to measure pleasure, happiness, pain and unhappiness;
- the problem of sacrificing individual interests to the whole.

Recent utilitarian theory

Bentham's and Mill's hedonistic account of utility no longer has currency in modern moral thinking, although, as a word of caution, some nurse authors persist in advocating the 'greatest happiness principle' in nursing ethics and nursing models of moral decision-making. The main reason for abandoning hedonistic utilitarianism has been its inadequacy to determine right action 'objectively'. The major alternative approach is 'preference utilitarianism', which views the maximisation of individual preferences as being of intrinsic value, rather than the maximisation of hedonistic pleasures or hedonistic states of affairs. As Beauchamp and Childress observe:

> what is intrinsically valuable is what individuals prefer to obtain, and utility is thus translated into the satisfaction of those needs and desires that individuals choose to satisfy.
>
> (Beauchamp and Childress 1989, p. 28)

By this view, preference utilitarianism as a moral theory translates into the demand that we ought in all circumstances to produce the greatest possible balance of 'value over disvalue' for all persons affected (Beauchamp and Childress 1994, p. 47). In other words, we ought in all circumstances to produce the greatest possible balance of individuals satisfying their preferences over individuals not satisfying their preferences. The problem of individuals asserting immoral desires or preferences is overcome by the claim that our commonsense and past experience will be enough to distinguish unacceptable desires which can be excluded 'on more general utilitarian grounds' (Beauchamp and Childress 1989, p. 29).

On the whole, preference utilitarianism is considered more satisfying, since its calculations are easier to work out. For instance, it takes little more than basic 'commonsense and careful deliberation' to determine an individual's preferences; it would take considerably more to determine an individual's internal experiences of pleasure and pain, if, indeed, these things can be determined at all.

Applying utilitarian theory

As with deontological moral theory, utilitarian theory can be applied either by separate evaluation of a given act (act-utilitarianism), or by an appeal to general rules (rule-utilitarianism). Each approach places different demands on the deliberating agent.

Act-utilitarianism demands that the deliberator considers the moral consequences of each particular act under scrutiny. The rightness or wrongness of the act in question is ultimately determined by the total goodness and badness of its particular consequences; that is, whether it alone maximises or minimises intrinsic value (Smart and Williams 1973, p. 4). Consider, for example, the case of a nurse involved in the care of the seriously injured motor vehicle accident victim whose neurological prognosis is uncertain. A person applying act-utilitarianism would, in this case, ask what good or bad consequences would result from this particular motor accident victim being resuscitated at all costs? The ultimate answer will depend on whether such an act in this particular case results in the maximisation of value over disvalue.

Act-utilitarianism, like act-deontology, has been severely criticised on much the same grounds: that it would commit an agent to unacceptable conclusions and may permit acts which ordinarily would not be permitted, such as lying or sacrificing innocent life.

Rule-utilitarianism, on the other hand, demands that the deliberator considers the moral consequences of generally observing a rule. In the example of the nurse involved in the care of a seriously injured motor accident victim, rule-utilitarianism would require the nurse to ask what good or bad consequences would result from the general rule that all motor accident victims with uncertain neurological prognoses must be resuscitated rigorously. The ultimate answer depends on whether as a general rule the unconstrained resuscitation of all accident victims results in the maximisation of value over disvalue.

Rule-utilitarianism has also been the subject of much criticism, with objectors arguing that it too could commit the deliberator to accept otherwise unacceptable conclusions such as lying or sacrificing innocent life. Another criticism is that rule-utilitarianism collapses into act-utilitarianism once the 'best consequences' are adhered to (Smart and Williams 1973).

Moral principles and moral rules

In completing our discussion of classical moral theory, we need to examine what gives moral theories their substance or their 'guts', and so we turn to moral principles and rules. Like the theories under which they operate, moral principles and moral rules are subject to philosophical controversy. Nevertheless, they have an important role to play in guiding moral behaviour and moral decision-making, as will become clearer in the chapters to follow. What, then, are some of the popular moral principles which people appeal to when attempting to solve moral problems? How do we know the difference between moral principles and moral rules as prescriptive action guides? The following sections attempt to answer these questions briefly.

Ethical principlism

General standards of conduct which make up an ethical system are known as moral principles. To say that a principle is 'moral' is merely to assert that it is a behaviour guide which 'entails particular imperatives' (Harrison 1954, p. 115).

Moral principles function by specifying that some type of action or conduct is either prohibited, required, or permitted in certain circumstances (Solomon 1978, p. 408). By this view, an action or decision is generally considered morally right or good when it accords with a given relevant moral principle, and morally wrong or bad when it does not. To illustrate how this works, consider the action of making a measurement using a ruler. If the line you have drawn measures the desired length of, say, 12 cm — as measured against your ruler — you would judge the length as 'correct'. If, however, the line you have drawn is only 10 cm long — not the desired 12 cm — you would judge the length to be 'incorrect'. By analogy, principles also function like rulers, insofar as they provide a standard against which something (in this case, actions) can be measured. For example, if an action fails to 'measure up' to the ultimate standards set by a given principle, we would judge the action to be 'incorrect' or, more specifically, morally wrong. If, however, an action fully measures up to the ultimate standards set by a given principle, we would judge the action to be 'correct' or morally right. So far, so good. The next question is: what are these moral principles against which actions can be measured?

Moral principles commonly used in bioethical discussions include the principles of autonomy, non-maleficence, beneficence, and justice. It is to examining the content, prescriptive force and application of these principles that this discussion now turns.

Autonomy

The term 'autonomy' comes from the Greek *autos* (meaning 'self') and *nomos* (meaning 'rule', 'governance' or 'law'). When the concept of autonomy is used in moral discourse, what is commonly being referred to is a person's ability to make or to exercise self-determining choice — literally, 'self-governing'. Included here is the additional notion of 'respect for persons'; that is, of treating or respecting persons as ends in themselves, as dignified and rational autonomous choosers, and not as the mere means (objects or tools) to the ends of others (Kant 1972; Benn 1971). The principle of autonomy, however, is a little different, and is eloquently formulated by Beauchamp and Walters as follows:

> Insofar as an autonomous agent's actions *do not infringe on the autonomous actions of others*, that person should be free to perform whatever action he or she wishes (presumably even if it involves considerable risk to himself or herself and even if others consider the action to be foolish).
>
> (Beauchamp and Walters 1982, p. 27, emphasis added)

What this basically means is that people should be free to choose and entitled to act on their preferences provided their decisions and actions do not stand to violate, or impinge on, the significant moral interests of others.

Both the concept and the principle of autonomy have important implications for nursing practice. For example, if autonomy is to be taken seriously by nurses, nursing practice must truly respect patients as dignified human beings capable of deciding what is to count as being in their own best interests — even if what they decide is considered by others (including nurses) to be 'foolish'. In short, nurses must allow patients to participate in decision-making concerning their care. Given this, it soon becomes clear that the whole practice of 'negotiated patient goals' and 'negotiated patient care' as advocated by contemporary nursing philosophy has its roots in the moral principle of autonomy, and the derived duty to respect persons as autonomous moral choosers. It is not derived merely from a concept of 'acceptable professional nursing practice'.

In application, the principle of autonomy would judge as being morally objectionable and condemnable any act which unjustly prevents rational and autonomous persons from deciding what is to count as being in their own best interests. The kinds of act which might come in for criticism here include, for example:

- treating patients without their consent;
- treating patients without giving them all the relevant information necessary for making an informed and intelligent choice;
- telling patients 'white lies' (such as telling a patient that 'the operation went well', meaning that there were no intra-operative or post-operative complications, but, in fact, a large inoperable malignant tumour was found);
- withholding information from patients when they have expressed a reflective choice to receive it;
- forcing information upon patients when they have expressed a reflective choice not to receive it; and
- forcing nurses to act against their reasoned moral judgments or conscience.

It should be noted, however, that while the moral principle of autonomy is very helpful in guiding ethically just practices in health care contexts, it is not entirely unproblematic. Indeed, its uncritical and culturally inappropriate application in some contexts may, in fact, inadvertently cause rather than prevent significant moral harms to patients, for reasons which are considered in Chapters 5 and 6.

Non-maleficence

The term 'non-maleficence' comes from the Latin *maleficent* — from *maleficus*, (meaning 'wicked', 'prone to evil'), from *malum* (meaning 'evil'), and *male* (meaning 'ill'). As a moral principle, *non-maleficence* (literally 'refuse evil'), prescribes 'above all, do no harm' which entails a stringent obligation not to injure or harm others. This principle is sometimes equated with the moral principle of 'beneficence' (considered below under a separate subheading) which prescribes 'above all, do good'. Trying to conflate these two obviously distinct principles under one principle is, however, misleading. As Beauchamp and Childress (1994, p. 190) explain, not only are these two principles obviously distinct (for instance, our obligation not to kill someone does seem qualitatively and quantitatively different from our obligation to rescue someone from a life-threatening situation), but it is important to distinguish between them so as not to obscure other important distinctions which might be made in ordinary moral discourse. One instance in which 'other important distinctions might need to be made' is in the case of where both principles might apply to a given situation, but where the strength of the respective moral imperatives of each may nevertheless differ significantly and thus might prescribe quite different courses of action. As Beauchamp and Childress point out:

> Obligations not to harm others are sometimes more stringent than obligations to help them, but obligations of beneficence are also sometimes more stringent than obligations of non-maleficence.
>
> (Beauchamp and Childress 1994, p. 190)

'Stringentness' thus stands as an important distinction that might be obscured if the principles of non-maleficence and beneficence were conflated into one single principle. Beauchamp and Childress (1994, p. 191) conclude, however, that generally 'obligations of non-maleficence are more stringent than obligations of beneficence', and, in some cases, may even override beneficence particularly in instances where beneficent acts, paradoxically, are not morally defensible (for example, depriving one's family of food for a week and failing to pay the rent [thereby increasing the risk of eviction] because of donating the household's weekly budget to charity).

Applied in nursing contexts, the principle of non-maleficence would provide justification for condemning any act which unjustly injures a person or causes them to suffer an otherwise avoidable harm (examples of which will be given in the chapters to follow).

Before continuing, some commentary is warranted on the notion of 'harm' and how it might be interpreted (given that it is open to a variety of interpretations). For the purposes of this text, harm may be taken to involve the invasion, violation, thwarting, or 'setting back' of a person's significant welfare interests to the detriment of that person's wellbeing (Feinberg 1984, p. 34; Beauchamp and Childress 1994, p. 193). Interests, in this instance, are taken to mean 'a miscellaneous collection, consist[ing] of all those things in which one has a stake' together with the 'harmonious advancement' of those interests (Feinberg 1984, p. 34). Interests are morally significant since they are fundamentally linked to human wellbeing; specifically, they stand as a *fundamental requisite* (although, granted, not the whole) of human wellbeing (Feinberg 1984, p. 37). Wellbeing, in turn, can include interests in:

> continuance for a foreseeable interval of one's life, and the interests in one's own physical health and vigour, the integrity and normal functioning of one's body, the absence of absorbing pain and suffering or grotesque disfigurement, minimal intellectual acuity, emotional stability, the absence of groundless anxieties and resentments, the capacity to engage normally in social intercourse and to enjoy and maintain friendships, at least minimal income and financial security, a tolerable social and physical environment, and a certain amount of freedom from interference and coercion.
>
> (Feinberg 1984, p. 37)

The test for whether a person's interests and wellbeing have been violated, 'set back', thwarted or invaded rests on 'whether that interest is in a worse condition than it would otherwise have been in had the invasion not occurred at all' (Feinberg 1984, p. 34). For instance, if a person (for example, a patient) is left psychogenically distressed (for example, emotionally distressed, anxious, depressed and even suicidal) or in a state of needless physical pain and/or disability as a result of his/her experiences (for example, as *a patient* in a given health care setting) our reflective commonsense tells us that this person's interests have been violated and the person him/herself 'harmed'. As the American philosopher, Joel Feinberg (1984), explains, the violation of a person's welfare interests renders that person 'very seriously harmed indeed' since 'their ultimate aspirations are defeated too'.

Beneficence

The term 'beneficence' comes from the Latin *beneficus*, from *bene* (meaning 'well' or 'good') and *facere* (meaning 'to do'). As already mentioned above, the principle of beneficence prescribes 'above all, do good', and entails a positive obligation to literally 'act for the benefit of others' *viz.* contribute to the welfare and wellbeing of others (Beauchamp and Childress 1994, pp. 259–60). Acts of beneficence can include such virtuous actions as: care, compassion, empathy, sympathy, altruism, kindness, mercy, love, friendship and charity. It is recognised, however, that bestowing benefits on others is not always without cost to the benefactor. Thus there are some limits to the principle; that is, it is not 'free standing' and its application can be appropriately constrained by other moral (for example, utilitarian) considerations. To put this another way, we are not obliged to act beneficently towards others when doing so could result in our own significant moral interests being seriously harmed or compromised in some way.

Although the notion of 'obligatory beneficence' remains a controversial one in mainstream moral philosophy (for instance, it is popularly accepted that we are not 'morally required to benefit persons on all occasions, even if we are in a position to do so'), there are nevertheless a number of conditions under which a person can indeed be said to have an obligation of beneficence and that this obligation might, sometimes, be overriding (Beauchamp and Childress 1994, pp. 262, 266). These conditions, devised by Beauchamp and Childress (1994, p. 266), are as follows:

> a person X has a determinate obligation of beneficence toward person Y if and only if each of the following conditions is satisfied (assuming X is aware of the relevant facts):
>
> 1. Y is at risk of significant loss of or damage to life or health or some other major interest;
> 2. X's action is needed (singly or in concert with others) to prevent this loss or damage;
> 3. X's action (singly or in concert with others) has a high probability of preventing it;
> 4. X's action would not present significant risks, costs, or burdens to X;
> 5. the benefits that Y can expect to gain outweigh any harms, costs, or burdens that X is likely to incur.

They go on to suggest that it is only when these conditions are satisfied that a person's 'general duty of beneficence' becomes a 'specific duty of beneficence' toward another given individual.

The principle stands to have an interesting and useful application in nursing practice. Consider the following case (personal communication; names have been changed).

Mrs Jones, a Jehovah's Witness, is admitted to an intensive care unit in a terminal condition, suffering from advanced hepatitis B and severe liver failure. She has a slow internal haemorrhage and is only semiconscious. Before her alteration in consciousness she had given her doctors a written statement specifically requesting that she not be given a blood transfusion under any circumstances. Upon her arrival in the unit, however, the attending doctor prescribes a unit of blood and requests that it be given immediately. Mrs Jones' husband and children are all present and, upon overhearing the doctor's request, become very upset. Mr Jones approaches the doctor and asks that his wife not be given the blood transfusion. He reminds the doctor that Mrs Jones has made explicit her wish not to have a blood transfusion under any circumstances. Nurse Smith, the registered nurse caring for Mrs Jones, hears the discussion and has to make a decision whether or not to intervene on her patient's behalf. In making her decision, Nurse Smith might appeal to the principle of beneficence in the following manner:

1. Mrs Jones, a terminally ill Jehovah's Witness, is at risk of suffering a significant loss (a violation of her spiritual values and beliefs) if she is given the prescribed blood transfusion;
2. action by Nurse Smith, the attending nurse, is needed to prevent Mrs Jones from experiencing the loss in question;
3. Nurse Smith's action of refusing to administer the prescribed transfusion would probably prevent Mrs Jones' loss;
4. Nurse Smith's action will not present a significant risk to her (for example, she will not lose her job);
5. the benefits gained by Mrs Jones outweigh any harms Nurse Smith is likely to suffer (given that Nurse Smith autonomously chooses to uphold Mrs Jones' interests, and does not stand to suffer any morally significant consequences of her actions).

In this particular case the nurse refused to give the transfusion which had been prescribed. When the doctor insisted that it be given, the nurse pointed out that the transfusion would probably be of no benefit to Mrs Jones, as she was clearly in the end stages of her disease — to put it bluntly, 'she was dying'. Nurse Smith then suggested to the doctor that perhaps he would prefer to administer the transfusion himself. Interestingly, the doctor declined this invitation, and the transfusion was not given. Mrs Jones died a short while later, without having to experience a needless violation of her expressed wishes, values and beliefs.

In summary, by this principle, any act which fails to address an imbalance of harms over benefits where this can be done without sacrificing a benefactor's own significant moral interests, warrants judgment as being morally unacceptable.

Justice

The principle of justice (its nature and content), unlike the principles above, is not so amenable to definition or quantification. As a point of interest, questions concerning what justice is and what its origins are have occupied the minds of philosophers for nearly three thousand years, and to this day remain the subject of intensive philosophical debate (MacIntyre 1988; Solomon and Murphy 1990). Significantly, the end result of this great philosophical debate has not been the development of a singular and refined universal theory of justice, but the development of a range of rival theories of justice — and, it should be added, a range of competing underlying subjectivities and perspectives supporting each of these respective theories (MacIntyre 1988). Different conceptions of justice (from the Latin *justus* meaning 'righteous') have included: justice as revenge (retributive justice — for example, 'an eye for an eye'); justice as mercy (Christian ethics); justice as harmony in the soul and harmony in the state (Pythagorean ethics, 600 BC–1 AD); justice as equality ('equals must be treated equally, and unequals unequally'); justice as an equal distribution of benefits and burdens (distributive justice); justice as what is deserved ('each according to one's merit or worth'); and justice as love (Rawls 1971; Outka 1972; MacIntyre 1985, 1988; Waithe 1987; Solomon and Murphy 1990; Singer 1991; Beauchamp and Childress 1994).

Given these different conceptions of justice, the problem arises of what, if any, conception of justice nurses should adopt? While it is beyond the scope of this text to answer this question in depth, there is nevertheless room to advocate at least two senses of justice which nurses might find helpful: (1) justice as fairness; and (2) justice as the equal distribution of benefits and burdens (Beauchamp and Childress 1994, p. 327). It is these two senses of justice which will now be considered.

Justice as fairness

Justice as fairness finds interpretation in terms of 'what is deserved'. Here, it can be said that:

> One acts justly toward a person when that person has given what is due or owed, and thus what he and she deserves and can legitimately claim.
>
> (Beauchamp and Childress 1989, p. 257)

If a person deserved something, justice is done when that person receives that particular something. Here, the 'something' may be either positive (a reward) or negative (a punishment). This view relies very heavily on an 'intuitive' sense of justice. For example, we may 'feel' it is unjust to punish or censure someone for a harm they did not cause, or not to punish someone for a harm they did deliberately cause. Likewise we may feel that it is unjust to reward someone for an accomplishment to which they contributed nothing, and yet not reward someone who contributed a great deal.

We do not need to look far in nursing practice to find sobering examples of where the principle of justice as fairness has been violated. Consider cases where nurses have been subjected to severe legal and professional censure on the basis of mistakes made by doctors (Johnstone 1994). The Somera case of 1929, cited in Chapter 3, involving a nurse who was fined and sentenced to prison after following an incorrect medical order, stands as an important example here (Grennan 1930). While it may well have been 'fair' that Somera was censured for her part in the administration of an incorrectly prescribed drug, it was hardly 'fair' that the doctor — who prescribed the drug, checked it with Somera, and administered it — was acquitted.

Other less dramatic examples involve cases where nurses have gained promotion or have secured employment on the basis of their claiming credit for the work of either their peers or their subordinates; at the other end of the continuum, some nurses have been denied promotion or employment because their superior has ignored, or refused for whatever reasons to recognise significant professional achievements the nurse applicant has in fact made. The story of 'Sally Trihard', a registered nurse who had difficulty getting a job because of a past difference of professional opinion with a charge nurse, is a case in point (Johnstone 1987, p. 41; see also 'A costly misjudgment', *Australian Nurses Journal* 1988 p. 3).

How, then, might we make choices on this view of justice? One possible approach which has received widespread attention is that discussed by the contemporary philosopher John Rawls, briefly mentioned earlier in this chapter. He argues, for example, that if parties are to exercise truly just or fair choices, they must choose from a hypothetically 'neutral' position, or from a position of what he describes as being 'behind the veil of ignorance' (Rawls 1971, p. 12). From such a position he argues:

> no-one knows his [sic] place in society, his [sic] class position or social status, nor does anyone know his [sic] fortune in the distribution of natural assets and abilities, his [sic] intelligence, strength, and the like ... [T]his ensures that no-one is advantaged or disadvantaged in the choice of principles by the outcome of natural chance or the contingency of social circumstances. Since all are similarly situated and no-one is able to design principles to favour his [sic] particular condition, the principles of justice are the result of a fair agreement or bargain.
>
> (Rawls 1971, p. 12)

While Rawls' view is problematic (for instance, it is open to serious question whether, in fact, all choosers are or could ever be 'similarly situated', as he assumes), it is nevertheless persuasive, particularly when considered in the light of broader philosophical demands which emphasise among other things that moral choice and judgment should be exercised from a position of impartiality and objectivity. However, whether in fact human beings are ever capable of exercising truly impartial and 'objective' choices — indeed, of choosing from behind that veil of ignorance — is a matter of great controversy. Despite its weaknesses, Rawls' justice theory helps us to come to terms with the notion of fairness and how it might be used in real life situations. It also alerts us to some of the potential difficulties of trying to determine and apply an uncontentious view of justice.

Justice as an equal distribution of benefits and burdens

A second sense in which justice can be used is that pertaining to 'distributive justice'; that is, an equal distribution of benefits and harms. By this view, all people are required to bear an equal share of their society's benefits and burdens. Such a view admits that all persons must have equal claims to liberty and opportunity, but in a way that is compatible with the claims of others. As well as this, there must be equal access (and opportunity to gain access) to positions of authority and power, and there must be an equal distribution of wealth and income. The only morally acceptable exception to this would be if an 'unequal distribution would work to everyone's advantage' (Beauchamp and Childress 1989, p. 269); or where an unequal distribution of benefits would be necessary so as to 'maximise the minimum level of primary goods in order to protect vital interests in potentially damaging or disastrous contexts' (Beauchamp and Childress 1989, p. 269). Simply put, inequalities in distributing benefits and primary goods are 'just' as long as this results in the least well-off (that is, those who are already disadvantaged unfairly) achieving a decent minimum level of wellbeing (that is, being advantaged by the benefits which have been conferred unequally). Given this view, 'injustice' finds interpretation as 'simply inequalities that are not to the benefit of all' (Rawls 1971, pp. 60–1).

As with the fairness sense of justice discussed earlier, we do not need to look far to find sobering examples in nursing where the principle of distributive justice has been violated. In many cases, nurses have had to (and continue to) bear unequal and intolerable burdens on account of certain inequities in the distribution of scarce health care resources. For example, historically nurses have had to endure poor and unsafe working conditions with a maximum of responsibility and a minimum of financial or personal reward (Johnstone 1994). Indeed, the historic 1986 nurses' strike for fifty days in the State of Victoria (Australia) was largely a protest by nurses against the decline in their work conditions and in standards of patient care, against heavy and diverse workloads, and against the tardy government response to their log of claims. (The issue of strike action by nurses is discussed in greater depth in Chapter 15.)

Another example illustrates that to deny the principle of distributive justice may have an immediate practical effect. Nurses can, for instance, be forgiven for feeling a powerful sense of injustice when a new piece of costly medical equipment or a considerable quantity of pharmaceutical supplies is purchased, while at the same time basic items of critical use in safe patient care and management are apparently lacking. It seems ludicrous, for instance, to allocate a considerable portion of a hospital budget to, say, antibiotics, but to cut back on the supply of items such as sterile surgical scissors and forceps — both of which are basic items necessary for aseptic wound packing and management. Such equipment will help to avoid unnecessary and prolonged wound infection which, if it was to occur, would result in the patient having to endure (unjustly) a prolonged stay in hospital.

In considering the fairness and the distributive senses of justice, it is instructive to note that both uphold two common minimal principles: formal equality ('equals must be treated equally, and unequals must be treated unequally'); and a mixture of autonomy and beneficence ('we all ought to bear certain burdens, usually of a minimal sort, for the common good') (Beauchamp and Childress 1989, pp. 256–306).

In calculating the balance or distribution of harms and benefits, notions of comparative and non-comparative justice are also used. Justice is 'comparative' when what a person deserves can be determined only by balancing the competing claims of others against the person's own claims (Beauchamp and Childress 1989, pp. 256–306). For example, whether a nurse qualifies for a job or a promotion will depend largely on the competing claims of the other applicants. If the other applicants are more qualified and more experienced, it seems reasonable to hold that they are more 'deserving' of the position being offered. Justice is 'non-comparative', on the other hand, when 'desert is judged by standards independent of the claims of others' (Beauchamp and Childress 1989, pp. 256–306). For example, a nurse who is guilty of breaching acceptable professional standards of conduct deserves to be censured, or even deregistered, if the breach of conduct warrants such an action; a nurse who is innocent of professional misconduct, however, does not deserve to be censured or deregistered. (See Beauchamp and Childress [1994, pp. 328–45] for a brief but comprehensive overview of the principle of formal justice; the material principles of justice; utilitarian, libertarian, communitarian and egalitarian theories of justice; and the 'fair opportunity rule'.)

Moral rules

Like moral principles, moral rules also have a place in making up a general overriding and prescriptive action-guiding system. And, like moral principles, moral rules function by specifying that some type of action or conduct is either prohibited, required or permitted (Solomon 1978, pp. 408–9). What distinguishes a moral rule from a moral principle is its structure and nature. Moral principles, for instance, tend to be regarded as providing the content of morality, and the bases or the 'parent' forms from which general moral truths (insofar as these can be determined) are derived. In application, moral principles incline more toward a general focus. Consider, for example, the broad moral principle of 'autonomy'. In general, the principle demands that rational persons should be respected as autonomous choosers, capable of judging what is in their own best interests. As such, rational persons should be free to act as they wish provided their actions do not violate the moral interests of others.

Moral rules, on the other hand, stand as being merely derivative of moral principles and theories and, in application, are much more particular in their focus. Although it is difficult to draw a firm distinction between moral rules and moral principles, it is generally recognised that moral rules have different force, sanctioning power, conditions of existence, scope of application, and level of concreteness from moral principles (Solomon 1978). An example of a moral rule would be the demand, say, to 'always tell the truth' or 'never tell a lie'. Thus, if a patient asks an attending health care professional a question concerning a diagnosis and proposed treatment, the health care professional could be said to be obliged to give the information the patient has requested. The apparent 'obligation' here finds its force not just from the moral rule 'always tell the truth', but from the moral principle of autonomy which demands that rational people be respected as autonomous choosers, and be given the information required to make an informed and intelligent choice.

Another example can be found in a set of rules that prescribe such things as 'do not kill others', 'do not cause pain and suffering to others', 'do not affect detrimentally the physical and mental health of others', and so forth. The apparent obligations here find their force not just from the rules stated, but from the moral principle non-maleficence which prescribes 'do no harm'.

In order for a particular moral rule (or set of moral rules) to be justified, it must be fully derived from and reducible to established parent principles of morality.

In summary, moral rules derive from moral principles, and as such have only prima-facie force (i.e. they can be overridden by stronger moral claims). Given their prima-facie nature, moral rules cannot override the moral principles from which they have been derived. To accept that they could would be to suggest, somewhat paradoxically, that derived rules could meaningfully conflict with parent principles — which, of course, is absurd. The question of moral rules is an important one for nurses, particularly as it relates to the broader issue of professional codes of conduct, an issue that will become clearer in the following chapters.

The issue remains, however, whether moral principles and rules provide an adequate theoretical framework for guiding moral conduct.

Moral rights theory

Moral rights theory, which is both deontological and modernist in nature, stands as an extremely popular and influential theoretical perspective in Western cultures. Evidence of this can be found in the vast array of contexts in which moral rights discourse has currency. For example, we see moral rights discourse in: statements on and bills of clients/patients rights, professional codes of ethics and conduct (for example, the International Council of Nurses *Code for Nurses* and supporting position statements), statutory authorities (for example, the various Australian state and territory Human Rights and Equal Opportunity Commissions), government inquiries (for example, the *Report of the National Inquiry into the Human Rights of People with Mental Illness* by Burdekin et al. 1993), in global declarations (for example, the Universal Declaration of Human Rights in 1948 [United Nations 1978]), and not least the plethora of literature on the subject (this present text being no exception). Despite postmodernist trends in ethics criticising modernist moral perspectives, it is unlikely that the influence of moral rights discourse will weaken in the immediate future. To the contrary, as marginalised and vulnerable groups of people discover through interpretation and social criticism their own inclusion under a moral rights schema that previously excluded them in favour of society's dominant elite, and through this discovery recognise the potential for moral rights discourse to be subversive of class and power (Walzer 1987, pp. 22, 27), it is probable that moral rights discourse will continue to increase in its influence. If nurses are to participate effectively in discourses on moral rights, it is, therefore, essential that they have some understanding of the theoretical underpinnings of a moral (and human) rights perspective on ethics. It is to providing a brief examination of moral rights theory that this chapter will now turn.

Rights

Moral rights (to be distinguished here from legal rights, institutional rights, civil rights, etc.) generally entail claims about some special entitlement or interest which ought, for moral reasons, to be protected. The kinds of interests for which protection might be sought include, for example, life, freedom, happiness, privacy, self-determination, fair treatment and bodily integrity. The language used in asserting rights typically involves expressions such as: 'I have a right to …', 'It is your right to …', 'They have a right to …', and so on.

There is no single thesis of moral rights. The following is a brief overview of better-known theories concerning the existence of moral rights and the conditions under which they can be validly claimed.

Based on natural law and divine command

Natural rights theory argues that certain entitlements are simply 'built into' the universe like the laws of gravity, and as such are neither the products of human invention nor the constructs of other moral theories (Martin and Nickel 1980). A variation of this thesis is that natural rights have been divinely ordained for all human beings. From both these points of view, since the laws of nature and the ordinances of God apply equally to all human beings, it follows that all human beings, young and old, male, female, transgender and intergendered (e.g. haemophrodites) unconditionally have natural rights.

Objections to this account of moral rights derive from those raised against a theological account of morality generally. For example, if it were shown that God did not exist, or that natural law did not exist, this account of moral rights would immediately collapse because its very foundation would be pulled out from underneath it. Another objection rests on the problem that natural rights essentially defy scientific verification.

Based on common humanity

Another popular natural rights thesis is that all human beings have rights simply by virtue of being 'human' and 'equal'. What is critical to this thesis is the notion that 'being human' is something over which we have no control; that is, we cannot choose to be either human or not human (Martin and Nickel 1980). In this sense, then, we can be said to enjoy a 'common humanity', a notion which Leah Curtin (1986) explores in her treatment of advocacy. This view of rights is vulnerable to the objection that not all human rights are natural rights. The human right to education, which is contingent on the availability of educational resources, is an example of a human right which is not a natural right. Likewise the rights to health care, legal representation and so on are human rights but not natural rights.

Another more serious problem is that given the recent advancements made in the field of genetic engineering, 'being human' may indeed be something over which we have control in the near future. Human genes have already been cloned onto animals (for example, pigs); it is not far-fetched to imagine that scientists will succeed (if they have not already done so) in cloning animal genes onto humans. Persons with a genetic makeup comprising both human and non-human genes could be said to be not 'fully human', at least, not in a 'speciesist' sense, just as someone who is part Greek and part Chinese is not 'fully Greek' or 'fully Chinese' in a racial sense. Were someone to be not 'fully human', their claim to moral rights on the basis of a *common humanity* would be cast in doubt.

Based on rationality

A Kantian thesis of natural rights holds rationality as being the sole basis upon which a right's claim can be made. In other words, only those people who are capable of rational, autonomous thought are entitled to claim moral rights. One disturbing consequence of this thesis is that any human being (or non-human being, for that matter) who is unable to reason is not regarded as having moral status. Such a view clearly excludes infants, brain-dead and intellectually disabled persons from having a just claim to moral rights. It might be tempting to dismiss this view as being merely an intellectual one, of interest only to moral philosophers. There is ample evidence, however, that this view is influential and enjoys considerable currency in the 'real world' of human affairs. (The most notable examples here can be found in the use of brain-dead persons as organ donors, and, more recently, the suggestion that live-born anencephalic babies and fetuses should be used as organ donors [Meinke 1989; Gillam 1989; Sanders and Moore 1991].)

Based on interests

The North American philosopher Joel Feinberg offers quite a different theory of moral rights. He argues that, in order for an entity to be able to claim rights meaningfully, that entity must have interests (Feinberg 1979). To have interests, the entity must be capable of being either benefited or harmed. In order to be either benefited or harmed, one must be able to experience pleasure and pain. In short, unless one has sentience one cannot have interests, and thus cannot be either benefited or harmed, and therefore cannot make claims.

This theory of moral rights can be expressed diagrammatically as shown in Figure 4.2.

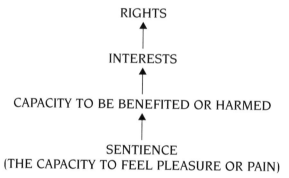

Figure 4.2 Feinberg's theory of moral rights

It can be seen that by this view it would be nonsense to assert, for example, that a rock has rights. Why? Because a rock does not have sentience and therefore cannot, strictly speaking, be benefited or harmed, and thus cannot meaningfully be said to have interests and hence rights. Those who value rocks (for example, conservationists, geologists, rock collectors) might be benefited or harmed by what happens to a rock, but it is not meaningful, philosophically speaking, to assert that a rock per se has rights. In contrast, any entity which can be shown to have sentience (that is, the capacity to experience pleasure or suffer pain) would, by this view, be entitled to be respected as having rights. Given this, it is clear that we can, for example, assert meaningfully that entities such as dolphins, puppies, kittens, horses, demented people and babies have moral rights.

Like Bentham, the founding father of utilitarianism, Feinberg sees the capacity to suffer, not reason, as the ultimate basis upon which a person's interest claims become the focus of moral action.

One shortcoming of this view is that agents must be able to represent their own interests. Feinberg (1979, p. 595) argues that, if agents cannot represent their own interests, they have no more rights than 'redwood trees and rosebushes'. Unhappily, the 'human vegetable', it seems, is no better off under an interests-based thesis of moral rights than it is under a thesis based on reason.

Feinberg does not, however, offer an adequate account of why entities must be able to 'represent their own interests', and why others (who are quite capable of making sound judgments about the moral interests of vulnerable persons and acting in a way to protect those interests) could not speak for them when they are unable or incapable of speaking on their own behalf. On closer analysis, there is room to suggest that an interests-based thesis of moral rights could even justify such acts involving, as it were, 'surrogate' representation.

Different types of rights

When speaking of moral rights, it is important to distinguish three different types which can be claimed: notably, inalienable, absolute and prima-facie rights.

Inalienable rights

An inalienable right is one which cannot be transferred under any circumstances. For example, if we accept the right to life as being an inalienable right, we are committed to accepting that it cannot be transferred to someone else or for some other cause under any circumstances. According to this view, sacrificing one's life either in suicide, martyrdom, or in an act of supreme altruism (for example, a mother sacrificing her life for her child) would be condemned as morally wrong. Of course, we may ask the question whether the right to life is an inalienable right.

Absolute rights

An absolute right, by contrast, is a right which cannot be overridden under any circumstances. For example, if we take the right to life as being absolute, we would be bound to respect it whatever the cost. By this view, any wilful taking of life, whether through war, self-defence, abortion, capital punishment, or any other act, would be morally wrong. Here the question arises whether the right to life really is an absolute right.

Prima-facie rights

A prima-facie right (from the Latin *primus*, meaning 'first', and *facies*, meaning 'face') is a right which may be overridden by stronger moral claims. For example, a patient's right to privacy may be overridden by the right to life in a cardiac arrest situation where the patient's body is exposed during the resuscitation procedure. In such an emergency, it would be a mistake for an ethicist to insist that the patient's right to privacy should take priority in the situation at hand.

Some argue against the notion of prima-facie rights by saying that if a right can be overridden it does not exist. Against such a criticism, Martin and Nickel (1980) comment:

> to describe a right as Prima Facie is to say something about its weight but not about its scope or conditions of possession ... Overridence depends on whether the case of conflict is central to the values that the right serves to protect or whether it is a marginal case and thus can be expected in all cases without great loss to those values.
>
> (Martin and Nickel 1980, pp. 172–4)

Making rights claims

Having a right usually entails that another has a corresponding duty to respect that right. As Feinberg (1978, p. 1508) explains, when people assert their moral rights, they assert a kind of 'moral power' over us which we feel constrained to respect. Where claims have a special convincing force they have a coercive effect on our judgments, which in turn make us feel driven to both acknowledge and support the interest claims being made as being genuine rights claims.

Rights which entail a corresponding duty are typically referred to as 'claims rights'. These rights can be either positive or negative, and can entail either a positive or a negative rights claim. Positive rights claims generally entail a correlative duty to act or to do, in contrast with a negative rights claim which generally entails a correlative duty to omit or to refrain (Feinberg 1978, p. 1509). For example, if a patient claims a right not to be harmed, this claim imposes a negative duty on an attending nurse to refrain from acts which may cause harm. On the other hand, if a patient claims a right to be benefited in some way, such as by having an intolerable pain state relieved, this imposes a duty on an attending nurse to perform the positive act of promptly administering an effective analgesic. If a person's rights claims are not upheld, or are infringed or violated in some way, that person generally feels wronged or feels a serious injustice has been done.

Correlative moral duties

As already discussed in the section on teleological theory (p. 82 of this chapter) moral duty (to be distinguished here from a legal duty, a civil duty, a professional duty, and so on) is an action which a person ought to do. In other words, it is a task or an action which a person is bound to perform for moral reasons. Bear in mind that a person can be bound to perform tasks for other reasons, such as legal reasons in the case of legal duties. In a rights view of morality, a moral reason is supplied by a correlative rights claim. This contrasts with a teleological ethical theory, in which duties are generated by respect for or consideration of some predicted moral consequence which ought to be furthered or upheld. Language used in identifying duties typically involves expressions such as: 'I have a duty to …', 'You have a duty to …', 'They have a duty to …', and so on. The critical task for moral agents is to decide just what one's duty is. This, of course, is contingent on correctly determining what is to count as an overriding moral reason for doing something or, as in the case of rights, correctly determining whether a given rights claim is genuine, and, further, whether the agent does in fact have a duty correlative to the claim in question.

Before moving on, the important task remains of clearing up some confusion which some nurses may have about their own rights and duties in relation to caring for patients. Consider, for example, a situation involving an abortion procedure. A nurse could reasonably claim either a right to refuse to participate in an abortion procedure or a duty to refuse. What is important here is to distinguish the basis upon which each claim might rest. If a nurse claims the *right* to refuse, this is fundamentally a claim involving the protection of *the nurse's own interests* (as opposed to the interests of the patient). The nurse might, for instance, have a religious-based conscientious objection to abortion and assert an entitlement to practise the tenets of that faith. A refusal based on a *duty* claim is significantly different, however. In this instance, the refusal is based more on the consideration of *another's interests*; that is, the interests of the patient or the fetus. Here the duty to refuse would derive from the broader moral duty to, say, prevent harm or to preserve life.

By this brief account it can be seen that to use the terms 'rights' and 'duties' interchangeably is not only incorrect, but misleading. When nurses speak of their *right* to, say, care for a patient in a certain way, it is quite possible they are really asserting that they have a *duty* to care for the patient in that way. This is just another example of an area where nurses need to improve understanding and use of moral language.

Problems with rights claims

In discussing rights it is important to keep in mind at least five central problems that can arise when dealing with rights claims. First, rights and interests can seriously compete and conflict with one another. For example, a patient's right to life could seriously compete or conflict with another patient's right to life in a situation involving scarce medical resources; or a nurse's conscientious refusal to assist with an abortion procedure could conflict with a patient's right to have an abortion and to receive care following the procedure. In such instances there may be no easy solution to the conflict of interests at hand.

Second, it may be difficult to establish the extent to which a person's rights claim entails a correlative duty. For example, if someone claims a right to life, who or what has the corresponding duty to respond to that claim? Does it fall to the health professional, or to family, friends, the hospital, the state, or another body? There may be no satisfactory answer to this question.

Third, there may be disagreement about which entities have rights. For example, some might rigorously argue that brain-dead people, anencephalic babies, the intellectually impaired and babies do not have moral rights, while others might just as rigorously argue that they do. Again there may be no happy solution to this type of disagreement.

Fourth, it may be very difficult to try and satisfy the rights claims of all people equally. For instance, if there is a genuine lack of resources, it may be impossible to satisfy all rights claims. Once again, we are left, unhappily, with an unresolved moral problem.

Fifth, and more seriously, is the controversial claim that moral rights theory is not a complete theory at all, but only 'a piece of a more general account of what makes a claim valid [and justified]' — a 'partial framework' as it were (Beauchamp and Childress 1994, pp. 76–7). By this view, rather than being a comprehensive theory, a moral rights perspective is at best only an account of 'minimal and enforceable *rules* that communities and individuals must observe in their treatment of persons' (Beauchamp and Childress, 1994, p. 76, emphasis added).

On account of these and other difficulties (not least, the inherent adversarial nature of rights claims and entitlements), some have sought to avoid a moral rights perspective altogether, or at least to 'replace the language of rights' (Beauchamp and Childress 1994, p. 77). (For example, when referring to people's moral entitlements, instead of using 'rights' language, some writers use such terms as 'interests', 'welfare', 'wellbeing', and so on.) Others, however, defend the use of rights language despite the theoretical weaknesses of a moral rights perspective. Beauchamp and Childress, for example, conclude:

> We suspect that no part of the moral vocabulary has done more to protect
> the legitimate interests of citizens in political states than the language of

rights. Predictably, injustice and inhumane treatment occur most frequently in states that fail to recognise human rights in their political rhetoric and documents. As much as any part of moral discourse, rights language crosses international boundaries and enters into treaties, international law, and statements by international agencies and associations. Rights thereby become acknowledged as international standards for the treatment of persons and for the evaluation of communal action.

(Beauchamp and Childress 1994, p. 77)

The issue of moral rights is an important one for nurses — particularly as the issue relates to patients' rights and the patients' rights movement. As this is an enormous issue on its own, it is considered separately in Chapter 8.

Revitalisation of other traditional perspectives on ethics

Over the past several decades, there has been mounting dissatisfaction among some moral philosophers in regard to the ability of dominant mainstream moral theories to provide an adequate account of moral conduct and the 'moral life'. For these philosophers, something has been 'missing' in the mainstream moral scheme of things which, unless addressed, could seriously undermine the entire project of ethics. This dissatisfaction has resulted in some significant developments. In the first instance, it has seen the revitalisation of at least two previously abandoned traditional approaches to ethics, namely: (1) virtue ethics, and (2) casuistry ethics (to be considered shortly under separate subheadings below). In the second instance, it has seen the emergence of novel perspectives on ethics; for example, (1) feminist ethics (considered as a separate topic in Chapter 5 of this text), (2) transcultural ethics (considered as a separate topic in Chapter 6 of this text), (3) communitarianism (which views 'everything fundamental in ethics as deriving from communal values, the common good, social goals, traditional practice, and cooperative virtues' [Beauchamp and Childress 1994, p. 77; see also Rasmussen 1990]), and (4) communicative or 'discourse' ethics (which relies on the insights gained not from thought experiments [as is characteristic of positivist moral philosophy], but through 'participation in communicative or discursive exchanges' [Benhabib and Dallmayr 1990, p. 2; Habermas 1990]). Regrettably, because of the complexity of communitarian and communicative ethics, and the limits of space in this present book (which prevents a coherent articulation of these respective ethical perspectives and the debates associated with them), a critical examination of these two latter perspectives and their relationship to the other perspectives considered in this text must be left for another time.

Meanwhile, it is to exploring the revitalisation of virtue ethics and casuistry ethics that the remainder of this chapter will now turn.

Virtue ethics

Virtue ethics (also known as character ethics) has an impressive history dating back to the ancient philosophical and theological texts of both Western and non-Western cultures (Kruschwitz and Roberts 1987; Pellegrino 1995). As Pellegrino

(1995, p. 254) writes, 'Virtue is the most ancient, durable, and ubiquitous concept in the history of ethical theory'.

Despite its durability, virtue theory has experienced a significant decline particularly within the field of Western moral philosophy. This decline can be traced to the rise of scientism. By the late seventeenth and eighteenth centuries, for instance, the 'Enlightenment project of finding a rational justification for morality' saw moralists look away from the law of God 'to actual, observable human nature for a justification of traditional moral norms' (MacIntyre — cited in Krushwitz and Roberts 1987, pp. 12–13). Although virtue ethics has still retained some considerable currency in some fields, for example, the medical profession up until as late as the 1970s (Pellegrino 1995, p. 264), and the nursing profession up until the present time *apropos* a nursing ethic of care (Johnstone 1993), its importance to and in mainstream moral philosophy has long been lost, having been seriously neglected by philosophers preoccupied with turning ethics into a science.

Significantly, over the past several decades, there has been a revival in virtue-based theories of ethics (Pence 1984; Pellegrino 1995). This revival (which has included both religious and non-religious approaches to virtue theory) has been driven by an increasing dissatisfaction and frustration among some philosophers with the otherwise narrow, abstract, impersonal and at times oversimplified approach of traditional theories of ethics, and the need to find an alternative approach that is more reflective of and responsive to the complexities of the moral life (Pence 1991; Pellegrino 1995). Of particular concern has been the questionable neglect within mainstream moral philosophy of considerations relating to the moral character of moral agents (persons who engage in moral actions). One aspect of this concern is expressed eloquently by Pence (1991), who, commenting on what he sees as 'a common defect in non-virtue theories', points out:

> On the theories of duty or principle, it is theoretically possible that a person could, robot-like, obey every moral rule and lead the perfectly moral life. In this scenario, one would be like a perfectly programmed computer (perhaps such people do exist, and are products of perfect moral educations).
>
> (Pence 1991, p. 256)

The idea that persons could function as 'moral robots' is both disturbing and unsatisfactory to virtue theorists, and, it might be added, to others who feel at least an intuitive unease about the prospect of morality being merely a matter of following a set of rules. We do seem to think, as Clouser (1995, p. 231) reminds us, that morality 'also encourages us to act in ways that go beyond what is required' — beyond a robot-like obedience to rules.

There does seem to be something 'missing' in the traditional picture of 'the moral life'. For virtue theorists, this 'something' is character. As Pence (1991) writes:

> we need to know much more about the outer shell of behaviour to make such [moral] judgments, i.e. we need to know what kind of person is involved, how the person thinks of other people, how he or she thinks of his or her own character, how the person feels about past actions, and also how the person feels about actions not done.
>
> (Pence 1991, p. 256)

Furthermore, there is a sense in which virtue theory is inevitable. As Pellegrino (1995) points out:

> One cannot completely separate the character of a moral agent from his or her acts, the nature of those acts, the circumstances under which they are performed, or their consequences. Virtue theories focus on the agent; on his or her intentions, dispositions and motives; and on the kind of person the moral agent becomes, wishes to become, or ought to become as a result of his or her habitual disposition to act in certain ways.
>
> (Pellegrino 1995, p. 254)

Virtue theory raises some important questions, namely: (1) what is virtue? (2) what constitutes a virtuous person? and (3) given virtue theory, does virtue ethics offer a plausible and viable alternative to traditional theories of ethics?

The notion of virtue

The term 'virtue' (from the Latin *virtus* meaning 'manliness', courage from *vir* meaning 'man') denotes the quality or practice of *moral excellence*. As an ingredient of moral theory, it can be defined as:

> a trait or character that disposes its possessor habitually to excellence of intent and performance with respect to the *telos* specific to a human activity. Virtue gives to reason the power to discern and to will the motivation asymptotically to accomplish a moral end with perfection.
>
> (Pellegrino 1995, p. 268)

Examples of the moral virtues include: care, compassion, kindness, empathy, sympathy, altruism, generosity, respectfulness, trustworthiness, personal integrity, forgiveness, friendship, love, wisdom, courage, fairness (justice), and so on (Blum 1980, 1994; Walton 1986; Krushwitz and Roberts 1987; Blustein 1991; Beauchamp and Childress 1994, pp. 67–8; Pellegrino 1995).

The virtuous person

The notions of 'virtue' and 'virtuous persons' are both universal constructs. As Pellegrino points out:

> Every culture has a notion of the virtuous person — i.e., a paradigm person, real or idealised, who sets standards of noble conduct for a culture and whose character traits exemplify the kind of person others in that culture ought to be or to emulate.
>
> (Pellegrino 1995, p. 255)

Such paradigm persons include: Buddha, Confucius, Jesus Christ and, more recently, the Catholic nun, Mother Theresa (see Vardey 1995), hailed for her charitable works in India.

The question remains: what is a virtuous person? In a purely virtue-based theory of ethics, morally exemplary (virtuous) persons (including moral heroes and moral saints), are generally distinguished from other persons who 'do their duty', that is, in a Kantian deontological (impersonal, impartial, universalistic rule-bound) sense (Blum 1988). In a purely virtue-based ethic, a virtuous person is taken to be 'the good person, the person upon whom one can rely habitually to be good and to do the good under all circumstances' (Pellegrino 1995, p. 254).

Blum (1988) takes the notion of virtuous persons even further to include what he calls 'moral heroes' and 'moral saints'. A moral hero, by his view, is someone:

- who brings about a great good (or prevents a great evil);
- who acts to a great extent from morally worthy motives;
- whose moral-worthy motives are substantially embedded in his or her own personal psychology;
- who carries out his or her moral project in the face of risk or danger; and
- who is relatively 'faultless' or has an absence of unworthy desires, dispositions, sentiments, attitudes.

(adapted from Blum 1988, pp. 199, 203)

A moral saint, in contrast, is not altogether different from a moral hero, except for one feature. According to Blum, moral saints share three features in common with moral heroes:

they are animated by morally-worthy motives, their morally-excellent qualities exist at a deep level of their personality or character, and they meet the standard of relative absence of unworthy desires.

(Blum 1988, p. 204)

The salient feature which distinguishes a moral saint from a moral hero, however, is that the moral saint exhibits 'a higher standard of faultlessness' *viz.* the absence of unworthy desires (Blum 1988, p. 204).

Virtue ethics: alternative to or component part of traditional theories?

Some virtue theorists have made the claim that 'a good theory of virtue could replace traditional deontological or utilitarian theories' (Pence 1984). Others, however, have dismissed such claims as implausible, taking the position that virtue cannot stand alone 'but must be related to other ethical theories in a more comprehensive moral philosophy than currently exists' (Pence 1984, p. 282; Pellegrino 1995, p. 254). In other words, virtue theory, at most, can function only as a *part* of an overall moral schema rather than being its whole (Pence 1984, p. 282). Beauchamp and Childress (1994), for example, doubt that a virtue theory of ethics is comprehensive enough to do the work of ethics on its own. Nevertheless they do regard the virtues as having 'a special place in the moral life' and one that is compatible with (if not perfectly corresponding to) — and mutually reinforcing of — traditional obligation-based theories (Beauchamp and Childress 1994, pp. 66–7). In sum, contrary to what appears to be the case, virtue ethics is not necessarily in competition with traditional obligation-based theories, such as deontology and teleology (consequentialism). Whether virtue ethics is as compatible with traditional obligation-based theories as Beauchamp and Childress claim, however, is another matter entirely, and regrettably one which is beyond the scope of this present work to examine. Nevertheless, there is room to make one or two concluding remarks.

Virtue ethics, like other traditional theories of ethics, is not free of difficulties. Key among these are: the 'circularity of justification' in virtue theory (virtuous persons do what is good, the good is what virtuous persons do); the inability of virtue theory to explain adequately its force as a moral action guide (*viz.* compared with other obligation-based theories that can rely the force of moral rules, principles and maxims to justify moral conduct); and the high expectations virtue theory imposes on people to be 'good' (while a good many of us can be conscientious in our actions, few of us can be 'exemplary' (Pellegrino 1995, pp. 262–3). These difficulties, however, may be more a product of the traditional modernist philosophical approach used to critically examine and raise objections to virtue theory, than a problem with virtue ethics itself. For instance, given the distinctive non-rational quality of the moral virtues, it seems odd to suggest that virtuous actions require 'justification' (how does one 'justify' an inclination to be kind toward another, or to be fair? how does one 'justify' an act of saintliness or heroism?); similarly, it seems odd to expect that virtue theory can be reduced to a set of justificatory rules, principles and maxims (noting that, what makes the virtues what they are is their spontaneous and unconditional expression *beyond* that otherwise required by rules, principles and maxims). There is room here to suggest that to 'justify' the virtues in a traditional rationalistic and reductionistic sense is to do violence to them and to all that they represent. Finally, it seems odd to suggest that expecting people to be 'decent' and 'morally excellent' human beings is 'too high an expectation'. Even in its most traditional sense, morality is precisely about expecting people to strive to achieve the ideal of morally excellent conduct. Virtue ethics is no different in this regard. That people may not achieve such an ideal is no reason to abandon ethics generally, and it is no reason to abandon virtue ethics in particular.

It is unlikely that virtue ethics will achieve full restoration in mainstream (modernist) moral philosophy. This is not to say, however, that it will not gain increasing currency as a bona fide theoretical perspective in this new age of multiple moral realities. As will be discussed in the following chapter examining feminist perspectives on ethics, virtue ethics has high prospects in other fields of ethical inquiry — not least, in the field of professional nursing ethics.

Casuistry ethics

Casuistry (from the Latin *casus*, meaning 'case') dates back to medieval and early modern moral philosophy. For the past 300 years, however, it has lain in a state of disrepute. Interestingly, over the last decade, it has been revitalised owing largely to a rediscovery of its practical usefulness in contemporary moral debate (Jonsen 1995). A re-examination of the history of casuistry has, to some extent, vindicated its resurgence (Jonsen 1995; Jonsen and Toulmin 1988). The question remains: what is casuistry and how does it differ from other traditional approaches to ethics?

It is more accurate to describe casuistry as an *approach* to practical moral decision-making, rather than as a moral theory per se. Unlike other traditional approaches to moral decision-making, casuistry takes as its starting point 'a case' rather than ethical theories and principles. The case, in this instance, is regarded as the 'base of moral perception, reasoning, and judgment' (Jonsen 1995, p. 250). Whereas traditional and contemporary obligation-based theories (for example, ethical principlism) involve the application of moral principles to cases, casuistry starts from cases and moves up to principles (Beauchamp and Childress 1994, p. 93). This activity of moving from cases to principles basically consists of 'thinking and talking about how the circumstances of this or that case of moral perplexity fit the general norms, rules, standards, and principles of morality' (Jonsen 1995, p. 237).

Pivotal to casuistry is the presentation and consideration of cases. *A case*, in this instance, can be defined as:

> a confluence of persons and actions in a time and a place, all of which can be given names and dates. A case ... is concrete as distinguished from abstract because it represents the congealing, the coalescence, or the growing together (in Latin, *concrescere*) of many circumstances. Each case is unique in its circumstances, yet each case is similar in type to other cases and can, therefore, be compared and contrasted.
>
> (Jonsen 1995, p. 241)

From a casuist perspective, the only way that appropriate moral judgment and practical moral decisions can be made is through 'an intimate understanding of particular situations and the historical record of similar cases' (Beauchamp and Childress 1994, p. 92). To gain this intimate understanding, casuists rely heavily on 'narratives, paradigm cases, analogies, models, classification systems, and even immediate intuition and discerning insight' (Beauchamp and Childress 1994, p. 94). The actual activity of moral decision-making, meanwhile, involves three key steps:

1. designating the topic;
2. describing and evaluating the circumstances/particulars of cases (who, what, where, why, when and where); and
3. comparing cases (seeking similarities as well as differences in circumstances).

> (adapted from Jonsen 1995, pp. 242–46)

In deciding cases, casuistry has no theoretical allegiances. While casuistry 'does need moral theory', as Jonsen (1995, p. 246) explains, 'only rarely must it have recourse to moral theory for resolution of a particular case'. Mostly, cases are settled by agreement among decision-makers after engaging in a process of 'reasoning with contingent facts and drawing plausible conclusions' (Jonsen 1995, p. 241).

Like other perspectives, casuistry is not without difficulties (for instance, there is no certainty that decision-makers will always reach agreement on a given case and/or will not be troubled by competing and conflicting judgments in given cases). Nevertheless, contemporary casuistry is seen to have made a significant contribution to moral philosophy by emphasising the importance of circumstances in moral deliberations, something that modernist moral philosophy historically has neglected. As Jonsen (1995) concludes:

> The value of casuistry lies in its effort to appreciate more fully the way in which circumstances play an intrinsic role in moral judgment and in its attempt to provide to the one making a judgment a sort of 'guided tour' through the complexity of circumstances.
>
> (Jonsen 1995, p. 249)

Beauchamp and Childress (1994) reach a similar conclusion. They write:

> Sensitivity to context and individual differences is essential for a discerning use of principles. Casuistry would be notable if for no other reason than its long history of attempting to deal with this problem.
>
> (Beauchamp and Childress 1994, p. 100)

Conclusion

In this chapter, brief attention has been given to examining the relationship between moral theory and ethical conduct. A distinction was made between traditional and non-traditional, modernist and postmodernist theories of ethics. The notion of moral justification and its role in moral decision-making was also examined. Attention then focused on examining a number of key theoretical perspectives underpinning and informing ethical practice, namely: deontology, teleology (consequentialism), ethical principlism, and moral rights theory. The revitalisation of two other (previously neglected) traditional theories of ethics was also considered, with particular attention being given to virtue theory and casuistry. While the views presented in this chapter are far from exhaustive, they are nevertheless sufficient for the purposes of this text, namely, to provide nurses with a working knowledge and understanding of the theoretical perspectives that can and have influenced the development and practice of nursing ethics in health care domains. Meanwhile, there remains the task of providing a brief examination of two new theoretical perspectives on ethics that have emerged over the past two decades. It is to fulfilling this task that the next two chapters will now turn.

Chapter 5

A feminist perspective on ethics and bioethics

Introduction

Over the past several decades, there has been mounting dissatisfaction among some moral philosophers in regard to the ability of dominant mainstream (modernist) moral theories to provide an adequate account of moral conduct and the 'moral life'. There has also been a commensurate dissatisfaction with mainstream bioethics and its apparent (in)ability to deal effectively with ethical issues in health care and related domains. As already discussed in the previous chapter, this dissatisfaction and other related responses has resulted in at least two significant developments in contemporary moral philosophy: (1) the revitalisation of previously abandoned traditional approaches to ethics, and (2) the emergence of novel perspectives on ethics. In the case of the emergence of novel perspectives, this has tended to be in direct response to what some see as being some of the fundamental and untenable flaws of a modernist approach to ethics and bioethics, namely, that:

- it is too abstract to be able to deal effectively with the concrete circumstances of life;
- it pays too much attention to upholding abstract rules and principles, rather than: (1) promoting quality relationships between people, and (2) upholding the genuine welfare and wellbeing of people;
- its practices have tended to privilege dominant groups over marginalised groups (more specifically, they have tended to privilege the interests and concerns of white middle-class able-bodied heterosexual politically conservative males at the expense of those deemed 'other', and hence inferior — for example, women and children, people of non-English-speaking and culturally diverse backgrounds, the disabled, gay men and lesbians, the poor, the uneducated, and so on);
- its emphasis on rational argument has tended to fuel rather than quell moral controversy, disagreement, and distress;
- its augmentative and adversarial approach has tended to divide rather than unite and reconcile people in common bonds.

The emergence and development of feminist ethics (and feminist bioethics) as a new approach to ethics, which to a large extent has been in response to the above 'flaws' of a modernist approach to ethics, is the subject of this chapter.

A feminist approach to ethics

Before beginning this discussion, some clarification is required on what constitutes a feminist approach to ethics and bioethics, and to settle some prevailing misunderstandings about the nature and project of feminist ethics generally and feminist bioethics in particular.

Feminist ethics is not, as some assume, merely women talking about ethics, or merely ethics discourse that focuses only on women's issues — although, feminist ethics does substantially involve both of these things (as one writer insists: 'feminist ethics *must* recognise the moral perspective of women [Sherwin 1992, p. 49, emphasis added]). In other words, feminist ethics is not a *separate* ethics or bioethics 'for women' (Wolf 1996a, p. 8). Neither is feminist ethics synonymous with an ethic of care (Wolf 1996a, p. 8) — although, feminist theorists have been at the forefront of advancing an ethic of care perspective. Rather, feminist ethics (and its counterpart, feminist bioethics) 'is the examination of all sorts of [ethical and] bioethical issues from the perspective of feminist *theory*' (Little 1996, p. 1). Feminist theory, in turn, can be described as:

> an attempt to uncover the ways in which conceptions of gender distort people's view of the world and to articulate the ways in which these distortions, which are hurtful to all, are particularly constraining to women.
>
> (Little 1996, p. 2)

A feminist theoretical perspective on ethics can thus be both useful and influential in a range of domains. As Little explains:

> feminist theory will be useful to disciplines whose subject-matter or methods are appreciably affected by such [harmful gender] distortions — and it will be useful in ways that far outstrip the particular policy recommendations that feminists might give to some standard checklist of topics. For one thing, feminist reflection may change the checklist — altering what questions people think to ask, what topics they regard as important, what strikes them as a puzzle in need of resolution. Or again, such reflection may change the analyses underlying policy recommendations — altering which assumptions are given uncontested status, which moves feel persuasive, what elements stand in need of explanation, and how substantive concepts are understood and deployed.
>
> (Little 1996, p. 2)

In understanding that feminist ethics is substantially ethics from the perspective of *feminist theory*, it is important to further understand that there are 'different sorts of feminism' (or *feminisms*, as some would say), that there exist different orientations within the overall category of 'feminism', and that there exist conflicts within and between some of these orientations (Wolf 1996b; Hekman 1995; Holmes and Purdy 1992; Sherwin 1992; Card 1991; Hoagland 1988). In speaking of feminist ethics or feminist bioethics then, what is in effect being referred to are feminist *perspectives* on or *approaches* to ethics/bioethics. Despite the rich multiplicity of views that characterise feminist ethics, however, as Sherwin (1996, p. 47) points out, it is nevertheless possible to identify some common themes. Some of these themes will be explored in this and subsequent chapters of this text.

Gender distortions in moral philosophy

Gender distortions and biases in mainstream philosophy are readily demonstrated.

Popular philosophy texts and standard reference texts (for example, encyclopedias and dictionaries of philosophy) make little reference, and in most instances none, to the philosophical contributions of women. This absence was highlighted some years ago by a seemingly trivial incident. In 1987 Dr Lynda Burns, an academic at Melbourne University, entered a 'Philosophy's Greatest Hits' competition, run by the university's philosophy department. Her entry was disqualified, because none of the female philosophers she named were in the required sources — specifically, the *Encyclopedia of philosophy* or the index of *Modern philosophical writings* (Hutton 1987, p. 20).

Another example (personal communication) of bias involved a female registered nurse who had successfully completed a first degree majoring in philosophy (with straight 'A' passes and the university prize for philosophy in her third year), and who transferred to another university to continue her studies. On her first visit to the philosophy department of the new university at which she was intending to study, and with which she had already been in contact by correspondence, a senior lecturer (male) approached her, inquiring: 'Who are you?'. After she introduced herself, the lecturer exclaimed: 'Oh yes. I've heard about you. The nurse …', and without another word abruptly walked off! Later she learned that this same lecturer had been overheard lamenting the increase in the number of female students enrolling in philosophy courses and declaring that it would mark the demise of philosophy as a sound and respectable discipline.

During my own university education in the early-to-mid 1980s, philosophy classes I attended were advised on more than one occasion that the reason the philosophical views of ancient and early women philosophers were not taught was because 'there were no women philosophers'.

The contributions of women to philosophy

Contrary to popular impressions, and despite the lack of visible evidence in standard philosophy texts, the contributions made by women to philosophy — and to moral philosophy in particular — have been substantial, with some of the earliest recorded contributions dating back to the early and late Pythagorean cults of the sixth century BC to the first century AD. The moral theories developed by Pythagorean women share a number of similarities with each other, in particular their emphasis on kindness, friendship, compassion, harmony, justice, care, wisdom, and the recognition of obligations incurred in immediate relationships (Waithe 1987, 1989a, 1989b, 1991).

The early Pythagorean philosopher Theano I emphasised the principle of *harmonia* (harmony) and the existence of a principled and harmonious universe. Immoral acts, by her view, are at serious odds with the principle of *harmonia* and stand to contribute to disorder and discord — in particular of the otherwise orderly and harmonious universe.

Theano saw women as those who bear the major responsibility for maintaining order, harmony and justice in the state. Her reasoning on this typically reflects Greek culture, both past and present. For Theano, the family or the home is a microcosm of the state: women's responsibility for maintaining harmony and order in the home extends to the maintenance of harmony and justice in the state. This responsibility is not merely 'natural', but requires a critically reflective approach. As Theano said, 'It is better to be on a runaway horse than to be a woman who does not reflect' (cited in Waithe 1987, p. 15).

Another accomplished personage during this period was Arete of Cyrene (fourth century BC). This remarkable figure succeeded her father as head of the Cyrenaic School of Philosophy. It is recorded that she taught natural science, moral philosophy and ethics for over thirty-five years and wrote at least forty books, including treatises on Socrates. It is also believed that she taught over 110 philosophers. On Arete's tomb is an epitaph calling her 'the splendour of Greece' with 'the beauty of Helen [of Troy], the virtue of Thirma, the pen of Aristippus, the soul of Socrates, and the tongue of Homer' (cited in Alec 1986, p. 26).

Following close in these women's footsteps was the ingenious Aesara of Lucania, a late Pythagorean who generated a comprehensive (familiar and intuitive) natural law theory of morality. Like Theano, Aesara saw the family as playing an important part in defining moral obligations. Her natural law theory views moral law as applying on three levels: individual or private, familial (one which emphasises the family), and social. These three levels are all characterised by the moral virtues of love, as defined in terms of compassion for others, kindliness, self-esteem, and a justice that is fair and considerate of special needs and concerns, including 'extenuating circumstances and reasons for non-compliance' (an individualistic sense of justice) (Waithe 1987, p. 23).

Another influential Pythagorean mother was Perictone I, who actively encouraged women to philosophise and to seek the virtues of justice and courage (Waithe 1987, p. 32). She had little regard for the 'ideal theories' of morality (theories which sought to prescribe how the world ought to be), emphasising instead theories which were well grounded in pragmatism and the social reality into which one is inescapably born. She insisted that the principle of harmonia was one that should be applied in the actual and concrete circumstances of life — the here and now — and not in the decontextualised, hypothetical and ideal fantasies of the imagination (Waithe 1987, p. 35).

Women have made important contributions to philosophy and moral philosophy in other eras as well, although, as Waithe (1987) makes plain, these contributions continue to be ignored in the 'standard' philosophical texts. In fact, as Waithe notes in her introduction, the accomplishments of over 100 women philosophers have been omitted from the standard philosophical reference works and histories of philosophy (see also Waithe 1989a, 1991).

In fifteenth-century Italy an academic by the name of Dorotea Bocchi succeeded her father as professor of medicine and moral philosophy at the University of Bologna (Alec 1986, p. 58). In seventeenth-century Germany, Elizabeth of Bohemia (1618–80), a close friend, colleague and confidante of the French philosopher Descartes, lectured in Cartesian philosophy at the University of Heidelberg (Alec 1986, p. 9). Descartes later dedicated his *Principles of philosophy* (1644) to her. In eighteenth-century England, Mary Wollstonecraft wrote the acclaimed *A vindication of the rights of woman* (1792), the first serious work on the subject. This book was later published in 1929 in an edition also featuring John Stuart Mill's *The subjection of women*, an essay written some sixty years earlier. Wollstonecraft believed that, if inequalities in society were to be eliminated, distinctions drawn on the basis of wealth, class and gender would have to be abolished.

Mill's essay on the subjection of women, although an enlightening and provocative study, is rarely, if ever, considered seriously in philosophy courses. Mill's essays *Utilitarianism* and *On liberty* regularly feature on reading lists for philosophy courses, but *The subjection of women* is conspicuous by its absence. Its radical position favouring the emancipation of women may account for this omission. Mill argues in *The subjection of women* that male power (the success of which derives from its professed benevolence) is the instrument of female oppression. He writes:

> ... power holds a smoother language, and whomsoever it oppresses, always pretends to do so for their own good: accordingly, when anything is forbidden to women, it is thought necessary to say, and desirable to believe, that they are incapable of doing it, and that they depart from their real path of success and happiness when they aspire to it.
>
> (Mill 1992, p. 266)

(It should be noted here that *The subjection of women* and other pro-women essays written by Mill benefited from the influence of his wife and probable collaborator, Harriet Taylor. Spender [1988, p. 188] writes, for example, that *The subjection of women* would probably not have been written without Harriet Taylor's influence, and, by Mill's own admission, certainly would not have taken the form that it did without her — and later her daughter's — collaboration.)

Perhaps one of the greatest omissions (and ironies) of all, however, is that the very notion of philosophy (from Greek *philosophus,* meaning 'lover or friend of wisdom') is itself rooted in that which may be described as the 'divinely feminine'. Matthews (1991), for example, suggests that originally a 'philosopher' was a lover of the *goddess* Sophia (the goddess of wisdom), not merely a lover of wisdom per se. She further suggests that it was only with the passage of time and the increasing influence of patriarchy that the 'goddess' reference got dropped from the definition and meaning of philosophy and philosopher, and the significantly abbreviated definition (that is of philosophy meaning the lover of wisdom) became commonplace.

This brief historical overview shows that contemporary feminist ethics is the product of an eventful and respectable history (or rather *herstory*), not of some 'fringe lunacy' recently invented, as some perhaps have believed. (For further commentary on the contribution of women to philosophy, see Waithe 1987, 1989a, 1991, 1995; McAlister 1989.) The rise and development of contemporary feminist moral philosophy and its relevance to nursing are now discussed as part of this historical framework.

The task of feminist ethics

In early feminist discourses on ethics, considerable attention is given to possible (irreconcilable) differences between male and female moral thinking. Among other things, it is contended that (white) male moral thinking has come to dominate Western moral philosophy, to the extent that the interests and sufferings of women have been rendered irrelevant and invisible (Mullet 1988, p. 109; see also Tronto 1993; Cole and Coultrap-McQuin 1992; Frazer et al. 1992; Holmes and Purdy 1992; Sherwin 1992; Card 1991; Porter 1991; Brabeck 1989; Hoagland 1988; Kittay and Meyers 1987). As a result, modern moral philosophy is incomplete and inadequate and therefore incapable of supplying the world with a substantive and adequate moral theory on how best to conduct its affairs. Further to this, feminists argue, modern moral philosophy, contrary to its claims, has not succeeded in supplying a sound, reliable and universal moral theory. At best, it has only given the world a system of competing and different theories, each of which offers a different view of life, a different set of action-guiding principles, and a different style of moral decision-making (Parsons 1986, p. 82). The failure of modern moral philosophy in this respect, together with its unfruitful preoccupation with attempting to find rational explanations for the nature of moral language and the logic of moral thinking, has led some feminist critics to accuse modern moral philosophy of being little more than 'a pale shadow of its former self' (Parsons 1986, p. 76).

The task of feminist ethics is twofold: first, to function as a moral critique; and, second, to operate as a 'substantive radical moral theory' (Morgan 1988, p. 161). As a moral critique, the task of feminist ethics is fourfold: first, to critically examine supposedly empirically grounded theories of human nature, particularly those which exclude women and other 'non-rational' beings; second, to generate new paradigms of moral thinking; third, to distinguish what constitutes a genuine moral dilemma in the concrete circumstances of life; and fourth to 'discover and render visible the hidden moral domains of women's lives while establishing women's claim to the full human spectrum of moral action and character, whether good or evil' (Morgan 1988, p. 161).

As a substantive radical moral theory, on the other hand, feminist ethics aims to challenge 'the model of the moral subject as an autonomous, detached, rational subject, often seeing this hypermasculinist ideal of the moral self as both psychologically and morally flawed' (Morgan 1988, p. 161). This model is replaced, in feminist theory, with a more pluralistic model of morality, and one which literally incorporates 'a sense of moral imagination, moral empathy, and moral feeling into an integrated, other-connected self' (Morgan 1988, p. 162).

Feminist moral theorists conclude that, unless the gender imbalance in modern moral thinking is redressed, and unless the 'genuine womanly virtues' are placed firmly back on the hypothetical 'moral map', the moral outlook for the world is bleak. Not only are the welfare and survival of women at stake in this instance, but the welfare and survival of all humankind. On this, Carol Gilligan concludes:

> The promise in joining women and moral theory lies in the fact that human survival, in the late twentieth century, may depend less on formal agreement than on human connection.

> (Gilligan 1987, p. 32)

Despite the persuasiveness of the feminist theorists' claims, some questions remain. Are there significant differences between male and female moral thinking? Is Western moral philosophy nothing more than a collective of male-gender-specific ideologies? If so, has this been seriously detrimental to the formulation and development of a reliable and substantive moral theory? It is to answering these questions that this chapter now turns.

The alleged difference between male and female thinking

The supposed difference between male and female thinking has been given considerable attention in philosophy by many notable male philosophers, including the ancient Greek philosopher Aristotle (384–22 BC), the moral theologian and scholastic philosopher Saint Thomas Aquinas (1225–74), the French political and educational philosopher Jean-Jacques Rousseau (1712–78), and the German philosopher Immanuel Kant (1724–1804).

Aristotle's writings clearly depict women as both rationally and morally inferior to men, and thus lacking any form of moral authority. In *The Politics* (1957), for example, Aristotle argued (or rather assumed, since he did not, in fact, put forward any systematic argument to support his position) that the male 'is more fitted to rule than the female, unless conditions are quite contrary to nature' (1259a37) and that, as head of the household, the male is rightly the source of virtue in his wife, children and slaves (1259b18–1260b24). The source of male virtue is thought to be the rational element of the soul, which, while present in the female, is 'ineffective' (1259b32). Aristotle required women to have virtue (especially the virtue of silence!), but only insofar as this is required by her master (or husband, as the case may be) to fulfil her function; even then, she is expected to have only little if any 'intellectual appreciation of its [virtue's] nature and reasons' (1259b32). As Morgan (1988) observes on this passage in *The Politics*, 'the most that a woman can aspire to, from a moral point of view, is to be aligned with a fully developed man of moral integrity, and to obey his commands silently' (p. 148).

In *Ethics*, Aristotle (1976, pp. 269, 276) again emphasised the moral differences between males and females, and the superiority of male virtues. Women are portrayed as congenitally defective in virtue (Aristotle 1976, p. 243), while a man of even modest rational competence is regarded as still being able to 'conduct himself virtuously' (Aristotle 1976, p. 334). To be governed by the senses, in Aristotle's view, is to be utterly 'brutish' (Aristotle 1976, p. 328) or, worse, 'incontinent'.

Aquinas, a thirteenth-century moral theologian and scholastic philosopher, also regarded women as being rationally and morally inferior to men. He argued:

> As regards the individual nature, woman is defective and misbegotten, for the active force in the male seed tends to the production of a perfect likeness in the masculine sex.
>
> (cited in Morgan 1988, p. 148)

Aquinas argued that women lacked the 'discretion of reason' and could only achieve, at best, moral mediocrity when and if they were in positions of authority. For this reason, Aquinas considered that women should be rightly denied 'full moral and religious personhood as priests' (Morgan 1988, p. 148).

Rousseau (1911, pp. 321, 325), like many of his colleagues, also held women to be morally different and inferior to men. In the celebrated *Emile*, women are expected not 'to complain of the inequalities of manmade laws', while men are expected not to regard their laws as 'equally binding' on both sexes (Rousseau 1911, p. 324). A husband who is faithless to his wife is merely wrong, while a wife who is faithless to her husband is positively evil, since 'she destroys the family and breaks the bonds of nature' (p. 324). (It is worth considering the parallels that could be drawn here with nursing: if a male doctor is 'faithless' to a female nurse and, for example, lowers her reputation in the eyes of a patient or colleague, he is 'merely wrong'; if a female nurse is 'faithless' to a male doctor, she is 'positively evil' and could be successfully sued for defamation or negligence, imprisoned, fined or deregistered [see also Johnstone 1994].) If a woman were to usurp the rights of a man, she would succeed only in asserting her inferiority (Rousseau 1911, p. 327). Superiority of women, meanwhile, can only be achieved through obedience (p. 335), a logic difficult to follow. (Compare this with the notion of the supremely 'good' nurse being the supremely 'obedient' nurse [Johnstone 1994, Chapters 5, 6].) In terms of developing morality, Rousseau claimed that a woman should merely observe the world and discover by her observations 'an experimental morality'; a man, on the other hand, should use his reason and reduce the experimental morality of women into a system (Rousseau 1911, p. 350). The underlying reasons for this are, of course, that women are not capable of theoretical reasoning or of shaping a systematic morality. Only men should undertake this task. (Again, in drawing parallels to nursing today, nurses are supposed merely to 'observe' and collect data, while the doctor puts it all together and makes the diagnosis — a practice regarded by many in the medical profession as a doctor's overriding prerogative in all medical, moral and even nursing matters [Johnstone 1994, Chapters 6, 7].)

The last philosopher to be considered here is Immanuel Kant. Like his predecessors, Kant saw women as incapable of theoretical reasoning, arguing that 'women's morality should essentially be one of sentiment, governed by irrational moral feelings of aversion and beauty' (cited in Morgan 1988, p. 149). Kant's moral scheme of things is one based firmly on rationality. By denying the rational capabilities of women, Kant succeeded in excluding them from any substantial involvement in the development of moral discourse and the moral life.

The views of these philosophers and others like them have been overwhelmingly influential both inside and outside moral philosophy. Outside moral philosophy, for example, women are still regarded as being rationally inferior to men and emotionally fickle, and thus quite unsuitable for positions of authority (Pateman 1989; Lloyd 1984; Jaggar 1983; McMillan 1982). Evidence of this can be found in the under-representation of women in government, business management, professorial chairs and the traditional professions, not to mention in positions of religious leadership.

Inside moral philosophy, on the other hand, gender dualism in moral thinking continues to be rigorously debated. Male moral thinking is described in terms of rational constructs and abstract moral principles, such as those of autonomy and justice; female moral thinking is described more in terms of non-rational constructs, notably feelings of care, empathy, compassion, love, sympathy and friendship.

The supposed gender dualism in moral thinking has received particular attention over the past few years, initially because of the celebrated Kohlberg–Gilligan debate. Lawrence Kohlberg, an internationally renowned moral developmental theorist, is credited with having laid the foundations of modern moral psychology (Flanagan and Jackson 1987, p. 622). His views have been influential on the development of moral education programs — including those in some United States schools of nursing (Berkowitz 1982; Bridston 1982). Carol Gilligan, Kohlberg's former collaborator, challenged the validity of Kohlberg's research and entered into a strenuous public debate, as a result of which Kohlberg modified some of his claims.

Kohlberg's theory is based on empirical research. It asserts that there are culturally universal stages of moral development through which moral reasoning progresses. The ultimate level, stage 6, embodies a Rawlsian ideal of justice, and represents the highest stage of moral development. Kohlberg (1981, p. 123) maintains that his research shows that there are 'no important differences in development of moral thinking between Catholics, Protestants, Jews, Buddhists, Moslems, and atheists'. Research carried out in third-world countries, including Mexico and Taiwan, indicated the same six stages of development, except that their progress was 'slower' (Kohlberg 1981, p. 23).

The six moral development stages identified by Kohlberg (1981, pp. 409–12) are summarised below.

Stage 1. *Punishment and obedience*: an egocentric view of the world, judging actions in terms of physical consequences rather than in terms of the psychological interests of others.

Stage 2. *Individual instrumental purpose and exchange*: a concrete individualistic perspective which takes into account the actor's pragmatic needs and instrumental intentions; conflicting interests and needs can be met through instrumental exchange of services or goodwill, or by fair dealing; the agent recognises that others have personal interests to pursue.

Stage 3. *Mutual interpersonal expectations, relationships, and conformity*: the perspective of individual relationships to other individuals, including the shared feelings, expectations, concerns, loyalties and trusts in these relationships; what is right is determined by what is expected by people who are close in the relationship, or by what is expected of someone in a particular role — for example, as brother, sister, or friend.

Stage 4. *Social system and conscience maintenance*: the perspective of 'the system', which judges actions on the basis of whether they conform to societal requirements and values, and other social conventions serving social order.

Stage 5. *Prior rights and social contract or utility*: a view of the individual as an objective, rational and impartial spectator who is aware of values and rights which exist prior to 'social attachment and contracts'; right is seen in terms of upholding basic rights, values and social contracts.

Stage 6. *Universal ethical principles*: a view of the world in terms of a higher order or transcendent morality, assuming that all humanity should follow universal ethical principles (in particular, the universal principle of justice); right is judged on the basis of whether actions accord with universal moral principles.

Stages 1 to 4 of Kohlberg's moral development levels do not involve principled reasoning and are regarded as the lower levels of moral development; agents who achieve these levels of development are regarded as morally undeveloped and morally immature. Stages 5 and 6, on the other hand, involve principled reasoning and are therefore regarded as the higher levels of moral development; agents who achieve these levels, in particular stage 6, are regarded as being morally developed and morally mature.

Berkowitz, an associate professor of psychology, was quick to embrace Kohlberg's theory to assess the moral development of nurses and to recommend educational strategies accordingly. Berkowitz argues that nurses should not be taught to be 'Kantian moralists', since it is 'unlikely' they could develop such a level of moral thinking. He contends that nurses could possibly reach Kohlberg's stage 3 of moral development, or even stage 4 (or at least progress towards it), but no more. Berkowitz concludes that 'nursing ethics curricula should therefore be tailored to initiate and consolidate stages 3 and 4 not ... stages 5 and 6' (1982, p. 38).

The comprehensiveness and reliability of Kohlberg's 'empirically based' moral development theory became the subject of much criticism, however, when his former collaborator, Carol Gilligan, revealed a major design fault in Kohlberg's moral judgment research, namely 'the use of all-male samples as the empirical basis for theory construction' (Gilligan 1987, p. 21). Kohlberg had in fact studied the same group of seventy-five boys at three-year intervals for a total of fifteen years, following them from early adolescence through to young manhood; he later generalised his findings to apply to females, which (predictably) showed females to be morally 'undeveloped' and 'immature' (Kohlberg 1981, p. 115; Gilligan 1987).

Upon realising that Kohlberg's research had not examined girls and women, Gilligan condemned it as inherently biased, pointing out that it could hardly be taken as 'representative' of human experience. (Mistaking the masculine bias as universally representative has been dubbed 'phallocentrism' in some circles [Braidotti 1986, p. 48].) On the basis of her own observations and research into the apparent gender differences between male and female moral reasoning, Gilligan also argued that, by eliminating women from the research samples, Kohlberg had eliminated a 'care focus' in moral reasoning, a principal ingredient in women's moral thinking (Gilligan 1987, 1982).

Irrespective of Gilligan's criticisms, Kohlberg's findings have essentially reinforced the popular myth that 'rationality' and reasoning by abstract principle are morally supreme, while 'feelings' or 'sentiment' are morally inferior. At least one author has defended Kohlberg and voiced scathing criticisms against Gilligan, claiming that Gilligan herself appeals to the same rational principles she has condemned in Kohlberg's analysis, and that her own theoretical stages of moral development are not very different from Kohlberg's (Broughton 1983). Another critic claims that 'looking more closely at Gilligan's research it is hard not to see there a methodology designed to exaggerate difference and to disregard similarity between men and women' (Segal 1987, p. 147). Nevertheless, the implications of Kohlberg's moral development theory are far-reaching: those (usually women) who base their moral judgments on non-rational considerations (for example, sentiment, care, friendship, 'the virtues') inevitably emerge as 'morally undeveloped' and thus 'morally immature', while those (usually men) who base their judgments on rational and universal ethical principles emerge as 'morally developed' and 'morally mature'. Women, once again, are portrayed as being incapable of authoritative moral reasoning.

Kohlberg accepted some of Gilligan's criticisms and eventually modified his claims, as already mentioned. He acknowledged the presence of a care perspective in people's 'higher order' moral thinking (Gilligan 1987, p. 22), although he maintained that an ethic of agape (Greek for 'love') 'still must rely on the stage 6 fairness principles to resolve justice problems' (Kohlberg 1981, p. 354). Gilligan's own research, meanwhile, suggests that, while a significant proportion (69 per cent) of both women and men can incline towards a dominant but alternating care and justice perspective in their moral reasoning, women are more inclined to include a 'care focus' in moral reasoning, and therefore that, if women are eliminated from a research sample, the 'care focus' will 'virtually disappear' (Gilligan 1987, p. 25).

Kohlberg's theory has also been criticised on more conventional philosophical grounds. Nicolayev and Phillips (1979), for example, have criticised his reliance on a dominant conception of morality and the connection he makes with a theory of increasing moral adequacy. They point out that there are many different ways of thinking about morality and about how different people should act in particular moral situations. How people view and think about moral issues is 'not necessarily committed to a developmental orientation, much less to the view that there are clear-cut stages of development' (Nicolayev and Phillips 1979, p. 232). They argue that there is absolutely nothing to suggest why Kohlberg's stage 6 of moral development should be considered superior to stage 5, stage 4, stage 3, stage 2, or stage 1 for that matter. A moral justification based on a principle of care could easily be just as compelling as a moral justification based on a principle of rational justice.

Crittenden (1979) has also been highly critical of Kohlberg's thesis. He openly disputes Kohlberg's account of justice and, in particular, its equation with morality. He contends that one of the major weaknesses of Kohlberg's position is his reliance on and endorsement of the views of 'certain distinguished ethical theorists' rather than on his own 'systematic exposition' (Crittenden 1979, p. 251). One unfortunate consequence of this debate for Kohlberg is that his account of justice is vulnerable to exactly the same criticisms as have already been made against the justice theorists he supports. Crittenden (1979, p. 259) has also disparaged Kohlberg's defence of what by all accounts is merely a 'particular moral system dominated by an interpretation of justice'. He further points out that there is nothing arbitrary or logically inconsistent in holding 'a plurality of ultimate moral principles' (Crittenden 1979, p. 258); something that Kohlberg's theory (and, in particular, its principle of justice-as-morality) seems to negate. In short, Kohlberg's theory of moral development wobbles on its inadequate account of the moral terms and concepts it inherently relies on, using interpretations that have been the subject of intense philosophical controversy, and that are by no means accepted as universally true. One important implication, of course, is that if the central moral concepts of Kohlberg's theory of moral development are not universally true, how can his theory itself be plausibly regarded as being universally true?

The abstract versus the real

Modernist moral philosophy is unequivocally based on rationality, and in particular on critically reflective or 'reasoned' abstract principles of conduct. Proponents of rationality fervently argue that reason is value-neutral or objective (unlike feelings, which are value-laden and subjective), and therefore stands supreme as an enlightened authority on how best to live and how best to conduct one's behaviour in a world of competing self-interest. The individual, insofar as he (and, less frequently, she) is capable of functioning as a self-governing or law-making 'agent', is the centre of moral endeavour and is free to pursue self-interest, constrained only by the 'significant moral interests of others'. The individual — or rather, the agent, as 'he' is now referred to — emerges as the objective and impartial spectator or 'ideal observer', choosing from behind a Rawlsian 'veil of ignorance'. Paradoxically, self-interest becomes interpreted as upholding the interests of others, which, in turn, reduces back to self-interest. In his celebrated essay *Utilitarianism*, Mill (1962) told us, for example, that if we maximise the general welfare, our own welfare will be enhanced in the process; the contemporary philosophers Rawls (1971) and Gauthier (1986) argue along similar lines.

Under the guidance of critically reflective moral principles, the person who was once an important member of a familial group, sharing the experiences, pains, joys, decisions and responsibilities of that group, is transformed into a solitary agent, operating alone towards achieving some ideal hypothetical good (Mullett

1988). Moral problems are no longer constructed in terms of care, responsibility and personal relationships, but in terms of abstract rights and duties and principles of conduct (Gilligan 1982). For example, the problem of a grief-stricken parent weeping over the brain death of an only son injured in a recent car accident is reconstructed into a detached and hypothetical problem of serving some ideal greater good. The parent is expected to be stoically and heroically detached from the parent–son relationship, and to consent to the son's vital organs being 'retrieved' or 'harvested' for transplantation into the worn-out body of some unknown other person. Coupled with this, the parent is supposed to feel virtuous for consenting to the desecration of that son's body and to feel guilty if consent is not given. Another example concerns the problem of whether an unsuspecting wife should be told that her husband has AIDS. The problem is not constructed in terms of 'care' for her as a person and as someone who is at risk of being seriously hurt, but is reconstructed in the rather abstract terms of an attending doctor being bound by the 'rational' principle of confidentiality, said to be 'implicit' in the professional relationship the doctor has with the patient, the AIDS infected husband. In this case, the attending doctor does not tell the unsuspecting wife of her husband's fatal diagnosis, even though the doctor knows that the couple have an active sex life and are planning a child. The doctor refuses to breach confidentiality because the patient specifically requests that his wife not be told of his AIDS diagnosis.

Sissela Bok (1980) cites a similar case, which occurred in 1904, where a physician refused to warn a prospective victim that her fiancé was a syphilitic, thereby risking both her and her offspring being exposed to the disease. Commenting on the case, the physician wrote:

> A single word ... would save her from this terrible fate, yet the physician is fettered hand and foot by his cast-iron code, his tongue is silenced, he cannot lift a finger or utter a word to prevent this catastrophe.
>
> (Bok 1980, p. 147)

Modern moral philosophy argues that the moral sentiments of sympathy, compassion, care and similar feelings are quite irrelevant to the moral worth of an action. The moral worth of an action is something that can be decided only by appealing to sound, critically reflective and universal moral principles, not mere sentiments. Even if an agent 'feels' bad, he or she must follow the dictates of reason; in short, the agent must free themselves from the corrupting influences of the passions and discover through reason alone the ideals of truth. If a man is to prove his moral integrity, he must act on reason alone — even if this means sacrificing those he loves. A classic example is the 'Abraham myth', discussed later in this chapter (Gilligan 1982, p. 104; Noddings 1984, pp. 40–6).

In many respects, feminist ethics is the antithesis of mainstream modernist ethics; in other respects, it stands as its happy companion — bearing in mind that not all moral philosophy falls under the same 'umbrella', so to speak. For example, the celebrated works of Bernard Williams (1972, 1981, 1985), Alasdair MacIntyre (1985), Michael Walzer (1987) and Lawrence Blum (1980, 1994), all contemporary male moral philosophers, all seriously challenge the adequacy and reliability of modernist moral philosophy. Each of these writers suggests that modern moral philosophy is in a state of crisis and that a radical new direction in moral thinking is required if this crisis is to be overcome. Admittedly, neither Williams nor MacIntyre nor Walzer nor Blum suggests that feminist moral theory indicates the direction needed. Nevertheless, their views are compatible with and supportive of a feminist critique of modern moral thinking, and, like feminist moral philosophy itself, stand to make a valuable contribution to the development of a more substantive moral theory generally. The moral views of the Austrian-born philosopher Ludwig Wittgenstein (1889–1951) are also enlightening, and, although not directly suggesting that modern moral philosophy is in crisis, they do recommend a radical change in moral thinking. The views of these philosophers are briefly considered shortly.

Feminist critique of modern moral philosophy basically examines the nature of rationality and its supposed supremacy as a moral guide, denies the sovereignty of the individual and the acceptability of the pursuit of self-interest, and resists the demands of abstract rules and principles. It has also sought to emphasise interdependent relationships (particularly those involving family and friends), to promote the values of sharing, empathy, nurture and caring, and to stress the importance of context and situational demands (Grimshaw 1986, p. 203; Walker 1992, p. 165). As well, feminist ethics argues that a substantive moral theory or ethic is one that should be well grounded in the 'concrete circumstances of life' and not the 'detached fantasies of the hypothetical ideal' (Perictone I, cited in Waithe 1987, p. 35; see also Harding and Hintikka 1983; Grimshaw 1986; Kittay and Meyers 1987; Code et al. 1988; Gatens 1986; Braidotti 1986; Noddings 1984; Andolsen et al. 1987; Hoagland 1988; Brabeck 1989; Porter 1991; Card 1991; Sherwin 1992; Holmes and Purdy 1992; Frazer et al. 1992; Cole and Coultrap-McQuin 1992; Tronto 1993). Provocative questions are raised about the reliability of a value-neutral account of rationality, and about why reason should be regarded as having any more authority in moral thinking than the moral sentiments of, for example, empathy, compassion, sympathy, kindness, friendliness or caring.

Moulton (1983), a feminist scholar, gives a persuasive account of how the notion of value-free reasoning has been thoroughly rejected in respectable scientific circles. She points out that there is now widespread recognition that the paradigms of beliefs about methodology and evaluation, acceptable methods of inquiry, and notions of scientific good — for example, of good questions to ask; satisfying theories to follow; questions that are felt to be 'more important' — all import value orientations, and are subject to change. She is careful to point out that this now accepted value-laden account of reasoning does not mean that scientific theories or paradigms descendent of reason are 'irrational or not worth studying', but that 'there is no simple universal characterisation of good scientific reasoning' (Moulton 1983, p. 152; see also Harding 1987, 1991; Code 1991). This implies that 'objective' scientific reasoning is really no more 'objective' than the subjectivity with which it has been chosen (Gatens 1986, p. 25; Rich 1979, p. 207; Jaggar 1983, p. 360).

The next step in Moulton's thesis is to argue that criticisms of the value-neutral account of reasoning in science apply equally to the value-neutral account of reasoning in philosophy (Moulton 1983, p. 152). The weak link in the supposed objective and value-free chain of Western philosophical thinking can be found in its paradigm of reasoning, notably the 'adversary paradigm', as Moulton calls it, which sees 'an unimpassioned debate between "adversaries" who try to defend their own views against counter examples and produce counter examples to opposing views' (Moulton 1983, p. 153).

The adversary method supposedly ensures that only the 'best' of philosophical theses survive, bestowing upon them in the process of public scrutiny the supreme seal of approval — notably, the stamp of 'proven objectivity'. On this philosophical presumption, Moulton makes the rhetorical point:

> since there is no way to determine with certainty what is good and what is bad philosophy, the Adversary Method is the best there is. If one wants philosophy to be objective, one should prefer the Adversary Method to other, more subjective, forms of evaluation which would give preferential treatment to some claims by not submitting them to extreme adversarial tests.
>
> (Moulton 1983, p. 153)

Moulton convincingly rejects the adversary paradigm by pointing out that what is wrong with its method is not just its role as *a* paradigm, but its role as *the* paradigm of philosophical reasoning. If it were merely one among many methods which philosophy could employ, 'there might be nothing worth objecting to except that conditions of hostility are not likely to elicit the best reasoning' (Moulton 1983, p. 153). But, as Moulton argues, 'when it *dominates* the methodology and evaluation of philosophy, it restricts and misrepresents what philosophic reasoning is' (p. 153, emphasis added).

There are other, non-adversarial modes of evaluating, reasoning about and discussing philosophy, but philosophers do not seem to recognise these. Neither has philosophy learned from its philosophical father, Socrates, whose method of philosophical reasoning encouraged dialogue and discussion, and carefully resisted ridiculing speakers who held opposing views (Moulton 1983, p. 156). For his academic style and approach to philosophy (an approach that I have found very successful even in the teaching of non-philosophical clinical nursing subjects), Socrates has been described in the Platonic dialogues as the 'wisest man on earth'. As Moulton points out, as a playful and helpful teacher, Socrates' aim 'is not to rebut, it is to show people how to think for themselves' (p. 157).

Moulton concludes that the adversary paradigm of philosophical reasoning has presented the world with distorted images about 'what sorts of positions are worthy of attention', and has fallen prey to the world view of the hypothetical adversary who fundamentally ignores the 'positions which make more valuable or interesting claims' (p. 158). The pessimism of Moulton leaves the lasting impression that perhaps modern moral philosophy as it has been commonly portrayed really has failed at its most basic task: to guide us as the 'lovers or friends of wisdom' to discover the truth about the world in which we live and how best to live the good life in that world.

Gibson (1976), a philosophy scholar, also launches a scathing critique on the value-neutral account of rationality. Her thesis argues that rationality cannot escape the influences of the social patterns and institutions around it, and that a value-neutral account of rationality is quite inadequate for dealing with this fact. She concludes that at best rationality should be regarded as a *value*, rather than as a *property* which all 'normal' people have (Gibson 1976, p. 193). Gatens (1986) argues along similar lines, saying that the male desire for objectivity (philosophy's sacred cow) 'is itself a subjective drive and this subjective drive throws into question the objectivity that many philosophers claim for their accounts' (Gatens 1986, p. 25).

Parsons (1986) formulates an imaginative and interesting critique on rationality and on what she sees as the rise and rule of 'rational imperialism'. Citing Mary Midgley's *Beast and man* (1980), Parsons points out that Western thinking on human nature has been 'hampered by dualistic thinking regarding our nature which has not allowed us to appreciate the fullness or complexity of both our inheritance and our possibilities' (Parsons 1986, p. 85). Referring to Midgley's views, Parsons (1986, p. 86) contends that, if reason is to occupy a fruitful position in our moral thinking, it should not be viewed 'as a colonial oppressor ordering the natives to behave in ways which have been designated for them extraneously, but rather as a "clever integrater"'. The real task of moral reasoning, Parsons suggests, is not to determine our human potential and desires, but to help us assess, organise, and express these more effectively. If moral reasoning is to fulfil its task, it needs to be viewed as a complex and interdependent concept, not a simple and independent one.

Another important philosophical notion to be criticised by feminist moral theory is the notion of the *individual agent* operating as a lone decision-maker in a hypothetical world comprised of philosophical fantasies about ideal moral truths. Important questions are raised concerning why modern moral philosophy has tended to neglect the intermediate region of family relations and relations of friendship which otherwise exist between the rationally self-interested agent and the collectively interested universal others (Held 1987, p. 117). Indeed, why has it also neglected the significant phenomena of caring, concern and sympathy which people feel for those with whom they have personal and closely entwined relationships?

Perhaps one of the most disturbing things about modern moral philosophy's neglect of the family and personal relations is that it appears to have been deliberate. Lloyd (1984, p. 75), for example, points out that the pride of classical philosophy derives from its success in achieving 'complete detachment from the complexities and participation of ordinary living'. This pride inevitably extended to classical moral philosophy, which has come to prize the self-conscious ethical life as being closely associated with 'breaking away from the family' (the family, of course, is regarded as being closely allied with 'particularity') (Lloyd 1984, p. 92). The need to 'break from the family' and to surrender the 'private' domain of domesticity for the 'public' domain of higher-order activities is well documented in both ancient and modern philosophical literature.

In part 4, book 3 ('Guardians and auxiliaries') of the celebrated *Republic*, Plato advocated that the state's rulers and auxiliaries must live a life of 'austere simplicity, without private property or family life'. And in part 6, book 5 ('Women and the family'), Plato advocated that women should receive the same physical and intellectual education as men — including being trained for war. This egalitarian view of the role of women is not without a price, however, as we shall soon see. Plato went on to assert that 'if men and women are to lead the same lives, the family must be abolished'. In its place would come the setting up of state nurseries which would be filled with the babies born of 'breeding rituals'. Plato saw the advantages of this system as being twofold:

> first, that it makes it possible to breed good citizens, and second, that it gets rid of the distracting loyalties, affections and interests of the family system.
>
> (Plato 1955, p. 211)

The influence of 'anti-family' sentiment is more subtle in later works, but is nevertheless there. John Stuart Mill, for example, advocated individual liberty, but failed to consider that the liberty he spoke of was not even a remote possibility for the women of his society, who were grounded by the responsibilities of children, and household management (a point made abundantly clear in Midgley and Hughes' interesting book *Women's choices* [1983]). More recently, Richard Hare (1981, p. 27), in *Moral thinking*, uses a provocative example in which he appears to adopt the position that breaking a promise to his children (for example, that he would take them on a picnic) is less odious than disappointing a lifelong friend who arrives unexpectedly from overseas and wishes to be shown around the Oxford colleges. After engaging in an elaborate philosophical argument on the philosophy of moral language, Hare concludes that breaking the promise he has made to his children (and thereby hurtfully disappointing them) is a matter only of regret, not of moral remorse (Hare 1981, p. 28). Thus the apparent conflict of duties raised by the unexpected visit of his overseas friend is rendered not to be a conflict at all. Hare therefore feels free to show his friend around the Oxford colleges without a flicker of remorse for the disappointment he has caused his children and without offering any acceptable alternatives to cancelling the picnic. (Another significant feature about Hare's position here is that it is so readily accepted by the philosophers who cite it.)

This 'breaking away from the family' and being freed from the 'distracting loyalties of family life' has been legitimised by the doctrine of decontextualisation. This doctrine holds, roughly, that if moral choices are to be objective (popularly regarded as one of the minimum requirements of sound moral decision-making) they should be made from the position of an 'impartial spectator' or, to borrow again from Rawls, from behind 'a veil of ignorance'. In other words, the decision-maker must transcend the boundaries otherwise imposed by context, and choose from a universal, objective, impartial and unbiased point of view, notably one guided by sound rational and universal moral principles. Since it is doubtful whether any chooser could successfully transcend his or her context, the doctrine of decontextualisation is less than compelling, however. Anthropologists, historians, political scientists, sociologists, psychologists, and, more recently, some philosophers, have made it abundantly clear that we are overwhelmingly the products of our culture and history in the broadest sense, irrespective of any prevailing ideal theory of morality (see, in particular, Marshall 1992; Elliott 1992; Singer 1991; Cortese 1990; de Bono 1990; Leininger 1990a, 1990b; Stout 1988, Walzer 1987). The notion that an individual (abstract agent, or otherwise) could genuinely operate in a value-void is quite implausible.

Even admitting the behavioural guiding force of rational moral principles does little to rescue the doctrine. As Grimshaw points out:

> principles invite contextualisation of judgments, consideration of the particular. To have principles is not to be inclined to ignore complexity; it is quite compatible with recognising that the judgment one made in a particular situation was so specific to that situation that other apparently similar situations might require a different one.
>
> (Grimshaw 1986, p. 208)

Neither does the doctrine of decontextualisation's promise of securing sound moral judgments stand to rescue it — a promise of which feminist moral theory is rightly suspicious. Gilligan (1987), for example, warns that decontextualisation, and the detachment from self and others it advocates, 'breeds moral blindness' and an intolerable indifference to the needs of others (p. 24). It advances an ethic that 'has become principled at the expense of care' (Gilligan 1982, p. 105), and that, by blinding itself to the actual harms of particular individuals, fails altogether in fulfilling its task. There is no better example of this than that supplied by the Abraham myth, referred to earlier. In this classical myth, the biblical character Abraham is prepared to sacrifice the life of his son for the principle of supreme truth (God) and as a demonstration of his integrity to the principles of his faith (Gilligan 1982, p. 104; Noddings 1984, pp. 404–6). Abraham's actions in this myth stand in stark contrast to those of the lowly woman who comes before King Solomon and refuses to sacrifice the life of her son, even for the principle of truth, and demonstrates her care by relinquishing the child to the other woman who has falsely claimed to be the boy's mother. Joining Gilligan in her selection of this example, Virginia Held (1987) exclaims:

> A number of feminists have independently declared their rejection of the Abraham myth. We do not approve the sacrifice of children out of religious duty. Perhaps, for those capable of giving birth, reasons to value the actual life of the born will, in general, seem to be better than reasons justifying the sacrifice of such life. This may reflect an accordance of priority to caring for particular others over abstract principle.
>
> (Held 1987, p. 126)

The principle of care, placed entirely in context, thus offers modern moral philosophy a new and vital direction of inquiry.

Feminist moral theory does not altogether reject modern moral philosophy, or the moral principles derived from it. It merely asks that the products of modern moral philosophy be examined more thoroughly and its demands applied more cautiously and caringly. In other words, feminist moral theory is not about 'getting rid of morality', but about deciding 'which rules we will have' (Midgley 1980, p. 299), how and by whom they should be interpreted, and when they should be applied. Neither is feminist moral theory about splitting morality into gender-linked categories; such a split would be not only 'irrational' (Midgley 1980, p. 355), but a great waste of 'human potential', and would result in the narrowing of everyone's life. Nothing positive is to be achieved by having the world hopelessly divided.

Gilligan (1987) reminds us that all human relations are, at some stage, characterised by equality and attachment, inequality and detachment, and therefore everyone is vulnerable to oppression and abandonment. This risk of oppression and abandonment, if nothing else, calls for a comprehensive behaviour guide — something which probably neither a rational principle of justice nor a feminist moral principle of care can supply on its own. What is needed are the moral principles of both justice and care, with each constraining the authority of the other (Flanagan and Jackson 1987, p. 635), or, more to the point, each being viewed as 'essential elements of morally right actions' (the Pythagoreans, for example, held that for an act to be moral it needed to be both just and caring) (Waithe 1989b, p. 5).

Feminist moral philosophy has yet to articulate a coherent and substantive moral theory. (For an instructive overview of diverse feminist perspectives in moral thinking, see Robb 1985.) The virtues of care, compassion, empathy, kindness, friendship and sympathy have been identified as valid components of a substantive moral theory, but have not as yet been sufficiently articulated, or integrated, to form an independent and substantive ethical theory as such. Similarly, modern moral philosophy has yet to develop a substantive moral theory capable of directing human activity onto a path of harmonious order.

Whatever its weaknesses, feminist moral theory has provided the basis upon which a substantive moral theory can begin to be constructed — a theory which takes into account the 'concrete circumstances of life', which resists giving more weight than is due to the abstract principles of a rationally constructed morality, and which fully recognises the dangers of a 'particular perspective' creating and forcing unnecessary and destructive dichotomies (Katzenstein and Laitin 1987, p. 264). It is a theory which recognises the strengths of both women's and men's moral perceptions. The strength of women's moral perceptions, in this instance:

125

lies in the refusal of detachment and depersonalisation, and insistence on making connections that can lead to seeing the person killed in war or living in poverty as someone's son or father or brother or sister, or mother, or daughter or friend.

(Gilligan 1987, p. 32)

The strength of men's perceptions, on the other hand, lies in commitment to promoting human welfare, questioning basic assumptions, refusing to be blinded by false ideals, and rediscovering the wisdom of their Socratic forefather.

If there is an ultimate lesson to be learned from feminist moral theory, it is this: it is not enough to just have a morality or a reliable moral theory; there must also be care for and concern about how it will operate, and what it will achieve, viz. its outcomes. Morality is precisely about caring for what happens in the domain of human living (Cole and Coultrap-McQuin 1992; Hoagland 1988; Fisher and Tronto 1990; Brabeck 1989; Baier 1985; Noddings 1984). Any moral system which fails to care is a system of which all decent human beings should rightly be suspicious.

Many issues have still to be addressed by feminist moral philosophy. Its pragmatic grounding has yet to confront the reality of a world which culturally values individuality, autonomy and reason; which, rightly or wrongly, has condoned the disintegration of the extended family; and which is beginning to condone the disintegration of the nuclear family. It also has yet to persuade those thoroughly indoctrinated with the faith of Western moral philosophy that philosophy has failed at its most basic task: 'to question one's basic assumptions thereby to discover the truth' (Waithe 1987), a situation made overwhelmingly evident by the consistent exclusion of women from centuries of philosophical debate and philosophy's history. More importantly, it remains the task both of feminist moral theorists and the dominant and powerful leaders of masculinist modern moral thinking to integrate the contributions of women successfully with those made by men, and vice versa. Moral philosophy will be all the richer and more substantial for it.

Male alternatives to modernist perspectives

In *Beyond good and evil*, Nietzsche (1972) declares that morality is nothing but 'a protracted audacious forgery' (p. 291). He is even less complimentary about the philosopher, describing him (sic) as a 'creature' around whom 'snarling quarrelling, discord and uncanniness is always going on' (p. 292), and who 'often runs away from itself, is often afraid of itself — but which is too inquisitive not to keep "coming to itself" again ...' (p. 292).

Some feminist moral theorists would undoubtedly feel vindicated by these passages. Feminist moral theory is not alone in its concern about the reliability and adequacy of modern moral philosophy and its methods, theories and conclusions. As already mentioned, a number of internationally reputed male moral philosophers share this concern, which indicates that in some respects feminist criticism of 'male' philosophy and moral philosophy has not always been fair. Some of these male philosophers, past and present, have unrelentingly pursued a course of 'moral radicalism', although their works have been aggressively criticised by philosophical peers, or simply ignored or dismissed as 'insignificant' or 'too trivial' to be worthy of attention. (Mill's *The subjection of women* [1929] is a case in point, as is the dismissal of some existential philosophy.)

The English philosopher Bernard Williams (born 1929) has written several books in which he discusses the crisis of modern moral philosophy and the need for a radical new direction in moral thinking. Among other things, he argues that philosophical questions take far too much for granted and that some moral theories 'may well turn out to be mere prejudices' (Williams 1985, p. 117).

In advancing his discussion, Williams challenges the assumptions of Kantian philosophy — in particular, that reason or rationality has supreme moral authority and is the basis of sound moral theory, and, second, that abstraction and decontextualisation of the individual is necessary in order to arrive at objective moral truths (Williams 1985, pp. 17, 28). In his critique of a Kantian approach to morality, Williams (1985, p. 17) argues that the assumption about rationality in ethics is 'at once very powerful and utterly baseless', and that its widespread acceptance is more a product of 'unblinking habit' than of reflective inquiry. He also takes the provocative step of condemning the Kantian abstraction of the individual as being both absurd and dangerous. The absurdity here derives from the ridiculousness of the abstract agent trying to 'model precisely the moral choice of a concrete agent' on the basis of what the concrete agent would choose had he (sic) made 'the kinds of abstractions from his [sic] actual personality, situation and relations which the Kantian picture of moral experience requires' (Williams 1981, p. 3). The danger of the Kantian abstraction, on the other hand, derives from its total misrepresentation of the issues at stake, distracting attention from moral responsibility in the process (Williams 1981, p. 19). Williams points out that just who acts in a given situation has enormous bearing on determining responsibility; by abstracting the individual and decontextualising the abstracted individual's actions, responsibility may become diffused (p. 4). Williams argues forcefully in favour of contextualisation, pointing out that, unless people have 'enough substance or conviction' in their lives, nothing will bind their allegiance to life itself (the pessimistic consequences of this being glaringly obvious). He writes:

> Life has to have substance if anything is to have sense, including adherence to the impartial system; but if it has substance, then it cannot grant supreme importance to the impartial system, and that system's hold on it will be, at the limit, insecure.
>
> (Williams 1981, p. 18)

The cultural, historical, social, political and religious reality of a particular ethical life is crucial to any ethical analysis of it, and to any ethical theory that might be generated for it. Williams suggests that, if modern moral philosophy persists in disregarding these variables, it does so at its own peril — whether philosophers wish to admit it or not, morality is not an invention of philosophy, but an outlook on life, of which almost all of us are a part (Williams 1985, p. 174).

Ethics for Williams is more than a matter of decision; it is also a matter of agreeing what to decide (1985, p. 170). We then have to go through an elaborate process of selecting and contrasting moral and factual knowledge, and then assimilating them (Williams 1972, p. 48). This process, however, also fundamentally involves 'caring about what happens' and not abandoning this care just because 'someone else disagrees with you' (Williams 1972, p. 48). Williams, like so many feminist moral theorists, views care as the fundamental and crucial common denominator of ethical and factual knowledge. To abandon care is to abandon morality, and to doom human welfare and survival. Since this is a supremely irrational outcome, there is room to suggest a very strong sense in which the sentiment of care is not the antithesis of rationality, but rather its counterpart.

The British philosopher Alasdair MacIntyre (1985, p. 256), a contemporary of Bernard Williams, also warns that modern moral philosophy 'is in a state of grave disorder'. This disorder, he suggests, is largely the product of barren armchair philosophy (MacIntyre 1985, p. ix), of misleading and betraying moral language (p. 4), and of a blind reliance on ideas that have claimed false independence from the cultural, social and historical milieus in which they have been generated (p. 11).

Like Williams, MacIntyre rejects the view of rationality as having supreme moral authority, and as offering a convincing escape from emotivism; that is, the view that moral utterances are really expressions of emotion and individual preferences. In his critique of rational morality and its activities, MacIntyre (1985, p. 9) raises the provocative question: 'What is it about rational argument which is so important that it is the nearly universal appearance assumed by those who engage in moral conflict?'. His short answer to this is that there is nothing compelling or important about it at all. If anything, the rational paradigm of moral argument is uncomfortably aligned with a 'disquieting private arbitrariness' (MacIntyre 1985, p. 8). What appears to be a 'rational' approach is not a rational approach at all, at least not in the genuine 'critically reflective' sense. Philosophical opponents enter into moral debates with their minds already firmly made up. Their lack of unassailable criteria to convince their opponents inevitably sees what should be an instructive and enlightening debate reduced to nothing more than a battleground characterised by dogmatic assertions and counter-assertions (MacIntyre 1985, p. 8). Small wonder, MacIntyre ponders, that 'we become defensive and therefore shrill' in our public arguments.

The conclusion of Macintyre's philosophy is pessimistic. He warns that we have entered a 'new dark age', and one which, unlike other dark ages, is *already* governed by the barbarians. This predicament, he argues, is every bit the product of our diminished moral consciousness and our failure to construct local forms of community 'within which civility and the intellectual and moral life can be sustained' (MacIntyre 1985, p. 263).

The theme of diminished moral consciousness is one also advanced by the contemporary philosopher Lawrence Blum. In *Friendship, altruism and morality*, Blum (1980) writes that modern Anglo-American moral philosophy has paid appallingly little attention to the moral emotions of sympathy, compassion and human concern, and to friendship 'as a context in which these emotions play a fundamental role' (p. 1). He writes further that the Anglo-American tradition within moral philosophy has not only ignored these moral emotions but has positively militated against their having 'any substantial role in the moral life' (p. 1).

Blum goes on to suggest that the moral emotions such as sympathy, compassion, friendship and altruism are just as valid, just as reliable, and have just as important a role to play in moral life as do rational constructs such as moral duty, impartiality, fairness or consistency. On this point, Blum (1980, p. 55) notes that 'impartiality, fairness, and justice are personal virtues, but they are merely some virtues among others. They are not definitive of moral virtue altogether'.

The ultimate finding of Blum's thesis is not just that moral emotions have a place in the moral scheme of things, but that it is good to have them. That is, being sympathetic, being compassionate, being friendly, being altruistic, and being concerned about other people are all *morally good* things to be. And, as moral behaviour guides, they are no less reliable and no more vulnerable to the corrupting influence of 'negative moods' than is a rationally inspired sense of duty (Blum 1980, p. 29).

Blum's presentation of a dynamic moral life resting firmly on a sustained concern for the wellbeing of others offers some hope of escaping MacIntyre's 'new dark age' and the tyranny of Kantian barbarians. The realisation of this hope, however, altogether depends on how enlightened people (and philosophers!) are prepared to allow their moral consciousness to become, and just how prepared they are to modify their attitudes and admit that possibly they have, after all, been mistaken in their beliefs.

Other modern moral philosophers are also beginning to change their attitudes and are beginning to refer and appeal to the moral emotions in their moral monologues. Engelhardt (1986, p. 71), for example, speaks of morality as 'a reciprocal web of sympathies'. Richard Hare (1981, p. 73) concedes that our moral thinking will be less than complete, and will even be faulty, if we do not 'put ourselves in the place of somebody who is suffering'. He also concedes that principles of altruism might, on occasion, be chosen as a means of keeping 'us away from the more seductive vice of selfishness', a view originally advanced by the great patriarch Aristotle (Hare 1981, p. 129).

One of the most dynamic radical views on ethics comes from the sensitive but controversial interpretation by James Edwards (1982) of the moral views of the famous and influential Austrian-born philosopher Ludwig Wittgenstein (1889–1951). Wittgenstein viewed the moral life not as something that can be reduced to abstract rules and principles, or deduced from some general theory, but as something which can only be achieved by upholding a transcendent *ethic of love* and by *actually living* 'a life devoted to direct action in service to others' (Edwards 1982, p. 228). Ethics is not a scientific curiosity, nor anything to do with a scientific approach to dealing with the problems of human conduct (Edwards 1982, p. 234). Rather, it is a matter of profound humanism, characterised by deep sensibility and interconnectedness with the real concrete world and the real living and breathing human beings in that world. To treat morality as 'a set of obstacles to be surmounted, or as a maze to be run, or as a set of tasks to be fulfilled, or as a set of decisions to be computed and taken' is to render it 'a sort of technical, even technologised problem', something which is truly horrible (Edwards 1982, p. 238).

Edwards argues that Wittgenstein held that theory had nothing to offer ethical reflection and in fact impeded the development of moral sensitivities and human understanding (1982, p. 98). For example, if we become obsessed with rational representations of the moral life and devote all our energies to rational reflection, we will quite simply lose sight of important human concerns and will not have the energy to 'love thy neighbour'. Instead of helping us to get on with the business of 'loving thy neighbour', reflection distracts our attention from this and plunges us into a total and fruitless preoccupation with questions such as: 'But who is our neighbour?' (Edwards 1982, p. 228). By the time we come anywhere near to an answer, if we come near to one at all, our neighbour will have long gone. The love of neighbours requires actual deeds, not fruitless theoretical reflection, and it requires 'that we abandon the global for the local, the abstract for the concrete, the wilful for the self-effacing' (Edwards 1982, p. 243). In short, love of neighbours requires a life devoted to the service of others.

Ethics is, in a Wittgensteinian sense, a commensurate of sound human understanding. To gain this sound understanding, however, we need to 'deliteralise' our perceptions of the world (Edwards 1982, p. 214). To achieve this deliteralisation of our perceptions of the world, we need to disengage from our idolatrous worship of naive realism and refrain from taking our rational representations of the world as being the realities themselves and allowing these, like idols, to govern our life and practices. If we do not disengage from this 'idolatrous dogmatism', as Edwards calls it, then we risk 'a debilitating loss of moral energy or the collapse of ethical sensibility into an arbitrary willing' (Edwards 1982, p. 223).

Interestingly, Wittgenstein (originally an engineer by profession) despised professional philosophy, and felt oppressed and conscientiously troubled by his own career as a professional philosopher (Malcolm 1958, p. 62; Edwards 1982, p. 228). He apparently broke away from philosophy, and returned only because 'he felt that he could again do creative work' (Von Wright 1958, p. 12). Wittgenstein basically believed that philosophy had 'therapeutic value' in that it could work to deliteralise our perceptions of the world in much the same way that poetry and the poetic image 'can help us to see through what we ordinarily see'; in other words, philosophy, like poetry, 'is a way of deliteralising and thus expanding our perceptions' (Edwards 1982, p. 213). Just as the poet can help us to see an image that we might ordinarily fail to see in our usual way of perceiving the world, so too does philosophy. Once we have experienced 'deliteralisation', and the perceptual expansion that comes with it, we will learn that the world is 'much richer than our everyday conceptions of it' and 'we can never be so complacent in our ordinary ways of seeing, feeling, and acting' (Edwards 1982, p. 213). Philosophy, like poetry, can help us to go beyond the 'cage of language', as Wittgenstein called it (1965, p. 12), and beyond our naive thought-representations of the world, to a more meaningful experience of life. Thus, when a person complains of a 'broken heart', we know, thanks to our expanded perceptions, that it is not a cardiologist who is needed, but the hand of human love and understanding.

Wittgenstein's academic life at Cambridge University was not typical of a professor of philosophy. He dissuaded his favourite students from becoming professional philosophers, declined professional association with philosophers, sought no wide recognition for his work (and in fact was greatly distressed that his work had emerged as virtually 'gospel' in philosophical circles), and resigned his chair of philosophy at an early opportunity (Malcolm 1958; Von Wright 1958; Edwards 1982). Interestingly, Wittgenstein was profoundly influenced by the works of Leo Tolstoy and sought to live the Tolstoyan ethic of 'love of neighbour, especially the poor and untutored; rejection of personal wealth and affectation; pursuit of simplicity' (Edwards 1982, p. 245). He gave away his large patrimony, lived and dressed frugally, spent six years teaching in the peasant schools of Lower Austria, worked as a gardener's assistant in a monastery and, during World War II, worked as a hospital orderly and laboratory assistant. Edwards (1982, p. 76) also recounts the touching story of how Wittgenstein repaired the steam engine of a wool factory and, in lieu of payment, directed the owners to distribute woollen cloth to the needy children of the village.

Edwards's rather saintly portrait of Wittgenstein, however, may not be altogether accurate. Other biographers describe Wittgenstein as a man of harsh and even violent temperament, and as someone who had enormous difficulty getting on with people; even his friends feared him and found it a great strain being with him (Von Wright 1958; Malcolm 1958). There is even some suggestion that he left teaching in the peasant schools of Lower Austria because of interpersonal conflict (Von Wright 1958, p. 10).

Whatever Wittgenstein's personal life was, he has undoubtedly left a valuable philosophical legacy. Drengson (1985) describes Wittgenstein's contribution to modern moral philosophy in this way:

> [he] sought to change sensibilities and engender a healthy human understanding. He offered not a theory, but a way of being in the world, not just another way of seeing, but a way of acting and appreciating, an attitude ...
>
> (Drengson 1985, p. 131)

The lesson of Wittgenstein's ethics is the reminder that what is crucial in ethical reflection 'is the quality of attention that comprises it'; as Edwards concludes:

> In reflecting upon the formulation and application of the ethical terms, principles and judgments of a person or culture, we can discriminate care from carelessness, patience from haste, scruple from self-interest, courage from fear, and the like; and these qualities of attention are just what is at issue.
>
> (Edwards 1982, p. 249)

The ultimate lesson, though, is that it is people who matter, not things, and it is the love of people that directs the moral life, not the love of abstract and decontextualised principles.

The rationality thesis and the role of emotion in moral decision-making

Recently, support for the feminist thesis regarding the need to have a radical change in thinking about ethics, and the role of rationality and 'pure practical reason' in moral decision-making, has come from an unexpected source. In a controversial book entitled *Descartes error: emotion, reason, and the human brain*, the renowned neurologist Antonio Damasio (1994) presents a persuasive account of the crucial role of emotion in moral decision-making. In his book, Damasio examines a number of case studies involving people who have suffered serious brain injuries. Significantly, his research has found that, under certain circumstances, just as *too much* emotion can disrupt reason, so too can *too little* emotion. Calling into question traditional accounts of the relationship between reason and emotion, Damasio (1994, p. 53) suggests that a reduction in emotion may, paradoxically, 'constitute an equally important source of irrational behaviour'. It can also give rise to annihilistic decision-making. On the basis of observations made of people with 'defective emotional modulation' (in particular, those who could be described as being 'flat' in emotion and feeling), Damasio concludes that there is a significant 'interaction of the systems underlying the normal processes of emotion, feeling, reason, and decision-making'; where the emotion centres of the brain are affected adversely, so too is a person's capacity to make important life-sustaining (moral) judgments (Damasio 1994, pp. 40, 54). Significantly, this is so even in the case of where a brain-injured person's basic intellect, language ability, attention, perception, memory and language remain intact. In sum, to borrow from Damasio, a decline in the emotions can and do result in serious 'decision-making failures'.

Drawing on his scientific findings, Damasio (1994) goes on to warn of the inherent dangers to personal and interpersonal human relationships, and to human survival, of adopting a purely rationalistic and rule-bound approach to moral decision-making. He writes:

> The 'high-reason' view, which is none other than the commonsense view, assumes that when we are at our decision-making best, we are the pride and joy of Plato, Descarte and Kant. Formal logic will, by itself, get us to the best available solution for any problem. An important aspect of the rationalist conception is that to obtain the best results, emotions must be kept *out*. Rational processing must be unencumbered by passion.
>
> (Damasio 1994, p. 171)

After outlining a step-by-step approach to 'pure' rational decision-making, Damasio continues:

> Now, let me submit that if this strategy is the *only* one you have available, rationality, as described above, is not going to work. At best, your decision will take an inordinately long time, far more than acceptable if you are to get anything done that day. At worst, you may not even end up with a decision at all because you will get lost in the byways of your calculations. [...] You will lose track. Attention and working memory have a limited capacity. In the end, if purely rational calculations is how your mind normally operates, you might choose incorrectly and live to regret the error, or simply give up trying, in frustration.
>
> (Damasio 1994, p. 172)

He concludes that experience with brain-damaged patients such as those considered in his book suggest that 'the cool strategy advocated by Kant, among others, has far more to do with the way patients with prefrontal damage go about deciding than with how normals usually operate' (Damasio 1994, p. 172).

In contrast, 'integrated' decision-makers will fare much better. This is because somatic markers ('gut feelings'/emotions) help improve both the accuracy and efficiency of the decision-making process. Damasio explains:

> [The somatic marker] focuses attention on the negative outcome to which a given action may lead, and functions as an automated alarm signal which says: Beware of danger ahead if you choose the option which leads to this outcome. The signal may lead you to reject, *immediately*, the negative course of action and thus make you choose among other alternatives. The automated signal protects you against future losses, without further ado, and then allows you to choose from among fewer alternatives. There is still room for using a cost/benefit analysis and proper deductive competence, but only *after* the automated step drastically reduces the number of options.
>
> (Damasio 1994, p. 173)

Given the findings of Damasio's research, and at the risk of stating the obvious, there is clearly considerable room to suggest, contrary to the modernist rationality thesis, that sound moral decision-making requires the resources and merging of — or more to the point, the synchronicity of — *reason* and *emotion*, and it should be added *intuition* (see also Little 1996, p. 13). Anything less could risk the practice of a dissociative and annihilist ethic — that is, an ethical perspective that justifies annihilistic (versus survival) type outcomes, such as those already being advanced in mainstream bioethics (for example, euthanasia and assisted suicide).

Mainstream bioethics and feminist bioethics

Despite the proliferation of feminist literature in recent decades, there exists a relative paucity of literature on the subject of feminist bioethics. There is some evidence to suggest that mainstream ('malestream') bioethics has, in fact, paid remarkably little attention to 'gender and feminist work', and up until recently, feminist scholars have stopped short of providing a thorough examination of 'bioethical problems with systematic attention to gender and feminist work' (Wolf 1996a, pp. 4–5). (The notion of 'malestream' moral philosophy has been influenced by the work of O'Brien [1981]; see also Sherwin [1992, p. 37].) As Wolf concludes, however:

> Bioethics cannot afford to overlook half the world, to ignore the pervasive effects of gender, and to avoid the feminist literature transforming the disciplines that make up this field.
>
> (Wolfe 1996a, pp. 32–3)

It might also be added that neither can the women who comprise half the world afford to overlook the way in which the world continues to ignore them; and, while possibly not wanting to be identified with feminism (as many women do not), they cannot avoid the important contribution that feminists are making in challenging and changing the status quo of a genderised world, and the genderised legal and ethical systems that have, for so long, regulated it in a manner that has been contrary to women's moral interests (Johnstone 1994). There is then a demonstrable need for a revitalised feminist agenda to advance feminist bioethics.

Parallels between feminist ethics and nursing ethics

Nursing ethics, while not a subcategory of feminist ethics, nevertheless shares a number of features in common with it. The most obvious starting point is the reality that nursing has historically been — and remains — a female-dominated profession, with between 94–97 per cent of nurses in English-speaking-countries being women. The dismissive way in which the moral authority, interests and concerns of nurses have been treated historically parallels in significant ways to the dismissive manner in which the moral authority, interests and concerns of women generally have been treated. For instance, just as women have historically been treated as being morally incompetent, and the moral inferiors and subordinates of men, so too have nurses been treated as being morally incompetent, and the moral inferiors and subordinates of (medical) men (for an in-depth discussion of this problem see Chapter 9, 'The legal invalidation of professional nursing ethics' in Johnstone 1994, pp. 251–67). Further, just as the moral concerns and viewpoints of women have tended to be marginalised, trivialised or invalidated, so too have the moral concerns and viewpoints of nurses tended to be marginalised, trivialised or invalidated (examples of which are given in Chapters 2, 11 and 12 of this text). Thus, although not always recognising it, nurses have had first-hand experience of the kinds of negative and harmful consequences that can flow from a constraining gender-distorted (maculinist/malestream) view of the world.

In terms of the actual nature of the respective perspectives of feminist ethics and nursing ethics, again there are some commonalities. For instance, like feminist ethics, nursing ethics is critical of the abstract, decontextualised and adversarial approach of modernist moral philosophy and its privileging of reason over other moral sentiments (including the moral virtues) as a guide to ethical conduct, its rejection of the moral significance and importance of 'relationship' between people, and its tendency to privilege the authority, interests and concerns of dominant groups over marginalised groups (for example, the privileging of medical concerns over nursing concerns). And, like feminist ethics, nursing ethics seeks to contribute to and expand the domain of mainstream bioethics (as derivative of modernist moral philosophy) by examining a range of issues from a distinctive (and otherwise marginal) perspective — in this case from the perspective of nursing theory and practice — and in so doing de-centring dominant discourses in the hierarchy of (bio)ethics discourses.

Another feature which feminist ethics and nursing ethics share is their respective appreciation of virtue theory (discussed in Chapter 4 of this text) — if not as an alternative to modernist mainstream ethics, then at least as something that has a 'special place in the moral life'. Although not always explicitly acknowledged, both feminist and nursing scholars have been participants in the revitalisation of virtue ethics. What is particularly tenable about virtue theory for both feminist ethics and nursing ethics is, of course, its recognition and advancement of the morally exemplary qualities: care, compassion, kindness, empathy, friendship, love and so forth, all of which are critical to maintaining quality relationships between people — a key concern of both feminist and nursing ethics. The advancement of an ethic of care as a component of feminist ethics and nursing ethics respectively stands as an important example of the substantive contribution that both feminist and nurse scholars have made to the revitalisation of virtue theory. As a point of clarification, however, (and as already pointed out in Chapter 2 of this text) although nurse theorists (like feminist theorists) have been at the forefront of advancing an ethic of care perspective, nursing ethics (like feminist ethics) is not synonymous with an ethic of care (see the working definition of nursing ethics on pp. 45–8 of this text).

Virtue theory, an ethic of care, and nursing ethics

Before concluding this chapter, some commentary is required on the restoration of virtue in nursing ethics, and the pertinence of an ethic of care to and in the therapeutic nurse–patient relationship.

In the preceding chapter (under the discussion on virtue ethics on pp. 102–6), it was claimed that a full restoration of virtue ethics in mainstream modernist moral philosophy was unlikely. This, however, should not be taken to mean that virtue ethics has no prospects. Certainly, in the case of health professional ethics (including nursing ethics), the prospects for virtue ethics is not only extremely promising, but probable (Pellegrino 1995, p. 266). One key reason for this can be found in the fundamental link between 'the virtues' and 'the right attitudes' or 'characterological traits' (for example, of care, compassion, empathy, presence) that are generally recognised as being both essential to and constitutive of a *healing* health professional–client (nurse–patient) relationship (Dossey 1991, 1993; Gaut and Leininger 1991; Peterson and Bossio 1991; Starck and McGovern 1992; Moore and Komras 1993).

Explaining why the ethics of the health professions stand to offer a particularly promising prospect for virtue ethics, Pellegrino (1995) writes:

> Unlike general ethics, professional ethics offers the possibility of some agreement on a *telos* — i.e. an end and a good. In a healing relationship between a health care professional and a patient, most would agree that the primary end must be the good of the patient. The healing relationship, itself, provides a phenomenological grounding for professional ethics that applies to all healers by virtue of the kind of activity that healing entails. In general ethics, on the other hand, at least at present, the analogous possibility for agreement on something so fundamental as the *telos*, end, or good of human life is so remote as to be practically unattainable.
>
> (Pellegrino 1995, p. 266)

Pellegrino (1995, p. 268–70) goes on to articulate seven virtues which he believes will define 'the "good" physician, nurse or other health professional' and which can be supplemented by other virtues:

1. fidelity to trust and promise (encompassing a recognition of the importance of trust to healing);
2. benevolence (noting that people seek to be helped, not harmed);
3. effacement of self-interest (to help protect patients against being exploited);
4. compassion and caring (so that patients can be assisted in their healing in the fullest sense);
5. intellectual honesty (to ensure competent practice);
6. justice ('removing the blindfold and adjusting what is owed to the specific needs of the patient, even if those needs do not fit the definition of what is strictly owed'); and
7. prudence (encompassing the qualities of practical wisdom and the ability to deal effectively with complexity).

Pellegrino's thesis holds a particular pertinence for nursing ethics *apropos* providing a justificatory framework for nursing moral decisions and actions, as will now be considered.

The agreed end or *telos* of the profession and practice of nursing is the promotion of health, healing and wellbeing, together with the alleviation of suffering, in individuals, groups and communities for whom nurses care. This end is a moral end, and one that carries with it a strong moral action guiding force for nurses insofar as it requires nurses to engage in the behaviours necessary to promote health, healing and wellbeing in people, and, when manifest, to alleviate their suffering. In light of these ends, and the nature of the means necessary to achieve them (that is, 'good' nursing care), nursing thus stands fundamentally as a benevolent (virtuous) activity, or, more precisely, a 'moral practice' that aims to discover (through assessment), make explicit and accomplish (through cooperation and negotiation) whatever is 'good' for (read as 'conducive to the health, healing and wellbeing of') the individuals, groups and communities for whose care nurses share responsibility (Gastmans et al. 1998, p. 58).

In speaking of 'good' nursing care, it is important to clarify that something much more than merely 'competent' nursing care is being referred to. Rather, it is competent care integrated with a 'virtuous attitude' of caring. As Gastmans et al. (1998) explain:

> It is only by integrating a virtuous attitude of caring with the competent performance of care activities (*caring behaviour*) that *good care* can be achieved ... Morally virtuous attitudes are an integral part of nursing practice, since this practice takes place within a human relationship where the nurse and the patient are the main actors ... This is in essence what is meant by caring behaviour: *the integration of virtue and expert activity.*
>
> (Gastmans et al. 1998, pp. 45, 53, emphasis added)

'Virtuous caring' is integral to 'good' (moral) nursing practice (and, by implication, nursing ethics) in at least two important ways. First, virtuous caring or 'right attitudes' (which include the behavioural orientations of compassion, empathy, concern, genuineness, warmth, trust, kindness, gentleness, nurturence, enablement, respect, mutuality, 'giving presence' (being there), attentive responsiveness, providing comfort, providing a sense of safety and security, and others) have all been thoroughly implicated as effective nursing healing behaviours in the alleviation of human suffering (hence the notions in nursing of *caring as healing* and *nursing as informed caring for the wellbeing of others*) (Oliver 1990; Connelly 1991; Geary and Hawkins 1991; Ching 1993; Larson and Ferketich 1993; Leftwich 1993; Swanson 1993; Taylor 1995). Such behavioural orientations have been demonstrated as making a significant and positive difference not only to a patient's existential sense of — and actual — 'wellbeing', but to the effectiveness of drugs, to wound healing, and even to survival itself (it is well known, for example, that premature newborns will 'fail to thrive' in the absence of attentive, 'high touch' and informed nursing care and may even die; similarly, it is known that adults who are deprived of meaningful care will fail to heal and may even die prematurely from life-threatening diseases) (Dossey 1991, 1993; Gaut and Leininger 1991; Peterson and Bossio 1991; Starck and McGovern 1992; Moore and Komras 1993; Kanitsaki 1996; Gastmans et al. 1998).

Second, 'virtuous caring' plays an important theoretical role in providing an account of moral motivation in nursing to act in beneficent ways. For instance, whereas in obligation-based theories the motivation to act morally is thought to be derived from a rationally appraised commitment to 'do one's duty', in the case of virtuous caring the motivation to be moral is derived from moral sentiment (for instance, caring about a thing in some way [Rachels 1988, p. 20]), specifically a nurse's affective involvement in (*viz. caring about*) the patient's wellbeing. The explanation of Gastmans et al. (1998) is worth quoting at length. They write:

> In addition to the collection and availability of relevant information [to plan and implement patient care], the caring nurse needs to be affectively involved in the patient's wellbeing. The caring nurse needs to be emotionally touched by what happens to the patient, both in a positive and a negative sense. The cognitive and affective dimensions of the virtue of care are not rightly understood as merely two separate *components* — a cognition and a feeling-state — added together, rather they inform one another. The (altruistic) virtue of care is more than a passive feeling-state that has a person in a state of woe as their object. The (altruistic) virtue of care involves an active, motivational aspect as well, relating to the promotion of beneficent acts aimed at helping the other person. In other words, the caring nurse must be motivated to respond to the appeal of the patient. Common to the altruistic virtue of care is a desire for, or regard for,

for, the good of the other (for his or her own sake). This desire prompts (intended) beneficent action when the nurse is in a position to engage in it.

(Gastmans et al. 1998, p. 54)

(Examples of the motivational aspect of virtuous nursing care are given in Chapter 7 of this text.)

Given this very brief account of nursing as 'moral practice' (Gastmans et al. 1998), it can be seen that the prospects of virtue ethics are indeed promising in nursing ethics. The agreed ethical standards of nursing require nurses to promote the genuine welfare and wellbeing of people in need of help through nursing care, and to do so in a manner that is safe, competent, therapeutically effective, culturally relevant, and just. These standards also recognise that in the ultimate analysis nurses 'can never escape the reality that they literally hold human wellbeing in their hands' (Taylor 1998, p. 74), and accordingly must act responsively and responsibly to protect it. These requirements are demonstrably consistent with a virtue theory account of ethics.

Also consistent with a virtue theory account of ethics is a nursing articulated 'ethic of care' regarded by many nurse theorists as the moral foundation, essence, ideal and imperative of nursing (Benner 1984; Watson 1985a, 1985b; Carper 1986; Roach 1987; Leininger 1988, 1990a, 1990b, 1991; Fry 1988a, 1988b, 1989a, 1989b; Benner and Wrubel 1989; Twomey 1989; Klimek 1990; Leininger and Watson 1990; Cooper 1991; Gaut and Leininger 1991; Gaut 1992; Brown et al. 1992; Hodge 1992a, 1993b; Bowden 1994). Despite this, there has been mounting criticism in recent years about the place of 'care' in nursing ethics. These criticisms have ranged from describing an ethic of care as being 'hopelessly vague' and as 'obscuring more than it promotes' (Allmark 1995), to rejecting that care is a virtue at all (Curzer 1993). Still others denigrate care as an untenable form of 'subjugation' of women on account of its apparent 'sexist service orientation' that could see women (nurses) carrying a disproportionate 'burden of care' in a society (or a system) that is, for the most part, *careless* (Puka 1989). In concluding this discussion, I would like to make a brief response to some of these criticisms.

Firstly, as just demonstrated, a reflective articulation of an ethic of care in relation to the moral ends of nursing helps to clarify the precise behaviours expected of a 'good' nurse. It not only prescribes 'do good', but it describes *what* those 'goods' are (the promotion of health, healing and wellbeing, and the alleviation of suffering), and *how* to achieve them (through an integration of expert and virtuous caring comprising a range of 'healing promoting behaviours'). Second, given the mutually beneficial nature of 'virtuous caring' (it has demonstrable positive outcomes for *both* the receiver and the giver of authentic virtuous care), there is room to suggest that 'caring' that is unjustly burdensome is not only *not* 'virtuous caring' but not ethical. Arguments against 'virtuous caring' are thus not correctly aligned at the right target; they are, as it were, 'attacking a straw man'. Thirdly, the criticisms are just plain unpersuasive. For instance, in the case of the criticism that an ethic of care could be unduly burdensome on women (nurses), it is not immediately clear why it would be any more burdensome than say an obligation-based theory of ethics. As the example of the Abraham myth (discussed earlier in this chapter) demonstrates, 'doing one's duty' can, in some circumstances, be an extremely burdensome thing to do and further may not be able to be done without sacrificing something of moral importance. Further, to suggest that nurses might in someway become enslaved or 'subjugated' by an ethic of care, seems to imply erroneously that (and, it must be added, perpetuate the patriarchal myth that) nurses *qua* nurses lack the discretion and moral competence necessary to *decide for themselves* what moral standards they will adopt and uphold; in short, it seems to suggest, incorrectly in my view, that nurses will just 'follow slavishly' an ethic of care. Finally, these criticisms seem to overlook that an ethic of care is, paradoxically, protective of its practitioners in that it rejects symbiotic (over) emotional involvement with 'the other', emphasising instead moral virtue (characterological excellence) as its foundation (Gastmans et al. 1998, pp. 54–7).

Conclusion

Feminist ethics is a new theoretical perspective that has emerged largely in response to the flaws and failings of modernist 'malestream' ethics which, historically, has not been responsive to the concerns and interests of women. A key task of feminist ethics and bioethics has been to examine all sorts of issues from the perspective of feminist theory.

Nursing ethics shares a number of features in common with feminist ethics and has much to gain by considering a feminist theoretical perspective. Significantly, nurse theorists have joined feminist theorists in being critical of the modernist approach to ethics and bioethics, particularly in regard to its advocacy of an augmentative application of abstract rules and principles. Although these commonalities are both strong and significant, nursing ethics is not a subcategory of feminist ethics. Nursing ethics stands as a discrete role-differentiated ethic.

Despite the flaws and failings of a modernist approach to ethics, it is important 'not to toss the baby out with the bath water'. Modernist ethical perspectives still promise some assistance in the world of everyday human affairs. For instance, as is still evident, moral principles and moral language are needed to: adjudicate rationality (however defined) (Moulton 1983); secure some reliability about what people can reasonably expect from each other (Williams 1985); help order our value priorities and remind us not to be capricious (Held 1987, p. 119); and to produce some stability in the interpersonal relations we have with people who otherwise have no personal connection with us (Flanagan and Jackson 1987, p. 633). Nevertheless, there is room for nurses to be cautious in their adoption and/or rejection of given competing moral theories, and the extent to which these can be reliably and helpfully incorporated into a coherent nursing perspective on bioethics.

In conclusion, MacIntyre's 'new dark age' governed by barbarians and Nietzsche's 'trembling creatures' all warn of the urgent need for a radical new direction in moral thinking. The direction this moral thinking should take is clear. It must strive to:

- rediscover the principle of *harmonia*, so well articulated by the ancient Pythagoreans, which, in their hands, once promised an achievable *balance* in the world of human affairs and a harmonisation of diversity;
- construct a theory which is firmly based and shaped by practice, viz. the concrete circumstances of life;
- recognise the importance of shared lived experience, context and the significance of interdependency;
- recognise the biases of its own tradition and be prepared to admit that its findings might sometimes be mistaken;

- recognise the relation of the individual to the group, and the shared responsibility all group members have for each other, as well as for achieving a broader spectrum of human welfare, wellbeing and survival; and
- accept that there are some things that cannot be rationalised and objectively defined, and that some of our most decent human acts might be beyond rational explanation — such as those performed out of love, care and friendship. To think of acts performed out of love, care and friendship in terms of abstract principle or duty is, to borrow from Williams (1981, p. 18), to think 'one thought too many'.

Chapter 6

A transcultural perspective on ethics and bioethics

Introduction

In this text the discussion of the theoretical perspectives underpinning our moral thinking in nursing would not be complete without some reference to and acknowledgment of the cultural specificity, or the (Anglo-American) 'ethnocentrism', of the moral perspectives being presented and its bearing upon the topics chosen, the questions asked, and the type of moral thinking used to consider these.

It is no coincidence that most of the issues considered and the views expressed in this text reflect the dominant cultural Western (Anglo-American) philosophical traditions that have constructed and informed them (hence the reference to *Western* moral thinking and philosophy throughout this text). And it is no coincidence either that even the previous chapter, which has as its focus a brief overview and examination of a feminist perspective on ethics and its critique of mainstream (malestream) bioethics, is also ethnocentric, having been informed by the now substantial body of Anglo-American feminist literature on the subject of ethics and moral conduct. One important reason why this ethnocentricism is not coincidental is that the discipline of ethics, as being considered here, is a product of the dominant cultural contexts from which it has emerged.

Given this, it can be seen that ethics (and its derivatives) can be described appropriately as having been 'culturally constructed' (Cortese 1990, p. 1) and that dominant views suggesting the *naturality, objectivity, rationality* and *universality* of established Western ethical thinking (its theories and principles) are not only misleading but false. (For a comprehensive and critical discussion of whether ethics is a human invention or a naturally occurring material fact interwoven into the fabric of the observable world, see McNaughton 1988; Brink 1989; Dancy 1993.) Indeed, it is evident that, contrary to the dominant views of mainstream Anglo-American moral philosophers, *culture exists logically prior to ethics, not the other way around.* To reject this view is to risk corrupting rather than preserving the integrity of our moral thinking, and, in the ultimate analysis, to undermine our ability to be moral in a world which is unequivocally multicultural in nature and outlook. To insist on upholding an ethnocentric and imperialist 'universal' world view of ethics would be not only to pervert morality and all that it has been constructed to protect, but to threaten the survival of morality itself, for reasons that will be considered shortly.

Leininger (1990), an American leader in transcultural nursing, has made the important claim that 'culture has been the critical and conspicuously missing dimension in the study and practice of ethical and moral [sic] dimensions of human care' (p. 49). She has also criticised nurse ethicists for their failure to recognise the important and significant role that culture plays in guiding moral judgments and behaviour in human care contexts; and she contends further that some nurse ethicists have even 'deliberately avoided' the concept of culture altogether, preferring instead to assume the universality of the ethical principles, codes and standards of human conduct that have become so prevalent in mainstream nursing ethics discourse (Leininger 1990, p. 51). Leininger concludes that, if nurses are to provide appropriate ethical care to individuals, families and groups of different cultural backgrounds, they must have knowledge of and the ability to uphold sensitively the culturally based moral values and beliefs of the people for whom they care (Leininger 1990, p. 52). On this point, she states:

> most assuredly, the evolving discipline of nursing needs an epistemic ethical and moral [sic] knowledge base that takes into account cultural differences and similarities in order to provide knowledgeable and accurate judgments that are congruent with clients' values and lifeways.
>
> (Leininger 1990, pp. 52–3)

Without this knowledge base, Leininger contends, it is not possible for nurses to make the 'right' decisions or to provide the 'right' (ethical) human care when planning and implementing nursing care (Leininger 1990, p. 64).

Questions remain, however: What is culture? and, further, What is culture's relationship to and role in ethics generally, and nursing ethics in particular? It is to briefly answering these questions that this discussion now turns.

Culture and its relationship to ethics

Culture is an extremely complex concept, and one that has been defined, interpreted and analysed from a variety of disciplinary perspectives (see, for example, Mead 1955; Sorokin 1957; Kluckholn 1962; Spindler 1974; Beals 1979; Bullivant 1981, 1984; Wuthnow et al. 1984; Fieldhouse 1986; Williams 1989; Helman 1990; Leininger 1991; Midgley 1991a; Kanitsaki 1993, 1994). Not surprisingly, this has seen the emergence of a number of rival theories and viewpoints on what culture is, and on what its relationship to and role in human affairs is or should be (Kanitsaki 1992, p. 5). Even anthropologists do not agree about how culture should be defined, interpreted and analysed (Kanitsaki 1989a, p. 11). Nevertheless, there is some agreement among scholars that culture is a human invention and one which is critical for human survival and the development of human potential (Kanitsaki 1989a, p. 11).

What then is culture? As already stated, culture has been defined, interpreted and analysed in a variety of ways. Cohen, for example, argues that:

> culture is made up of the energy systems, the objective and specific artefacts, the organisations of social relations, the modes of thought, the ideologies, and the total range of customary behaviour that are transmitted from one generation to another by a social group and that enables it to maintain life in a particular habitat.
>
> (Cohen 1968, p. 1)

Bullivant argues along similar lines, adding to the description of culture that it is something which:

> can be thought of as the knowledge and conceptions embodied in symbolic and non-symbolic communication modes about the technology and skills, customary behaviours, values, beliefs, and attitudes a society has evolved from its historical past, and progressively modifies and augments to give meaning to and cope with the present and anticipated future problems of its existence.
>
> (Bullivant 1981, p. 19)

A more accessible description of culture, however, and one which is very helpful to this discussion, comes from an Australian leader in transcultural nursing, Olga Kanitsaki. Kanitsaki describes culture as follows:

> Culture includes a particular people's beliefs, value orientations and value systems, which give meaning, logic, worth and significance to their existence and experience in relation to both the universe and other human beings. These value orientations, value systems and beliefs in turn shape customs and traditions, prescribe and proscribe behaviour, determine the structure of social institutions and power relations, and identify and prescribe social relations, modes and rules of communication, *moral order*, and, indeed, the whole spirit and web of meaning and purpose of a given group in a particular place and time. Culture thus reflects the shared history, traditions, achievements, struggles for survival and lived experiences of a particular people. Its influence extends over politics, economics, the development and use of technology, the boundaries and meaning of class, the determination of gender roles, and so on.
>
> (Kanitsaki 1994, p. 95, emphasis added)

Unfortunately, it is beyond the scope of this text to discuss the concept of culture at the level and depth it warrants, and its consideration must be left for another time. Nevertheless, there is room to emphasise the point that, regardless of the competing theories on what culture is, it is clear that it (culture) plays a fundamental and critical role in shaping people's values, beliefs, perceptions and knowledge about the world within which they live, that it influences people's behaviour and generally gives logic and meaning to a whole way of life in that world, and that it ultimately provides the 'blueprint' for their (human) survival in that world (Kanitsaki 1992, p. 5). It is also clear that culture's relationship to and role in ethics (including its relationship to the theoretical underpinnings and practical application of ethics) cannot be plausibly denied. One does not have to be a distinguished cultural anthropologist to recognise and accept the critical link between culture and people's moral values, beliefs, perceptions and knowledge of what constitutes morally right and wrong conduct. As Mary Midgley points out, the 'communication explosion' has meant, among other things, that:

> virtually everybody, even in quite remote corners of the world, now grows up with the background knowledge that there are many ways of life deeply different from their own — a kind of knowledge which once used to be quite rare.
>
> (Midgley 1991a, p. 72)

Similarly, nearly all of us know that there are in the world many people whose moral values and beliefs are radically different from our own (Midgley 1991a,

p. 72). And we also know that in any one society there is likely to be a diversity of valid moral schemas (moral pluralism), and that this has created the possibility for, and the actuality of, irreconcilable moral disagreements, examples of which are given throughout this text (Elliott 1992, p. 32). Questions arising here include: What, if any, is the best way to respond to the problematic of moral pluralism? and, more specifically, How should nurses respond to the challenge of what can be appropriately referred to as transcultural ethics? It is to briefly answering these questions that this discussion now turns.

The nature and implications of a transcultural approach to ethics

It is not the purpose of this text to advance a substantive theory of transcultural ethics or cultural relativism, or to provide an in-depth study of the ethical concepts, theories and practices of different cultural groups. Such a task is beyond our present scope, and requires much more space than it is possible to provide here. (See, meanwhile, Cortese 1990; Leininger 1990; Singer 1991; Midgley 1991a; Elliott 1992; Marshall 1992; Macklin 1998.) Nevertheless, it is important to have some understanding of the nature and implications of transcultural ethics (a form of ethical pluralism), and of how nurses might respond better to the challenges it poses.

One central point that needs to be thoroughly understood is that, while all societies have some sort of moral system for guiding and evaluating the conduct of their members, the moral constructs of one culture (for example, North American or English culture) cannot always be applied appropriately or reliably to another culture — at least not without some modification (Silberbauer 1991, p. 15). Further, language usage alone, and the difficulties encountered in reaching accurate culturally thick (rich) translations of accepted moral terms and concepts, may even make meaningful moral discourse across cultures impossible (Stout 1988). These points have, however, been largely overlooked by modernist (Anglo-American) moral philosophers, who have tended to support an imperialist model of morality — that is, that their way of moral knowing and thinking is not only superior but 'right', and is thus something to be applied (read imposed) universally on to others whose moral systems they have judged to be inferior — even 'savage' (Midgley 1991a, p. 78).

As already argued, this is an inadequate and fraudulent approach to moral thinking and conduct, and one which should be questioned. Nevertheless, this does not mean that Anglo-American modernist moral philosophy itself should be abandoned. To the contrary — its rich traditions offer us important insights into our own culture-specific moral values and beliefs about how to be moral beings. We must, however, pay much greater attention to the influences of the primary organising principle of morality, namely, culture. We also need to recognise that, while it is true that all cultures have some 'priority rules', or principles for arbitrating between conflicting obligations and duties, just what these rules and principles are, how they are defined and interpreted, when they will be applied, and who ultimately applies them (and to what end) will, contrary to an imperialist model of ethics, vary across — and even within — different cultures (Midgley 1991b, p. 11). In short, morality will be expressed differently cross-culturally and intra-culturally.

An interesting example of the different ways in which morality can be expressed cross-culturally or even intra-culturally can be found in the case of small-scale and large-scale societies. In small-scale or traditional societies, for example, morality tends to be viewed as a *process* — as a means to an end — and is expressed through the *quality of relationships* (characterised by upholding values such as friendship, loyalty to kin, empathy, altruism, familial trust, and so on), rather than a deontological adherence to abstract principles. Silberbauer explains:

> Morality is less of an end in itself but is seen more clearly as a set of orientations for establishing and maintaining the health of relationships. Morality, then, is a means to a desired, enjoyed end.
>
> (Silberbauer 1991, p. 27)

This view is in sharp contrast to that upheld by large-scale (non-traditional or industrialised) societies, in which relationships are less proximate, less intense and less significant, both at the individual and the societal level. Here morality is viewed as an end in itself rather than as a means to an end, and is expressed by adherence to rules (viz. adjudicating the conduct between strangers) rather than by and in the quality of relationships per se. On this point, Silberbauer explains:

> Morality certainly provides a set of orientations and thus helps to create and maintain coherent expectations of behaviour, but operates *impersonally* in that there is not the same capacity for negotiation. Morality thus tends to be valued more as an end in itself and less as a means to an end.
>
> (Silberbauer 1991, p. 27, emphasis added)

To illustrate the different ways in which small-scale and large-scale societies might each express their different moralities, Silberbauer (1991) uses the simple example of the relationship between a bus-conductor and a passenger. He suggests that, in large-scale societies, where relationships tend to be 'single-purpose and impersonal', the relationship between a bus-conductor and a passenger would be of limited importance, and would probably manifest itself quite differently than it would in a small-scale society, where relationships were more proximate, multi-purpose and personal. He points out:

> how different it would be if the conductor were also my sister-in-law, near neighbour and the daughter of my father's golfing partner — I would never dare to tender anything other than the correct fare. In a small-scale society every fellow member whom I encounter in my day is likely to be connected to me by a comparable, or even more complex web of strands, each of which must be maintained in its appropriate alignment and tension lest all the others become tangled. My father's missed putts or my inconsiderate use of a motor-mower at daybreak will necessitate very diplomatic behaviour on the bus, or a long walk to work and a dismal dinner on my return.
>
> (Silberbauer 1991, p. 14)

A less masculinist and more relevant example here can be found in the comparison of nurses working in large city-based university teaching hospitals with those who work in small, close-knit 'outback' country communities. It has been my experience that nurses working in small rural or remote ('outback') country communities (where 'everyone is known to everyone') are far more vulnerable to putting local community members 'off-side' by offending an individual member of that community than are nurses working in large city-based university teaching hospitals. In this instance, we could speculate that nurses working in small country-based community nursing care settings might put more weight on *preserving the quality of relationships* in that community than on *upholding abstract moral principles*. Conversely, nurses working in large and impersonal communities may put greater emphasis on upholding abstract principles of conduct than on preserving the quality of relationships with 'strangers' whom they are unlikely to encounter more than once during their working lives.

Bear in mind, however, that this is only an example, being used here to help clarify Silberbauer's point. In reality it is likely that nurses express morality both as a process (as a means to an end) and as an end in itself. Whether this is so, and the extent to which it is so (that is, where the balance lies), may depend ultimately on the nature of the context they are in — whether it is characterised by personal or impersonal relationships. When it is considered that it is not contradictory to view the maintenance of quality relationships as an important moral end in itself (not just a means to an end), there is room to suggest that the distinction Silberbauer makes may, in the final analysis, be overstated.

Despite this observation, Silberbauer is correct to point out that abstract moral principles do not always have currency in some cultural or social groups, and that, even if there do exist some commonly-accepted standards of moral conduct, we cannot assume that these standards will be expressed or applied uniformly across, or even within, different cultural groups. A good example of this can be found in the wide and popular acceptance of the moral principles of autonomy, non-maleficence, beneficence and justice, which are considered in Chapter 4. These principles are referred to and used widely in mainstream bioethics discourse (see in particular Beauchamp and Childress 1994), and are viewed popularly as 'self-standing conceptual systems by which we can impose some sort of order upon ethical problems' (Elliott 1992, p. 29). But, as Elliott correctly points out, what proponents of this view tend to overlook is that in reality, ethics does not stand apart. It is one thread in the fabric of a society, and it is intertwined with others. Ethical concepts are tied to a society's customs, manners, traditions, institutions — all of the concepts that structure and inform the ways in which a member of that society deals with the world (Elliott 1992, p. 29).

He goes on to warn that, if people forget this inextricable link between ethics and culture:

> we are in danger of leaving the world of genuine moral experience for the world of moral fiction — a simplified, hypothetical creation suited less for practical difficulties than for intellectual convenience.
>
> (Elliott 1992, p. 29)

A poignant example of the inaccuracy and fraud of viewing moral principles as self-standing conceptual systems rather than as ethical concepts tied to a particular tradition (culture) can be seen in the way in which the principle of autonomy tends to be interpreted and applied in professional health care contexts. As stated in Chapter 4, the concept of autonomy refers to an individual's *independent* and *self-contained* ability to decide. As a principle, autonomy prescribes that an *individual's rational preferences* ought to be respected even if we do not agree with them — and even if others consider them foolish — provided they do not interfere with or harm prejudicially the significant moral interests of others.

At first glance, this articulation of the concept and principle of autonomy appears unproblematic. And it is probably true that most nurses familiarising themselves with the moral nature and application of the principle of autonomy value the 'right' to make their own self-determining choices, and would probably feel a strong sense of outrage if their considered wishes were overridden arbitrarily by another. They may also share a strong conviction that patients should always be informed about their diagnoses, and about the details of their proposed treatment and care, and that it would be a gross violation of patients' rights not to accept or facilitate patients' self-determining choices regarding their own care and treatment options. In most cases, this position would probably be a demonstrably justifiable one to take. It would, however, be a grave mistake to accept the concept and principle of autonomy (as articulated above) as holding *universally*; that is, without exception. Consider the following.

Earlier in this text, it was pointed out that definitions of ethical terms and concepts can be 'ethically loaded', and hence can themselves be an important influence on how a moral debate or analysis might be conducted and what the outcomes of a given debate or analysis might be. This is true even (or perhaps especially) in the case of moral principles — the moral principle of autonomy being a case in point. It will be noted, for example, that even the definition of the concept and principle of autonomy reflects the dominant cultural values of the highly individualised large-scale Western Anglo-American culture from which it has arisen (Marshall 1992). Of particular importance to this discussion are the italicised terms *individuals, independent, self-contained*. Here the ethical loading clearly rests on respecting individualism, independence, and isolation (insulation) from one's social 'connectedness'. (As a point of interest, in contemporary Italian culture the notion autonomy [*autonomia*] is often used synonymously for isolation [*isolamento*] [Surbone 1992, p. 1662].) For people who hold these values, this ethical loading is not a major problem. But for people who do not hold or share these values — who may, for instance, subscribe to the values of collectiveness, interdependence, and social connectedness (context) — it is open to serious question whether the concept and principle of autonomy as popularly defined and applied in mainstream bioethics discourse could, or indeed should, be given any currency in mediating the relationships, and the responsibilities within those relationships, of people who do not subscribe to the values embraced by autonomy as described.

To illustrate the kinds of moral problems that can arise as a result of applying the principle of autonomy in an abstract, universal and context-independent way rather than in a substantive, context-dependent, culture-specific way, consider the case of Mr G (taken from Johnstone and Kanitsaki 1991). Mr G, an elderly Greek who spoke no English, was admitted to hospital for investigations, and was later diagnosed as having cancer of the lung. Mr G had a number of other health problems, including a mildly debilitating hemiplegia — although he could move about with assistance. Before his admission into hospital, Mr G was totally dependent on and cared for by his family.

When radiological and laboratory tests confirmed the provisional medical diagnosis of a malignant lung tumour, Mr G's physician arranged for an interpreter to come to the ward and through him informed Mr G directly that he had cancer of the lung. In this instance, it was the physician's personal policy to be candid with his patients, and inform them according to what he judged to be 'their right to know and be informed', as prescribed by the moral principle of autonomy. Unfortunately, in this case, although well intended, the physician's approach was culturally inappropriate, and had the undesirable moral consequence of causing the patient and his family otherwise avoidable suffering (Johnstone and Kanitsaki 1991).

A mainstream ethical analysis of the physician's actions in this case would probably support the view that informing the patient of his cancer diagnosis was a 'morally right' thing to do. And, interestingly, when I present this case to students (nursing and medical students alike), most contend that the physician's actions were not only morally correct but *praiseworthy*, given the reluctance by many doctors to be candid with their patients about diagnostic, care and treatment matters of this nature.

From a cultural perspective, however, the physician's actions can be shown to be not only mistaken but morally harmful, for reasons that will now be explained. In this case it would have been more culturally appropriate and morally beneficial had the physician communicated the cancer diagnosis to the patient's *family* rather than to the patient himself (see also Kanitsaki 1993, 1994). This is because, as Johnstone and Kanitsaki point out, during a health crisis, patients like Mr G who are of a traditional (rural, small-scale societal) cultural background, tend to prefer:

> the close involvement of their family and value the supportive, protective and therapeutic role that the family can and does play when one of its members is ill or suffering ... Indeed, the involvement of the patient's family is an essential and integral part of the therapeutic relationship and of the process required to uphold the patient's best interests.
>
> (Johnstone and Kanitsaki 1991, p. 280)

By not recognising the protective authority of Mr G's family to decide '*if, when, how and by whom* the diagnoses should be disclosed to Mr G', the physician inadvertently 'pointed the bone' at his patient and thereby undermined rather than promoted Mr G's autonomy. The reasons for this are complicated, but important. Kanitsaki (1989a) explains that for many rurally-based Greeks who emigrated to Australia during the 1950s and 1960s the very word 'cancer' carries a whole range of negative connotations and thus is something never to be mentioned, since to do so would be to risk stimulating the *nocebo phenomenon*. The nocebo phenomenon (from the Latinate *noceo*, 'I hurt', and the Greek *nosis*, 'disease') is defined by Helman (1990, p. 257) as 'the negative effect on health of beliefs and expectations — and therefore the exact reverse of the "placebo" phenomenon' (see also Dossey 1982, 1991; Weil 1983; Chopra 1989; Moyers 1993). Kanitsaki (1989a, p. 46) explains that during the 1950s and 1960s, rural Greece had virtually no hospitals, and that if people required treatment for serious illness they would have to travel great distances to the nearest cities. She goes on to point out that, because of this, as well as because of a scepticism about scientific medicine's ability to treat diseases effectively, people from rural areas would seek hospital treatment only as a last resort. As Kanitsaki explains:

> the reluctance to frequent doctors and hospitals was exacerbated by a general dislike of hospitals, rumours about the lack of nursing care and unkind nursing staff, and a fear of cities generally. Pressures of local work demands, a lack of economic resources, and the probability of having to travel alone and thus without the protection, support, and physical presence of the family, also militated against scientific medical services being used by rural community members.
>
> (Kanitsaki 1989a, p. 47)

As a result of this reluctance — and, indeed, inability — to access scientific medical services, many people suffering from cancer-related illness did not receive the optimal treatment available, and as a result frequently died painful and agonising deaths (Kanitsaki 1989a). And it is the memories of these kinds of cancer-related deaths that many rural Greek immigrants have brought with them to Australia. Kanitsaki explains (personal communication) that many Greek immigrants of this background simply do not have any experiential knowledge of, or even a conception of, the kind of treatment and care that is available in Australia today; thus, even mentioning the word 'cancer' is sufficient to trigger in ill persons an overwhelming sense of hopelessness which ultimately finds its expression in their losing their will to live. Under these circumstances, to tell such patients, 'You've got cancer' — no matter how benevolent the intention in doing so — would probably be sufficient to trigger the nocebo phenomenon, resulting ultimately in the ill person's premature death (Kanitsaki, personal communication).

The way to avoid this disastrous situation is for the patient to be spared the information likely to stimulate the nocebo phenomenon, and for the patient's family to be respected as having the authority to decide — in the moral interests of and for the wellbeing of their sick loved one — *whether, when, where, how and by whom* information about the diagnosis of a serious illness and poor prognosis will be given (Kanitsaki, personal communication). A major *moral* motivation for this, Kanitsaki explains (personal communication), is to avoid undermining the sick person's hope (about getting better and being able to go on living a meaningful life), and thereby to maximise the person's ability to continue making important life-interested choices; that is, to maximise the person's autonomy. In sum, maintaining hope is the linchpin to promoting autonomy. This is because, without hope there is simply *nothing left to choose for* (Kanitsaki, personal communication). Interestingly, current research has shown that, even in contemporary Greek society, truth telling about a diagnosis of serious life-threatening illness is still viewed by many rural Greeks as something 'undesirable', on the grounds that it could undermine hope and the will to live (Dalla-Vorgia et al. 1992).

It should be noted that this moral world-view is not held exclusively by Greeks of rural or traditional cultural backgrounds. People of other traditional cultural backgrounds also believe that in some circumstances patients should not be told that they have a serious life-threatening illness, and that to do so would be sufficient to trigger the nocebo phenomenon (see, for example, Surbone 1992; Macklin 1998). The following anecdote shows this. The case concerns an elderly non-English-speaking Italian man who, like Mr G, had emigrated to Australia in the 1950s. He was admitted to hospital for tests which later confirmed a cancer diagnosis. Although the man's family explicitly requested that their father not be given any information about the test results if they were positive, an interpreter was called in their absence and the man was told of his cancer diagnosis and poor prognosis. This information caused the man to become extremely distressed and, as his son commented later, 'the life just went out of his eyes and we knew he would die very soon'. The son, who was Australian-born and a qualified pharmacist, decided in consultation with the rest of his family to remedy the situation. This he did by contacting Italian-Australian friends who worked as doctors at the hospital where his father was a patient and arranging for all his father's tests to be repeated. His friends agreed to explain to his father that the tests needed to be repeated because 'there had been a terrible mistake' and that 'his earlier tests results had got mixed up with someone else's'. They later returned to tell the man that his tests showed he in fact did *not* have cancer. The son explained that his father was told he still needed medical treatment, but that he would 'be all right'. Ultimately, the family took their father home and cared for him. He continued to live beyond the time limit suggested by his poor prognosis and, in fact, was still alive at the time the anecdote was being shared. The son attributed this to the fact that they were able to convince their father all was not hopeless, which in turn had the effect of restoring his will to live. In short, the son's actions reversed his father's sense of hopelessness, and thus promoted rather than undermined his father's autonomy.

Interestingly, when I have shared this anecdote with students, many are appalled at the blatant deception that was employed in this case. Others, however, notably those whose parents are from rural Greece or Italy, have expressed enormous relief at the insights this and other cases like it have given them. One postgraduate nursing student, for example, commented (personal communication):

> I've always felt that if either of my parents should get cancer they should be told their diagnosis. But when speaking of this issue, my mother — who is Italian — has always insisted, 'No! You must not allow that to happen'. My Australian side of me tells me it is wrong not to tell them. But now I can see it would be wrong *to tell* them, and that my mother is right. I can live with this now. It is such an enormous relief. I am no longer in a dilemma. Thank you.

The comments of this student are included here because, among other things, they demonstrate the very practical help that adopting a transcultural view of ethics can offer; they help to support the view that, by tying ethical views to the cultural traditions that inform them, we will be in a much better position to embrace morality as an experience rather than as an abstraction (Marshall 1992, pp. 53–7), and to avoid falling prey to the unhelpful, idle fantasies of moral fiction which, as Elliott (1992, p. 2) suggests, are suited more to the purposes of intellectual convenience than to resolving genuine practical difficulties in the concrete circumstances of life. The student's comments and, indeed, the anecdotes themselves also show, to borrow from Cortese (1990, p. 157) that 'relationships ... are the essence of life and morality', and that to view morality simply as conceptions of abstract reified rational principles is 'to remove us from the real world in which we live, and separate us from real people whom we love' (Cortese 1990, p. 157). The lesson to be learned here is that, unless we embrace morality as an experience rather than as an abstraction, what we will end up with is only a concept of morality and not morality itself. And, borrowing again from Cortese (1990, p. 158), unless we have a 'deep sense of relationship, we may have a conceptualisation of the highest level of justice, but we will not be moral'. The point being that without relationships, justice — morality — 'contains no system of checks and balances. It becomes primarily an end in itself without regard to the purpose of morality' (Cortese 1990, p. 158).

Although only the principle of autonomy has been considered here, the other principles considered in Chapter 4 (non-maleficence, beneficence and justice) could all be examined along similar lines. We could, for example, ask in regard to each of these principles: From whose perspective are these principles to be meaningfully and appropriately defined, interpreted, analysed and applied? In the case of non-maleficence, for instance, meaningful questions can be asked about what constitutes a 'harm' in a given culturally-constructed clinical context? By whose standards and cultural perspectives is the notion of harm to be measured and evaluated? Likewise for the principles of beneficence and justice.

Where then does this leave the role of moral principles and culturally different moral schemas in our nursing ethics discourse? In answering this question, it might be useful at this point to consider the problematic of diversity or pluralism in moral values and moral world views.

Moral diversity and the challenge of moral pluralism

Earlier, it was asserted that the world in which we now live has become unequivocally multicultural in nature and outlook, and that this has brought with it a diversity or pluralism of moral values and beliefs. Some fear that this diversity or pluralism of values may be 'the barrier to agreement' (Elliott 1992, p. 32), and, hence, the catalyst to producing a world hopelessly divided by radical and destructive moral disagreement. Others reject moral pluralism outright on the grounds that, in their view, it is 'just another name for confusion' (Stout 1988, p. 1). Moral diversity need not lead to destructive disagreement, however, nor to blinding confusion. Indeed, as is well recognised within the discipline of moral philosophy, moral disagreement has historically been the beginning and the development of moral thinking, not its end or disintegration (see also Stout 1988; Benhabib and Dallmayr 1990). Further, as Mary Midgley correctly points out, 'nobody is infallible; and for that reason many different points of view are needed' (Midgley 1991a, p. 83).

What must also be recognised and understood here is that a diversity of values and beliefs is the key to morality's survival; it prompts critical reflection, rather than uncritical acceptance, and in so doing invites constant revision and creative refinement. Moral diversity also helps to ensure that no one moral point of view dominates; in short, it helps to prevent what might otherwise be termed 'moral fascism'. Meanwhile, its emphasis on understanding difference rather than striving for uniformity will help to ensure that the moral systems we end up embracing will be of a nature that is truly responsive to the lived realities and experiences of all human beings, not merely those of a select few whose positions of power have enabled them to manipulate morality into a tool for repressing unwanted truths and legitimating further the authority of moral imperialists who would impose their values on others as a means of maintaining rather than challenging their cultural hegemony.

Adopting a transcultural approach to ethics can be beneficial in a range of ways. Among other things, at a global level, it can enable cross-cultural interactions that 'build bridges of understanding between persons and cultures that make cooperation possible and conquest unnecessary' (Fasching 1993, p. 6). It can also help to avoid the perils of 'moral suprematism' such as those which have been amply exemplified during wartime (see, for example, Fasching 1993). For instance, during the second world war, the world bore witness to Nazis believing in 'their own moral superiority (supported by ultimate justification)' and the consequential rendering as mute 'all opposing views' (Gergen 1994, p. 113). As Gergen points out in relation to this historical period:

> Had the means been available much earlier for an unobstructed interpretation of meaning systems — Nazi, Jewish, Christian, Marxist, feminist, and the like — one must imagine that the consequences would have been far less disasterous.

> (Gergen 1994, p. 113)

We thus stand warned that what is sometimes presented as *the* 'superior morality' might well prove to be little more than 'the morality of the superior' (meaning the extremely powerful and the dominant), with little to recommend itself to 'the other', rendered by it (the 'superior morality') as having only inferior moral status, or worse, as having no moral status at all (as indeed happened in the case of Nazi characterisations of the Jews) (Bauman 1993, p. 228).

At a more local level, a transcultural approach to ethics can enrich greatly our moral view of the world and the various relationships (including nurse–patient relationships) we experience within it. In the case of the nurse–patient relationship, however, a transcultural approach to ethics may not only enhance the moral quality but also the therapeutic effectiveness of that relationship (most notably through avoiding the harmful consequences of the nocebo phenomena [Kanitsaki 1996]), and hence the moral ends of nursing itself (referred to in the previous chapter).

An important lesson for nurses here is, I believe, that moral diversity is not something to be feared, but something to be embraced as a means of challenging our complacent thinking about the moral world we live in, and of improving our understanding of and ability to experience both ourselves and others as moral beings who have a mutual interest in living a worthwhile and meaningful life. Further, whether we wish to admit it or not, as Elliott point out:

> Moral disagreement will be with us as long as there is disagreement about what way of life is best for human beings. It is not at all obvious that this is a question that is answerable, even in principle. There may be no best life, only better and worse lives. And if morality is tied to a form of life, then it is a mistake to think that we can eliminate moral differences without eliminating the differences in cultures, and in individuals, to which morality is tied.
>
> (Elliott 1992, p. 35)

Elliott goes on to make the additional point that:

> Though the biological characteristics humans share will mean that some lives, and some features of lives, are necessarily good or bad for human beings, there is no compelling reason, universally applicable, for adopting any one particular sort of life over all others — even if we had the choice, which we do not. For this reason, we should expect diversity in the sort of lives that people live, as well as the moral differences that inevitably follow.
>
> (Elliott 1992, p. 35)

Problems associated with a transcultural approach to ethics in health care

Before concluding this discussion, it is important to acknowledge that upholding a transcultural view of ethics can sometimes be extremely difficult, and may give rise to serious dilemmatic situations for health care professionals — nurses included. For instance, it is not uncommon for nurses to encounter a situation in which a patient requests one thing and his or her family requests another. A typical scenario is as follows.

A patient from a traditional cultural background (for example, Greek or Italian) discloses to an attending nurse: 'If my test results come back positive and I have cancer, I want to be told. I know my family has told you not to tell me, but I must ask you not to take notice of them. *I* want to know. And that is the end of the matter'. The family, meanwhile, may request: 'If our father's test results come back positive and he has cancer, under no circumstances is he to be told. We know him. Such news will kill him. You must give *us* the information and we will deal with it. This is family business and that is the end of the matter'. Usually, the attendant nurses in these kinds of situations are desperate to do what is best for all concerned, but are troubled about how to decide what, in fact, *is best* for all concerned. Typically, the questions they ask include: 'Who do I listen to — the patient, or the family? How best can I serve the patient's interests given that the family just might be right — that is, the information might "kill him"? What should I do?'. Just what attending nurses ought to do, all things considered, might not be as problematic as at first it appears to be. Consider the following.

In responding to the kind of scenario just outlined, it is vitally important that nurses do not *stereotype* people of different cultural backgrounds and assume that 'all immigrants' *ipso facto* practice traditional live-ways, or that 'all immigrants' *ipso facto* practice a family-centred (versus an individualistic) model of informed decision-making in health care contexts. Many immigrants to a host country assimilate to the mainstream culture of their new country, and have internalised very effectively the core cultural values of the (new) mainstream culture. Immigrants to Australia are no exception in this regard. Thus, when a 'new Australian' (as immigrants to Australia have been known in the past) makes an explicit request to the effect 'If my test results come back positive and I have cancer, I want to be told', it is highly probable that not only does he or she mean it, but will also be able to deal with it in a culturally adapted way. In such instances, there is no question that the nurse's primary responsibility is to initiate steps to ensure that the patient's request for information is honoured. Where then does this leave the family's request?

Giving primacy to the patient's request for information does not mean that the family's request has no bearing on the matter or should be ignored altogether (see, for example, Kuczewski 1996). To the contrary. The family's request is just as deserving of consideration as is the patient's — not least because *they too* are experiencing the health crisis of their loved one. What differs, however, is the way in which nursing and medical staff might respond to a family's requests. Kanitsaki, for example, advises (personal communication) that after securing consent from the patient, the following actions might alleviate the situation considerably:

- inform the family that the patient has explicitly requested to be told the details of a diagnosis, and that the doctors and nurses have a legal and moral obligation to honour this request;
- express understanding of the pain of the situation, and acknowledge that the family is only trying to do what is 'good and right' for their loved one;
- invite the family to be present when the information is to be given to their loved one;
- negotiate a plan of care that, in the event of a 'bad' diagnosis, all parties can be mutually supported; for example,

  1. it might be necessary to arrange for the family to meet with the attending physician on a regular basis in order to obtain and discuss details of their loved one's health status and progress;
  2. it might be necessary to organise culturally relevant help (for example, counselling — noting, however, that it might be necessary not to call it

'counselling' for cultural reasons) to assist family members and their sick loved one to re-establish communication patterns that the 'telling, not telling' scenario has possibly disrupted, and consequently left each family member feeling alienated from each other.

In most instances, a 'commonsense' approach to managing individuals and families experiencing grief crises will result in satisfactory outcomes and a 'therapeutic partnership' between lay and professional (nursing) carers.

Another kind of problem that is not uncommon in nursing care domains involves extended-family members visiting in contravention of hospital visiting rules; for example, visiting outside of a hospital's regulated visiting hours and/or in numbers in excess of the usual two-visitors-per-patient visiting rule. In regard to the latter, this is seen as problematic by nurses since it sometimes compromises the privacy entitlements of other patients — especially when the presence of a large number of extended-family members creates undue conversational 'noise'. It is also seen as problematic by nurses since it is not uncommon, over the duration of their visit and/or the patient's hospital stay, for different family members to ask the same nurse the same question about the health condition of their loved one. Nurses not infrequently cite being frustrated at repeatedly being asked the same question by different family members as, among other things, this is commonly seen by nurses to embarrass their already strained 'time resources' to attend other patients. All things considered, however, this problem is also not as problematic as at first it might appear to be and is amenable to remedy.

In addressing this kind of problem it is important for nurses to understand that 'presencing' by extended-family members is a crucial component of the lay-therapeutic relationship (Kanitsaki 1989a, 1989b, 1993, 1994, 1996). By being 'present', family members believe they are contributing to the healing process by 'giving strength' to their loved one. Significantly, it is not uncommon, especially in the case of seriously ill patients, to see family members strategically placed around the bed of a sick person, for example, with one family member touching the head, another the left hand, another the right hand, another the left foot, and another the right foot of the ill person. This 'touching' (often manifest as massage of a given part of the body or the sprinkling of healing waters over the part) is an important component of the process of giving 'healing energy' to the ill person and to assist them to 'get well'. The loved one, meanwhile, generally regards the presence of his or her family member as an indication of their 'caring'. To ask family members to leave under these circumstances thus stands as a major violation of the lay-therapeutic relationship, and it is understandable that extended-family members might react 'badly' to a nurse's directives to 'be considerate' of other patients and to observe the 'two-visitors-per-patient' rule. The question to arise here is: How can nurses best manage the situation?

Key to the effective management of extended-family visiting is for nurses themselves to understand the lay-therapeutic (healing) nature of this visiting, as well as the crucial role it also plays as a 'quality assurance' check of the care a loved one might be receiving. For instance, the repeated questioning of nursing staff by family members is an attempt to secure as much information as possible about the care of their loved one, which can subsequently be interrogated by family members for its consistency, accuracy and hence reliability (Kanitsaki 1989a, 1989b, 1993, 1994, 1996). Obviously, if six family members ask the same nurse the same question, yet receive six different answers, they would have grounds to be suspicious about whether their loved one was, in fact, receiving optimal care. Similarly, if their repeated requests for information are met with annoyance or hostility by nurses, this could be construed as meaning that the nurses 'do not care' and, again, that their loved one is not receiving optimal care. This, in turn, could result in the family removing the loved one from a given location of care and taking them elsewhere for care — even overseas (Kanitsaki 1989a, 1989b, 1993, 1994, 1996).

There are a number of strategies which nurses might use to help remedy a situation such as this. These include:

- asking the family to nominate a spokesperson for the family and for a primary nurse to agree to meet with this person, as required, to answer any questions the family might have;
- advise the family (in non-serious cases) of the constraints under which nurses are forced to operate and explain the need for considering the interests of other patients;
- in the case of seriously ill patients, move the patient to a single room so that the lay-therapeutic relationship can be expressed as fully as is possible under the circumstances (adapted from Kanitsaki 1989a, 1989b, 1993, 1994, 1996).

Feedback from nurses over the years has indicated that the implementation of these and related kinds of strategies have been very effective in maximising the quality of care experienced by patients (and their chosen carers) of culturally diverse backgrounds, and improving nurses' job satisfaction when involved in the care of such patients.

The third and final kind of problem to be considered here, and which nurses not infrequently have to deal with, concerns the codified demand on nurses to respect certain religious and traditional practices of patients. The nature of the problem is as follows.

The International Council of Nurses (1973) *Code for Nurses* (included as Appendix I to this text) prescribes that 'the nurse, in providing care, promotes an environment in which the values, customs and spiritual beliefs of the individual are respected'. The *Code of Ethics for Nurses in Australia* (included as Appendix III to this text) likewise prescribes that 'Nurses respect persons' individual needs, values and culture in the provision of nursing care'. The nursing ethics codes of other countries carry similar provisions. The problem for nurses, however, is that some religious and traditional practices either pose a threat or are actually harmful to patients — the case of female genital mutilation being an obvious example here. In such instances, nurses are troubled by what appears to be two conflicting demands: on the one hand, to respect the patient's cultural values and beliefs; and yet, on the other hand, to protect the patient from harm. This dilemma is compounded by postmodernist requirements to explain: 'harm' by *whose standards*? 'harm' by *whose world view*?, and to demonstrate that the apparent moral dilemma at issue is not merely a creation of 'moral ethnocentrism' or 'cultural (moral) imperialism' (James 1994).

This kind of problem is enormously complex, and requires a much deeper examination than is possible here. Further, addressing this kind of problem requires a deep understanding of the cultural complexities and dynamics informing the practices at issue. Nevertheless, at the risk of oversimplifying the issue, I offer the following comments.

Most nurses would agree, I believe, that they have at least a prima facie obligation to respect the cultural practices of their patients. More specifically, they would probably accept that:

> Intolerance of another's religious or traditional practices that pose no threat of harm is, at least, discourteous and at worst, a prejudicial attitude. And it does fail to show respect for persons and their diverse religious and cultural practices.
>
> (Macklin 1998, p. 7)

This does not mean, however, that nurses are obliged — either on the basis of the above view or of the nursing profession's formally adopted code of ethics — to tolerate, *without reflective judgment*, all religious and cultural practices of their patients. There are a number of reasons for this. Firstly, to borrow from Macklin (1998, p. 17), we can 'be respectful of cultural difference *and at the same time acknowledge that there are limits*' (emphasis added). Second, the 'limits' to our obligation of respect can be discerned by a critical examination of: (1) the internal cultural justifications and considerations raised in support of a given 'harmful' religious or traditional practice; and (2) external viewpoints (that is, from other cultural groups) about the 'harmfulness' of the practice (recognising here that culture is not static and can change in positive ways when exposed to relevant influences). Thirdly, we are not obliged to be respectful of practices which, when examined comparatively from an intra-cultural and cross-cultural perspective, are themselves disrespectful and oppressive of persons.

The question remains, however, of how these considerations might apply to the case of requests being imposed on nurses to assist with medical procedures that are culturally prescribed, but nevertheless judged by nurses to be 'harmful' to persons? Let us consider a possible answer to this question in relation to the practice of female genital mutilation, taken here as referring to a traditional procedure (as opposed to a medically therapeutic procedure, say for cancer) that may involve 'only' a clitoridectomy, or may include (as well as the removal of the clitoris) the excision of parts of the labia minoria or the removal of virtually all of the external female genitalia (James 1994, pp. 6–7).

Transcultural ethics and the case of female genital mutilation

It is estimated that the practice of female genital mutilation (usually performed on girls between the ages of 7 days and 15 years [Robson 1994, p. 15]) has affected more than 134 million women worldwide (Gilmore nd; Walker and Parmar 1993). In 1998, an information letter distributed by Amnesty International Australia estimated that during any one twenty-four hour period, 6000 young girls will undergo 'the knife' believing that 'they will become more feminine, clean and obedient' (Gilmore nd).

There are a number of internal cultural justifications offered for the brutal practice of female genital mutilation; these include 'appeals to custom, religion, family honour, cleanliness, esthetics, initiation, assurance of virginity, promotion of social and political cohesion, enhancement of fertility, improvement in male sexual pleasure, and prevention of female promiscuity' (Sherwin 1992, p. 62). Significantly, most of these justifications do not stand up when considered from an internal cultural perspective.

Firstly, although practised by Muslims, Christians, Jews and animists alike, female genital mutilation as such is not supported by any formal doctrine of religion. Rather, its support 'can be attributed, at least partly, to the manipulations of knowledgeable, male religious elites' who continue to this day to perpetuate 'false understandings among their followers' that the procedure is a religious requirement rather than an inherited custom (James 1994, p. 10). Perhaps an important lesson for nurses here is to ascertain whether a given questionable 'cultural' practice does in fact have the legitimacy being claimed.

Secondly, there is ample evidence to show that the practice of female genital mutilation fails to achieve a large number of the outcomes for which it is thought to be internally justified, namely: the promotion of family honour, cleanliness, aesthetics, assurance of virginity, promotion of social and political cohesion, enhancement of fertility, and the prevention of female promiscuity. Research has shown that the negative health effects of the procedure far outweigh the supposed benefits. As James explains:

> Typically, for those undergoing the process, the operation results in severe pain, shock, infection, difficulty urinating and menstruating, malformation and scarring of the genitalia, physical and psychological trauma with sexual intercourse, bleeding, increased vulnerability to the AIDS virus, difficulty with childbirth, increased risk of sterility and infant mortality. There is also the risk of death to the female from the direct effects of the operation ... Fear, anxiety, pain, scarring and emotional trauma from circumcision combine to produce severe psychological disturbance and sexual dysfunction in many women subject to the procedure.
>
> (James 1994, pp. 8–9)

It is also known that the procedure does not 'assure virginity' or prevent 'female promiscuity'.

Thirdly, it is wrong to assume that female genital mutilation is unanimously supported in the countries and cultures where it is practised. For instance, many internal sub-cultural groups of the cultures believed to support female genital mutilation are actively working for the eradication of the practice (James 1994; Walker and Parmar 1993). The workings of these groups have included the development of local community health education programs, the production of film documentaries, and political lobbying (James 1994; Walker and Parmar 1993). There is also an increasing religious tolerance in some countries for supporting an international human rights approach to help eradicate the practice. James (1994, p. 24) writes, for example, that there is some suggestion 'Islam would be favourable to international human rights protection based on the equality of women and the moral wrongness of discrimination on the basis of sex' since in Islam, 'piety alone was to be the final test of a person's worth — woman or man'.

Another important consideration is that many cultural groups and countries condemn the practice of female genital mutilation (and the cultures that support it) on grounds of human rights violations; in some instances, countries have even outlawed the practice (for example, the United Kingdon) (James 1994; Robson 1994). In Australia, girls facing 'female circumcision' have been regarded as 'at risk' by child protection agencies and placed under supervised care (see, for example, the 1994 case of an eighteen month supervision order granted by a Victorian court for the protection of two children aged 21 months and 3 years [Saunders 1994, p. 2]). Amnesty International, among other organisations, has also been at the forefront of campaigning against female genital mutilation, and the contravention of children's rights and the rights of women 'to equality, integrity and health' that the procedure constitutes. In 1994, the Australian Medical Association called on the federal government to outlaw female genital mutilation in Australia (Robson 1994). These and other groups have presented substantive evidence supporting the harmful nature of the practice and the need for its eradication.

To some, the activities of powerful Western lobby groups like medical associations or international human rights organisations might seem little more than 'Western cultural imperialism' or an instance of the 'morality of the superior' being imposed as *the* 'superior morality'. There is room to suggest, however, that to characterise the moral activism of these and like groups as 'moral ethnocentrism' or 'cultural (moral) imperialism' is rather hollow. The millions of females who have suffered as a result of this practice might have quite a different view. And I wonder what the answer would be if these women were asked the question: 'If there was another way — a way that would enable you to function fully as respected members of your society *without* the need to undergo genital mutilation — would you still submit to such a procedure?'. But then, for many women, this question would be redundant, since being mutilated was never a matter of 'real' choice for them. And currently, for 6000 girls per day, it still is not — notwithstanding the powerful enculturation process that occurs in young girls from the day they are born to accept the practice as 'normal' and to submit to it else risk the shame, stigma and social ostracism that would inevitably follow should they refuse. As Boulware-Miller (1985 — cited in James 1994) explains:

> The stigma associated with not being circumcised attaches early, virtually compelling a choice to undergo the operation.
> An un-excised, non-infibulated girl is often despised, ridiculed and referred to as *el beydourha meno* ('who wants her?') and *el beyaresha meno* ('who marries her?').

(Boulware-Miller 1985, cited in James 1994)

The activism of a range of groups (not just one cultural group) aimed at eradicating female genital mutilation at the very least draws attention to the need to question and to call into question things as they are. It reminds us that while culture can provide a group with a 'blue print for life', it can also be imprisoning, oppressive, cruel, and provide a 'blue print for death'. In such instances, 'minding our own cultural business' (viz. 'looking the other way' and allowing mutilating traditions to arbitrarily supplant moral considerations of human wellbeing) can be just as 'imperialistic' (viz. exercising supreme authority) as 'making other people's cultures our business'. To borrow from popular feminist thought: if it is males who are being mutilated, the world acknowledges that it has a major crisis of human rights violations on its hands. But when it is females who are being mutilated, the world turns away saying: 'its culture, and we shouldn't interfere'.

The activism of external cultural groups reminds us of both the possibility and the importance of making *critical discretionary judgments* about the kinds of religious and traditional practices which we, as health care professionals, ought and ought not to respect. This critical discretionary judgment may, however, rest less on questions of 'tolerance' (including the problematic questions of intolerance and over-tolerance), than on questions of culturally informed critical reflection grounded in the lived experiences of those who suffer demonstrably and intolerably on account of cultural practices that no longer serve the survival and prosperity interests of the group if, indeed, they ever did. By engaging in such critical reflection we should be able to discern the practices against which our conscientious objection, at least, is warranted if not our fully committed collective activism aimed at their eradication.

When discerning and focusing on 'harmful' traditional and religious practices, however, it is important that we do not become distracted from our original project of improving understanding and informed tolerance of cultural diversity, or the merits of a transcultural approach to ethics. Every culture has its 'down side' *apropos* upholding questionable and possibly harmful traditional values, beliefs and practices. Furthermore, just because a certain behaviour is seen to be characteristic of a given culture, it does not follow that the behaviour in question is either accepted or regarded as being acceptable by all members of that culture. For instance, child abuse and domestic violence are characteristics of Australian society and culture; aside from the perpetrators of such abuse and violence (religious elites among them), the Australian people would, I suggest, firmly reject any notion that such abuse and violence is culturally accepted and acceptable.

The above considerations are all important and need to be taken into account when 'reading the cultural world' and drawing upon it for cues to guide our moral actions both as individuals and as professionals. But most important of all, they remind us of the need to remain committed to acquiring and maintaining a deep understanding of the cultural complexities and dynamics that inform the range of practices which people from different cultural groups may observe, and the potential for disagreement (both from within and outside of those cultural groups) about the moral acceptability of those practices.

Conclusion

Transcultural ethics, like feminist ethics, recognises the inherent difficulties associated with genuine moral problems in human life being 'confronted as abstraction rather than experiential realities' (Marshall 1992, p. 52), and affirms that, if moral abstractions are to count for anything, they must be brought 'back to earth' (Stout 1988, p. 8). It also recognises the inability of abstract and decontextualised moral thinking to provide concrete answers to complex questions concerning a range of human experiences. Key among these experiences are: human pain and suffering, intense and sometimes conflicting human emotions, ambivalent and ambiguous human relationships, and, not least, differing cultural world views about the value and meaning of life — all of which often (too often) have to be dealt with in the face of overwhelming uncertainty, the unpredictability of probable outcomes (positive and negative), fallible modes of communication, and the fallibilities of decision-makers (Stout 1988; Cortese 1990; Marshall 1992; Elliott 1992).

Unlike other moral critiques, however, transcultural ethics offers an optimistic outlook. Its suggestion that acceptance of — and achieving a harmony of — moral diversity offers the key to sustaining the existence and purpose of morality provides an important basis upon which we can all develop, not just our moral thinking and sensibilities, but our ability to actually be moral in a world characterised by diverse and competing valid world views. This is not merely compromise, as some might believe, or even tolerance — the blinded eye of an indiscriminate mind (see Wolff et al. 1969; Midgley 1991a). Nor is it confusion. Rather, it is celebration. In particular, it is the celebration of the 'other' as different, but not inferior or fallacious or superstitious — as having something worthwhile to share, not as being something worthless to be marginalised, trivialised and ignored. If we accept this, we will all be in a much better position to judge what is really unethical as opposed to being merely disliked; what is truly wrong, as opposed to being merely unfamiliar and strange; and what is really confusion as opposed to simple misunderstanding of another's moral language with which we are not familiar (Stout 1988). This insight is, among other things, what we stand to gain by embracing a diversity of moral values and beliefs as being the beginning of morality and not its end.

In conclusion, I should like to list a number of questions nurses ought to ask when making moral decisions about the nursing care of people from diverse cultural backgrounds. Borrowing from Kanitsaki:

- Is my understanding of this person's values and value systems such that it entitles me to override her or his family's requests or instructions?
- Can I by way of a third party (such as an interpreter) really ensure that my interventions will result in benefits not harms to that person?
- Are my values and frame of reference the only ones which warrant overriding consideration in this relationship?
- How do I know my judgments in this relationship are morally and culturally appropriate? In short, how do I know I am right?

(Kanitsaki 1989b, p. 70)

By asking these and similar questions, and by seeking the 'right' answers to them, nurses will demonstrate successfully that they are able to embrace morality as something more than a set of abstract self-standing principles. They will also demonstrate that, in the ultimate analysis, it is people and relationships that count — not a blind deference to rules, which, when stripped of their cultural content and context, become little more than intellectual curiosities empowered by arbitrary will, incapable of responding to the lived realities and needs of human beings who have been born into circumstances which are very often beyond their control. Embracing this approach will also remind us that:

any theory of ethics is, in the end, only as plausible as the complete picture of the world of which it forms a part.

(McNaughton 1988, p. 41)

160

Chapter 7

Moral problems and moral decision-making in nursing

Introduction

Nurses, like other health professionals, encounter many moral problems in the course of their everyday professional practice. These problems range from the relatively 'simple' to the extraordinarily complex, and can cause varying degrees of perplexity and distress in those who encounter them. For instance, some moral problems are relatively easy to resolve and may cause little if any distress to those involved; other problems, however, may be extremely difficult or even impossible to resolve, and may cause a great deal of moral stress and distress for those encountering them. Sometimes, as discussed in Chapter 1 of this text, a failure to remedy moral problems can also result in violence.

Nurses, like other health care professionals, have a fundamental and unavoidable moral responsibility to be able to identify and respond effectively to the moral problems they encounter (whether 'simple' or 'complex'), and, where able, to employ strategies to prevent them from occurring in the first place (otherwise known as 'preventionist ethics' [see Johnstone 1998, pp. 71–96]). In order to be able to do this, however, nurses must first be able to distinguish moral problems from other sorts of problems, and to be able to distinguish different types of moral problems from each other. It is to advancing knowledge and understanding of the different kinds of moral problems (as distinct from other kinds of problems, for example practical or clinical problems) that nurses might encounter in the course of their day-to-day practice — and how best to decide when encountering these problems — that provides the focus for this chapter.

Distinguishing moral problems from other sorts of problems

All health care professionals encounter a variety of problems in the course of their everyday practice, and nurses are no exception. And it is probably the case that most of these problems have a moral dimension to them. This does not mean, however, that all problems that have a moral dimension are *moral problems* per se. Part of the clue to making this distinction lies in the degree to which the moral dimension of a given problem might be deemed 'weightier' and thus *prima facie* as 'overriding' of the other dimensions of the problem, and the

161

kinds of solutions that might be fruitfully employed to resolve the problem. Consider the following example.

A patient is in severe and intolerable pain due to not receiving pain medication. Nevertheless, while this is a problem and one which clearly has a moral dimension, it is not immediately evident that the problem is a 'full-blown' moral problem per se requiring moral analysis, debate and possibly the intervention of an 'ethics expert' or ethics committee. Further analysis is required. It might be, for instance, that the patient's pain management has, for some reason, been neglected. What is required in this instance is a competent and compassionate clinical assessment of the patient and the swift administration of needed analgesia. The problem may thus be correctly characterised as a 'technical problem' requiring and resolvable by a 'clinical solution'. It might also be, however, that the patient is in pain due to her refusing pain relief on religious grounds. In such an instance even the most competent and compassionate of clinical assessments will not necessarily result in the identification of a satisfactory solution to the problem of the patient's pain since the obvious 'clinical solution' (that is, of giving analgesia) is precluded by the moral demand to respect the patient's autonomous wishes. The problem may thus be correctly characterised as a moral problem (not merely a clinical problem) since:

- the patient's moral interest and wellbeing are at risk (if her autonomous wishes are respected, she will suffer the harm of intolerable pain; conversely, if her pain is alleviated by the administration of analgesia, she will suffer the harm of having her autonomous wishes violated);
- the nurses' moral interests and wellbeing are at risk on account of the moral distress they experience at their genuine inability to maximise the patient's moral interests; and, finally,
- assistance is required to help attendant nurses to answer the question: What should we do?

To help clarify the basis upon which the above distinction has been made, the following framework is offered. It is generally accepted that something involves a (human) moral/ethical problem where it has as its central concern:

- the promotion and protection of people's genuine wellbeing and welfare (including their interests in not suffering unnecessarily);
- responding justly to the genuine needs and significant interests of different people; and
- determining and justifying what constitutes right and wrong conduct in a given situation (Frankena 1973; Blum 1980, 1994; Amato 1990; McNaughton 1988; Singer 1993; Beauchamp and Childress 1994; Bond 1996).

The nursing profession is fundamentally concerned with the promotion and protection of people's genuine wellbeing and welfare, and in achieving these ends, responding justly to the genuine needs and significant interests of different people. The nursing profession is, therefore, fundamentally concerned with 'moral problems' as well as other kinds of problems (for example, technical, clinical, legal, and so forth).

In order to deal with moral problems appropriately and effectively it is evident that nurses need to know, first, what form a moral problem might take and how to recognise it; and, second, how best to decide when dealing with them. It is to answering these questions that this discussion now turns.

Identifying moral problems in nursing

Moral problems can emerge in many forms: they can be of a somewhat 'unglamorous' nature, as in cases involving a decision about whether to restrain a happily demented elderly person who keeps wandering unaided from her bed and risks debilitating injury if she falls; or they can be of a somewhat 'exotic' nature, as in cases involving abortion, organ transplantation and experimental medicine. Our concern in this chapter, however, is not with these more practical and secondary bioethical problems but with the more fundamental and primary problems of how bioethical issues are perceived (i.e. whether they are perceived correctly, if at all), and how bioethical problems are dealt with (i.e. whether they are dealt with appropriately and effectively, or whether they are simply dismissed as being too difficult, and not dealt with at all).

Unfortunately, it is beyond the scope of this text to give the discussion that is warranted to the issue of identifying and resolving moral problems. Nevertheless, it is hoped that the following discussion will help to clarify and rectify some of the common misconceptions nurses have had about what moral problems are and how they might be best dealt with.

1. Moral unpreparedness

The first type of moral problem to be considered here is that of general 'unpreparedness' to deal appropriately and effectively with morally troubling situations. What invariably happens here is that a nurse (or other health professional) enters into a situation without being sufficiently prepared to deal with the moral complexities of that situation specifically. The nurse (or other health professional) may lack the requisite moral knowledge, moral imagination, moral experience and moral wisdom otherwise necessary to be able to deal with the moral complexities of the situation at hand (this could also count as *moral incompetence* or *moral impairment* [Johnstone 1998]). When eventually faced with a particular moral problem, the nurse acts in bad faith by pretending that the situation at hand is one which can be handled 'with one's given moral apparatus' (Lemmon 1987, p. 112). The room for moral error here, needless to say, is very considerable.

To illustrate the seriousness of moral unpreparedness, consider the analogous situation of clinical unpreparedness. A nurse who is not educated in the complexities of, say, intensive care nursing, but who is nevertheless sent to 'help out' and care for a ventilated patient in intensive care, would not only be inadequate in this role, but could even be potentially dangerous. Such a nurse would not have the learned skills necessary to detect the subtle changes in a sedated patient's condition — changes indicating, for example, the need for more sedation, or the need to perform tracheal suctioning, or the need to increase the tidal volume of air flow or oxygen administration. Neither would this nurse be able to distinguish the many different alarms that can go off on the high-tech equipment being used to give full life support to the patient, or to detect any malfunctioning of this sophisticated equipment. Without these skills, a nurse working in intensive care would be likely to place the life and wellbeing of the patient at serious risk.

The argument of the seriousness of unpreparedness also applies to the complexities of sound ethical reasoning and ethical health care practice generally. Such a nurse, left to deal with a morally troubling situation, would not only be inadequate in that role but, as the intensive care example shows, his or her practice could be potentially hazardous. Without the learned moral skills necessary to detect moral problems and to resolve them in a sound, reliable and defensible manner, an unprepared nurse, no matter how well intentioned, could fail to correctly detect moral hazards in the workplace, and therefore fail to act or respond in a way that would prevent a moral calamity from occurring.

The kinds of moral calamities or near calamities that can occur as a result of nurses' (and doctors', and other allied health professionals') moral unpreparedness to deal appropriately and effectively with moral problems in professional practice are well illustrated by the numerous anecdotal case studies and other factual legal case studies discussed in both the nursing and bioethical literature. The 'unfortunate experiment' at Auckland's National Women's Hospital, discussed in Chapter 2, is an important example here. The moral unpreparedness of nurses and doctors alike resulted in an unchecked violation of patients' rights for over twenty years. Some women have been left permanently scarred — both emotionally and physically — as a result of this experiment; and still other women have needlessly lost their lives. Had the doctors and nurses witnessing the 'unfortunate experiment' been better prepared to deal with the moral complexities involved, the moral calamity that followed could have been prevented.

An important Australian example of the kind of moral calamity that can occur as a consequence of nurses' and others' moral unpreparedness to respond effectively to moral problems in health care contexts can be found in the human tragedy involving Sydney's Chelmsford Private Hospital. In this case, many people were left permanently damaged and scarred — some even died — as a result of receiving deep sleep therapy (DST) prescribed by Dr Harry Bailey, a consultant psychiatrist, who later suicided in connection with the scandal that was eventually uncovered (Bromberger and Fife-Yeomans 1991; Rice 1988). It is now known that approximately one thousand patients were 'treated' with DST at this hospital. It is also known, as revealed as early as 1977 by the current affairs television program '60 Minutes', that many of these patients did not receive the standard of care and treatment they were entitled to receive. Among other things — including the deaths of seven people between 1974 and 1977 — the '60 Minutes' program revealed that 'recognised standard precautions for the safety of patients were not taken; and that patients received the treatment without their consent' (Bromberger and Fife-Yeomans 1991, p. 142). In the Chelmsford Royal Commission that was eventually established in 1988 to 'examine the provision of Deep Sleep Therapy and the administration of Chelmsford Private Hospital', it was confirmed that:

> The signature of some [consent] forms were obtained by fraud and deceit. Some were signed by people whose judgment was compromised by drugs. Some patients were even woken up from their DST [Deep Sleep Therapy] treatment to complete their authorisation. Other patients were treated contrary to their express wishes and some were treated despite the fact they had specifically refused the treatment.
>
> (Commissioner Slattery, cited in Bromberger and Fife-Yeomans 1991, p. 171)

Nursing care was also seriously substandard. In one notable case, the nursing care had been so negligent that a patient developed severe decubitus ulcers between her knees, which became 'glued' together as though they had been skin-grafted. The former patient recalled:

I was having hallucinations about a lot of coloured ribbons and trying to climb out through them finding the world again. I woke up in a bath tub and two nurses were bathing me. I felt really dirty. One of the nurses said, 'My God, look at her knees.' I looked down and they were joined together. The nurses gently pulled them apart.

(Bromberger and Fife-Yeomans 1991, p. 94)

Bromberger and Fife-Yeomans (1991, p. 94) comment that the patient 'still retains the scars on the inside of her knees'.

Another example of the substandard nursing care that was provided (or more to the point, *not* provided) can be found in the experiences of another patient, Barry Hart, outlined in the following statement read to the New South Wales Parliament in 1984:

Basic, commonsense nursing practice was ignored. Patients were sedated for ten days and given no exercise during this period. They were incontinent of faeces and urine most of the time and were left lying incontinent of faeces until they woke up.

There was no attempt to maintain a fluid balance. Patients wet the bed and remained lying in the urine until the sheets were changed. The staff made an approximation of whether the patients were actually passing urine (i.e. a fluid output) by seeing how wet the bed was.

(cited in Rice 1988, p. 47)

One of the troubling things about the whole Chelmsford scandal is that rumours about Dr Bailey's unscrupulous practices had been circulating for years, yet nothing was done about it (Bromberger and Fife-Yeomans 1991, p. 176). Equally disturbing is the fact that it was not until 1988 — twenty-four years after the investigated death of the first 'deep sleep' patient, and only after 'treatment' had led to the deaths of twenty-four patients — that a Royal Commission was set up to investigate the allegations concerning the blatant patient abuse that was subsequently proved to have occurred at Chelmsford Private Hospital (Bromberger and Fife-Yeomans 1991, p. 162). Significantly, in the Royal Commission of Inquiry that was conducted, and in the report on its findings, it was revealed that between 1963 and 1979 only *two* nurses took action in an attempt to expose the unscrupulous practices they had observed (*Report of the Royal Commission into Deep Sleep Therapy* 1990, p. 127). As in the case of the 'unfortunate experiment', there is room to speculate here that had nursing personnel been better prepared to recognise and respond effectively to violations of professional ethical standards, the trauma and suffering experienced by the patients at Chelmsford could have been reduced considerably, if not avoided altogether.

Not all moral calamities occurring in health care contexts are as ethically exotic as those that occurred in the 'unfortunate experiment' and the Chelmsford Private Hospital cases, however. Moral calamities can and do occur on a much more commonplace level in the health care arena. Consider, for example, the common but morally odious practice of withholding nourishing tube feeds from severe stroke patients. Wilson-Barnett (1986) cites the heart-rending case of a 66-year-old man who had suffered several strokes and as a result had been left paralysed, aphasic, depressed and suicidal. After two months of rigorous medical and nursing care, a medical decision was made to discontinue his nourishing tube feeds and to commence a three-hourly regime of restricted water. The fluid regime was not sufficient for his needs, however, and he became severely dehydrated. As his condition deteriorated, he began to pass only small quantities of offensive urine and, despite full nursing care, became malodorous and halitotic. Because of his terrible smells, few people entered his room. A senior student nurse involved in caring for him was very distressed about his discomfort, but relayed her distress only to other nurses. Her concerns were not relayed to the patient's attending physician, and she felt unable to approach him herself. (In fact, in accordance with hospital norms, students at that time were not generally encouraged to approach senior doctors.) After ten days of existing in a dehydrated, anuric, malodorous and halitotic state, the patient died. The student nurse meanwhile continued to suffer on account of what she perceived as her dismal failure to maintain her patient's dignity and to 'speak up on his behalf' (Wilson-Barnett 1986, p. 125).

Registered nurses all know that this type of scenario is common, and may occur in a ward not once but a dozen times, and in a hospital not once but a thousand times (see, for example, Lynn 1989). What may not be so well appreciated, however, is that the kind of suffering that occurs in these and similar scenarios is very often unnecessary and preventable. Had the participants in Wilson-Barnett's example been better prepared as moral negotiators and moral mediators, the simple remedy of giving more water to the stroke patient might have been quickly and simply advocated. Instead, all involved were hopelessly paralysed by their moral ignorance and unpreparedness, and as a result both the patient and the student nurse suffered needlessly. Other registered nurses who have had experiences similar to those of the student nurse in this example have carried the guilt incurred by their experiences for years. When discussing their experiences in educational forums I have conducted, they have broken down and cried — mostly because of the relief of at least being able to discuss their experiences openly and in a non-judgmental environment.

2. Moral blindness

A second type of problem that nurses very often encounter is that of what I shall call 'moral blindness'. A morally blind nurse (or other health professional) is someone who, upon encountering a moral problem, simply does not see it as a *moral* problem. Instead, they may perceive it as either a clinical or a technical problem. Carlton (1978, p. 10) argues, on the basis of her field research, that there is a tendency by many health professionals (particularly doctors) 'to translate ethical issues into technical problems which have clinical solutions'.

Moral blindness can be crudely likened to colour-blindness. Just as a colour-blind person fails to distinguish certain colours in the world, a morally blind person fails to distinguish certain 'moral properties' in the world. Perhaps a better example can be found by appealing to a set of imageries commonly associated with Gestalt psychology and theories on the nature of perception. What I particularly have in mind here are the two drawings which are popularly presented in psychology texts to demonstrate certain perceptual phenomena, including perceptual organisation and the influence of context on the way in which an object is perceived.

The first of these drawings (Figure 7.1) depicts what initially appears to be a white vase or goblet against a black background; after a more sustained glance, the drawing changes (or rather, one's perception 'shifts') and what is perceived instead are two black facial profiles separated by a white space. Some people see the alternating vase–face images relatively quickly and easily, while others struggle to shake off what for them remains the dominant image (i.e. *either* the vase *or* the faces).

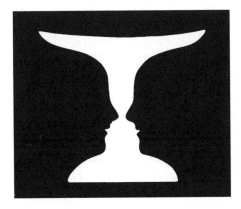

Figure 7.1 Reversible figure and background

(reproduced with permission from R. L. Atkinson, R. C. Atkinson and E. R. Hilgard, *Introduction to psychology*, 8th edn, Harcourt Brace Jovanovich, New York, 1983, p. 139)

The second ambiguous drawing (Figure 7.2) depicts what can be seen as either an unsophisticated-looking old woman or a very sophisticated-looking young woman. As with the vase–face drawing, some people see the alternating old woman–young woman images relatively easily, while others literally get 'stuck' with a dominant perception of *either* the young woman *or* the old woman.

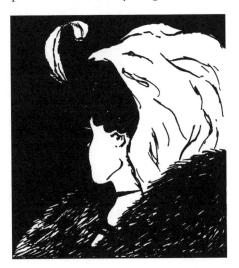

Figure 7.2 Ambiguous stimulus

(reproduced with permission from R. L. Atkinson, R. C. Atkinson and E. R. Hilgard, *Introduction to psychology*, 8th edn, Harcourt Brace Jovanovich, New York, 1983, p. 139)

Psychologists claim, however, that people's perceptions can be altered by context — in this instance, by showing photographs before the ambiguous drawings are viewed. They claim that, on an initial viewing of this drawing, 65 per cent report seeing the young woman first. If subjects are shown photographs of an old woman before seeing the drawing, however, almost all see the old woman first.

The same 'reversals' can be achieved by conditioning subjects with photographs to see the young woman first (Atkinson et al. 1983, p. 147).

I am not here attempting to present an elaborate theory of moral perception but merely trying to illustrate what I believe is a common and a potentially morally dangerous phenomenon in health care contexts: that of impaired moral perception. There is, I think, some room to suggest that health professionals (including nurses) are so dominated and conditioned by the 'clinical imagery' around them that, when they do encounter a bona fide moral problem, it is very often perceived not as a *moral* problem per se, but as a *clinical* or a *technical* problem and, as such, one requiring a clinical solution, not a moral solution. Some health professionals have a healthy perception of the alternating moral–clinical images depicted by a given scenario; many, however, remain stuck with a dominant *clinical image* and just simply do not see the alternative *moral image*, which for them is less discernible. One unfortunate consequence of this, of course, is that *technically correct* decisions are made at the expense of *morally correct* decisions.

The extent to which clinical perceptions and judgments dominate over moral perceptions and judgments is well illustrated by the common hospital practice of ordering 'Not For Resuscitation' (NFR) on hopelessly or chronically ill patients. It is probably true to say that many doctors and nurses perceive NFR practices as involving a *clinical issue*, not a *moral issue*, and, as such, one to be rightly decided by doctors, not ethicists. The clinical–moral Gestalt problem became particularly clear to me at a nursing law and ethics conference in 1988. After presenting a paper on the nature and moral implications of NFR orders, I was approached by several registered nurses with what has now become a familiar and distressing comment: 'My God! I had never thought about it [NFR] as a *moral* issue before ... What have I done?'. The issue was taken up by the media (see Miller 1988, 1989; Schumpeter 1988; Craig 1989; *Upfront* 1988); other nurses wanted to challenge or attack the view that NFR directives involve moral decisions. The Victorian State President of the Australian Medical Association, Dr Bill McCubbery, was prompted to respond to the issue, and is reported as saying that 'NFR decisions had to depend on professional judgment' (Schumpeter 1988, p. 21); the failure to mention 'moral judgment' is, I think, illuminating.

The clinical–moral Gestalt shift that has occurred in those who have been persuaded that current NFR practices have a profound *moral* dimension as well as a clinical dimension has been, for me, an interesting phenomenon to observe.

Other equally persuasive examples of the extent to which clinical perceptions and judgments dominate over ethical perceptions and judgments can be found in sociologist Wendy Carlton's work, '*In our professional opinion ...': the primacy of clinical judgment over moral choice* (1978), in which she details a number of persuasive anecdotal case studies collected while doing field research in a university teaching hospital. One case study, which has already been briefly mentioned in Chapter 3, concerns an 11-year-old Down's syndrome child who had been admitted to hospital for a hysterectomy. It will be recalled that most of the doctors and nurses involved in the case were appalled that this child was being considered for such a radical operation, yet felt that they could not go against the consulting physician's decision. Interestingly, the moral problem posed by this case was not resolved by open and honest moral debate among those involved, but by the anaesthetist declaring that because of a pre-existing heart condition the child was unfit for a general anaesthetic and surgery. As Carlton (1978, p. 37) points out, the child's heart condition conveniently 'allowed the sidestepping of ethical concerns in favour of sound clinical reasons against surgery'.

The issue of 'moral blindness' among nurses is an important and far-reaching one, and, as with the problem of moral unpreparedness, risks the realisation of otherwise avoidable moral harms. I do not believe that this problem is insurmountable, however. Just as subjects can be 'conditioned' to see the old woman rather than the young woman in the ambiguous drawing shown in Figure 7.2, so too can nurses, doctors and allied health professionals be 'conditioned' to see the moral dimension of an ambiguous scenario which can be perceived as involving either a moral problem or a clinical or technical problem. The critical question here, however, is: What kind of conditioning should nurses and others be given to ensure that they do experience a Gestalt clinical–moral shift in their professional perceptions?

Whatever the answer is to this question, the unhappy reality remains that, unless nurses, doctors and other health professionals remedy their 'moral blindness', they will never be in a position to identify and respond effectively to morally iniquitous practices in health care settings. It hardly needs pointing out that the possible consequences of this 'moral disability' could be extremely tragic, and could result in avoidable human suffering like that which occurred in the cases of the 'unfortunate experiment' and the Chelmsford Private Hospital.

3. Moral indifference

A third type of problem which nurses may encounter is that of 'moral indifference'. Moral indifference is characterised by an unconcerned or uninterested attitude toward demands to be moral; in short, it assumes the attitude of 'why bother to be moral?'. The morally indifferent person is someone who typically refrains from expressing any desire that certain acts should or should not be done in all comparable circumstances (Hare 1981, p. 185). An example of a morally indifferent nurse would be a nurse who is both unconcerned about and uninterested in alleviating a patient's pain, or is unconcerned about or uninterested in the fact that an NFR (Not For Resuscitation) directive or an order to perform ECT (Electroconvulsive Therapy) has been given on an unconsenting patient, or is unconcerned about and uninterested in any form of violation of patients' rights, for that matter. As well as this, a morally indifferent nurse would probably refrain from expressing a desire that anything should or should not be done about such situations.

The problem of moral indifference in nursing is well captured by Mila Aroskar (1986) in her illuminating article 'Are nurses' mind sets compatible with ethical practice?'. Aroskar (1986, p. 72) cites the findings of a study done in the late 1970s which showed that nurses tended to defer to institutional norms 'even when patients' rights were being violated'. She also points out that, despite the North American nursing profession's formal commitment to ethical practice (as manifested, among other things, by its formal adoption of various codes and standards of practice), arguments are still widely heard among nurses that 'ethical practice is too risky and requires a certain amount of heroism on the part of nurses' (Aroskar 1986, p. 69). Although Aroskar is writing from a North American point of view, her words apply equally to many nursing care contexts outside the United States of America.

The retreat by nurses into moral indifference, while not condonable, is understandable. The North American legal cases of *Tuma v Board of Nursing of the State of Idaho* (1979), *Warthen v Toms River Community Memorial*

Hospital (1985) and *Free v Holy Cross Hospital* (1987) stand as sobering reminders of the kinds of difficulties nurses might find themselves in when attempting to conduct morally responsible, professional practice, and the ultimate price that can be paid for taking a firm moral stand (see also Johnstone 1994, Chapter 9). In the *Tuma case*, a registered nurse by the name of Jolene Lucile Tuma, a clinical teacher, had been involved in caring for a patient by the name of Grace Wahlstrom who had been suffering from leukemia for a number of years. Mrs Wahlstrom asked Tuma to discuss with her possible alternative (unorthodox) treatments to chemotherapy, which Tuma agreed to do. The patient's family, however, took exception to Tuma giving Grace Wahlstrom the information she had requested, and immediately informed the consulting physician. Upon being contacted by the patient's family, the physician asked for Tuma's name. Two weeks later, despite receiving chemotherapy, the patient died. The physician meanwhile reported Tuma's actions to the state board of nursing, and she was subsequently deregistered. The ground for her deregistration was that she had 'interfered with the physician–patient relationship', and thus was guilty of 'professional misconduct'.

Tuma took her case to the Supreme Court and appealed against the state board's decision to deregister her. Although Tuma won her case, the publicity given to it had effectively ruined her professional nursing career, and she 'felt it unwise' to resume her nursing practice (King 1985, p. 162; see also Johnstone 1994, Chapter 6). It is perhaps worth noting here that Tuma did not win her case on grounds of the legitimacy of the relationship she had with her patient (and of legitimately meeting her patient's expressed needs and considered wishes in that relationship), but on a technical point of law pertaining to the state nursing board's failure to make explicit just *what* constituted an 'interference with the physician–patient relationship', and, further, that interference with the physician–patient relationship constituted 'unprofessional conduct' (Johnstone 1994, Chapter 6).

In the *Warthen case* (already briefly mentioned in Chapter 2, pp. 19–20) a registered nurse by the name of Corinne Warthen was dismissed after refusing to dialyse a terminally ill bilateral amputee patient. It will be recalled that Warthen cited 'moral, medical and philosophical objections' to performing the procedure, since it was causing the patient more harm. In the legal case that followed, the court did not accept her defence, and Warthen lost her appeal against what she argued was an 'unfair dismissal'.

Finally, in the American legal case *Free v Holy Cross Hospital* (1987) (also briefly mentioned in Chapter 2, pp. 20–1) a nurse was dismissed for insubordination because she refused to evict a seriously ill and bedridden patient from hospital. It will be recalled that at one point the nurse was instructed to remove the patient 'even if removal required forcibly putting the patient in a wheelchair and leaving her in the park' (*Free v Holy Cross Hospital* 1987, p. 1189). It will be further recalled that the nurse took the case to court, arguing that her dismissal was unfair. In defence of her actions, Free argued that to evict the patient would have been:

> in violation of her ethical duty as a registered nurse not to engage in dishonourable, unethical or unprofessional conduct of a character likely to harm the public as mandated by the *Illinois Nursing Act*.
>
> (*Free's case* 1987, p. 1190)

The court hearing the case did not accept Free's defence, however, and she lost her fight to be reinstated.

The difficulties nurses often face when trying to deliver ethically responsible nursing care are worldwide. We all know (and, no doubt, have even personally experienced at some stage) the forces that can be brought to bear upon a nurse who takes a moral position which conflicts with established hospital norms and etiquette. The degree to which many professional nurses feel intolerably burdened in their efforts to deliver ethical nursing practice has been made clear to me by comments made at a number of nursing ethics seminars and in-service lectures I have given in Australia. For example, in two separate incidents, registered nurses openly broke down and cried in a room full of people when relating morally troubling experiences they had each personally had. In one of these incidents the registered nurse told of how she had been ordered to administer large and potentially lethal doses of narcotics to an unconscious, terminally ill patient. Upon performing a thorough pain assessment of the patient in question, however, she judged the prescribed analgesia regime to be excessive, and concluded that giving the amounts ordered would almost certainly hasten the patient's death. She reasoned further that giving the prescribed analgesia regime would, in this instance, be tantamount to committing murder. The dilemma for her was that she had 'not been trained to kill people', and yet here she was being expected to do just that. When she voiced her concerns to a senior nurse administrator, she was strongly criticised and accused of being personally and professionally 'immature' — a view which the prescribing doctor also came to share. The nurse was told that, if she persisted in her objection to administering the prescribed analgesia regime, she would have to leave her job (Johnstone 1987, p. 30).

Other sobering examples of the kinds of difficulties nurses can face when taking a moral stand on a nursing matter can be found in Chapter 14 in the discussion on Not For Resuscitation directives, and in Chapter 15 in the discussion on conscientious objection.

It is then perhaps understandable (be it so not excusable) that nurses become morally indifferent to the violations of patients' rights and other unjust practices in health care domains. The reality is that both legal and institutional constraints may make it very difficult for nurses to act morally. The price paid for acting morally or for taking a moral stand can be intolerably high, as we have seen. What this signifies, however, is not that nurses should abandon the demands of morality; rather, they should seek ways in which morality's demands can be safely and effectively upheld (see, for example, Johnstone 1998).

4. Amoralism

A fourth type of moral problem which nurses might encounter, and which is similar to moral indifference, is that of 'amoralism', which is characterised by an absence of moral concern and a rejection of morality altogether (a position significantly different from *immoralism*, [discussed below] which accepts morality, but violates its demands). An amoral person is someone who refrains from making moral judgments and who typically rejects being bound by any of morality's behavioural prescriptions and proscriptions. If an amoralist were to ask: 'Why should I be moral?', it is likely that no answer would be satisfactory. (For a helpful response to the question 'Why should I be moral?', see Nielsen 1989.)

A nurse who is an amoralist would reject any compulsion to behave morally as a professional. For example, the amoral nurse might reject that there is any moral compulsion to alleviate a patient's pain even though it was possible to do so, or not to violate a patient's rights. The amoral nurse would also probably claim that it does not make any sense even to speak of things like a patient's pain or its relief, or the violation of a patient's rights, in terms of being 'good' or 'bad'; for the amoral nurse, moral language itself has no meaning. The amoralist's position in this respect is analogous to the atheist's rejection of certain religious terms. The extreme atheist, for example, would argue against uttering the word 'God', since it refers to nothing and therefore has no meaning. Such an atheist might also claim that there is no point in engaging in a religious debate on the existence of God, since there is just nothing there to debate. To try and debate the existence of God would be like trying to debate the existence of 'a black cat in a darkened room when there isn't one!'. The amoralist may argue in a similar way in relation to the issue of morality.

It can be seen that the amoralist's position is an extreme one, and one which is very difficult to sustain. (Even thieves, who may appear amoral, act on the 'moral' assumption that it is good/right to steal.) Perhaps the most approximate example that can be given here is that of psychopaths or frontal lobe damaged persons who simply lack all capacity to be moral (see Damasio 1994). If amoralism is encountered in health care contexts, it is likely that very little can be done, morally speaking, to deal with it. The only recourse in dealing with the amoral health professional would be to appeal to non-moral censuring mechanisms such as legal and/or professional disciplinary measures (see, for example, Johnstone 1998).

5. Immoralism[1]

At its most basic, immoral conduct (also known as moral turpitude and moral delinquency) can be defined as any act involving a deliberate violation of accepted or agreed ethical standards. Moral turpitude (a notion which has received more stringent attention in the United States of America than in Australia) has been defined specifically as:

> anything done knowingly contrary to justice, honesty, principle, or good morals ... [or] an act of baseness, vileness or depravity in the private or social duties which a man [sic] owes to his fellow man [sic] or to society in general. The term implies something immoral in itself.
>
> (*Seary v State Bar of Texas* — cited in Freckelton 1996, p 142)

Moral delinquency, in turn, is taken here as referring to any act involving moral negligence or a dereliction of moral duty. As in the above definitions, moral delinquency in professional contexts entails a deliberate or careless violation of agreed standards of ethical professional conduct.

Accepting the above account, an immoral nurse can thus be described as someone who knowingly and wilfully violates the agreed norms of ethical professional conduct or general ethical standards of conduct towards others. Judging immoral conduct, by this view, would require a demonstration that the accepted ethical standards of the profession were (1) known by an offending nurse, and (2) deliberately and recklessly violated by that nurse. There are many

---

1. Adapted from Johnstone, M-J (1998). Determining and responding effectively to ethical professional misconduct in nursing: a report to the Nurses Board of Victoria. Melbourne. Section 6: Responding effectively to breaches of ethical standards of conduct in nursing, pp. 71–96.

'obvious' examples of immoral conduct by nurses. These include: the deliberate theft of patients/clients money for personal use (see, for example, Chapell 1994, p. 29); the sexual, verbal and physical abuse of patients/clients (see, for example, *Nexus* 1996, p. 7; Kent 1990, p. 20); xenophobic behaviours (including racism, sexism, ageism, homophobia and a range of other unjust discriminatory behaviours [see, for example, O'Hanlan et al. 1997; Stevens and Herbert 1997; Johnstone and Kanitsaki 1991]); participation in unscrupulous research practices (see, for example, Vessey 1994; Coney 1988), and so on.

It should be noted that regardless of whether an act involving the violation of agreed professional or general ethical standards results in a significant moral harm to another, it would still stand as an instance of immoral conduct. For example, a nurse who knowingly and recklessly breaches a patient's/client's confidentiality would have committed an unethical act even if the breach in question did not result in any significant moral harm to the patient/client.

6. Moral complacency

A sixth type of moral problem nurses can encounter is that of 'moral complacency', defined by Unwin (1985, p. 205) as 'a general unwillingness to accept that one's moral opinions may be mistaken'. It could also be described as a general unwillingness to 'let go' one's own point of view as the *only point of view*, or to put one's own point of view alongside other views as *just one of many to be compared, contrasted and considered*. Again, we do not need to look far to find examples of moral complacency in health care contexts.

I recall being approached by a gerontology clinical nurse specialist lamenting the 'short-sightedness' of some of her students, who were of the view that elderly people in residential care homes should be resuscitated in the event of cardiac arrest, and that the blanket NFR status given to all elderly residents upon entering a residential care home was both immoral and illegal. The nurse specialist was insistent that the students were morally wrong, and was clearly disturbed and outraged by their position.

In my response to her, I enquired concerning the discussion she had with her students whether anyone had thought to ask the elderly residents what their preferences were — whether, in the event of cardiac arrest, *they* wished to be resuscitated or not? It should be noted that elderly people entering a residential care agency are almost invariably asked whether upon their death they wish to be cremated, or where they wish to be buried; they are not generally asked whether they wish to be resuscitated if and when they cardiac arrest. The nurse specialist became obviously agitated by my question, and exclaimed: 'Surely it is ludicrous to ask all elderly residents whether they wish to be resuscitated!'. After I had expressed my disagreement and pointed out the minimal requirements of the moral principle of autonomy, the nurse specialist retorted: 'Would you really expect us to ask each and every resident whether they wish to be resuscitated? It's ludicrous! It's silly! It's unnecessary ...'. To this retort, I reminded the nurse specialist that elderly residents are already asked whether they wish to be cremated or where they wish to be buried upon their death so what was so difficult about asking them whether they wish to be resuscitated? The nurse specialist was still unconvinced, and persisted in rejecting the view I was putting to her. She further maintained that it was right and proper that all elderly residents should be uniformly labelled NFR upon admission to a residential nursing care home. Even the thought that such a practice was tantamount to mass passive involuntary euthanasia failed to move her. The attitude of the nurse specialist in this anecdote is an example of moral complacency.

Like moral unpreparedness and moral blindness, moral complacency is, I believe, something which can be rectified by moral education and moral consciousness raising. The objective of taking this action would be, of course, to produce in the morally complacent person the attitude that nobody can afford to be complacent in the way they ordinarily view the world — least of all the moral world. This is particularly so in instances where *other* people's moral interests are at stake. It is a grave mistake to assume that our moral opinions are 'right' *just because* they are our own opinions. As ethical professionals, our stringent moral responsibility is to *question* our taken-for-granted assumptions about the world, and not to presume their inviolability.

7. Moral fanaticism

A seventh type of moral problem which may be encountered by nurses, and which is similar in many respects to moral complacency, is that of 'moral fanaticism'. The moral fanatic is someone who is thoroughly 'wedded to certain ideals' and uncritically and unreflectingly makes moral judgments according to them (Hare 1981, p. 170). Richard Hare's celebrated case of the fanatical Nazi is a good example here (Hare 1963, Chapter 9). The fanatical Nazi in this case stringently clings to the ideal of a pure Aryan German race and the need to exterminate all Jews as a means of purging the German race of its impurities. The Nazi falls into the category of being a 'fanatic' when he/she insists that, if any Nazis discover themselves to be of Jewish descent, then they too should be exterminated along with all the rest of the Jews (Hare 1963, pp. 161–2).

Examples of moral fanaticism abound in health care contexts. The surgeon who repeatedly operates in order to 'save life' regardless of a dying patient's wishes to the contrary, or regardless of the suffering it causes, is an important example here. Morally fanatical doctors in this instance might further boost their position by claiming that it is a supremely moral one. The maintenance of absolute confidentiality, even though harm might be caused as a result, is another good example. So, too, is the example of a doctor or a nurse forcing unwanted information on a patient in the fanatical belief that all patients must be told the truth, even if the patient in question has specifically requested not to receive the information.

In the case of moral fanatics, an appeal to overriding considerations or principles of conduct would not be helpful (Hare 1981, p. 178). As with the amoralist, the problem of the moral fanatic in health care contexts is likely to have disappointing outcomes. In the final analysis, it may be that other (non-moral) mechanisms will have to be appealed to in order to resolve the moral problems caused by moral fanaticism; for example, it may be necessary to seek the adjudicating involvement of a public advocate, a court of law or a disciplinary body.

8. Moral disagreements and controversies

A eighth type of moral problem nurses will very often encounter is that involving 'moral disagreement' — concerning, for example, the selection, interpretation, application and evaluation of moral standards. Milo (1986) identifies two fundamental types of moral disagreement: internal moral disagreement and radical moral disagreement.

Internal moral disagreement

Three forms of internal moral disagreement can occur. The first of these involves a fundamental conflict about the force or priority of accepted moral standards. For example, two people may agree to common moral standards but disagree about what to do when these standards come into conflict. Milo (1986, p. 455) argues that the disagreement here is not necessarily attributable to 'any disagreement in factual beliefs or to bad reasoning', but to a disagreement in *attitude* (see also McNaughton 1988, pp. 17, 29). Consider the following hypothetical example to illustrate Milo's point.

Two nurses might both accept a moral standard which generally requires truth-telling, but may disagree on when this standard should apply. Nurse A, for instance, might favour (that is, have a 'pro-attitude' towards) telling the truth to patient X about a pessimistic medical diagnosis. Nurse B, on the other hand, might not favour (i.e. might have a 'con-attitude' towards) telling the truth to patient X about this diagnosis and prefer a pro-attitude to avoiding unnecessary suffering (e.g. as a result of a nocebo effect that might be inadvertently stimulated upon learning about the diagnosis). It is not that these two nurses have different criteria of relevance, as such, but rather have *different principles of priority* (Milo 1986, p. 457).

A second type of internal disagreement centres on what are to count as acceptable exceptions and limitations to otherwise mutually agreed moral standards. As Milo explains, we generally accept that moral standards are limited by other moral standards, as well as by the competing claims of self-interest. (Morality does not usually expect us to risk our own lives or our own important moral interest in morally troubling situations.) People might agree that as a general rule we ought all to make certain modest sacrifices in terms of our own interests (a minimal requirement of justice), but may disagree 'about what constitutes a modest sacrifice' (Milo 1986, p. 459). In many respects this type of disagreement could be loosely described as a disagreement in interpretation of an accepted moral standard. Consider another example.

Two nurses might agree that patients' rights should not be violated. Nurse A might further hold that, in situations involving violations of patients' rights, a nurse should act — even if this means threatening the nurse's job security (which nurse A views as a modest sacrifice). Nurse B, on the other hand, might agree that nurses should in principle act to prevent a patient's rights from being violated, but disagree that nurses should do so if they stand to lose their jobs as a result (something which nurse B views as an unacceptable and extreme sacrifice). What these two nurses are essentially disagreeing about is not the moral standard per se (that nurses should act to prevent violations of patients' rights), but about when morally relevant considerations can be and cannot be overridden by self-interest. In disagreements like this, and where the disagreement is based on preferences rather than attitude, there may well be no happy solution, a situation which Milo calls a 'moral deadlock' (1986, p. 461).

A third and final type of internal moral disagreement centres on the selection and applicability of accepted ethical standards. This kind of disagreement has nothing to do with whether a standard can be overridden by other considerations, but concerns whether it should have been selected or appealed to in the first place.

For example, two nurses may agree that killing an innocent human being is wrong. They may disagree, however, that abortion is wrong. Nurse A, for example, might argue that, since the fetus is not a human being, abortion does not entail the killing of an innocent human being and therefore is not wrong. Appealing to a moral standard prohibiting the killing of innocent human life would then, for nurse A, be quite irrelevant. Nurse B, on the other hand, may argue that the fetus is a human being, and therefore abortion, since it entails killing an innocent human being, is absolutely morally wrong. Appealing to a moral standard prohibiting the killing of innocent human life would then, for nurse B, be supremely relevant. The disagreement between these two nurses hinges very much on a disagreement about the moral relevance of the facts on what constitutes a human being.

Radical moral disagreement

Milo (1986) identifies two types of radical moral disagreement: the first type he calls 'partial radical moral disagreement', and the second type 'total radical moral disagreement'.

In cases of *partial radical moral disagreement*, dissenting parties might agree on some criteria of relevance but not all. For example, a nurse might argue that directly killing terminally and chronically ill patients with a lethal injection is morally wrong, whereas merely 'letting nature take its course' or 'letting patients die' is not morally wrong. Another nurse might agree that directly killing terminally and chronically ill patients is wrong, but thoroughly disagree that merely 'letting patients die' is less morally offensive. Here there may be no court of appeal to reconcile the distinction between direct 'killing' and merely 'letting die'. In this case, partial radical disagreement is very similar to internal moral disagreement. It may be very difficult to distinguish between the two, a point which Milo reluctantly concedes.

In cases of *total radical moral disagreement*, disputants do not agree on any criteria of relevance, and do not share any basic moral principles. For Milo (1986, p. 469), this is 'the most extreme kind of moral disagreement that one can imagine'.

An example of total radical moral disagreement would be where two theatre nurses radically disagree with each other about the moral acceptability of organ transplantations. Nurse A argues that retrieving or harvesting organs from so-called 'cadavers' is an unmitigated act of murder, since the person whose organs are being retrieved is not yet fully dead. (Nurse A, in this instance, rejects brain-death criteria as indicative of death.) Nurse A also argues that, even if the potential cadaver is restored to nothing more than a persistent vegetative state, and even if another person may die as a result of not getting a life-saving organ transplant operation, this does not justify violating the sanctity of life of the potential organ donor. The death of another person through not receiving a new organ, while 'unfortunate', cannot be helped. Such are the tragic twists of life.

Nurse B, on the other hand, argues that retrieving organs is nothing like murder since, among other things, the person is already dead. (Nurse B, in this instance, totally accepts brain-death criteria as indicative of death.) Nurse B also totally rejects a 'sanctity of life' view, arguing that it has no substance; only quality of life considerations have ethical meaning. Nurse B further argues that, even conceding the unreliability of brain-death criteria as indicative of death, retrieving the organs is still morally permissible, since the donating person can at best look forward only to a 'vegetative existence' and one devoid of any 'quality of life' (which is cruel and immoral), whereas an organ recipient could look forward to a renewed quality of life.

In the dispute between nurse A and nurse B, resolution is unlikely. As Milo points out, in total radical disagreement the disputants reach a total and irreconcilable impasse. The possibility of this situation occurring in health care contexts is, I believe, something which needs to be taken very seriously, and which has important implications for conscientious objection claims (an issue that is given separate consideration in Chapter 15 of this text).

It should be clarified here that, while moral disagreements can certainly be problematic (particularly if a person's life and wellbeing are hanging in the balance, and an immediate decision is needed about what should be done), these need not be taken as constituting grounds upon which morality as such should be viewed with scepticism or, worse, rejected altogether. As Stout (1988, p. 14) argues persuasively, the facts of moral disagreement 'don't *compel* us to become nihilists or skeptics, to abandon the notions of moral truth and justified moral belief'. One reason for this, he explains, is that moral disagreement is, in essence, just a kind of moral diversity or, as he calls it, 'conceptual diversity' (Stout 1988, pp. 15, 61). While moral disagreement may rightly challenge us to 'meticulously disentangle' diverse and conflicting moral points of view, it does not preclude or threaten the possibility of moral judgment per se, either within a particular culture or across many cultures (Stout 1988, p. 15).

In the previous chapter, it was argued that moral disagreement has historically been the beginning of critical moral thinking, not its end. Given this, there is room to suggest that we should be very cautious in accepting Milo's pessimistic conclusions about the irreconcilability of radical moral disagreement. Instead, we should look towards a more optimistic solution, and view such disagreements as an important and necessary opportunity for 'enriching [our] conceptions of morality through comparative inquiry' (Stout 1988, p. 70), and thereby augment our collective wisdom about what morality is, and what it really means to *be* moral in a world characterised by individual and collective (cultural) diversity. In the ultimate analysis, the solution to the problematic of moral disagreement may not be to engage in adversarial dialogue (fight/litigate), or even to negotiate a happy medium between conflicting views (compromise). Rather, the solution may be, to borrow from Edward de Bono (1985), to engage in 'triangular thinking'; to engage in moral disagreement, not as a judge or as a negotiator, but as a 'creative designer' who is able to escape the imprisonment of the positivist logic and language that is so characteristic of mainstream Western moral discourse, and to engage in moral disagreement as someone who is able ultimately to resolve the conflicts and disagreements which others have long since abandoned as hopeless and irreconcilable impasses. Such an approach, however, requires not just an ability to think about new things, but, to borrow from Catharine MacKinnon (1987, p. 9), 'a new way of thinking'.

9. Moral dilemmas

Another significant moral problem to be considered here (and one which has been widely discussed in both nursing and bioethical literature) is that of the proverbial 'moral dilemma'. Broadly speaking, a dilemma may be defined as a situation requiring choice between what seem to be two equally desirable or undesirable alternatives; it may be crudely described as an 'awful feeling of being stuck'. A moral dilemma, however, is a little different, and can occur in one of several forms.

First, a moral dilemma can occur in the form of *logical incompatibility* between two different moral principles. For example, two different moral principles might apply equally in a given situation, and neither principle can be chosen without violating the other. Even so, a choice has to be made. Consider the case of a nurse who accepts a moral principle which demands respect for the sanctity of life, and who also accepts another moral principle (non-maleficence) which demands that persons should be spared intolerable suffering. Now, imagine this nurse in the situation of caring for a terminally ill patient who is suffering intolerable and intractable pain. In this situation, if the nurse accepts the sanctity of life principle, the administration of the large and potentially lethal doses of narcotics that might be required to relieve the patient's intolerable pain would probably be prohibited. On the other hand, if the non-maleficence principle were followed, the nurse might be required to administer the potentially lethal doses of narcotics, even though this could hasten the patient's death. In this situation, the nurse is unavoidably confronted with the profound and troubling dilemma that to uphold the sanctity of life principle could violate the non-maleficence principle, but to uphold the non-maleficence principle could violate the sanctity of life principle. The ultimate question posed for the nurse in this situation is: Which principle ought I to choose?

The options open to the nurse are:

- to modify the principles in question so that they do not conflict (i.e. by adding 'riders' to them);
- to abandon one principle in favour of the other;
- to abandon both principles in favour of a third (for example, autonomy and respect for the patient's rational wishes, or compassion).

It should be noted that none of these options is free of moral risk.

A second type of moral dilemma is that involving *competing moral duties*. Consider the following case. A nurse working in a specialised unit is assigned a patient with a known history of drug addiction, and is instructed to chaperone the patient when there are visitors to make sure that illicit drugs are not 'slipped in'. The nurse, however, believes that the duty to protect this patient from harm (such as might occur from receiving illicit drugs) competes with the duty to respect the patient's privacy. The question for the nurse in this scenario is: Which duty ought I to fulfil?

In another case, a nurse is assigned a patient of traditional Greek background who has recently been diagnosed with metastatic cancer. The doctor has ordered that the patient not be told his diagnosis. The patient, however, keeps asking the nurse and his family for information about his diagnosis. The family knows the diagnosis, but wants the doctor to tell the patient. Here the nurse is caught between a duty to tell the truth to the patient, and a duty to respect the wishes of the family. The nurse is also bound to follow the doctor's orders (although the question of whether there is a *duty* to follow them is another matter). The question for the nurse in this scenario is, again: Which duty ought I to fulfil — my duty to the patient or to the family, or to the doctor, or to whom?

Philosophical answers to questions raised by a conflict of duty are varied and controversial. In *The right and the good*, W. D. Ross (1930) argues that duties are prima facie or 'conditional' in nature. Thus, when two duties conflict, we must 'study the situation' as fully as we can until we are able to reach a 'considered opinion (it is never more) that in the circumstances one of them [the duties] is more incumbent than any other' (Ross 1930, p. 19). Once we have worked out which of the conflicting duties is the more 'incumbent' on us, we are bound to consider it our prima facie duty in that situation. Richard Hare (1981, p. 26), however, takes quite a different view. He argues that, if we find ourselves caught between what appear to be two conflicting duties, we need to look again. For it is likely that, in the case of an apparent conflict in duties, one of our so-called 'duties' is not our duty at all; we have only mistakenly thought that it was. In other words, what happens here is that one of the two apparently conflicting duties is eventually 'cancelled out', so to speak.

Williams (1973) disagrees. While he believes that one of the conflicting *oughts* has to be rejected (but only in the sense that both conflicting duties/oughts cannot be acted upon), he does not agree that this means that the duties or oughts in question do not apply equally in the situation at hand, or that one of the conflicting duties must inevitably be 'cancelled out'. To the contrary: our reasoning may assist us to deal with a conflict of duty and may assist us to find a 'best' way to act, but this does not mean that we abandon one or other of the duties in question. How do we know? Even after making a choice between two conflicting duties, we are still left with a lingering feeling of 'regret'. And it is this very feeling of regret which tells us that we have not altogether abandoned or 'cancelled out' the duty we decided could not, in that situation, be also acted upon.

In the drug addict case, we might well side with Richard Hare and unanimously agree that the nurse is mistaken in a belief that there is an overriding duty to respect the patient's privacy, and that clearly the primary duty is to prevent the patient from suffering the harms likely to be incurred by the administration of illicit drugs. But here the question arises: Is it really a nurse's duty to act as a kind of police warden? What if the patient is not receiving any form of therapy for the immediate drug addiction problem, and is at risk of developing severe and life-threatening withdrawal symptoms? How is the nurse's duty to 'prevent harm' to be regarded in this instance? Does cancelling out one of the conflicting duties here relieve the moral tension created in this scenario? Or is there more to be achieved by exploring ways in which they can be reconciled with each other?

In the cancer diagnosis case, we might unanimously agree that the nurse's primary duty is to the patient, and that any apparent duty owed to the family is not a bona fide one (after all, does not the moral principle of autonomy demand respect for the patient's rational wishes in this scenario?). Placed in a cultural context, however, the scenario takes on a whole new dimension. As Kanitsaki (1988, 1989, 1993, 1994) points out, and as was considered briefly in Chapter 6 of this text, families from a traditional cultural background very often play a fundamental and highly protective role in mediating the flow of information to a sick loved one. To ignore a family's request in such a situation could be to risk terrible violence to the wellbeing of the patient. Where this is likely, it is imperative that the nurse works closely with the family and ensures that the transfer of information to the patient is handled in a *culturally appropriate manner*. While the family may be perceived as 'interfering', in reality it may be providing an important and key link in ensuring that the patient's wellbeing and moral interests are fully upheld. Cancelling out one of the duties in this scenario is unlikely to relieve the moral tension generated by the patient's request for and the doctor's refusal to give the medical information on the patient's diagnosis. Had the only criterion for action been what superficially appeared to be a primary duty to the patient, the nurse may have unwittingly facilitated the flow of information in a culturally *inappropriate* and thus harmful manner. By reconciling the apparent conflict in duties, and by working closely with the family, however, the nurse is able to facilitate the flow of information to the patient in a culturally appropriate and thus less harmful manner. In this instance, by fulfilling the duty owed to the family, the nurse could also succeed in fulfilling the duty owed to the patient.

It might be objected that the examples given here do not involve difficult cases, and that the required choices are relatively easy to make. But even if we admit 'hard cases', Hare's position is somehow unsatisfactory, as is his argument that when there is an apparent conflict in duties, it is likely that one of the duties involved is not our duty at all. There is, I believe, always room to question how we can ever be really sure that a 'cancelled' duty was not our duty in the first place. The cancer diagnosis case, I think, illustrates this point well. Ross's and Williams's positions, on the other hand, remind us that matters of moral duty are never clear-cut; and, further, that we always have to be very careful in our appraisal of given situations and in the choices we make regarding to whom our moral duties are owed and what our moral duties actually are.

A third kind of moral dilemma, and one closely related to a dilemma concerning competing duties, is that entailing *competing and conflicting interests*. Here the question raised for the moral observer is: Whose interests ought I to uphold?

Consider the following case. A clinical teacher on clinical placement at a residential care home was informed by a student that an elderly demented resident had been physically and verbally abused by one of the ward's permanent staff members, as witnessed by the student. The clinical teacher was temporarily undecided about what to do. It was a very serious matter — and, indeed, a very serious accusation — but it would be very difficult to prove. If the incident was not reported to the home's nursing administrator, the staff member concerned would probably continue to abuse the home's residents. If the incident was reported, there was a risk that the interests of both students and the school of nursing could be threatened. (The home's administrator might, for example, refuse to continue allowing students to be placed at the home for the purposes of gaining clinical experience.) The dilemma for the clinical teacher was whether or not to report the matter and thereby protect both the students' and the school's interests in having continued clinical placements, or to report the matter fully, whatever the consequences to the school and the students, and thereby protect the residents' interests.

The teacher and the student mutually agreed that the matter was too serious to ignore and decided they would risk the consequences of reporting the incident. The exercise, as feared, proved extremely distressing and painful for both the student concerned and the clinical teacher. The accused staff member denied having abused the elderly resident, and in turn accused the student of lying and of being the one who had really committed the abuses. The opinion of the patient could not be sought, as the elderly resident concerned was demented. Fortunately, the matter was eventually resolved to everyone's satisfaction. The administrator took the allegation seriously and, later, took the initiative to emphasise to *all* staff the importance of protecting and upholding residents' rights. The student was reassured that she had done the 'right thing', and that she had fulfilled her professional and moral obligations both (i) in *reporting* the incident, and (ii) in the *manner* in which she had reported it (i.e. she had followed proper processes). The clinical supervisor and administrator reached an agreement that any matters of concern discussed during clinical teaching placements be referred directly and immediately to the administrator for action.

The staff member who was the subject of the unsubstantiated allegation was counselled in confidence by the administrator.

A fourth type of dilemma is taken from a feminist moral perspective, and is described by Gilligan (1982, 1987) in terms of being caught between attachments to people and trying to decide upon ways that will avoid 'hurting' each of these 'attached people'. Gilligan uses the example of a woman contemplating an abortion; she argues that generally a woman faced with having to make a choice in this situation 'contemplates a decision that affects both self and others and engages directly the critical moral issue of hurting' (Gilligan 1982, p. 71). Here the question to be raised in contemplating a difficult choice is: How can I avoid hurting the people to whom I am attached?

It might be objected here that Gilligan's sense of 'hurt' and 'avoiding hurt' is not very different from the general moral principle of non-maleficence and its demand to avoid or prevent 'harm'. While I concede that 'hurt' is a type of harm, there is a subtle distinction between 'hurt' in the sense that I think Gilligan is using it and 'harm' in the abstract sense that modernist philosophy uses it. It is important to draw a distinction between these two notions so as not to obscure other important distinctions which can be drawn in our moral discourse. Let us examine this point a little more fully.

The sense in which 'hurt' is being used here is not simply 'physical', but rather existential, spiritual, and even 'soulful' or 'soul-felt'. There is even room to make the radical claim that the notion of 'avoiding hurt' is not being asserted as a *principle* as such, but more as an *attitude*, and one which reminds us that we need to take very special care in our selection, interpretation and application of general moral principles in our everyday personal and professional lives. In short, it is an attitude which serves to *mediate* the use of more general moral principles. Consider, for example, the demand to 'avoid hurt' in a situation involving a patient who has yet to be told an unfavourable medical diagnosis. The demand to 'avoid hurt' reminds us that it is not enough just bluntly to *give* the patient the diagnosis (as may otherwise be required by the moral principle of autonomy), but that it must also be given in a caring, compassionate and culturally appropriate manner. Furthermore, it is not clear to me that the principle of non-maleficence fully captures the demand to be caring, compassionate and culturally appropriate in manner when performing such an unpleasant task as giving someone an unfavourable medical diagnosis. And in some instances, taken to its extreme, the principle of non-maleficence might even instruct that the diagnosis should not be given at all. 'Avoiding hurt', on the other hand, recognises that the information that needs to be given could be 'harmful' and is probably 'hurtful', but that there is a way of *lessening* if not *avoiding* this harm and hurt. To illustrate this point, consider the following case (told to me by a nursing colleague).

A young doctor walked into a patient's room, stood at the end of the bed, and in full view and hearing distance of other patients in the room, and without greeting the patient or smiling, stated abruptly: 'We've looked at your throat and the lump you have there is cancer'. Without another word, the doctor then briskly walked off. The patient had previously expressed a desire to know the diagnosis when it was available, so in many respects we could conclude that the doctor acted 'ethically' in that the patient's wishes had been respected and the requested information had been relayed to the patient. What is evident in this case is that the doctor had not considered ways to give the information less 'hurtfully' — or, if such ways had been considered, they were certainly not heeded. For example, the doctor might have at least greeted the patient, used a friendlier tone of voice, drawn the curtains around the patient before speaking, sat down on a chair to be at the same level as the patient, and stayed long enough to allow the patient to ask questions, which the patient stated later would have been desirable. If the doctor felt inadequate to deal with this situation, it might have been advisable to wait until a colleague or a nurse was available to accompany him. Or, more simply, the doctor should have passed the task over to someone else who was more experienced and better prepared to deal with the situation. By using such an abrupt manner, the doctor not only failed to 'avoid hurt', but exacerbated it. To make matters worse, the diagnosis given to the patient later turned out to be incorrect. At the time of learning that in fact there was no cancer, the patient was still in a state of psychological shock. This could have been avoided had the situation been handled more compassionately and caringly, and with an attitude intent on 'lessening hurt'. Within the same week, two other patients confided in my colleague that they had undergone similar experiences with the same doctor.

Of course, doctors are not the only ones guilty of hurt-causing attitudes. I have seen many instances (far too many, in fact) where nurses have likewise failed to avoid or to lessen the hurt of a given situation. I recall the tragic case of a middle-aged man who was dying from advanced cancer. A close friend and members of his family were greatly distressed about his deteriorating condition, and even accused the nursing staff of 'trying to kill' their loved one by giving him morphine for his pain. On one occasion the nursing staff observed the family friend clutching his friend and pleading with him not to accept the morphine injections, telling him: 'Don't you see, they are killing you! They are killing you! You don't have to have them ...'. The nursing staff tried to get the friend to leave, but he refused to go. When he became abusive, the nursing staff contacted a hospital security officer, and he was forcibly removed. There is, I believe, room to speculate about this case: had the friend's grief been properly addressed by the nursing staff, and the dynamics and benefits of effective pain management fully explained to him, both he, and the patient, the patient's family and attending nursing staff would have been spared the 'hurt' that this most unpleasant situation caused.

These two cases demonstrate that 'avoiding hurt' is not something that can be fully directed or achieved by an abstract moral principle. Rather, it requires that we draw very heavily on our past experience, knowledge, intuition, feelings, and interpersonal skills, as well as on a thorough and systematic analysis of the facts of the situation at hand.

10. Moral stress, moral distress and moral perplexity[2]

It has long been recognised that nurses experience moral stress, moral distress and moral outrage during the course of their work (see, for example, Jameton 1984; Andrews and Fargotstein 1986; Wilkinson 1987/88; Cahn 1989; Andersen 1990; Corley and Raines 1993). Defined as 'the psychological disequilibrium and negative feeling state experienced when a person makes a moral decision but does not follow through by performing the moral behaviour indicated by that decision' (Wilkinson 1987/88, p. 16), moral stress/distress can arise in a number of

---

2. Adapted from Johnstone, M-J (1998). *Determining and responding effectively to ethical professional misconduct in nursing: a report to the Nurses Board of Victoria.* Melbourne. Section 3: 'Defining ethical professional misconduct in nursing', pp. 17–28.

situations. Jameton (1984, p. 6) points out, for example, that nurses experience moral distress when they know the right thing to do, 'but institutional constraints make it nearly impossible to pursue the right course of action'. In such instance, unchecked moral stress and distress can turn into moral outrage which can, in turn, compound the original distress. Andersen explains:

> Moral outrage is a product of the emotional turbulence, pain, incredulity, indignation, and rage that ... occurs when a logical attempt to solve a moral problem results in denial of the problem and an assault on the nurse's integrity by those who have sacrificed their integrity and the welfare of patients to preserve the status quo of submarginal performance. The psychobiological remnants of moral distress are then compounded by the experience of moral outrage.
>
> (Andersen 1990, p. 9)

Moral distress can also follow from moral perplexity, taken here to be a state of moral confusion or bewilderment that arises when a person is faced with a morally problematic situation, recognises it (the situation) as being morally problematic, has the resources for dealing with it, but genuinely does not know what is the right thing to do. Nurses can and do suffer moral perplexity when confronted with a range of moral problems (examples of which are given in this text). Perhaps among the most perplexing of moral problems faced by nurses are those otherwise known as moral dilemmas and moral disagreements (just discussed above). These problems can be particularly perplexing in instances where it becomes apparent that, due to a variety of reasons, they may not be or indeed are not amenable to resolution. Since I have discussed the problem of moral stress/distress in nursing extensively elsewhere (Johnstone 1998), I will not venture any more on the topic here.

Moral decision-making — a systematic approach

Many nurses respond to moral problems with a 'gut response'. Needless to say, this is no more appropriate than it would be to respond to *clinical problems* with a 'gut response'. Does this mean that gut feelings have no part to play in clinical or moral decision-making? To the contrary. As we all know, many of our clinical findings are inspired by an intuition that 'something is not quite right with a patient', or that 'there is something wrong with the patient'. But the point is, when we have these 'clinical intuitions' we do not just leave it at that. We systematically set about to get more concrete data so as to obtain a more complete picture of what is going on. We may, for example, ask the patient how they are feeling, check the patient's vital signs, examine the patient's drug sheet and check which drugs have been administered, ask the opinions of others involved in caring for the patient, and so on. On the basis of the data collected, we then proceed to diagnose the problem, formulate objectives, plan a course of action, implement the plan of action, and evaluate the outcomes. This systematic approach (generally called the *nursing process*) is now taught to and used by nurses around the world in their clinical nursing practice.

Moral problems can be dealt with and solved in much the same way. In short, moral problems, like clinical problems, can be dealt with by a systematic decision-making process. It should be cautioned, however, that there is no *one* right way of going about solving moral problems. The following five-step process is merely one among many which might be used by nurses (see, for example,

Bergman's [1973] model of ethical decision-making, and Curtin and Flaherty's [1982] model for critical analysis). Nevertheless, since nurses are already familiar with the nursing process, I would suggest that the model of moral decision-making I propose is one which nurses would find relatively easy to use.

A moral decision-making model

A moral problem can be approached by way of a five-step process:

1. assessing the situation;
2. diagnosing or identifying the moral problem(s);
3. setting moral goals and planning an appropriate moral course of action;
4. implementing the plan of moral action;
5. evaluating the moral outcomes of the action implemented.

This model may be expressed diagrammatically as shown in Figure 7.3. The following is a somewhat simplistic hypothetical case study to illustrate how this model can be applied to clarify the nature of and solve a moral problem. The case involves Mrs A, a patient who has been diagnosed as having advanced cancer, but has not been told her medical diagnosis.

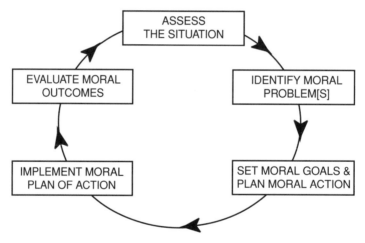

Figure 7.3 Moral decision-making model

1. Assessing the situation

To make decisions with insufficient knowledge is to risk making serious errors. Making moral decisions without first obtaining the relevant information about a point of moral controversy is likewise to risk making serious errors; it is also likely to reduce the possibility of moving closer to negotiation and resolution of moral disagreement. The first step towards solving a moral problem, as with any problem, is to fully assess the problem and the factors establishing it. What the nurse first needs to do, on being alerted to the possibility that a moral problem is at hand, is to bring together all the relevant facts of the matter as well as all the relevant ethical information. Here facts and ethical information count as *relevant* if it appears that they will make a difference and will probably influence a person's ultimate choice. The information collected should include at least the following. (The hypothetical case of Mrs A is used to illustrate each point.)

1. *A detailed description of the facts of the matter.* Mrs A has recently been diagnosed with advanced cancer. The diagnosis is correct, but little can be done for her, medically speaking. Mrs A does not know that she has cancer. She has expressed a desire to know the findings of recent tests and what her medical diagnosis is; she has said there are matters in her life which are outstanding. Dr X, Mrs A's surgeon, has not told Mrs A her diagnosis.

2. *A detailed description of the factors establishing the facts.* The reason Mrs A does not yet know she has cancer is that her doctor, Dr X, has ordered that she not be told her diagnosis. Dr X has given no reason for withholding this information from Mrs A. Dr X typically withholds information of this nature from his patients, for reasons unknown to nursing staff.

3. *The points of view of those who stand to be affected by any decisions made.* Mrs A repeatedly asks to be told her diagnosis, and states she does not care *who* gives it to her — she 'just wants to know'. The nurses caring for Mrs A have to give untruthful answers to her questions, and believe this is wrong, on grounds that she has a right to be told the truth. The nurses also believe that they are bound to follow Dr X's orders. (Whether this belief is correct is another matter, and one which will also need to be subjected to moral scrutiny.) The nurses unanimously agree that Mrs A is the sort of person who will be able to cope with her diagnosis, and that she should be told what is wrong; Mrs A's children also want to know their mother's diagnosis, and furthermore, they want their mother to know what it is.

4. *Selection of a preferred ethical perspective (theory) to underpin moral decisions and actions.* To counter the risks associated with using one's 'ordinary moral apparatus' and personal moral viewpoints for dealing with moral complexity, the selection of a preferred theoretical perspective in ethics is warranted. Choices can be made from the range of perspectives considered in Chapters 4, 5 and 6 of this text. For instance, attending nurses might choose ethical principlism to guide their moral decision-making in this scenario. This might include consideration of the following moral principles: *autonomy*, which would demand respect for Mrs A's expressed preferences (for example, to be told her diagnosis); *non-maleficence*, which would demand that Mrs A be protected from otherwise avoidable harms (for example, of non-disclosure about her medical diagnosis); *justice*, which would demand that Mrs A should not carry a disproportionate burden of suffering (for example, on account of not having her expressed preferences respected when these preferences could be respected without causing an undue burden of suffering to others). Alternatively, nurses might opt for a transcultural approach to ethics, taking as their starting point a thorough cultural assessment of the patient and the relevant cultural meanings of the situation which might have an important bearing on moral decision-making *apropos* providing information to Mrs A on her medical diagnosis.

5. *Clarification of definitions of moral principles and moral terms used.* It should be noted here that in some instances clarifying the definition and content of given moral terms and principles may be enough to settle a misunderstanding involving a moral problem.

6. *Prediction of possible consequences of the current position and an estimation of the probability that these consequences will occur.* Mrs A will not have time to adjust to the altered circumstances of her life. Mrs A and her family will carry an intolerable burden of anxiety at not knowing what is going on,

while attending nurses will also carry an intolerable burden of having to lie to Mrs A and of not being able to fulfil their professional responsibilities to her. Mrs A will be prevented from setting in order the outstanding matters in her life before she dies, and this will have predictably undesirable consequences. On the basis of past experience, and given the nature of her tumour and its advancement, it is likely that these consequences will eventuate.

7. *Prediction of possible consequences of appealing to adjudicating moral principles, and an estimation of the probability that these consequences will occur.* The possible consequences of upholding the principle of autonomy are that Mrs A is told her diagnosis, and the family can begin to support their mother and can start the grieving process. The nurses can better support Mrs A and her family in coming to terms with the cancer diagnosis, and no longer have to feel guilty at not telling her the truth. Mrs A can begin to settle the outstanding matters of her life before she dies. On the basis of past experience, it is likely that these outcomes will be achieved; it is also likely that other predicted harms will be avoided.

8. *Availability of alternatives.* Mrs A has another consulting physician caring for her who could also tell her the diagnosis. The hospital has a patient's advocate on staff who could initiate action likely to result in the patient being told her diagnosis. The hospital has a newly established hospital ethics committee set up to deal with 'hard cases'. The hospital has access to the facilities of the public advocate, which other hospitals have successfully used in the past in similar situations, and which have resulted in the patients concerned being told their diagnoses. The charge nurse has in the past, without serious consequences, overridden Dr X's orders and told requesting patients their diagnoses.

9. *Availability of resources.* There are enough members of staff to support Mrs A in coming to terms with her diagnosis. The ward has a single room available which Mrs A can move into if she wishes and be more private with her family. Mrs A is a religious person, and the hospital chaplain is also available to comfort her.

10. *Clarification of personal values and beliefs.* The people involved in the scenario clarify personal values and beliefs, including their own selection, interpretation, weighting and application of given moral principles and their compatibility with those of other people. Dr X is appealing to the principle of non-maleficence, which he interprets as requiring that Mrs A not be given the 'harm-causing' information regarding her diagnosis. The patient, her family and the attending nurses are all appealing to the principle of autonomy which emphasises that Mrs A's wishes must be respected and that she should be told her diagnosis even if this stands to cause her 'harm'. (The risk of being harmed is one she is entitled to take.)

11. *Assessment of the moral competence of the ultimate decision-maker and dissenting decision-makers.* It is extremely important to establish whether moral decision-makers have: (i) mastery of the requisite knowledge and skills, and (ii) soundness of moral judgment otherwise necessary for making sound moral judgments and decisions (Johnstone 1998, p. 20). Decision-makers must know not just *that* something is the right thing to do (*moral knowing that*) in this case (for example, inform Mrs A of her diagnosis), but also to know *how* (in a performative sense) best to do it (*moral knowing how*). Here it is important to understand that merely having an 'epistemology' of ethics may not be sufficient in a given scenario to resolve the moral problem at hand; decision-makers also need 'practical know-how' *apropos* applying the theoretical knowledge they have

(Johnstone 1998, pp. 53–5). This 'practical know-how' may need to include skills for dealing with interpersonal conflicts (akin to family therapy), such as: 'reframing, reconstructing narratives, and shifting from conflict to metareflective postures' (Gergen 1994, p. 112).

12. *Select and clarify key information for guiding decision-making.* The decision-makers should clarify:

- which features of a given situation are morally significant — that is, Mrs A has not been told her medical diagnosis when she has explicitly requested to be told;
- which aspects of a given situation need to be morally justified — that is, why Dr X has ordered that Mrs A not be told her diagnosis, or why Mrs A's family and attending nurses believe she should be told her diagnosis;
- where the onus of justification lies — that is, in light of the compelling moral nature of Mrs A's autonomous wishes, the onus of justification for withholding the information falls on Dr X;
- just what is to count as a justification — that is, whether it is to be personal taste, habit and/or convention, or something more substantial, such as that supplied by critically reflective moral analysis; and
- whose justification should be given the most weight and on what grounds — that is, the doctor's, the patient's, the family's, or the nurses'.

As with making a clinical assessment, having collected all the relevant information (including both subjective and objective data), and, of course, validated these, the nurse will then need to set about organising or 'clustering' the data into patterns and filling in any gaps where information appears to be lacking. On the basis of the clustered data, the nurse can then proceed to identify the specific moral problem or problems at hand.

2. *Diagnosing or identifying the moral problem(s)*

Nurses need to be open-minded about the precise nature of the problem at hand when diagnosing or identifying a supposed moral problem. The possibility always exists that the nurse might be mistaken, either factually (clinically or technically) or morally in their initial assessment of a situation. For instance, what might at first appear to be a 'moral problem' may turn out not to be a moral problem at all, but merely a problem of poor communication, misunderstanding, misinterpretation of the facts, ignorance of legal law or institutional policy, inappropriate legal law, inadequate institutional policy, or cultural unawareness. In such instances, it is likely that the problem at hand is one to be settled by education, psychology, law or some other mechanism, rather than by moral reasoning. If the nurse is satisfied that the problem at hand is more than merely practical, it becomes necessary to make a more definitive 'moral diagnosis'. The possibilities, as we have learned, are numerous and can include one or a combination of the following:

- moral unpreparedness;
- moral blindness;
- moral indifference;
- amoralism;
- immoralism;
- moral complacency;
- moral fanaticism;

- moral disagreement (e.g. internal moral disagreement, partial radical moral disagreement, and total radical moral disagreement);
- moral dilemmas (e.g. conflicting moral principles, conflicting moral duties, conflicting moral interests, conflicting personal responsibilities, and the effort to avoid hurt to those with whom one has 'attachments');
- moral stress, moral distress, and moral perplexity.

Once the nurse has made a 'moral diagnosis', the moral goals can be formulated and a moral course of action planned to achieve those moral goals.

Before continuing, it is worthwhile at this point to try and formulate a diagnosis of the moral problem in the case of Mrs A. On the surface it would appear that there are several problems at hand, including:

- moral unpreparedness (on the part of the nurses to deal with the situation at hand effectively and appropriately);
- moral complacency (on the part of Dr X, who appears to be unwilling to accept that he could be mistaken in his view that Mrs A should not be told her diagnosis);
- moral disagreement between Dr X, Mrs A, Mrs A's family and attending nurses about the priority of the given moral principles of non-maleficence and autonomy and, further, about how each of these should be interpreted and applied.

3. Setting moral goals and planning an appropriate moral course of action

Just as nursing diagnoses direct the planning of client-orientated nursing care and the setting of client-orientated health goals, so too do moral diagnoses direct the setting of moral goals and the planning of moral action. Unlike nursing diagnoses, however, the plan of action with regard to each possible moral problem is likely to be very similar. In the case of moral problems, for example, a combination of strategies will probably be required. This will involve a mixture of *moral education* (informal, formal, or both); *moral coordination* (individual or collective); *moral cooperation* (among those involved in a given scenario, as well as relevant others outside the scenario); *moral negotiation* and *moral persuasion* (again with all those involved); and, as a last resort, *mechanisms of non-moral enforcement* (particularly in instances where moral coordination, cooperation and negotiation break down) (Johnstone 1998). In choosing strategies, the decision-maker again needs to be very mindful of the possibility of making moral errors, and needs constantly to be justifying and validating the decisions being made along the way.

In the case of Mrs A, it is likely that all those involved need to be educated about the moral dimensions of the situation. For example, Dr X needs to be made aware that his values and preferences are causing serious 'hurt' to his patient and her family, and are also forcing the nurses into an intolerable position — both morally and professionally. Mrs A and her family need to be made aware of the difficulties facing the nurses, and of why the nurses believe they cannot just go ahead and tell Mrs A her diagnosis. The nurses need to come to some understanding about whether in fact they are 'prohibited' from telling the patient her diagnosis, and, if so, to work out which alternatives are available to them to get the information to Mrs A; the nurses also need to be educated about what role they can play in terms of getting medical information to patients who request it.

The priority, as I see it, is to seek prompt communication and negotiation with Dr X — after all, he too has significant moral interests at stake, which must also be considered. If the nurse succeeds in bringing Dr X to the negotiating table, but still fails to obtain his understanding and cooperation, or if she fails to bring Dr X to the negotiating table at all, then there is no alternative but to go outside the immediate doctor–patient and doctor–nurse relationship and seek cooperation from others who can assist; for example, the charge nurse, the doctor's superior, the hospital's patient advocate, the hospital ethics committee, the public advocate, or, as a last resort, the courts. The coordinator or coordinators of the strategies being used must take great care to avoid 'hurting' those involved, including Dr X and, in particular, Mrs A.

Before moving on, I would suggest that the most important strategies to be used in resolving moral problems are those of *education, mediation* and *negotiation.* Often merely learning of new information or new facts about a given matter may make it possible to move closer towards negotiation and resolution of disagreement. And negotiation and reaching an agreement on a common set of principles or on the concepts and definitions of moral language may also come some way towards settling moral disagreement. Other strategies which might be employed include trying to persuade a dissenting party by using examples and counter-examples, or more simply by exposing the inadequacies and unexpected consequences of an argument being used (Beauchamp and Walters 1982, pp. 4–6). Mechanisms of enforcement (such as the law, the courts, or professional disciplinary measures) should be used only as a very last resort — for the simple reason that, once mechanisms outside moral reasoning and moral negotiation are appealed to, the matter ceases to be a problem solvable by voluntary moral means and becomes — undesirably — a problem that can now be solved only by some form of force.

4. Implementing the plan of moral action

Once the nurse has formulated a plan of moral action, it is then possible to implement it. For example, the nurse may embark on a detailed educational strategy, assist in the coordination of a strategy aimed at resolving a moral problem at hand, engage in certain moral negotiations, seek cooperation with morally significant others, or, if all else fails, appeal to some outside mechanism necessary to achieve the desired moral outcomes.

In the case of Mrs A, the nurse would go ahead and seek negotiation with Dr X, or, if attempts to do so failed, embark on some other planned course of action aimed at ensuring that Mrs A receives the information about her diagnosis as she wishes.

In summary, what the nurse chooses to do here is to engage in the moral actions that have been chosen, or refrain from the immoral actions that have been identified and rejected.

5. Evaluating the moral outcomes of the action implemented

After implementing the planned moral course of action, the nurse should evaluate whether the projected moral goals and the desired moral outcomes have been achieved. The kinds of questions the nurse might ask here include those listed below.

- Has my action or strategy achieved the desired moral outcome? If not, why not?

- Was all the relevant information included in the original analysis of the moral problem?
- Was the original moral diagnosis correct?
- Was the moral reasoning used in identifying and planning a moral course of action sound?
- Was the chosen theoretical stance used appropriately and correctly? Was it adequate for the purposes chosen?
- Were the correct ethical principles selected?
- Were the selected moral principles interpreted and weighed correctly?
- Was there sufficient agreement between dissenting parties on the selection, interpretation and application of given moral principles?
- Was there sufficient agreement between dissenting parties on chosen definitions of moral terms and concepts?

It can be seen that, in attempting to answer these questions, the nurse would need to repeat the whole moral problem-solving process.

Returning one last time to the Mrs A case, the questions which would need to be asked in an effort to evaluate whether the moral plan had been successful or not would be, among others, the following.

- Has Mrs A been told her diagnosis? If not, why not?
- If so, did Mrs A suffer, as Dr X feared she would, by receiving the diagnosis? If so, why?
- Did any other undesirable moral consequences occur as a result of implementing the moral plan of action? If so, why?

Moral decision-making — an experiential approach

A major problem for the nursing profession is that not all of its members have had the opportunity to study nursing ethics at a formal educational level. This has sometimes meant, as previous examples have already demonstrated, that nurses have not always been well enough prepared to detect, and respond effectively and appropriately to, moral problems arising in or as a result of the delivery of nursing care to patients.

Consideration of this problem raises at least two critical questions. First, is it always the case that nurses who lack a formal education in nursing ethics (in particular, its theoretical underpinnings, the nature and use of a systematic approach to moral decision-making, specific ethical issues in nursing practice, and so on) are incapable of ethical professional conduct when planning and implementing nursing care? Second, if not, then to what extent, if any, should nurses allow their thinking and conduct to be driven by an abstract and systematic approach to moral deliberation such as that advocated by mainstream bioethics. Let us now examine these two questions.

A calculus of experience as a guide to moral conduct

The first question to be addressed here is whether nurses who have not had the benefit of a formal education in nursing ethics, or indeed bioethics, are capable of acting morally when planning and implementing nursing care. From anecdotal evidence, the short answer to this seemingly trite question is quite obviously, yes. As the following anecdotes will show, even without a formal education on moral theory, on the nature and use of a systematic approach to moral decision-making, and on specific ethical issues in nursing practice, nurses are still capable of making sound moral judgments and of acting in morally sound ways.

The ability of experienced and expert nurses to make impeccable moral judgments has become increasingly apparent to me recently while I have been exploring the issue at nursing ethics seminars and workshops. At one seminar, for example, a nurse, a bioethicist and a medical doctor (who was also a philosopher) agreed to sit on a panel and present a personal response to a real-life case scenario, which they had been given beforehand. They also agreed to receive and respond to questions from the exclusively nursing audience which had been invited to attend. As the evening progressed, many other actual case scenarios were presented by individual nurses in the audience. All the cases shared involved extremely delicate and morally complex situations. As the nurses shared their experiences, it became increasingly apparent to the panellists and others present that, without exception, each of the nurses involved had acted in a morally impeccable manner. Despite the nurses' expressed concerns that perhaps they could have been 'more moral', careful moral analysis showed that their decisions and actions had been quite faultless.

Upon leaving the seminar venue, I asked the bioethicist whether she could explain how the nurses sharing their experiences could have got it so 'right', given that, as had been confirmed at the time, none of them had ever studied or read articles on bioethics or nursing ethics. She replied that it seemed 'beyond an immediate explanation', and that she would 'have to think about it'.

Other seminars have been equally illuminating. For example, at a seminar on ethical issues in clinical nursing practice, at which I was a principal speaker, an experienced intensive care nurse asked for advice on 'what more she could have done' in the situation which she then related as follows.

She had been involved in the care of a middle-aged woman who, after suffering a massive myocardial infarction, had been admitted (deeply unconscious) into the local intensive care unit. The woman had been intubated before admission to the unit, and was placed immediately on a respirator. A few days later the medical hopelessness of the patient's condition was confirmed, and a medical decision was made to remove the artificial life-support system that was sustaining her life.

The woman's husband, who had been present most of the time since his wife's admission, objected strongly to this decision, however, and became very aggressive towards the medical and nursing staff. He also threatened to sue the hospital. Recognising the husband's reaction as a manifestation of extreme grief, the intensive care nurse approached the woman's adult children, who were also present, and, in a private setting, discussed with them what *they* thought should or could be done to help their father deal with the situation better. The children were unanimous that what was required was 'extra time' — specifically, that the removal of the life-support system be delayed so that they could console their father and help him to see that the situation really was 'hopeless'; that, tragic as it was, nothing further could be done. Upon learning of the family's wishes, the nurse offered to act as a mediator between them and the medical staff, to herself remove the life-support from their mother at the appropriate time, and to seek support for their wishes from the attending medical staff. This the family accepted. Over the next hour, the nurse was able to fulfil her role as 'mediator', and succeeded in obtaining full support from the medical staff involved in the case. This support included the medical staff agreeing to the nurse deciding when

191

and how to remove the life-support system from the patient. As a result of this mediation, extra time was 'bought', and the woman's husband and children were able to come to terms with the tragic decision that had been made. The family were all able to sit with the woman as the nurse progressively turned off the artificial life-support system. Later, the husband returned to the intensive care unit and thanked the nurse for her intervention.

Upon hearing this anecdote, my initial thought was, 'How could I possibly give this nurse any advice?'. It was evident to all present that the nurse had acted with extreme sensitivity, and that her actions were morally beyond reproach. As with the nurses at the seminar referred to earlier, it was later confirmed that this nurse had never read anything about or studied 'ethics'. Thus, again, the question arose: How did this nurse get it so 'right'?

It could be objected here that the nurse's actions in this case were not so remarkable, and that any experienced nurse in a comparable situation would probably have acted as this nurse did. This, however, is questionable. It will be recalled that, in the earlier discussion on moral dilemmas, a distraught visitor mourning the deteriorating condition of his friend was removed forcibly from the hospital after nursing staff called a hospital security officer to evict the man from the hospital premises. There is room to speculate here that, had the nurse in the previous example been involved in this scenario, the outcome might have been quite different. Meanwhile, we could ask: How did the nurses in the distraught visitor's case get it so 'wrong'?

There are many reasons and theories advanced by, among others, psychologists, anthropologists, sociologists, theologians and philosophers, about why some people are able to behave morally when others are not, or are able to behave more morally than others who, in the ultimate analysis, prove morally 'weak-willed'. Unfortunately, since it is not the purpose of this work to advance or elaborate a theory on moral motivation, consideration of these reasons and theories must be left for another time. Nevertheless, there is at least one nursing-specific factor that has an important bearing on the moral motivations, sensibilities and abilities of nurses, and that warrants some consideration here, and that is nurses' actual clinical practice and, more specifically, the 'virtuous caring' nature of the nurse–patient relationship (discussed previously in Chapter 5 of this text). (See also Yarling and McElmurry 1986; Cooper 1988, 1990, 1991; Packard and Ferrara 1988; Twomey 1989; Bishop and Scudder 1990; Benner 1991; Gaut and Leininger 1991, Bowden 1994; Gastmans et al. 1998).

Unlike the relatively detached and decontextualised activity of modernist moral philosophy (see Chapter 4 of this text), clinical nursing practice, and the lived realities of the nurse–patient relationship, offer nurses:

- 'hands-on' (lived) experience in detecting and recognising, engaging with, and responding directly to the suffering of their patients;
- developing the ability to make fine discretionary moral judgments about whether a patient's wellbeing is being violated or is at risk of being violated;
- building up a repertoire of possible actions that can be effectively deployed to alleviate patients' suffering in appropriate ways; and
- developing effective ways in which nurses' perceptions, and the morality of their judgments and actions, can be validated.

Over time this lived experience can contribute to the development and refinement of nurses' perceptual apparatus (Benner 1984, 1991; de Bono 1990). This, in turn, can enable them to develop the 'background' patterns necessary to perceive correctly the moral dimensions of human suffering (Amato 1990), and to act appropriately to try and alleviate human suffering when it is encountered. In other words, nurses' vast experience as clinical practitioners can enable them to develop exquisite experience-based knowledge on what constitutes right and wrong conduct in regard to human suffering in nursing care contexts. This, in turn, can enable nurses to fine-tune their moral perceptions and moral intuitions, and concomitantly enhance their ability to make the fine discretionary moral judgments that are so often required to ensure appropriate ('right') moral behaviour during moments of human crisis, which are characterised all too frequently by intense and sometimes overwhelming feelings of fear, anxiety, loneliness, uncertainty, ambivalence, pain (at all physical, emotional, spiritual and psychic levels), hopelessness, helplessness, despair, and a deep and abiding sense of vulnerability.

It might be objected here that if *experience* is *all* that is required in order to develop moral sensibilities and moral attunement to people and their suffering, why is it that some nurses lack the ability to behave in morally acceptable ways? Why, for instance, do some experienced nurses seem blind to the suffering of their patients, or, when suffering is detected, seem quite unable to respond to it appropriately and effectively? Why are some nurses apparently indifferent to the wellbeing of their patients, or oblivious to the factors that may be threatening it? For example, many of the Brown Sisters of Nazi Germany (referred to in Chapter 2 of this text) were 'experienced' and even 'expert' nurses, yet demonstrably immoral practitioners. Drawing on this extreme — although real — example, clearly much more than *mere experience* is required in order to develop one's moral sensibilities, and, indeed, the ability to *be* moral. The question remains: Just what is required to develop these things?

The question of whether moral sensibilities ('virtue') and the ability to *be* moral can be taught is as old as Western moral philosophy itself, and, to this day, remains the subject of much controversy (a point I shall return to in the final chapter of this text). Despite the controversy, however, there does seem to be at least one factor that is crucial to a person's ability to be moral, and that is the level of personal commitment a person makes, or is prepared to make, to carefully chosen moral values (see also van Hooft 1987; Roach 1987). In the case of nursing, of particular importance is the nurse's commitment to 'virtuous caring' and to protecting the genuine welfare (as opposed to merely upholding the rights) of people made vulnerable by their health crises.

As discussed in Chapter 3 of this text, *care* has long been recognised, albeit controversially, as the moral ideal, essence and foundation of nursing and, as discussed in Chapter 5 of this text, 'virtuous caring' is demonstrably linked to the promotion of human welfare and wellbeing in nursing care contexts. Whatever the controversies surrounding the notion of virtuous care as providing a basis and framework for moral conduct in nursing, it is anecdotally evident that it has played an important and influential role in ensuring the realisation of morally just outcomes in nursing care contexts. For example, it was through a guiding framework of care that the experienced intensive care nurse referred to earlier was able to perceive the reaction of her patient's distraught husband not as aggression, nor as a threat to be removed forcibly by a hospital security officer, but as an expression of profound grief and vulnerability warranting a compassionate and understanding response. This is in sharp contrast to the case discussed earlier involving a visitor, it will be recalled, whose distress at the sight of his dying friend was perceived by attending nurses not as a reaction of grief, but as an act of unprovoked aggression — a threat — to be removed quickly and forcibly, without compassion and without any understanding of the sense of despair or hopelessness the visitor was experiencing. An important lesson here is that virtuous caring cannot only motivate moral action, but can assist the actor to perceive correctly an instance of human suffering (this may present as little more than 'a look of suffering' on a patient's face or a 'look of sadness' in their eyes), to decide how, if at all, to respond to the suffering that has been detected in another, and to decide when, where and by whom the suffering should be responded to.

Should nurses study moral decision-making?

The brief attention which has been given here to speculating about the experiential factors that may have been instrumental in guiding nurses to act morally has probably raised more questions than it has answered; it has also certainly illuminated the need for extensive empirical research on the subject. Nevertheless, the examples given are quite sufficient to demonstrate that there are in existence factors and means other than abstract moral principles and moral theories which can guide nurses in their moral deliberations, and enable them to make the exquisite moral judgments that they are often required to make in the course of their everyday practice. One question that now arises is: If nurses can be moral without studying moral theories, and without developing a systematic approach to moral decision-making, should educational programs and initiatives in this area be abandoned? Do nurses really need to study ethics as it is now commonly being taught in nursing courses around the world?

The short answer to this question is that we should be very careful not to 'throw the baby out with the bath water'. While abstract moral principles and theories have their limitations, they can nevertheless be extremely helpful in guiding nurses' perceptions of what constitutes right and wrong conduct — particularly in uncertain situations involving 'strangers', or patients with whom nurses have not yet had the opportunity to develop — or have been unable to develop — the level of intimacy required to achieve the degree of empathy necessary to inform and enable correct moral judgments to be made about whether the patient's wellbeing is being upheld or violated. Moral principles and theories can provide a quantifiable measure against which nurses can evaluate their actions in instances where they are just not sure about whether they have done or are doing the 'right' thing. Significantly, when I have asked nurses for their opinions on the value of their learning about the theoretical underpinnings of modernist moral philosophy and bioethics, including the nature and application of the abstract moral principles of autonomy, non-maleficence, beneficence and justice, their responses have tended to be unanimous. Firstly, the view is commonly expressed that 'it has been a relief' to learn about the four moral principles cited above, since it has provided something for them (the nurses) 'to hang their hats on'. The nurses often explain that these principles provide a useful framework in terms of which they can make sense of and, more importantly, justify their past moral actions. As a point of interest, it is not unusual for nurses to comment: 'I thought I did the right thing in such-and-such a situation, but I was never sure. Now I feel much more confident, and in a better position to justify to others why I did what I did.' Secondly, the view is commonly expressed by nurses that, upon learning of the theoretical underpinnings of Western moral thinking, they feel they can be more confident and courageous in taking the action that may be necessary to remedy moral problems that may occur at some future point in time in their places of work.

It is perhaps not surprising that nurses have responded in the way just described. With careful questioning, it soon becomes apparent that many nurses are already subscribing to the moral values and standards that have been formalised by the abstract moral principles of autonomy, non-maleficence, beneficence and justice. This I have been able to demonstrate repeatedly by the simple exercise of asking nurses whether they have ever given a wrong drug to a patient, and, if so, how they felt about it. Almost without exception, the responses have tended to be: 'I felt dreadful', 'I felt awful', 'I was devastated', and so on. When pressed to explain why they felt like this, again the responses have tended to be unanimous: 'Because I could have killed the patient', or 'Because the patient could have been harmed'. And when pressed to explain further why this mattered — that is, why did it matter to them particularly whether a patient was harmed — the nurses' responses again have tended to be unanimous: 'Because it is wrong'. At first glance, these responses might not seem very significant. But, on closer examination, what is highly significant is that the main concern of these nurses has been for the wellbeing of their *patients*, not themselves. Indeed, it has not been until after the above kinds of views have been expressed that, upon further prompting, the nurses concerned started to cite other, more self-interested, reasons why they were upset about their drug administration error; for example, 'I felt stupid', or 'I don't like making mistakes'; and then, finally, because they realised that their error could have resulted in some sort of disciplinary action against them if harm to the patient had occurred. From other examples and the responses to them, it has become apparent to me that nurses also subscribe to the values that have been formalised by the other moral principles of autonomy, beneficence and justice.

Although the examples given above are only anecdotal, they are nevertheless substantial enough to show that, in the ultimate analysis, nurses might not rely on experience alone or on one particular moral framework (for example, virtuous caring) for guiding their moral actions, but may in fact subscribe to a variety of frameworks (for example, virtuous caring *as well as* internalised moral principles). And they also show that, in practice, what nurses are faced with when dealing with moral problems is not a competitive struggle between a principle-orientated ethic and an ethic of care, as some have suggested, but a 'creative tension' between these two mutually-enhancing guiding moral frameworks (Cooper 1991). Either way, it is evident that greater attention must now be given to exploring the critical relationship — and the creative tension — between moral reasoning, emotion and intuition, and their vital influence on guiding nurses' thinking, perceptions and values about what constitutes right and wrong conduct, and hence their overall experience as 'morally mature' and wise practitioners. And much greater attention must be given to investigating generally the 'phemonenology of ethical expertise' (Dreyfus and Dreyfus 1991) and the experiential as well as the theoretical underpinnings of the demonstrable ability of nurses to be moral in situations where it is not always easy to decide what is the morally correct thing to do — even for accomplished moral philosophers.

Conclusion

Moral problems invariably involve multifaceted and complex human beings who have very real feelings and moral interests, and who are more often than not faced with very real and significant threats to these moral interests and, ultimately, their wellbeing. Dealing effectively with moral problems in nursing care domains is thus not an easy task and, among other things, requires a deep and informed understanding of the complexities and 'messiness' of human life.

Nurses are not immune from the many and complex moral problems that plague health care domains. As in the case of other professional–client relationships, no nurse–patient relationship occurs in a moral vacuum or is free of moral risk. Nurses have the capacity (whether by act or omission) to harm as well as benefit their patients. Nurses therefore need to be especially vigilant in regard to both their own and other's capacity to harm the significant moral interests and wellbeing of patients, and to take appropriate action to prevent such harms from occurring — even those which might be deemed 'inadvertent' and 'accidental'. To be effective in preventing moral harms occurring in nursing care domains, it is imperative that nurses have an informed knowledge and understanding of the nature of moral problems and the various forms in which they can manifest. This chapter has sought to provide such knowledge and understanding.

When dealing with moral problems it is important for nurses to remember, meanwhile, that sometimes it may be difficult to take the 'morally correct' action because of various institutional and legal constraints. As has already been discussed and demonstrated in this text, nurses can suffer enormously if they take a firm moral position in relation to a clinical nursing or controversial medical matter. Life can be made 'hell' for nurses if they do not conform to the status quo, and in many instances they have no choice but to 'voluntarily' resign. Victimisation, as we well know, is often difficult to prove; a nurse may be left with a good career in shreds (see Johnstone 1994, 1998). One of the troubling things about this situation for nurses is that this reality is often perpetrated by other nurses (in particular senior clinical nurses and nurse administrators).

Despite the difficulties that nurses face when attempting to deal with moral problems and make difficult moral decisions, various approaches are possible to achieve a morally tolerable clinical reality. In concluding this chapter I should like to make a number of recommendations.

1. Nursing management must provide a clinical environment that is more conducive to open and honest debate on bioethical issues affecting nursing practice and standards of nursing care.
2. Nurse practitioners must themselves create and demand opportunities for formal discussion of the many ethical issues that derive from clinical nursing practice (see the notion of 'ethical rounds', in Davis 1982 and moral incident stress debriefing, in Johnstone 1998).
3. Nurses must familiarise themselves with the legal acts and statutes governing their practice, and which may impinge on ethical nursing practice.
4. Nurses must lobby for law reform in areas which are intolerable to accountable and ethically responsible nursing practice.
5. Nurses must familiarise themselves with the written policies of their employing institutions, and seek changes to those policies that are obstructive to ethically responsible and accountable nursing practice.

6. Nurses should seek membership of a professional nursing organisation and actively work towards improving the nursing profession.
7. Individual nurses must lobby their professional organisations to formulate positions on, and to address the ethical issues that are found to be particularly troubling in, nursing practice (for example, giving information to patients, conscientious objection claims, unethical conduct by nursing and medical colleagues) — if nurses' professional representatives are not aware of an issue, they are powerless to effect any positive and helpful changes.
8. In extreme cases, nurses must be prepared to seek legal advice.

Moral problems are a fundamental and integral part of nursing practice, in much the same way that clinical problems are. If we do not address these moral problems, and, more importantly, address them competently, we risk a number of undesirable moral consequences, including:

- the enforcement of morally unsound decisions and actions;
- a failure to prevent moral harm;
- the actual causing of hurt and moral harm;
- the creation of moral conflict;
- the unjust imposition of our personal values on others ('moral bullying'); and
- the abdication of our broader moral responsibilities ('moral buck-passing').

Caring for our patients — caring for people — is not just a task; it is itself a virtuous moral ideal of nursing (Watson 1985, pp. 58, 63). If nurses are to uphold this ideal — and uphold it well — they must include a sound and experientially-based moral point of view in their clinical nursing practice. As well as this, they must be able to function as competent moral problem-solvers and decision-makers, and truly make a difference in terms of promoting and protecting the welfare and genuine moral interests of all those for whom they care.

Chapter 8

Patients' rights to and in health care

Introduction

In July 1987, the Melbourne *Age* carried a front-page report headed 'AMA will consider secret AIDS tests', in which it was revealed that New South Wales doctors had 'been testing selected patients for AIDS without their consent or knowledge' (Conley 1987, p. 1). A little over a year later, a front-page report in the Melbourne *Herald* claimed that 1 500 Aborigines on Palm Island had been tested for AIDS (Miller 1988). It was alleged in this report that, while consents had been obtained for taking a 'blood test' (screening was also being carried out for diabetes and other diseases), there was doubt about the quality of these consents. A senior Aboriginal Commonwealth officer was reported as saying that the quality of the informed consent was only '50–50 at best' (Miller 1988). Equally disturbing was the report's allegation that there had been serious breaches of confidentiality regarding five Palm Islanders who had been found to be HIV-positive.

On 27 January 1985, John McEwan, an Australian water skiing champion, was left a ventilator-dependent quadriplegic after a diving accident at Echuca, Victoria. Throughout his hospitalisation, he repeatedly asked to be allowed to die. At one point he went on a hunger strike and instructed his solicitor to draw up a 'living will', which stated 'that he did not wish to be revived if and when he fell into a coma' (*Request to die* 1985, p. 2). According to media reports, this led to a psychiatrist certifying him as rationally incompetent. The psychiatrist's judgment was revoked a few days later, however, when John McEwan 'agreed to end his hunger strike and accept a course of antidepressants' (*Bioethics News* 1985, p. 2).

A little over a year after his accident, and despite still being ventilator-dependent, John McEwan was discharged home. The round-the-clock day care he required was given by family members and friends who had received special training in how to care for him. In the weeks following his discharge from hospital, John McEwan continued to express his wish to be allowed to die (Social Development Committee 1987, pp. 310–11). This prompted the general practitioner who was medically responsible for him to inform the senior nursing assistant that:

> John McEwan at his own request could come off the ventilator from time to time but had to be reconnected if he became distressed *even if it was against his own wishes.*
>
> (Social Development Committee 1987, p. 312, emphasis added)

199

During one incident, while at home, John McEwan was observed to be angry at having been reconnected to the ventilator against his wishes. And in another incident shortly before his death, he talked openly with his general practitioner about 'hiring someone to blow his [John McEwan's] brains out or kill him as he felt his wish to die was being frustrated' (Social Development Committee 1987, p. 316). There was no reason to suspect that John McEwan's wishes were irrational. Before his accident he had been a committed sportsman. I have been told informally that sport was not merely an interest to him, but a passion and an obsession. Thus, for him, the life of a helpless quadriplegic was intolerable.

At four o'clock in the morning on 3 April 1986, John McEwan was found dead by his nursing attendant. At the time of discovery he was disconnected from his ventilator.

More recently, in what has been described by media commentators as 'the first case of its kind' in North America, a patient sued his treating physician for 'keeping him alive' against his expressed wishes and for not offering him an 'elective demise' (Reed 1996, p. 14). The patient in this case was a 66-year-old man who had been diagnosed with amyotrophic lateral sclerosis, a degenerative nerve disorder. Despite having made a 'living will' that clearly stated his wishes 'not to be attached to a respirator' should his condition deteriorate, the patient was nevertheless placed on an artificial life support machine when he began experiencing breathing difficulties. As a result of this paternalistic medical decision, he has been left totally dependent on 24-hour nursing care, depleted of his life-savings, and deprived of what he regarded as a 'dignified death' (Reed 1996, p. 14). The patient's life expectancy was estimated at the time of the report to be between five to ten years.

A little over one year later, in New Zealand, a case of a very different kind unfolded. In this case, a man suffering from an end-stage illness, was denied kidney dialysis treatment on 'economic grounds' (Field 1997, p. 10). Outraged by the hospital's decision not to treat their father, and in a desperate bid to secure life-saving treatment for him, the man's family applied to the New Zealand Court of Appeal to intervene. The Court is reported as ruling, however, that the hospital managers 'did not need to resume kidney dialysis treatment' (Field 1997, p. 10). In response to the case, the then associate Health Minister was reported to have said that 'health rationing was now a fact of life'. It was subsequently observed that:

> Although formal rationing has not previously been acknowledged here [New Zealand], from July every New Zealander referred for surgery in the public health system will be scored for points on clinical and social criteria to determine when they will be treated.

> (Field 1997, p. 10)

These reports on secret AIDS testing, inadequate consent practices, breaches of confidentiality, treating patients against their will, and denying patients life-saving treatment for economic reasons are just some among many examples of patients' rights violations occurring in health care contexts. In Chapters 2, 3 and 7 of this text, several other examples of patients' rights violations have been given, and the chapters to follow will provide still more.

The issue of patients' rights

People requiring or receiving health care are not, and never have been, obliged to be the passive recipients of unnegotiated care. Yet the more we examine the realities of health care practice and the way our health care institutions and services operate, the more apparent it becomes that the rhetoric surrounding the idealism of people's rights to and in health care does not match the reality. As the bioethics, legal, professional and lay literature, and our own everyday experience, make plain, people continue to be denied equitable access to the quality and quantity of health care they need; they continue to be denied the opportunity to make informed choices about their care and treatment options; and they continue to be harmed physically, psychologically, spiritually and morally as a result of unscrupulous or at least morally questionable practices in our health care services and institutions. This is an appalling indictment, not just of 'the system', but of the health care professionals who comprise it and, more specifically, of their culpable lack of ability and moral commitment to remedy it.

Over the past decade, the issue of patients' rights has received considerable attention both in Australia and overseas. There exists a vast body of literature on the subject, and there has been a proliferation of dramatised accounts of people's 'life stories' both in books and films (see, for example, Gilmour 1992; Gilbert 1997). There have also been significant policy and law reforms in the area of patients' rights, for instance, in relation to:

- clarifying people's common law right to refuse orthodox medical treatment;
- the lawful appointment of 'surrogate decision-makers' (persons with 'medical power of attorney') in the case of patients who become incompetent to decide their own medical treatment;
- formulating 'living wills';
- the right to an 'assisted death';
- the establishment of institutional-based ethics committees (IECs) and 'client support' persons;
- the establishment of statutory health services complaints mechanisms;
- the role of a public advocate in the case of disagreement about treatment decisions;
- the development of public consumer advocacy groups;
- the establishment of national ethics committees and commissions (in Australia known as the Australian Health Ethics Committee [AHEC]).

Despite these important innovations, however, the area of patients' rights remains problematic.

The Consumers' Health Forum (1990) points out, for example, that the Australian legal system has not been responsive to protecting the needs of health care consumers. In its report on the *Legal Recognition and Protection of the Rights of Health Consumers*, it states:

> For some consumers the diversity of the Australian legal system has provided some benefits. Unfortunately, for the majority it has been far more effective in creating an inequitable and unresponsive legal maze. As it currently stands:
>
> - there is no comprehensive, consistent, consumer-orientated health law that recognises individual consumers' and the community's health and wellbeing as a fundamental objective;
> - there is no clear direction for consumers as to how they should act, how others should act, and what redress they have if things go wrong (their

rights depend upon which State consumers live in or even whether they attend a public or private health facility); and

- the interests of bureaucrats and professional groups are better reflected in existing law than the interests of consumers and the community in such matters as information, participation, accountability and openness.

(Consumers' Health Forum 1990, pp. 1–2)

The issue of patients' (clients') rights is of obvious importance to and in the nursing profession. If nurses are to respond effectively to this issue, however, they need to have knowledge and understanding of, first, what patients' rights are, and second, how these rights can best be upheld. It is to advancing an understanding of these matters that this discussion will now turn.

What are patients' rights?

To put it simply, patients' or clients' rights are merely a subcategory of human rights. Statements of patients' or clients' rights are merely statements about particular moral interests that a person might have in health care contexts and that require special protection when a person assumes the role of a patient or client. Referring to this particular set of interests in terms of 'patients' rights' or 'clients' rights' serves more the purposes of convenience and manageability than those of philosophy. For example, when the notion patients' rights or clients' rights is used, we know immediately what kind of context and what kind of rights claims are likely to be encountered. The notion of patients' rights or clients' rights in this instance immediately 'sets the scene', or identifies the domain of concern. In the case of human rights language, the scene that is set is much broader. Some might consider human rights language in health care contexts to be somewhat cumbersome to manage. This is not to say that it would be inappropriate to use the notion of human rights in health care contexts; quite the reverse is true. In many respects, using human rights language might be more compelling and more effective in drawing attention to and demanding respect of the deserving moral interests of people in health care domains.

It is perhaps important to clarify that patients' rights statements tend to include a mixture of civil rights, legal rights and moral rights (see Appendixes II, IV and V). Popular examples of patients' rights include: a right to health care, a right to be informed, a right to participate in decision-making concerning treatment and care, a right to give an informed consent, a right to refuse consent, a right to have access to a trained interpreter, a right to know the name and status of attending health professionals, a right to a second opinion, a right to be treated with respect, a right to confidentiality, a right to bodily integrity, the right to compensation in the case of unlawful injury, a right to the maintenance of dignity, and many others. Many of these rights statements derive from the broader moral principles of autonomy, non-maleficence, beneficence and justice, already discussed in this text. Unfortunately there is insufficient space here to discuss every type of patients' right that has been formulated at some time or another. For the purposes of this discussion, attention is given to only five broad categories of rights, under which many other narrower rights claims fall. These category claims include the rights to health care, to make self-determining choices (informed consent), to confidentiality, dignity, (including the right to die with dignity), and to be treated with respect.

1. The right to health care

The right to health care (taken here in its broadest sense, and not to be confused with *medical* care) is complex and controversial. As well as being a sensitive moral issue, it is also a highly charged political issue, as ongoing debates on health care resource allocation make plain.

Bioethicists have yet to find a happy medium between the many competing and conflicting views on the subject. Some philosophers argue that health care is something all people are equally entitled to receive, regardless of the cost. Where human life is at stake, they contend, decisions should not be constrained by economic considerations (Brody 1986); if more money is required, the solution is relatively simple: redirect society's resources (for example, away from gross expenditures on arsenals of arms and other life-threatening instruments of war). Others argue that it is implausible and impossible to provide a high standard of health care to all persons equally. At best, all that people can reasonably claim is a 'decent minimum' of health care, as measured in terms of the amount necessary to secure a minimally decent or 'tolerable' life (Fried 1982; Buchanan 1984; Engelhardt 1986, p. 336). Still others argue that there is no such thing as a right to health care. One philosopher even claims that it is *immoral* to speak of health care as a 'right' (Sade 1983), and another that the expression 'a right to health care' is nothing but a 'dangerous slogan' (Fried 1982).

Charles Fried (1982, p. 400) makes the interesting and, if taken from the perspective of medical treatment, I think correct claim that the 'impossible dilemma posed by the promise of a right to health care' is really nothing more than a product of 'our culture's inability to face and cope with the persistent facts of illness, old age, and death'. He goes on to assert controversially that:

> Because we are little able to come to terms with the hazards which illness proposes, because the old are a burden and an embarrassment, because we pretend that death does not exist, we employ elaborate ruses to put these things out of the ambit of our ordinary lives.
>
> (Fried 1982, p. 400)

Whether the right to health care is a bogus claim or a dangerous slogan or a cultural quirk will, however, depend very much on how the notion of 'health care' is interpreted. I suspect that many philosophers' criticisms derive from their erroneously equating 'health care' with 'medical care'. Since medical care makes up only a small proportion of overall health care, it is obviously not synonymous with health care. Once the notion of 'health care' is understood in more holistic terms, the right to such care may not seem so outrageous or fraudulent or even culturally odd as a claim. Every culture has its way of dealing with sickness, illness, pain and suffering, and of caring for the sick. Not every culture embraces Western scientific medicine as the most effective way of dealing with sickness and related illness experiences, however. And thus not every culture is posed with the dilemma of economic restrictions on resource allocation; this, I suspect, is what lies at the root of the debate about whether people have a right to health (viz. medical) care. Once health care, in its more holistic sense, is seen as an important means of promoting a person's *total* (and not merely physical) wellbeing, it becomes increasingly difficult to deny that claims to it are valid and morally justified. What makes a claim to health care compelling is precisely that, once it is accepted, it has the moral power to prescribe actions to relieve the distressing symptoms caused by disease and illness, to promote human wellbeing (a moral end) and, indeed, to promote human life itself (also a moral end). If we deny entitlements to health care, we must also deny entitlements to a range of other interests, including those of life, happiness and even the exercise of self-determining choices.

It is beyond the scope of this text to deal with the many arguments and counter-arguments raised in response to the question of whether people have a right to health care. What is of concern here is to clarify the *nature* of the claim to *a right to health care*, and what might be meant by such a claim.

People's entitlement to receive health care first received global recognition with the signing of the United Nations Declaration of Human Rights on 10 December 1948. Article 25 states:

> Everyone has the right to a standard of living adequate for the health and wellbeing of himself [sic] and his [sic] family, including food, clothing, housing and medical care and necessary social services, and the right to security in the event of unemployment, sickness, disability, widowhood, old age or other lack of livelihood in circumstances beyond his [sic] control.
>
> (United Nations 1978, p. 8)

It is worth noting here that the right to health care embodied by this statement extends far beyond a claim of mere *medical* care, and embraces a more holistic interpretation of health care.

Since the signing of this declaration the question of the right to health care has taken on a new meaning, and has emerged largely as a result of what people perceive to be an 'unjust or unfair state of affairs' involving present structures of health care, which are seen as diminishing and even eliminating possibilities for the enhancement of the quality of human life and for human life itself (McCullough 1983).

In speaking of the right to health care, it is important to distinguish at least three different senses in which it can be claimed: that is, the right to equal access to health care; the right to have access to appropriate care; and the right to quality of care.

The right to equal access to health care

The right to equal access to health care raises questions of distributive justice and of how benefits and burdens ought to be distributed. It also raises questions of whether people or institutions can be found morally negligent for failing to provide equal access to health care for persons requiring it. Responses refuting this sense of a right to health care typically centre on such arguments as: 'there is not a 'bottomless pit' of health care resources, and somebody has to do without'.

Specifically, the 'scarce resources, but unlimited wants' argument tends to be constructed as follows:

1. the demand for health care has outstripped supply;
2. this is fundamentally because health care resources are limited;
3. different people have different health needs, and different views on how existing resources should be used to meet these needs;
4. it is true that existing health care resources can be used in alternative ways; and
5. nevertheless, health care resources are limited, so it is not possible to satisfy everybody's needs and wants (Johnstone 1990, p. 3; see also Council for Science and Society 1982; Fuchs 1983, p. 4).

The ultimate conclusion drawn from these premises — the 'bottom line', so to speak — is that, inevitably, choices will have to be made. In particular, borrowing from Sheehan and Wells (1985, p. 59), choices will have to be made about:

1. the conditions for which scarce resources should be made available; and
2. the priority with which given conditions should be treated.

It remains an open question, however, whether we have to accept the premises of this 'scarce resources, but unlimited wants' argument, and, further, whether we have to accept its apparent 'inevitable' conclusions. As I have argued elsewhere (Johnstone 1990), it is far from clear that we do have to accept them — particularly when the politics of health care resource allocation is considered fully, including the vested and powerful interests that the whole health care economics debate is serving. Further, it is also open to serious question whether we are obliged to accept that economic principles ought to supplant morality as the ultimate test of conduct, as an economic rationalisation approach to health care dictates. Human life is not something that can be reduced, like an object, to mere economic worth, and as moral beings we ought to resist attempts to do so; if we do not resist, we risk seeing 'worthless' human beings denied the health care entitlements they would otherwise be entitled morally to receive.

The arguments of economic rationalism are less than convincing when considered in relation to the demands of morality. On a more practical level, they are also less than convincing when considered in the light of the wastage that occurs in high-tech health care contexts (particularly hospitals) and the misallocation of health care resources generally. Consider, for example, the once routine usage in many hospitals of the seemingly inexpensive oxygen humidifier used on patients receiving oxygen by nasal cannula. Research done in the United States has shown that humidifying oxygen administered by nasal cannula has no therapeutic value and unnecessarily adds to hospital costs and expenditure (Campbell et al. 1988). Despite these research findings, many hospitals continued to advocate the routine use of humidification on patients receiving nasal oxygen. It is not insignificant that, in the United States alone, the manufacture of bubblejet humidifiers during the 1980's was an 18-million-dollar industry (Campbell et al. 1988, p. 293).

The cost-effectiveness of medical technology is already a subject of much controversy, both in Australia and overseas. Bates and Linder-Pelz (1987), for example, argue that since the 1980s it has become increasingly evident that damages inflicted by some medical technology by far outweigh many of the expected benefits, a problem which they see as being largely attributable to the lack of adequate evaluation of technology before its widespread acceptance (p. 124). Mulley (1984) also raises questions about the appropriateness of the high costs incurred by running technology-dependent intensive care units, given that the effectiveness of intensive care units is as yet unproven. Suspicion also surrounds the cost-effectiveness of highly priced diagnostic machinery. Rice (1988), for example, cites a research study conducted over a six-year period at Westmead Hospital, Sydney, in which the cases of 218 women who had attended the hospital for mammography were examined. The researchers discovered that in 95 (44 per cent) of these cases, the mammogram failed to detect an existing tumour (Walker and Langlands 1986, pp. 185–7; Rice 1988, p. 15).

Similar claims about the apparent unreliability of mammograms have also been made by medical authors. Mendelsohn (1982, pp. 109–10), for example, cites a screening program conducted over a three-year period between 1973 and 1976.

Of the 1800 cases of cancer detected, 48 were found to be cases of mistaken diagnosis, and of these 37 had resulted in the needless removal of breasts. Mendelsohn (1982, pp. 110–11) argues further that routine mammography for women under 50 years of age is actually 'potentially dangerous' to health, and can, ironically, predispose to iatrogenic breast cancer later in life. Following numerous studies, and warnings to a United States congressional subcommittee, routine mammography in women under the age of 50 years was finally abandoned by the National Cancer Institute (NCI) and the American Cancer Society (ACS) (Mendelsohn 1982, p. 110).

Other medical authors have claimed that, in 5–69 per cent of cases, mammography can yield false negative results, leading to failure to diagnose cancerous conditions:

> In one study of 48 'negative' mammograms of women who later turned out to have breast cancer, one-third had cancers that were clearly visible on the X-rays, but had been overlooked or misread by the X-ray personnel or physicians.
>
> (Inlander et al. 1988, p. 106)

These and other examples raise serious questions about the wisdom of spending vast amounts of money on equipment that cannot be relied upon to give accurate results.

The issue of medical technology aside, the cost-effectiveness of medical treatment itself is also open to dispute. Kerr (1987), for example, makes the controversial claim that 75 per cent of patients who see a doctor 'receive no benefit whatsoever from medical treatment' (p. 10). He also cites the findings of a Melbourne study revealed by the comments of Dr J. L. Frew, Chairman of the Victorian State Committee of the Royal Australasian College of Physicians, during an address at an annual meeting of the Australian Association of the Ethical Pharmaceutical Industry, which indicate that 10–15 per cent of patients admitted to hospital are suffering from iatrogenic illness; i.e., illness caused by previous medical treatment (Kerr 1987, p. 8). Commenting on the issue of how many people are in fact made worse by medical treatment, Kerr further states:

> Unremarkably enough, no precise figures are available on this subject. The information which medical practitioners are required to furnish to the Department of Health does not include an item such as 'The number of patients whom I made worse last month'.
>
> (Kerr 1987, p. 9)

It can be seen that the issue of resource allocation goes far beyond the simple question of merely how to allocate dollars and cents. It involves much broader questions of how to measure quality of life, efficacy of health care and medical treatment, and quality of care, and of how to calculate cost-effectiveness, as well as complex socio-cultural questions pertaining to power, politics, elitism and greed (Johnstone 1990; see also David Lindorff's controversial and provocative text *Marketplace medicine: the rise of the for-profit hospital chains* [1992]).

Unless nurses address these other broader questions — both academically and professionally — they will never be in a position to offer a convincing account of why *health care* (whatever form this may take), not merely medical care, needs to be better recognised and why it must be more appropriately funded. A strong stand must be taken on the need to recognise and to fund *health care* better, and there is considerable scope to suggest that it would be very appropriate for the nursing profession to lead such a stand. More than this, the nursing profession has a moral obligation to lobby effectively for the community as a whole, and the individuals who comprise it, to have better access to holistic health care, and not merely to scientific medical care.

The right to have access to appropriate care

The right to have access to appropriate care is a second sense in which a right to health care can be claimed. This sense raises important questions concerning the cultural relativity or ethno-specificity of care and its ability to accommodate people's personal preferences, health beliefs, health values and health practices. Failing to provide health care in an appropriate manner can have disastrous consequences (clinically, legally and morally). For example, Kanitsaki (1983; 1988a) offers a thought-provoking case study concerning an elderly woman of Greek origin who had been admitted to hospital for the treatment of a chronic leg ulcer, with a view to amputation. In this case, the woman's doctor and attending nursing staff viewed amputation as being the 'treatment of choice', whereas the elderly woman viewed this treatment option as being both personally abhorrent and culturally taboo; she would rather die than have the amputation. Fortunately, thanks to a sympathetic charge nurse who had a cultural understanding of the woman's plight, alternative remedies were tried and the woman's leg eventually healed.

Many other examples can be given here. The holistic health movement has posed all sorts of new dilemmas for the scientific health professional, particularly in instances where patients prefer to try scientifically 'unproven' vitamin or herbal remedies, meditation, and other therapeutic agents for serious diseases, rather than risk the known and unpleasant side effects of more orthodox medical treatments. To some extent this type of problem has been overcome by health professionals combining orthodox and unorthodox treatments (for example, performing surgery as well as administering vitamin and herbal therapies, or administering orthodox drugs as well as performing spinal manipulation, acupuncture and acupressure, facilitating meditation, and the like) — something which once would have been poorly tolerated in the domains of scientific Western medicine (see also Moyers 1993; Dossey 1991; Chopra 1989).

Another aspect of 'appropriate care' entails patients having access to people (lay, folk and professional) of their own choosing. It also includes patients' entitlements to seek a second medical opinion, to refuse a recommended medical therapy or folk therapy, to choose an alternative health therapy, to be surrounded by family and friends, to have unrestricted visiting rights, and to decline to be 'ordered' to do anything they do not wish to do (including getting out of bed, having a shower every day, and taking prescribed medication). As the Australian Consumers' Association (1988, p. 16) correctly points out, patients do not need a doctor's or nurse's 'permission' (to be distinguished here from *advice*) for anything!

If nurses are to respond to this sense of a right to health care, they need to gain knowledge and understanding of their patients' health beliefs and health practices and to negotiate ways in which these can be accommodated and met appropriately.

The right to quality of care

A right to quality of care is the third and final sense in which the right to health care can be claimed. This sense raises questions concerning the accountability, responsibility and competency of health professionals and health care providers, and about the standard of care that is actually delivered. Not only are practical and technical skills at issue here, but also attitudinal factors such as a health care provider's attitude towards patients as human beings with needs and interests, who are entitled to participate in decision-making concerning their care. A claim to receive quality care also raises questions concerning what should be done in the case of the 'impaired professional' (Somerville 1986) — someone who functions below an otherwise acceptable professional standard.

Quality health care as a right is an ambiguous and complex notion. Nevertheless, an attempt must be made to understand and use it in a meaningful way. This can be achieved by appealing to the agreed standards of the profession, experience, commonsense (for example, concerning the distinctions that can be readily made between 'quality care' and 'substandard care'), formal quality assurance processes, formal measures of patient outcomes, and the like. The task for the nursing profession is to ensure that health care delivery never falls to a level that compromises patient safety and wellbeing; nurses in many parts of the world have already demonstrated their willingness to take strike action when patient safety is compromised by substandard conditions and resources.

Challenges posed by the right to health care

It can be seen that all three senses of the right to health care pose a significant challenge to the nursing profession. As far as the right to equal access is concerned, nurses have much to contribute. Nurses know very well the areas in which access to health care has effectively been denied to people, and why (for example, lack of appropriate resource allocation, inappropriate structuring of health care delivery, obstructive institutional policies and legal laws, language and cultural barriers). Despite their knowledge and experience in relation to these matters, however, nurses are more often than not excluded from participating in important policy making and resource allocation initiatives in the health care arena. Nurses are not usually consulted on how and where the health dollar should be spent or on how health care services should be structured and could be improved.

As a point of interest, nurses comprise 70 per cent of health care workers. Yet they have next to no say in the overall management of the health industry or the health care arenas in which they work. The moral as well as professional implications of this situation are serious. What is particularly of concern is that the exclusion of nurses from top-level decision-making and policy formation effectively prevents them from fulfilling their broader moral responsibilities towards the community at large in terms of ensuring its access to appropriate and quality health care services. The lesson to be gleaned from this observation is clear: nurses must directly participate in high-level decision-making concerning health care matters, an imperative already well argued for by Paul Gross (1985) over a decade ago. If nurses fail to influence policy and decision-making, the prospects for patients' rights, not to mention the nursing profession's ability to promote and protect these, will remain pessimistic.

The right to health care, in the senses pertaining to both appropriate health care and quality health care, also poses significant challenges to the nursing profession, in terms not only of its own standards, but also of those applied in health care contexts generally. If the nursing profession is to succeed in providing appropriate nursing care (a subcategory of health care), it needs to pay careful and continuous attention to developing its curricula and to ensuring that its members are educationally prepared to meet and to respond to the needs of society, and in particular the needs of the culturally and individually diverse people comprising it. As well as this, the nursing profession must pay careful attention to developing reliable mechanisms for guiding its members in their attempts to deliver safe, therapeutically effective, culturally appropriate and morally accountable care, and for censuring those of its members who fail to do so (Johnstone 1998).

Nurses, individually and collectively, have a moral responsibility to respond to the serious threats mounting against a person's right to health care; they must therefore develop a well organised and effective lobby to champion a more balanced approach to resource allocation and a more balanced approach to the structuring of health care facilities generally. Nurses also have a moral responsibility to inform the community at large of its entitlements to, in and against health care, and to educate the community that the 'technologically big' is not necessarily the 'health care best'.

2. The right to make informed decisions

Traditionally, doctors have assumed ultimate decision-making authority in health care contexts. The notion of 'doctor knows best' has been, and in many instances continues to be, widely accepted by the lay community. Unfortunately, as numerous anecdotal case studies show, doctors have not always used their authority wisely, much less to the benefit of their patients' interests. In some instances (as happened in the John McEwan case cited at the beginning of this chapter), doctors have made and implemented decisions against their patients' expressed and considered wishes.

The role and authority of the doctor as ultimate decision-maker is, however, being increasingly questioned by the laity, academics, consumer rights groups, other health professionals and governments. In King et al. (1988), the conceptual underpinnings of physician authority are critically examined and successfully challenged. The unanimous conclusion of all twelve contributors to this volume is that it is no longer appropriate or necessary for doctors to be 'the captain of the ship', a metaphor borrowed from American legal law and used to describe the doctor as being in charge of 'the clinic, the operating theatre and the health care team'.

Of all the patients' rights which might be claimed in a given health care context, none is perhaps more threatening to the power and authority of attending health professionals (including nurses) than the patient's right to make informed choices about his or her care and treatment. This might help to explain why, despite the apparent success of the patients' rights movement over the past decade, the right of patients to give an informed consent to care and treatment continues to be violated at many levels. For example, over the past five years I have conducted a number of workshops and seminars addressing ethical issues in nursing. Disturbingly, nurses attending these educational activities have consistently identified the following problems in relation to consent to treatment practices:

- patients signing consent forms without having any comprehension of what it is they are consenting to;
- nurses assuming incorrectly that treating doctors have explained a recommended medical procedure or treatment to a patient/relatives before obtaining the patient's consent;
- relatives/chosen carers being upset at discovering that a recommended medical procedure had not been properly explained to a loved one before being performed;
- signed consent forms being treated as generic, that is, as signifying a consent to 'anything deemed necessary' during the period of hospitalisation;
- patients giving consent to a particular procedure being performed, only to discover later that a different procedure was performed without any 'real choice' being given (for example, the patient may have consented to having a biopsy *only*; upon recovery, however, he or she finds that radical surgery has been performed);
- verbal consents being obtained from relatives/chosen carers over the telephone in situations which are not of a true 'emergency' nature (for example, where there has been a last minute cancellation from a private list and a bed has become vacant for a new elective surgery patient);
- consents being obtained from people of non-English-speaking backgrounds without the assistance of qualified health interpreters;
- patients consenting to a procedure, knowing what the procedure involves, but having no knowledge of associated risks or potential adverse side effects of the procedure in question;
- consent being obtained from patients after they have received a pre-medication or when they are under the influence of alcohol or other mind-altering drugs; and
- procedures performed without consent being obtained from the patient at all.

In disclosing these problems, the nurses have also expressed considerable distress at what they see as their inability 'to do anything about the problem'.

The issue of informed consent has obvious implications for nurses, not least on account of them being at the forefront of receiving requests from patients and relatives for 'information'. As well, nurses are at the forefront of being expected to take appropriate action when patients' information needs are not being met and/or when their (the patients') entitlements in regard to consent practices are unjustly violated. It is therefore important that nurses have a thorough understanding of the nature and function of informed consent, as well as their responsibilities as nurses in relation to facilitating a patient making informed choices about recommended care and treatment options. It is to exploring these two issue that this discussion will now turn.

What is informed consent?

The doctrine of informed consent, although having a profound ethical dimension, is essentially a legal doctrine developed partially out of recognition of the patient's right to self-determination and partially out of the doctor's duty to give the patient 'information about proposed treatment so as to provide him or her with the opportunity of making an "informed" or "rational" choice as to whether to undergo the treatment' (Robertson 1981, p. 102).

In distinguishing the differences between a legal and a moral approach to informed consent, Faden and Beauchamp (1986) explain that the legal law's approach to informed consent 'springs from pragmatic theory', which focuses more on a doctor's duty to disclose information to patients and not to injure them. By contrast, moral philosophy's approach to informed consent 'springs from a principle of respect for autonomy that focuses on the patient or subject, who has a right to make an autonomous choice' (Faden and Beauchamp 1986, p. 4).

Whether such a clear-cut distinction can be drawn between a legal and a moral approach to informed consent is a matter of some controversy, however. The moral demand to respect autonomy is clearly the prime motivator of the doctor's duty to disclose information, and the moral principle of non-maleficence the prime motivator of the doctor's duty not to injure or harm patients. It seems that, while the moral and legal approaches to informed consent can be loosely distinguished, they are nevertheless inextricably linked. It is this linkage which highlights the other important functions, besides the promotion of patient autonomy, that the application of the doctrine of informed consent also serves, namely those of protecting patients, avoiding fraud and duress (i.e., as occurs when information is not disclosed), of encouraging self-scrutiny by health professionals, of promoting 'rational' and systematic moral decision-making, and of involving the public 'in promoting autonomy as a general social value and in controlling biomedical research' (Capron 1974).

The need to revise current consent to treatment procedures in Australia is long overdue. Despite popular medical opinion to the contrary, current consent procedures are inadequate and are open to abuse. (see, for example, the AMA's reported comments in Schauble and Willox 1987, p. 19). Nurses witness consent abuses in hospital contexts almost every day, and are sometimes unwitting (sometimes witting) accomplices to these abuses. For example, I have been told of several instances in which nurses have been 'ordered' by an operating surgeon to obtain the written consent of a patient who has already been given a pre-medication and who is drowsy and awaiting transfer to the operating theatre. In each instance, the fact that consent given under the influence of sedating or narcotic drugs is legally invalid seems to have been largely ignored by the surgeons in question. In one case, the gynaecologist 'ordered' a registered nurse to obtain the signature of a non-English-speaking and already pre-medicated woman on whom he was about to perform a dilatation and curettage (D&C) of the uterus. However, there was some suggestion that the gynaecologist also intended to sterilise this woman, and the nurse involved in the case was deeply concerned that the matter of surgical sterilisation had not been properly discussed with the woman. Further, the patient was in no state to give a valid consent, since she was very drowsy from the effects of her pre-medication. As well, no interpreter was immediately available to transmit to the woman the information she needed in order to give an informed consent. On the basis of her assessment of the situation the registered nurse refused to comply with the gynaecologist's order. Upon hearing her refusal the gynaecologist became abusive and was overheard to yell at her. Fortunately, other nurses on the ward came to her defence and supported her decision not to seek the woman's signature. Needless to say, the woman did not go to theatre that day.

The Victorian organisation Health Call (1987) cites an even more alarming case, which is worth quoting at length here, since it is very similar to the case just discussed and serves to show that this kind of case is by no means unique.

> Four weeks prior to giving birth a 26-year-old woman, pregnant with her fourth child, attended an antenatal appointment with her Medical Specialist.
>
> The physician initiated a discussion about sterilisation during which the woman made it quite clear to him she had no wish to undergo sterilisation.
>
> On admission to hospital for a caesarean section the woman was approached by nursing staff and asked to sign a form consenting to sterilisation and the caesarean section. The woman again made a clear verbal statement refusing sterilisation.
>
> After undergoing the caesarean section the woman was informed by the Medical Specialist that a tubal ligation had been performed. The woman asked the doctor why he had performed the procedure despite her consent not having been given. He replied: 'In my medical opinion you should not have any more children'.
>
> (Health Call 1987, p. 5)

These two cases are in no way isolated examples. Kanitsaki (1992), for example, cites the case of a 66-year-old Greek woman ('Mrs G') who had been admitted to hospital for elective surgery to treat a kidney disorder. As in the previous cases, informed consent was not obtained. Describing the circumstances surrounding the failure to obtain an informed consent from this woman, Kanitsaki writes:

> The morning of Mrs G's operation arrived, and it was observed by the nurse who was to prepare her for theatre, that Mrs G's consent form was not signed. The nurse reported this to the charge nurse who rang the relevant doctor to come and obtain Mrs G's signature on the consent form. The surgical registrar arrived, and in an irritable tone asked 'why this was not done the day before'. The nurse remarked that Mrs G only spoke a few words of English, and would need an interpreter to explain to her what she was signing and why. The doctor replied 'I know. But I have no time to wait. It will be alright'. He then proceeded to instruct Mrs G how to sign the consent form. Mrs G sat up in bed, however, and looking puzzled, uttered 'Me no understand. Me no understand'. The doctor then proceeded to pick up Mrs G's hand, placed a pen into it, and by holding and directing her hand, made a cross on the consent form. Once this was achieved, the doctor gently touched Mrs G's hand and said 'Good. Good'. He then left the ward.
>
> (Kanitsaki 1992, pp. 2–3)

While women feature large in allegations of consent abuses, they are of course not the only ones to fall victim to unscrupulous consent-to-treatment practices and related patients' rights violations. In one extraordinary case, which occurred in 1986, a 35-year-old man had been admitted to a major city hospital for a surgical fusion of his cervical spine. He was a self-employed carpenter, who had worked hard to build up his small business. Worried about the risks associated with the procedure for which he had been admitted, the man asked an attending junior registered nurse what the risks were of being left a quadriplegic following a cervical spinal fusion. In response to this question, the nurse informed the patient that he really needed to discuss the matter with his doctor, and that she would contact him to come and answer any questions. The patient at this point informed the nurse that his brother was a doctor and had advised him to ask the operating surgeon a number of questions pertaining to the procedure, including the question just ventured about the risk of quadriplegia.

A short time later the ward's junior medical resident came to see the patient to answer his questions. The patient was not, however, satisfied to discuss the matter with the junior resident, and asked to see the consulting surgeon. Three days later the surgeon walked briskly into the patient's room and, without greeting him by name, asked in a stern tone of voice: 'What is all this nonsense going on?'. The patient calmly replied that he had been informed by his medical brother that there was a significant risk of being left a quadriplegic following surgery to the cervical spine and that he simply wanted some reassurance that the risk was minimal. The surgeon replied curtly 'it's not worth worrying about' and further that the procedure was 'perfectly safe'. The patient then asked the surgeon whether he would be doing the operation *personally*. To this the surgeon replied, again in a curt tone of voice, 'you will be operated on by *whoever* is available — probably my registrar'. This is not an uncommon occurrence in Australian hospitals, and in fact the consent forms signed by patients generally carry explicit wording to the effect: 'No assurance has been given to me that the operation will be performed by any particular practitioner' (see Figure 8.1).

The man became very concerned upon receiving this piece of information, and insisted that, as he had been admitted under the surgeon Mr X, surely he had a right to be treated by Mr X, and surely Mr X had an obligation to treat him? To this the surgeon replied: 'As a Medicare patient, the answer is no. You are only entitled to be treated by whoever is available'. The surgeon then went on to inform the patient that either he accept that the registrar would be performing the operation, or else he was free to discharge himself.

Despite the severe neurological symptoms he was experiencing in his arm (including a loss of function and muscle wasting) the patient discharged himself. The matter was reported to the nursing supervisor who just shrugged, raised her eyebrows, and stated: 'there is nothing we can do ...'. None of the nurses involved in this case felt they could intervene on the patient's behalf. Their main reason was that they feared the wrath of the surgeon, who had a reputation for being 'abusive and difficult'.

Strong objections might be raised against the examples given here. A typical response may be: 'Of course the actions of the doctors in these examples deserve universal condemnation. But these are, after all, "one off" examples ...'. I would suggest that any number of experienced nurses could show that the examples given here are not 'one off'. Consider, for example, the 948 unconsenting women and the unconsenting parents of the 2200 newborn baby girls involved in the National Women's Hospital 'unfortunate experiment' in New Zealand, or the unknown number of unconsenting women patients used as teaching objects when under general anaesthetic specifically to teach medical students how to perform vaginal examinations (Bone 1987; see also Chapter 2).

CONSENT FOR OPERATION AND ANAESTHETICS

I, ... of ....

.... hereby consent to
undergo

the submission of my (child)/(ward) .... to undergo

the operation of ....

the nature and purpose of which have been explained to me by

Dr/Mr ....

I also consent to such further or alternative operative measures as may be found appropriate during the course of the abovementioned operation, and to the administration of general, local or other anaesthetics for any of these purposes.

No assurance has been given to me that the operation will be performed by any particular practitioner.

Date .... Signed ....
*Patient/Parent/Guardian

I confirm that I have explained the nature and purpose of this operation to the *patient/parent/guardian.

Date .... Signed ....
*Medical/Dental Practitioner

*Delete as appropriate

Figure 8.1 Typical consent form for operation and anaesthetics procedure
(from J. Fordham, *Doctor's orders or patient choice*, Leo Cussen Institute, Melbourne, 1988, p. 68)

One reason why consent practices in Australia and New Zealand are less than desirable is the model they are based on. Unlike the United States and Canada, which use a *reasonable patient standard* model of consent (emphasising trespass and battery), Australia and New Zealand use a *reasonable doctor standard* model (emphasising negligence and malpractice). Understanding the difference between these two models is important to any debate on informed consent, and I will briefly outline them here. (For a more detailed discussion on the legal aspects of informed consent to medical treatment, see Andrews 1985; Faden and Beauchamp 1986; Law Reform Commission of Victoria et al. 1987; Wallace 1991; Staunton and Whyburn 1997; Kirby 1995.)

In the *reasonable doctor standard* model of consent, a consensus of reasonable and established medical opinion provides the 'objective' measure. On the basis of this model, a doctor has the duty to use reasonable skill and may *withhold* information if, in the doctor's opinion, its disclosure would be injurious to the patient. If patients are to successfully sue for damages on account of a failure to disclose information relevant to the consent process, they have to show, first, that the doctor failed to provide information and advice to a patient that accords with the 'practice existing in the medical profession' (Law Reform Commission of

Victoria et al. 1987, p. 8), and, second, that injury was suffered as a (causally) *direct result* of this negligence. In establishing whether the doctor did in fact use 'reasonable skill', the law would appeal to the *reasonable doctor standard* model and would ask what most or many reasonable and competent doctors in a given particular branch of medicine would do and say in such circumstances; that is, what would be considered 'accepted medical practice' in this situation? If there were conflict, the answer to this question would be sought from an expert medical witness, or witnesses, who would testify what they, as reasonable and competent doctors in a particular branch of medicine, would probably do or say in the circumstances under question. For example, the question of whether a doctor should have disclosed to a patient a 0.1–0.2 per cent risk of quadriplegia in cases involving cervical spinal surgery would ultimately be decided on the basis of whether *other* reasonable and competent doctors in the field usually disclose this information. If it could be established that other reasonable doctors do not disclose to their patients a 0.1–0.2 per cent risk of quadriplegia in cases involving cervical spinal surgery, it is likely that a doctor who failed to disclose such information to a patient would *not* be found negligent or causally responsible for the patient's injuries in the case of a material risk manifesting itself (such as quadriplegia).

In the *reasonable patient standard* model, on the other hand, the standard is set 'by reference to hypothetical behaviour of adult, competent people in the sorts of situations which are presented to courts and other tribunals for decision' (Law Reform Commission of Victoria et al. 1987, p. 8). On the basis of this model, a doctor has the duty to *disclose* to the patient all the information necessary to making an intelligent and 'rational' choice (including information pertaining to small material risks). For example, consider the hypothetical case of a patient who has suffered the complication of quadriplegia following a cervical spinal fusion. Consider further that the patient claims that, had information been given about the associated risk of quadriplegia, the operation would never have been consented to in the first place. The famous *Sidaway case* provides a good and thought-provoking example of this kind of situation (Law Reform Commission of Victoria et al. 1987, pp. 3–4, 37–9; Andrews 1985, p. 14). In the hypothetical case, the question of whether a doctor should have disclosed to the patient a 0.1–0.2 per cent risk of quadriplegia in cases involving cervical spinal surgery would ultimately be decided on the basis of whether:

1. the information that was withheld was critical to the patient's making an intelligent choice;
2. the information would have caused the patient to make a different choice had she or he been informed of the associated risks before giving consent;
3. the patient's desire to know of the given associated material risks was consistent with the desires of a hypothetical reasonable and competent adult; and
4. the risk was considered to be severe (i.e. the injury, were it to occur, would be of a serious nature; quadriplegia in this instance is clearly 'severe' viz. 'of a serious nature').

If it could be established, in this instance, that the patient would not have consented to the procedure, and that the patient's declining to give consent would have been consistent with what a hypothetical reasonable and competent adult would do in a similar situation, then the patient's original consent would be vitiated and the doctor would be found guilty of trespass and battery.

Both models depend on the further consideration of a patient's rational or legal *competence* — a matter that, rightly or wrongly, the courts ultimately decide (the question of patient competency will be considered later in this discussion).

The issue facing us is whether we should totally abandon the reasonable doctor standard model in favour of the reasonable patient standard model, or whether we should opt for some middle ground between the two. There is some suggestion that this middle position has already been opted for in one or two Australian court cases (Russell 1987, p. 18); however, further legal opinion would be necessary to explore the issue in more depth.

Whatever the legal considerations and arguments for or against these models, from a moral point of view (and, indeed, a pragmatic point of view) neither is free of difficulties. It takes little imagination to see how the reasonable doctor standard can be unreliable. As books, articles, anecdotal case studies and media commentaries make plain, doctors are on the whole loath to testify against their colleagues. A Sydney developmental physician and advocate, Dr Cary Ooi, has even alleged that many of the so-called 'expert witnesses' provided by the Medical Defence Union of the United Kingdom (whose Australasian Secretariat is based in Sydney) give false and fraudulent testimonies in a bid to support colleagues brought before the courts for negligence or malpractice claims. In his unpublished paper 'Paediatrics — a new version', Dr Ooi argues that medical fraud occurs on an international scale and 'there is evidence that it is committed quite often without shame or effective sanction' (p. 1). He has also commented elsewhere that in one court case 'the evidence of a UK trained general nurse and midwife was completely ignored by the learned judge, and the false medical testimony of a paediatrician-defendant was accepted without thought that it was served by self-interest' (personal communication, 1988). The implication of this situation for the nursing profession is self-evident, and supports the view that judges/the courts have little regard for a nursing perspective on professional, clinical or moral matters (see in particular Johnstone 1994). Commenting on Australia's medical defence unions, Stephen Rice (1988) writes:

> the medical defence unions operating in Australia claim they do not object to their members testifying against colleagues. But they stress to members in newsletters: — 'Avoid unnecessary criticism of the work or conduct of other practitioners.'
>
> (Rice 1988, p. 124)

Rice also cites the experience of a Sydney solicitor (and former legal secretary of the Australian Medical Association) who, when addressing a medico-legal seminar organised by the AMA, was unable to find *one* doctor in the audience who was prepared to give evidence against another doctor at a court hearing. Rice comments further: 'Even with his impeccable contacts in the medical community, he [the solicitor] has discovered it is not easy to find willing witnesses' (p. 124).

The reasonable patient standard, however, can also be unreliable. For example, who is to say what is to count as a 'reasonable' patient, hypothetical or otherwise? Are we really expected to believe and accept that an abstract 'hypothetical reasonable and competent adult' — divorced from any cultural, social, historical and spiritual context of living — is able to represent reliably and truthfully what an actual person whose 'reasonableness' is at issue would ultimately desire? What one patient might consider *reasonable*, another might equally reject; and vice versa. The case of Jehovah's Witnesses and their well recognised refusal to accept life-saving blood transfusions is a point in question. It is not difficult to imagine a 'reasonable patient' of the Jehovah's Witness faith refusing a blood transfusion against an overwhelming body of public opinion that such a refusal was 'unreasonable' and even 'crazy'. In the case of culturally different persons, as in the Kanitsaki (1983) example of the elderly Greek woman who refused amputation of her leg, it is not difficult to imagine a 'reasonable patient' of a traditional and non-scientific cultural background refusing scientific medical treatments against an overwhelming body of public opinion that such a refusal would be 'unreasonable' and even 'odd'.

In dealing with these and other difficulties, as well as with other more general objections which may be raised against the doctrine of informed consent, it is important not to lose sight of the various theoretical perspectives underpinning and justifying the right of people to make informed choices about their care and treatment. For instance, key to both the legal doctrine and moral right of informed consent is (i) the liberal democratic notion of the *sovereignty of the individual*, and (ii) ethical principlism, considered under separate subheadings below.

Informed consent and the sovereignty of the individual

Informed consent rests heavily on the view that the individual is sovereign alias the *sovereignty of the individual*. This highly individualistic notion characterises the person (patient) as a solitary competent individual who possesses 'a sphere of protected activity or privacy free from unwanted interference'; by this view, although 'influence is acceptable', coercion in any form is not (Kuczewski 1996, p. 30). Kuczewski explains that:

> Within this zone of privacy, one is able to exercise his or her liberty and discretion. Within this protected sphere take place disclosure, comprehension, and choice, which express the patient's right of self-determination ... The person is opaque to others and therefore the best judge and guardian of his or her own interests. Although the physician may be the expert on the medical 'facts', the patient is the only individual with genuine insight into his [sic] private sphere of 'values'. Because treatment plans should reflect personal values as well as medical realities, the patient must be the ultimate decision-maker.
>
> (Kuczewski 1996, p. 30)

One serious and significant implication of this view is that the patient's family, friends and/or chosen carers (acknowledging here that not all patients have families or, if they do, desire the involvement of their families) are conceived 'as comprising competing interests'; they are also seen as having no entitlements whatsoever in regard to any consent to medical treatment processes that the 'sovereign individual' might otherwise engage in (Kuczewski 1996). This may help to explain some of the tensions examined previously in Chapter 6 of this text on transcultural ethics *apropos* family members of traditional cultural backgrounds seeking active participation in consent to medical treatment processes and the reluctance by some doctors and nurses to involve these family members in such processes.

Bioethicists are, however, beginning to rethink their traditional opposition to the involvement of family or chosen carers in consent to treatment practices. There is increasing recognition that illness can seriously undermine the patient's capacity to make prudent self-determined choices (autonomy) and to be an effective judge and guardian of his or her own self-interests. This has been matched by an increasing questioning of the traditional legalistic approach to informed consent that, among other things, presupposes that the values of the 'sovereign individual' are well-developed, fixed and adequate to the task of choosing between difficult treatment options, and that all the chooser needs in order to make an informed choice is 'information' (Kuczewski 1996).

Increasingly, family members and chosen carers are seen as having a vital role to play in consent processes. By being intimately acquainted with ('knowing well') the patient, family members or chosen carers are able to provide appropriate and meaningful feedback to their loved ones, and to generally assist in 'reality testing' their loved one's choices and the values, beliefs (new and old), and deliberations influencing these choices. In sum, the involvement of family members and/or chosen carers in consent to treatment processes can play a vital role in restoring the otherwise diminished autonomy of their sick loved ones (Kuczewski 1996). Furthermore, by fulfilling this role, they are also able to strengthen the bonds of their relationship with the patient and with each other — in short, to express their care of and for each other.

The ultimate conclusion of this new approach is this: we need to reconceptualised informed consent as a *shared* rather than as an *individual* decision-making process (Kuczewski 1996).

Informed consent and ethical principlism

Informed consent also rests heavily on ethical principlism (discussed in Chapter 4 of this text), both for its content and justification as an action guide. The principles of particular importance here include those of:

- *autonomy* — which demands respect for patients as self-determining choosers, and justifies allowing them the option of accepting risks;
- *non-maleficence* — which demands the protection of patients from battery, assault, trespass, exploitation, and other harms that may result from inadequate or inappropriate consent processes (including the inadequate or inappropriate disclosure of information);
- *beneficence* — which demands the maximisation of patient wellbeing via consent processes;
- *justice* — which demands fairness and that patients not be unduly or intolerably burdened by consent processes.

It should be noted that while autonomy is *a* value underlying the doctrine of informed consent it is not *the* value, nor an *absolute* value. As Faden and Beauchamp (1986, p. 18) point out, at best autonomy is only a prima facie value, and to regard it as having overriding value would be both historically and culturally 'odd'. This is not to say that autonomy does not have a significant place in a moral approach to informed consent. It merely means that it does not have a sole place, and can be justly restricted by other competing moral principles, such as those already mentioned.

Having now reviewed the function and theoretical underpinnings of informed consent, let us proceed critically to examine the constituents and nature of informed consent.

The elements of an informed and valid consent

It is generally recognised within bioethics that disclosure, comprehension, voluntariness, competence and consent itself form the analytical components of the concept of informed consent (Faden and Beauchamp 1986, p. 274).

Morally speaking, for a consent to be regarded as informed, it must satisfy a number of criteria, including those relating to the *informational* aspect of the consent and those relating to the *giving of consent* itself. Beauchamp and Childress (1989, pp. 74–119) argue that for consent to be informed: there must be a *disclosure* of all the relevant information (including both benefits and risks); the patient must fully *understand* (comprehend) *both* the information which has been given *and* the implications of giving consent; the consent must be voluntarily given (i.e. the patient must be free of coercion or manipulation); and, lastly, the patient must be competent to consent (i.e. be both 'rational' and prudent). Faden and Beauchamp (1986) argue along similar lines, but recommend what they believe are less 'overdemanding' and more plausible criteria, notably:

> (1) a patient or subject must agree to an intervention based on an *understanding* of (usually disclosed) relevant *information*, (2) consent must not be controlled by influences that would engineer the outcome, and (3) the consent must involve the intentional giving of *permission* for an intervention.
>
> (Faden and Beauchamp 1986, p. 54)

It needs to be noted that patients frequently do not realise that in giving consent they are not merely acknowledging the receipt of information concerning a recommended medical treatment or procedure, but are also actually *giving permission* to an attending health professional to go ahead and perform the treatment or procedure in question.

Faden and Beauchamp's theory of informed consent is probably one of the most comprehensive and convincing to date, and one which, although written from the cultural perspective of the United States, deserves to be given serious attention by those furthering the informed consent debate in Australia, New Zealand and other common law countries. As well as advancing their ethical theory, these authors also make a number of useful practical suggestions on how informed consent practices could be made more 'workable'.

It should be noted that the doctrine of informed consent has been the subject of much controversy, most notably amongst health professionals. Popular objections include:

- obtaining an informed consent is unacceptably time-consuming;
- when patients are told the information they need to know, they forget it;
- most patients do not want to know all the details of the risks and benefits associated with a recommended medical treatment or procedure, and forcing information on them would be just as paternalistic as withholding it;
- most patients would not understand the information required to make an informed choice;
- giving information to patients can be harmful (for example, they might refuse a life-saving procedure or drug because of a negligible risk); and
- informed consent is impractical and thus unworkable.

Despite their popularity, however, these and similar objections are difficult to sustain in the face of research findings, anecdotes and professional experience. For example, it is well recognised that people in stressful and unfamiliar situations are vulnerable both to information overload and short-term memory loss (Faden and Beauchamp 1986, pp. 324–5; Robinson and Merav 1983). The stress of being admitted to hospital; of coping with feelings of pain, fear and anxiety; of being separated from the familiarity of one's home, family and friends;

the general disruption of one's life, not to mention the effort required to adapt to a new (hospital) environment characterised by strange smells, sights, noises, tastes, routines, faces, procedures and sensations — all contribute, predictably, to lessening an individual's capacity to pay attention to and to recall information that has been disclosed. It is small wonder that patients forget. Information overload and short-term memory impairment in turn compromise the individual's actual understanding of information received.

To complicate matters, health professionals seeking consent or giving information do not always manage their encounters with patients very well (see, in particular, the example given in Chapter 7, under the sub-heading 'Moral dilemmas'). Some use a hurried, uninterested and sometimes positively intimidating approach when seeking a patient's consent. (Significantly, this has been the subject of formal complaint to the Victorian Health Services Commissioner [*Victorian Health Services Commissioner Annual Report 1991*]; see also Spitzer 1988.) When seeking consent from a patient, health professionals too often give little attention to controlling their tone of voice, choosing a suitable time and place to approach the patient, ensuring privacy, using the appropriate body language and facial expressions, choosing the right words, avoiding complicated jargon, sitting at the patient's level, and so on. I can recall many instances in my career of doctors standing at the end of the bed looking down on the patient lying in bed when offering an explanation of an impending procedure. No doubt the doctors in question regarded their towering position as being perfectly 'natural', and probably even now would consider nothing wrong with it. What some doctors do not seem to appreciate, however, is that standing above a patient in that manner can be very intimidating and can serve more to hinder the communication process than to enhance it. In such situations, patients may find it extremely difficult to ask the questions they really want to ask. Of course, many doctors do sit down, do face the patient at a mutually agreeable level, and are unafraid to touch their patients in a gesture of reassurance and care; unfortunately this is not the general rule.

When dealing with non-English-speaking patients, these problems are considerably worse. For example, health professionals may shout unnecessarily (a problem which also sometimes occurs when they are dealing with blind or physically handicapped people who nevertheless have perfect hearing), or they may use inappropriate body language and facial expressions, use the wrong intonations in speech, or use terms which cannot be readily interpreted into the patient's spoken language.

As far as patients who do not want to know the details of an impending medical procedure are concerned, there are few who seem to fit into this category. In some instances patients have declined information (on the basis of personal and cultural health beliefs and practices), but even then only certain select pieces of information have been declined; in these instances, patients have not voiced a blanket and unconditional rejection of all relevant information. In many instances, what has superficially appeared to be a 'refusal' was in fact more a demand that the information be given in a culturally appropriate manner (Kanitsaki 1988b). If, however, patients do make an informed refusal to receive certain relevant pieces of information, and on reflection are not open to changing their minds about receiving the information in question, then to give this information to the patients would certainly count as a paternalistic act, as Vandeveer (1980) and Kanitsaki (1988b) have already contended elsewhere (the subject of 'paternalism' will be considered shortly below).

The objection that patients would not be able to understand the necessary information in order to make an intelligent and informed choice is also difficult to sustain. It is sometimes difficult to avoid the impression that the claim that a patient cannot understand is more an assumption than a matter of sound deliberation and determination. Buchanan (1978, p. 386), for example, argues that to assume a patient would not understand given information is to make a 'dubious and extremely broad psychological generalisation', which, of course, ordinary doctors and nurses are not particularly qualified to make. Faden and Beauchamp (1986) also argue that most patients are able to understand the information given to them, and, what is more, that a patient's level of understanding can be ascertained and measured.

Even if patients do not fully understand the information given, this does not always imply that it is the fault of the patient. A patient's inability to understand is probably attributable just as much to a doctor's or a nurse's inappropriate behaviour and communication as it is to a patient's cognitive inability (Roth et al. 1983, p. 176). The onus then is on consent seekers to improve their approach to patients, and to presume a patient's *ability* to understand information rather than an inability to understand. On this point Muyskens argues:

> as in a court of law in which one's innocence is presumed until proven otherwise, the client's ability to comprehend and understand what is going on and to be able to make judgments based on the data must be presumed until firm evidence establishes the contrary.

> (Muyskens 1982, p. 119)

Just as there is no compelling evidence to suggest that patients would not understand information disclosed to them about a proposed medical procedure, there is no compelling evidence to suggest that patients would be unduly injured or harmed by disclosures. Bok (1980), for example, cites studies which show that very few patients withdraw their consent when informed of material risks or other so-called 'harmful' pieces of information concerning a proposed medical procedure. She further contends that in fact 'it is what patients do not know but vaguely suspect that causes them corrosive worry' (Bok 1980, p. 234).

Buchanan (1978) is even more scathing in his criticism of the 'information causing harm' objection, arguing that it reeks of nothing more than wide and unfounded 'psychiatric generalisations', which, again, ordinary doctors and nurses are simply not qualified to make. He argues further that even qualified psychiatric specialists would probably find it very difficult to judge correctly whether a patient would be significantly harmed by disclosure.

The 'information causing harm' objection, of course, also ignores the moral point that, even if a patient refused to undergo a recommended medical procedure on the basis of information received about certain material risks, this is, after all, something which any competent patient is morally entitled to do — whatever the risks involved and regardless of what others might think of their refusal. At best, all attending health professionals can morally do is to persuade patients *non-coercively* about the known benefits of undergoing a given medical procedure; but they are not entitled to interfere with the patient's choice if such persuasion fails (Faden and Beauchamp 1986).

Even if critics concede that these objections cannot be sustained, the objection still remains that informed consent procedures are impractical because they are unrealistically and unacceptably time-consuming. It is quite true that obtaining a voluntary consent (i.e. one free of coercive or manipulative influences) and a truly informed consent from a patient will take more time than the type of consent that is likely to be obtained in an 'assembly line' approach. But, then, so it should take more time. Health professionals *should* take more time (and as much as is required) to interact and communicate with their patients in a way that facilitates making informed choices and realising morally acceptable outcomes. If health professionals really do care about the wellbeing of their patients, there can be no excuse whatsoever for denying patients the time needed to deal with an anxiety, to answer a worrisome question, or to be reassured. Patients must have sufficient time to make an adequate decision and must have sufficient time to contemplate viable and real alternatives; anything less will result in information overload and will undermine their ability to make voluntary and informed choices (Faden and Beauchamp 1986, p. 326).

The so-called problem of 'time constraint' may be only a pseudo-problem. In some respects it may even be an *excuse* — to avoid respecting patients as autonomous choosers; to restrict and constrain the role of patients in decision-making concerning their own care; to avoid the intrusion of patient authority into physician authority — in short, an excuse to maintain the status quo and to avoid doing what is morally just.

In a culture so heavily dominated and constrained by considerations of 'time', it is very easy to accept 'time constraint' as a valid excuse for abrogating one's moral responsibilities. This, however, is not acceptable morally. There are ways around the difficulties posed by time constraints, and these must always be fully explored. In the case of informed consent, the one possible solution is to involve others in the business of information transfer to and sharing with patients. As considered above, these 'others' could include family and/or chosen carers.

While it is obviously and properly the responsibility of treating doctors to obtain informed consents to treatment from the patients they are treating, there is nevertheless considerable room to suggest that a collaborative approach to meeting patients' information needs would contribute substantially to maximising the patients' moral interests. Rightly or wrongly, nurses already play a major although unacknowledged role in meeting patients' information needs. This situation has arisen for many reasons, including the reality that treating doctors sometimes fail to meet the information needs of their patients — even when specifically requested to do so, either by patients themselves, or by nurses, or even by other doctors. In situations like this, an attending nurse is often the only immediately available person patients have to turn to in order to obtain the information they want. Indeed, nurses are very often the ones whom patients ask directly about what to expect of a given or pending medical procedure or treatment. (The experience of Ann Oakley, the internationally reputed English medical sociologist, considered in the final chapter of this book, is a case in point.) In such instances, nurses can find themselves in a very difficult situation — particularly if an attending doctor will not respond appropriately to a patient's request for information, as happened in the case of the man scheduled for spinal surgery, given earlier, and in Ann Oakley's case to be cited later. The nurses' dilemma is compounded by the fact that they know they can contribute a great deal to allaying patient anxiety related to knowledge deficits concerning proposed and rendered medical care and treatment options, but do not have the legitimated authority to undertake this role. Thus, if and when they are giving information to patients about medical treatments, nurses know they are 'taking a risk', since this could be construed as 'interfering with the physician–patient relationship' — as, indeed, happened in the *Tuma case* (see Chapter 7; see also Johnstone 1994).

Studies have also shown that nurses can greatly assist patients in coming to understand their illness experience and physician directives given during medical consultations (Uyer 1986). One study also shows that the task of giving information to patients and satisfying patients' information needs is *'impossible* without systematic collaboration between medical and nursing staff' (Engstrom 1986, emphasis added). It is clear that this is a matter which requires much greater attention than it has been given up until now.

A second obvious strategy which could be used to help resolve the time constraint problem is to restructure the time frame itself during which consents are usually sought. In elective admissions, consents are usually sought on the day before or evening before (or, as we have seen, even the minute before!) a scheduled medical or surgical procedure. The moral disadvantages of this are obvious. As Faden and Beauchamp ask:

> who would want, on the eve of surgery after having disrupted one's life, gathered one's courage, and entered the hospital, to change one's mind? And thus who would want to pay attention to information that challenges the wisdom of the decision?
>
> (Faden and Beauchamp 1986, p. 325)

The 'night before' time frame is hardly conducive to patients exercising voluntary and informed consent. One possible solution here would be to give patients all the 'usual' information during a pre-admission clinic a week or so before the procedure. In this way, patients would have time to go home, contemplate the information received, discuss it with family and friends, formulate any further questions they would like to ask, or even change their minds and decline the recommended therapy or procedure if they so desired. If patients were allowed time to reflect on the information given to them, not only would their consents to treatment be of better quality, but so too would their decisions to enter hospital.

The time factor involved in obtaining consent is crucial to the realisation of morally just outcomes. If sufficient time is not allocated for the purposes of gaining a patient's consent, a very real risk exists that the voluntary and informed nature of the consent will be seriously compromised, thus having the domino effect of violating underlying moral principles such as autonomy, non-maleficence, beneficence, and justice. In other words, a complete moral collapse of the situation could occur. In emergency or life-threatening situations, of course, it is not always possible to seek an informed consent and it could be hazardous to try and do so. The law recognises that in emergency or life-threatening situations consent can be 'waived'; morality likewise recognises situations in which consent can be justly waived.

The challenge to doctors and nurses and other health professionals is to restructure their thinking on informed consent, and to view it as something which 'should help overcome the inclination that many people have to yield compliantly to proposals from powerful authority figures' (Faden and Beauchamp 1986, p. 372). Faden and Beauchamp (1986, p. 305) argue that the questions that all health professionals and policy and law makers should be asking are not what patients should be told or even who should tell them, but 'What can professionals do to facilitate obtaining informed consents based on substantial understanding?', or 'How can professionals enable patients and subjects to make informed autonomous choices?'.

If informed consent procedures are to work and to achieve their desired ends, a number of other practical considerations need to be attended to. First, consent forms must be made available in the patient's own language. Where this cannot be done, the patient must be given access to a *trained health interpreter*. To illustrate the need, although over 25 per cent of Victoria's population are from non-English-speaking backgrounds, in 1988 fewer than twenty-nine full-time health interpreters were employed by the Victorian Central Health Interpreters Service. I was told by a coordinator from the Interpreters Service that, while interpreters had completed a general interpreters course, they had not been specially trained as health or medical interpreters. She further commented that the supply of health interpreters at the time was grossly inadequate to meet the demand of non-English-speaking patients. As an example, it was reported to me by a colleague that when she sought from the Central Health Interpreters Service the services of an Arabic-speaking interpreter (the patient was due to go to theatre the next day), she was informed that there was a six-week waiting list. Currently, the situation is in fact worse than it was a few years ago. The economic rationalisation of interpreter services in hospitals has in some instances seen a return to the situation of the 1950s, during which a lack of appropriate interpreting services risked the health and lives of immigrants who could not speak English (Johnstone 1991).

It is often the practice to ask cleaners or orderlies or kitchen hands who speak languages other than English to interpret for a non-English-speaking patient (see also Stone 1991, p. 4). This practice is, however, wholly undesirable. First, orderlies and cleaners and kitchen hands are not trained as interpreters and thus may seriously misinterpret the information being relayed, or may give their own assessment of and interpretation of a question being asked. For example, Olga Kanitsaki (who is Greek-speaking) describes a case involving a Greek-speaking patient. In this case, a cleaner called in to interpret for the doctor exclaimed to the patient, in Greek, 'Well, if you only have a headache why don't you take an aspirin? What did you come into hospital for? Why are you bothering the doctor?' (personal communication).

Another problem here, and one often overlooked by health professionals, is that orderlies and cleaners and kitchen hands do not have a professional relationship with the patient; thus, involving them as interpreters is tantamount to breaching confidentiality. Who is to know whether these 'informal' interpreters will keep confidential the information disclosed during an interpreting session? Since they are not bound by any professional code of ethics, they may not fully appreciate their moral responsibilities not to disclose the confidential information they have become privy to while acting as interpreters.

A second practical consideration is that patients' consent must be continuously *re-evaluated* so as to check whether their original consent still holds. This is particularly crucial in situations involving 'Not For Resuscitation' directives or refusal to consent to given life-saving therapies. In some instances, the terms of a patient's original consent may need to be modified. It has been asserted informally by those working in the area that the term 'informed consent' should be abandoned in favour of the term 'informed decision-making'. The rationale given is that the notion of *informed consent* has an air of finality about it — that is, once consent has been obtained that is the end of the process. With the notion of *informed decision-making*, however, the connotations are quite different. In contrast, it has an air of 'open-endedness' about it — of a process that is *ongoing*. Given this, it is thought, the notion of informed decision-making, unlike the notion of informed consent, seems to invite the continuous re-evaluation of any decisions made about care and treatment options. This change in thinking, however, has yet to be reflected fully in literature on the subject.

A third consideration is that patients must be informed of their entitlement to *refuse* a recommended medical or nursing procedure, and the opportunity to refuse must always be present without prejudice to the patients. Fourth, patients must be kept up to date on the relevant details pertaining to their cases. Details which are not readily understood should be explained (in understandable language), and reinforced through planned patient health education programs (something that nurses are educationally prepared to undertake).

Lastly, health professionals need to remind themselves constantly that many factors can deter patients from exercising informed and voluntary choices, including, but not limited to, fear of victimisation. For example, patients may fear that if they refuse to give consent to some aspect of the proposed procedure they may be victimised by being denied other forms of treatment or by being verbally and emotionally abused. Other factors include: feelings of guilt where patients might feel, for example, that somehow they ought to give consent for the sake of their families (see Roberts, 1987); fear of unknown outcomes, as happened in the cervical spinal fusion case cited earlier; frank disagreement and value conflict, where patients might refuse simply because they do not agree with a given recommended medical therapy and would prefer to try an alternative health modality; pain or grief states which can cloud patients' prudence; 'rational incompetence', and an associated inability to exercise self-determining choices; and incompetent or impaired health professionals who may, for instance, be poor communicators, have poor interpersonal skills, be rushed or hurried, or lack the relevant information to give to the patient.

Before concluding this discussion two further issues remain to be addressed — the problem of the so-called 'rationally incompetent' patient and medical paternalism.

The problem of rational competency

The issue of competency is controversial and complicated. There is no substantial agreement on the characteristics of a 'competent person' or on how 'competency' should be measured. To complicate this matter further, there is also no substantial agreement on what constitutes *rationality* (as already discussed in previous chapters).

Roth et al. (1983) argue that the concept of competency is not merely a psychiatric or medical concept, as some might assume, but is also fundamentally social and legal. They warn, however, that there is no magical definition of competency, and that the problems posed by so-called 'incompetent' persons are very often problems of personal prejudices and social biases, or of other difficulties associated with trying to find the 'right' words.

The critical issue in developing tests of competency is how to strike a happy balance between serving a rationally incompetent person's autonomy and also serving that person's health care, nursing care and medical treatment needs. Also of critical concern is finding a competency test which is comprehensive enough to deal with diverse situations, which can be applied reliably, and which is mutually acceptable to health care professionals, lawyers, judges and the community at large.

Roth et al. suggest that competency tests proposed in the literature basically fall into five categories:

1. evidencing a choice;
2. 'reasonable' outcome of choice;
3. choice based on 'rational' reasons;
4. ability to understand;
5. actual understanding.

(Roth et al. 1983, p. 173)[1]

The test of *evidencing a choice* is as it sounds, and is concerned only with whether a patient's choice is 'evident'; that is, whether it is *present or absent*. For example, a fully comatose patient would be unable to evidence a choice, unlike a semi-comatose patient or a brain-injured person, who could evidence a choice by opening and shutting their eyes or by squeezing someone's hand to indicate 'yes' or 'no'. The *quality* of the patient's choice in this instance is quite irrelevant. One problem with this test, however, is whether, say, the blinking of a patient's eyes can be relied upon as evidencing a choice; in a life and death situation one would need to be very sure that a patient's so-called 'evidencing a choice' is more than just a reflex.

The test of *reasonable outcome of a choice* is again as it sounds, and focuses on the *outcome* of a given choice, as opposed to the mere presence or absence of a choice. The objective test here is similar to that employed in law, and involves asking the question: What would a reasonable person in like circumstances consider to be a reasonable outcome? The reliability of this measure is, of course, open to serious question — as previously objected, what one person might accept as reasonable another might equally reject.

The test of *choice based on rational reasons* is a little more difficult to apply. Basically, it asks whether a given choice is the product of 'mental illness' or whether it is the product of prudent and critically reflective deliberation. A number of objections can be raised here. For example, contrary to popular medical opinion, there is nothing to suggest that a person's decision to suicide is always the product of mental disease or depression. A patient could without contradiction 'rationally' choose to suicide as a means of escaping an intolerable life characterised by suffering intractable and intolerable pain. Alternatively, a depressed and so-called 'irrational' person might refuse a particular psychiatric treatment, such as psychotropic drugs, electroconvulsive therapy, or psychosurgery, out of a very 'rational' and well-founded fear of what undesirable effects these treatments might ultimately have.

The test of *ability to understand*, on the other hand, asks whether the patient is able to comprehend the risks, benefits and alternatives to a proposed medical procedure, as well as the implications of giving consent. Here objections can be raised concerning just how sophisticated a patient's understanding needs to be. The problem also may arise of patients perceiving a risk as a benefit. Roth et al. (1983, p. 175), for example, cite the case of a 49 year-old woman psychiatric patient who was informed that there was a one in three thousand chance of dying from ECT. When told of this risk she replied, happily: 'I hope I am the one!'.

---

1. From L. H. Roth, A. Meisel and C. W. Lidz, Tests of competency to consent to treatment, *American Journal of Psychiatry* 134 (4), 1977, pp. 279–84. Copyright © 1977, The American Psychiatric Association. Reprinted by permission.

The fifth and final competency test is that of *actual understanding*. This test asks how well the patient has actually understood information which has been disclosed. This can be established by asking patients probing questions and inviting them to reiterate the information they have received. On the basis of educated skill and past experience, the health professional is usually able to ascertain the level at which the patient has understood the information received and what data gaps or misunderstandings remain.

Whatever the patients' competency to decide and quality of their autonomous choice may be, any duty of respect owed would still ultimately depend on the demands of other competing moral considerations, as already discussed. Thus, what may appear to be a dilemma involving whether to respect a patient's autonomy may not in fact be a dilemma at all. For example, if an elderly demented patient keeps wandering aimlessly from his bed, and is at risk of falling and fracturing his hip, overriding considerations do exist which would justify interfering with the choice to wander. If, after careful analysis of all available alternatives, the only way to stop this elderly patient from sustaining a fractured hip is to restrain him, it may well be that the use of a comfortable restraining device is the morally compelling option in this case. If, however, the elderly person is not at risk of falling and sustaining a fractured hip, and his wandering is merely an 'inconvenience' to staff, the solution might be better found in securing door locks so as to prevent the patient from wandering out onto the street where there is a very real risk of injury — say, of being hit by a car. This solution is already employed in a number of residential care homes which have installed combination locks on all their doors; only those residents who know the combination of the locks on the doors can freely come and go. Either way, entitlements and corresponding duties in the case of 'rational incompetence' must ultimately be determined by critical reflection and not, as can happen, by misguided or unfounded assumption.

It should be noted that competency is a key issue not just in psychiatric nursing, but in any health care context where judgments of competency are critical to deciding: (1) whether a patient can or should decide and/or be permitted to decide for herself or himself, and (2) the point at which another or others will need to or should decide for the patient — that is, become what Buchanan and Brock (1989) term *surrogate decision-makers*. The question remains, however, of how these things can be decided in a morally sound and just way. This question becomes even more problematic when it is considered that patients deemed 'rationally incompetent' can still be quite capable of making self-interested choices, and, further, that the choices they make — even if 'irrational' — are not always harmful.

Commenting on the moral standards which should be met when deciding whether to respect or override the expressed preferences of a patient deemed 'incompetent', Buchanan and Brock (1989) argue that it is important to be clear about what statements of competence refer to. They argue, for instance, that statements of competence usually refer to a person's competence to *do something* (in this instance, to *choose and make decisions*); by this view, competence is, therefore, 'choice and decision-relative'. Given this, determining competence in health care contexts fundamentally involves determining a person's ability to make particular choices and decisions under particular conditions (Buchanan and Brock 1989, pp. 311–65).

An important problem particularly in psychiatric contexts is that severe mental illness can significantly affect the capacities needed for competent decision-making (for instance, understanding, reasoning, and applying values), and hence the ability generally of severely mentally ill persons to make sound decisions about their own wellbeing — including the need for care and treatment (Buchanan and Brock 1989). For example, as Buchanan and Brock comment:

> a person may persist in a fixed delusional belief that proferred medications are poison or are being used to control his or her mind. Such delusions or fixed false beliefs obviously may also impair a person's capacity to reason about whether hospitalisation and treatment will on balance serve his or her wellbeing. Severe mental illness can also affect and seriously distort a person's underlying and enduring aims and values, his or her conception of his or her own good, that one must use in evaluating hospitalisation and treatment for an illness.
>
> (Buchanan and Brock 1989, p. 318)

It is precisely in situations such as these that attending health care professionals need a reliable framework within which to decide how best to act — notably: (1) whether to respect a patient's preferences even though the patient is deemed 'incompetent', or (2) whether to override patients' preferences in the interests of protecting or upholding what has been deemed by *others* to be in the patient's overall 'best interests'. Just what such a framework would — or indeed should — look like, is, however, a matter of some controversy. Nevertheless, as Buchanan and Brock's substantive work *Deciding for others: the ethics of surrogate decision-making* (1989) has shown, it is possible to devise at least a prima facie working framework to guide professional ethical decision-making in this sensitive, complex and problematic area. Specifically, Buchanan and Brock (1989) suggest that the whole issue hinges on:

1. setting and applying accurately standards of competency to choose and decide; and
2. achieving a balance between (i) protecting and promoting the patients' wellbeing (human welfare), (ii) protecting and promoting the patients' entitlement to and interest in exercising self-determining choices, and (iii) protecting others who could be harmed by patients exercising harm-causing choices.

In regard to setting and applying accurately standards of competency to choose and decide, Buchanan and Brock suggest that, among other things, ethical professional decision-making in this problematic area should be guided by the following considerations:

> No single standard of competence is adequate for all decisions. The standard depends in large part on the risk involved, and varies along a range from low/minimal to high/maximal. The more serious the expected harm to the patient from acting on a choice, the higher should be the standard of decision-making capacity, and the greater should be the certainty that the standard is satisfied.
>
> (Buchanan and Brock 1989, p. 85)

In other words, the extent to which an attending health care professional is bound morally to respect the choices of a person deemed 'rationally incompetent' depends primarily on the severity of the risks involved to the patient if her or his choices are permitted. The higher and more severe the risks involved, the higher and more rigorous should be the standards for determining the patient's decision-making capacity, and the more certain attending health care professionals should be that the patient has met these standards. This framework is expressed diagrammatically in Figure 8.2.

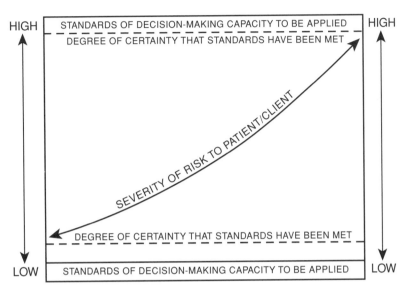

Figure 8.2 Assessing risks and permitting choices of patients deemed 'rationally incompetent'

For example, if a patient with severe mental illness chooses to refuse hospitalisation, the extent to which an attending health professional is obliged morally to respect this choice will depend on how severe the risks to the patient are of not being hospitalised— for instance, whether a failure to hospitalise the patient will result in her or him suiciding, or will result only in her or him being left in a state of moderate, although not life-threatening, depression. In the case of suicide risk, the grounds for not honouring a patient's choices do seem at least prima facie stronger than possible grounds for overriding the choices of a patient who is only moderately depressed. (Whether or not the risk of suicide does provide strong grounds for overriding a patient's choices to refuse hospitalisation and treatment is another question, however, and one which is considered separately in Chapter 13 of this text.)

While Buchanan and Brock's (1989) framework appears hopeful, it is not free of difficulties. For instance, there remains the problem of how to determine what is a harm, what is a low/minimal and high/maximal risk of harm, and who properly should decide these things — the answers to which involve complex value judgments. Consider, for example, the following case (personal communication).

An involuntary psychiatric patient refuses to take the psychotropic medication he has been prescribed. (For a helpful discussion on this problematic issue, see Feather 1985.) In defence of his refusal, the patient argues 'reasonably' that the adverse side effects of the drugs he is being expected to take are intolerable, and that he would prefer the pain of his mental illness to the intolerable side effects of the drugs that have been prescribed to treat his mental illness. Staff on the ward in which he is an involuntary patient are divided about what they should do. The more experienced staff in this case insist that the patient should be given his medication forcibly by intramuscular injection. They argue in defence of this decision that the patient's condition is deteriorating rapidly, and that if he does not receive the medication prescribed he will 'spiral down into a psychiatric crisis' (in other words a total exacerbation of his condition), which would be even more intolerable and harmful than the unpleasant side effects he has been experiencing as a result of taking the psychotropic drugs in question. They make the additional value judgment that it would be 'better' for the patient if his psychiatric condition was prevented from deteriorating, and that their decision to administer his prescribed medication forcibly against his will is justified on these grounds.

The less experienced staff on the ward disagree with this reasoning, however, and argue that, even though the patient's psychiatric condition is deteriorating, and this is a preventable harm, the patient is nevertheless able to make an informed choice about this and therefore his wishes should be respected. In defence of their position, they argue that the patient's complaints are justified — the adverse side effects of his psychotropic drugs have indeed been 'awful', and are commonly experienced by other patients as well; and that he has experienced a decline in his psychiatric condition before, and hence knows what to expect. Further, they argue, if he is given the medication against his will, an even greater harm will follow: specifically, he will trust the nursing staff even less than he does already, and will be even less willing to comply with his oral medication prescription than he is now.

In this case, the more experienced staff outnumbered the less experienced staff, and the patient was held down and forcibly given an intramuscular injection of the medication he had refused. Later, after recovering from this incident, the patient was, as predicted by the less experienced nursing staff, grossly mistrustful of the nursing staff on the ward, and even less willing to comply with his oral medication orders. His requests for different and less drugs, and more counselling, went unheeded.

This case scenario demonstrates the difficulties that can be encountered when accepting/rejecting a patient's ability to choose and decide care and treatment options, and deciding when and how to override a patient's preferences. Not only is there the problem of how to determine accurately what a harm is and how a given harm should be weighted morally when evaluating whether a patient's choices should be respected or overridden; there is the additional problem that attending health care professionals may disagree radically among themselves about how these things should be determined — to a point that may even cause rather than prevent harm to the patient, as happened in this case. What else then should health care professionals do?

One response is to insist on the development of reliable (research-based) criteria for deciding these sorts of problematic issues. The need to do this becomes even more acute when the problem of determining and weighting harms is considered in relation to the broader demand to achieve a balance between protecting and promoting the patient's wellbeing, protecting and promoting the patient's autonomy, and protecting others who could be harmed if a mentally ill person is left free to exercise harm-causing choices (as happened in the *Tarasoff case*, to be considered later in this chapter).

Just what these criteria should be, however, and how they should be applied, is an extremely complex matter, and one that requires much greater attention than it is possible to give here. Nevertheless, Buchanan and Brock (1989) provide an important starting point by identifying the following three factors which should be (and are already being) taken into consideration when deciding whether to override a mentally ill person's choices, namely (1) whether the person is a danger to herself or himself; (2) whether the person is in need of care and treatment; and (3) whether the person is a danger to others. In regard to the consideration of being a danger to self, Buchanan and Brock (1989, pp. 317–31) correctly argue that what is needed are stringent criteria of what constitutes a danger to self; in the case of the need for care and treatment, that what is needed are stringent criteria for ascertaining deterioration and distress; and in the case of harm to others, that what is needed are stringent criteria of what constitutes a danger to others. And while applying the criteria developed may inevitably result in a health care professional assuming the essentially paternalistic role of being a surrogate decision-maker for a given patient, this need not be problematic provided the model of surrogate decision-making used is *patient centred* — that is, committed to upholding the patient's interests and concerns insofar as these can be ascertained (something which was not done in the case given above).

A patient-centred model of surrogate decision-making, in this instance, would have as its rationale *preventing harm to patients*, and would embrace an ethical framework which is structured 'for deciding *for* patients for *their benefit*' (Buchanan and Brock 1989, pp. 327, 331). This is in contrast with a non-patient or 'other'-centred decision-making model, which would have as its rationale *preventing harm to others*, and which embraces an ethical framework 'for deciding *about* others for *others' benefits* (Buchanan and Brock 1989, pp. 327, 331). It should be noted, however, that these two models are not necessarily mutually exclusive and indeed could, in some instances, be mutually supporting (a man contemplating a violent suicide involving others is not only a danger to himself but to the innocent others he plans to 'take with him'). Just which model or models are appropriate, and under what circumstances they should be used, will, however, depend ultimately on the people involved (and the relationships between them), the moral interests at stake, the context in which these moral interests are at stake, the resources available (human and otherwise) to protect and promote the moral interests that are at risk of being harmed, and, finally, the accurate prediction of possibilities and probabilities in regard to the achievement of desirable and acceptable moral outcomes. This, in turn, will depend on the competence, experience, wisdom and moral integrity of the decision-makers, and the degree of commitment they have to: (1) ensuring the realisation of morally just outcomes, and (2) protecting and promoting the wellbeing and moral interests of those made vulnerable not just by their mental illnesses, but by the inability of their caregivers to respond to the manifestation of their illnesses in morally sensitive, humane, therapeutically effective and culturally appropriate ways.

Paternalism and informed consent

The word *paternalism* comes from the Latin *pater* meaning 'father', and literally means 'in the manner of a father, especially in usurping individual responsibility and the liberty of choice' (*Collins English Dictionary* 1995). In the bioethics literature, paternalism has been defined in a variety of ways. Literature published in the early 1970s, for example, defined paternalism (construed as a principle viz. the *Paternalistic Principle* [Beauchamp 1980, p. 98]) as:

> the interference with a person's liberty of action justified by reasons referring exclusively to the welfare, good, happiness, needs, interests or value of the person being coerced.
>
> (Dworkin 1972, p. 65)

Subsequently, paternalism was defined more specifically as:

> interference with a person's freedom of action or freedom of information, or the deliberate dissemination of misinformation, where the alleged justification of interfering or misinforming is that it is for the good of the person who is interfered with or misinformed.
>
> (Buchanan 1978, p. 372)

A further modification in definition resulted in the suggestion that for an act to be paternalistic:

> There must be a violation of a person's autonomy ... There must be a [sic] usurpation of decision-making, either by preventing people from doing what they have decided or by interfering with the way in which they arrive at their decision.
>
> (Dworkin 1988, p. 123)

A more recent definition of paternalism holds it to be:

> the intentional overriding of one person's known preferences or actions by another person, where the person who overrides justifies the action by the goal of benefiting or avoiding harm to the person whose will is overridden.
>
> (Beauchamp and Childress, 1994, p. 274)

Early literature on the subject distinguished between two types of paternalism: (1) harm paternalism, and (2) benefit paternalism (Beauchamp 1978; Beauchamp and Childress 1994). *Harm paternalism* (underpinned by the principle of non-maleficence) was thought to be justified where it had as its objective protecting individuals from self-inflicted harm. In contrast, *benefit paternalism* (underpinned by the principle of beneficence) was thought to be justified where it had as its objective securing a good or a beneficence that an individual would not otherwise get — for example, because their liberty is limited. These two forms of paternalism were, in turn, categorised still further, with the following distinctions being made: (1) strong paternalism and (2) weak paternalism, considered below.

In the case of *strong paternalism*, it was thought to be 'proper to protect or benefit a person by liberty-limiting measures *even when his [or her] contrary choices are informed and voluntary* (Beauchamp 1978, p. 1197). An example of 'strong paternalism' would be where a consultant physician refuses to release a competent although seriously ill patient from hospital even though the patient has requested discharge and knows the potentially fatal consequences of his/her request.

Strong paternalism is in contradistinction to *weak paternalism* where interference with an individual's conduct is only justified in cases where that person's conduct is 'substantially nonvoluntary or when temporary intervention is necessary to establish whether it is voluntary or not' (Feinberg 1971, pp. 113, 116). In short, where a person's autonomy has been compromised in some way (e.g. as a result of pain, drug ingestion, psychogenic distress, physical trauma to the head that interferes with memory, and the like), it is acceptable to paternalistically override a person's choices or restrain their liberty of conduct. This form of paternalism has been widely accepted in law, medicine and moral philosophy (Beauchamp 1995, p. 1915). An example of 'weak paternalism' would be where an attending health care professional attends the scene of a motor vehicle accident and picks up an injured, partially coherent victim and takes him/her to hospital even though the victim has refused an ambulance (Beauchamp 1995, p. 1915).

As a point of clarification, it should be noted that harm paternalism is thought to be easier to justify and uphold than benefit paternalism. One reason for this is that it was (and is) generally thought, controversially, that we have a greater duty to avoid harm than to promote good — which may not always be within our capacity in given contexts and thus not something for which we could be held morally responsible for not doing. If it was our duty to do or promote good — even where we lacked the resources to do so — this would risk us being condemned as 'unethical' for not doing something that we could not do anyway, which would be untenable.

However defined or conceptualised, it should be noted that *paternalism* remains morally controversial since it always entails *the choices or actions of one person being overridden by another without consent.* Even if a person's stated preferences do not originate from a substantially autonomous and authentic choice, 'overriding his or her preference can still be paternalistic' (Beauchamp 1995, p. 1915). This is because, even in the case of 'diminished autonomy', persons (for example, young children, the intellectually disabled and the mentally ill) can still be capable of exercising self-interested choices. It is against this backdrop then that a key question arises, namely: Is paternalism ever justified? and if so, under what conditions?

Is *paternalism justified*?

The literature reveals at least three possible answers to the question of whether paternalism is justified:

  (i) pro-paternalism (always justified);
  (ii) anti-paternalism (never justified); and
  (iii) prima-facie paternalism (sometimes justified).

These three possible answers are discussed below.

Pro-paternalism (always justified)

Pro-paternalism positions hold that paternalism is always justified to 'protect individuals against themselves' (Hart 1963, p. 31). This position is supported by an appeal to either of the principles of human welfare, beneficence (e.g. as in the case of overriding the harmful choices of children) and/or 'rational consent' (meaning consent that 'would otherwise have been given'; in this instance, paternalism is thought to be justified as a kind of 'social insurance policy' for our own protection (Beauchamp 1995, p. 1916). Further, it is held that sometimes an immediate act of paternalism may, paradoxically, protect a person's 'deeper autonomy', for example, such as in the case of someone who is depressed and suicidal (Beauchamp 1980, 1995). Justificatory considerations for strong paternalism, include the following conditions:

  - no acceptable alternative to the paternalistic action exists;
  - risks to the person that are introduced by the paternalistic action itself are not substantial;
  - projected benefits to the person outweigh risks to the person;
  - any infringement of the principle of respect for autonomy is minimal.

(Beauchamp 1995, p. 1917)

Anti-paternalism (never justified)

Anti-paternalism positions hold that paternalism is never justified. This is because paternalism always involves a violation of moral rules, for example, that we ought to respect people's choices even if we do not agree with them, provided they do not harm others; the individual is sovereign and any coercion or interference with their self-determining choices is morally unacceptable. Acts of paternalism also violate a person's privacy and fail to treat them as the moral equals of others (Childress 1982, cited in Beauchamp 1995, p. 1916).

Prima-facie paternalism (sometimes justified)

Prima-facie paternalism (also known as ambivalent-paternalism) holds the position that paternalism is sometimes justified, though severely limited. Any action of coercion against or interference with another's conduct carries a heavy burden of justification. Paternalism is only justified where:

(i) 'the evils prevented from occurring to the person are greater than the evils (if any) caused by violating the moral rule';
(ii) 'it is universally justified under relevantly similar circumstances always to treat persons in this way' (Gert and Culver 1976).

These three positions may be expressed diagrammatically as shown in Figure 8.3.

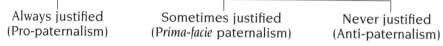

| Always justified | Sometimes justified | Never justified |
| (Pro-paternalism) | (*Prima-facie* paternalism) | (Anti-paternalism) |

Figure 8.3 Three positions on paternalism

Despite the apparent differences between these three positions, however, there is some agreement between the positions of 'weak paternalism' and 'anti-paternalism'. These are:

(i) it is justifiable to interfere in order to protect persons against harm from their own substantially non-autonomous decisions; and
(ii) it is unjustifiable to interfere in order to protect persons against harm from their own substantially autonomous decisions.

(Beauchamp 1995, p. 1917)

One reason for this closeness in position is that, as some contend, 'weak paternalism' is not really paternalism at all since it cannot be substantively distinguished from anti-paternalism. In the ultimate analysis both rest on the principles of beneficence and non-maleficence, and both reject strong paternalism (which justifies overriding strongly autonomous choices). However, when it is considered that even strong paternalism rests on the principles of beneficence and non-maleficence, the differences between all three positions may, in the end, be overstated.

Applying the 'Paternalistic Principle' in health care

Applying the 'Paternalistic Principle' in health care contexts, is not clear-cut and indeed raises a number of important questions, such as: How are we to justify overriding another's choices? What constitutes beneficial and harmful outcomes for the patient? What constitutes a patient's 'best interests'? How are we to measure the quality of another's autonomy and autonomous choices? Do people have the right to refuse life-saving/enhancing treatment? What if treatments are 'harmful'?

The abuses of paternalistic decision-making and the rise of individualism and 'patients' rights' in the 1970s and 1980s saw a backlash against paternalism in health care. The past two decades have, however, seen a tempering of this rejection. As Beauchamp concludes:

> Paternalism seems likely to continue to be a viewpoint that will gain or lose adherents as the issues and larger social context shift. We may never again see the concentrated flurry of scholarly interest in this subject that was exhibited from the mid-1970s to the mid-1980s, but paternalism is not likely to be an issue that will soon disappear.
>
> (Beauchamp 1995, p. 1920)

Informed consent and nurses

The discussion given here on informed consent (and its counterparts, competency and paternalism) is less than complete; much more can be said on the matter. Nevertheless, in the light of what has been discussed it is quite evident that nurses have much to contribute to the informed consent debate. Further, it is evident that the nursing profession needs to pay much greater attention to the doctrine of informed consent and its moral implications for nurses — not least the duties it imposes on nurses to obtain patients' informed consent to *nursing* care and procedures. It is perhaps important to emphasise that, although the doctrine of informed consent has traditionally been discussed primarily in regard to medical treatment and care, the underlying moral values, moral principles and moral requirements of this doctrine apply equally to other kinds of health care practices and procedures, including nursing care and procedures. The point is, of course, that nurses are no less exempt than are any other health care professionals from the moral standards governing consent procedures, including the demands to:

- disclose all relevant information necessary for making an informed choice about proposed nursing cares and procedures;
- ensure that the patient understands the information received and the implications of giving consent;
- ensure that the consent is given voluntarily (that is, that nurses do not coerce or manipulate the patient into giving consent); and
- ensure that the patient has the capacity to make an informed choice, and, if not, that any surrogate decision-making on the patient's behalf is in accordance with rigorous moral standards.

The nursing profession can obviously do much more than it has done up until now to challenge the status quo in regard to the informed consent issue. Specifically, the nursing profession could develop a systematic program to confront the many issues raised by the informed consent debate, and to develop ways in which these issues could be addressed constructively. For instance, nurses could:

- work closely with other groups (including health consumer groups) to ensure that the informed consent debate is kept firmly on the public agenda;
- organise a nursing action lobby group to push for positive changes to current consent practices which do not protect or promote patients' interests and entitlements in regard to making informed choices about proposed medical and psychiatric treatments and nursing cares;

- work for the development of sound, reliable and flexible institutional health care policies that are responsive to meeting the information needs of patients, and that can be appealed to in order to adjudicate troubling situations in which patients' information needs are not being met by an attending health care professional; and
- work to secure the legal, moral and professional freedoms necessary to encourage patients to ask questions about proposed medical and psychiatric treatments, nursing cares and other health care procedures, and to ensure that patients receive the information they need in appropriate ways so they can make informed and therapeutically beneficial choices.

By working to achieve these and like changes, the nursing profession will not only demonstrate its commitment to promoting and protecting the entitlements of patients to make informed choices about their care and treatment options, but also its commitment to upholding the view that patients are not — and never have been — obliged to be the passive recipients of unnegotiated care.

3. The right to confidentiality

The principle of confidentiality has long been recognised as an important guide to action in health professional–client relationships. This principle is recognised in law as well as in ethics. In so far as the law is concerned, Wallace (1991) explains:

> It is unlawful for any person to disclose any information relating to patients, except with their consent, when required by law, or to lessen a serious threat to the life and health of the individual.

(Wallace 1991, p. 146)

The moral position on confidentiality is very similar to the legal position, as will now be shown.

There are widely divergent views among health professionals and patients/clients about the nature and 'bindingness' of confidentiality (Winslade 1995, p. 454). For example, the International Council of Nurses (ICN) *Code for Nurses* (1973) states: 'the nurse holds in confidence personal information and uses judgment in sharing this information' (see Appendix I). By contrast, the *International Code of Medical Ethics* (1983) states: 'A physician shall preserve absolute confidentiality on all he [sic] knows about his [sic] patient even after the patient has died' (p. 6).

The principle of confidentiality (traditionally upheld by a variety of professional groups, including priests, doctors and lawyers, and more recently nurses and other allied health workers) demands roughly that information gained in a professional–client relationship must be kept secret, even when its disclosure might serve a greater public good. Both real and hypothetical cases, however, have exposed the inappropriateness and moral unacceptability of holding confidentiality as being an *absolute* principle (i.e. it may not be overridden under any circumstances). (It will be noted that confidentiality is held to be absolute by the *International Code of Medical Ethics*, but, not by the ICN *Code for Nurses* — something which immediately raises the prospect of moral disagreement between these two professional groups and the possibility of significant moral conflict.)

In cases where innocent victims stand to be significantly harmed by a failure to disclose, the demand to breach confidentiality becomes morally compelling. This was the view taken in the United States legal case *Tarasoff v Regents of the*

University of California (1974), the subject of Dennis Daley's (1983) thought-provoking article 'Tarasoff and the psychotherapist's duty to warn'. The case involved a university student, Prosenjit Poddar, who had met and fallen in love with a young woman, Tatiana Tarasoff. Unfortunately, Tarasoff did not share Poddar's feelings, and told him so. Consequently, Poddar became very depressed and sought psychiatric help on a voluntary outpatient basis at the Cowell Memorial Hospital at the University. During a consultation with his psychologist, Dr Lawrence Moore, Poddar revealed that he seriously intended to kill Tarasoff. After receiving this information the psychologist wrote to the campus police and informed them that Poddar was 'at this point a danger to the welfare of other people and himself', also pointing out that Poddar had been threatening to kill an unnamed girl who he felt had 'betrayed him' and had 'violated his honour' (Daley 1983, p. 243). The psychologist then went on to ask the police for assistance in detaining Poddar for psychiatric assessment. Daley writes that the campus police detained Poddar 'but released him when he appeared rational and promised to stay away from Tarasoff' (p. 235).

Following this, Poddar's psychologist was directed by a superior to take no further action and to destroy his client's records (a practice which is sometimes followed by psychologists, psychotherapists and psychiatrists in order to ensure confidentiality). Two months later, as he had threatened to his psychologist, Poddar carried out his intention and killed Tarasoff with a butcher's knife.

Daley (1983) notes that neither the girl nor her parents were warned of Poddar's threat. It seems that none of the psychotherapists involved considered it part of their professional morality to warn the victim. Even the California Supreme Court acknowledged recognition of the general rule that 'there is ordinarily no duty to control the conduct of another or to warn those endangered by such conduct' (Daley 1983, p. 235). However, the Supreme Court also recognised certain exceptions to the general rule, and its final decision in the *Tarasoff case* imposed a new duty to warn upon doctors and psychiatrists under its jurisdiction. The psychiatric profession 'reacted with alarm' to the California Supreme Court's ruling, claiming that it would 'cripple the use of psychotherapy by destroying the confidentiality vital to the psychiatrist–patient relationship' (Daley 1983, p. 234).

The *Tarasoff case* raises interesting and thought-provoking questions about the nature and force of the principle of confidentiality and the extent to which health professionals are really bound by it.

In general the demand to keep secret information disclosed in a professional–client relationship is thought to derive from the broader moral principles of autonomy, non-maleficence, justice and the obligation to keep one's promises. In the case of autonomy, it is held that individuals are entitled to choose who should have access to information about themselves, as well as what information should be disclosed, if any. Non-maleficence, on the other hand, demands that people are entitled to be protected from the harms that might flow from disclosure (which, as we know, can be both considerable and intolerable). And justice demands that a person, about whom 'private' information is known, deserves to be treated fairly. Promise keeping, simply put, demands that 'added respect is due for that which one has promised to keep secret' (Bok 1980, p. 149), although it is generally recognised that a promise to do morally evil things is either not binding at all or 'deficient in its binding power' (Freedman 1978, p. 12).

In health care contexts, the supremacy of the principle of confidentiality is thought to be particularly justified on grounds that it is crucial to preserving the fiduciary (trust) nature of the doctor–patient relationship, and any other health professional–patient/client relationship, for that matter (Beauchamp and Childress 1989, p. 4). If patients/clients can trust their attending health professionals to keep secret certain information disclosed in the professional relationship, it is thought that patients/clients will be more likely to reveal information crucial for making a correct assessment/diagnosis, and thus a correct prescription of care and treatment.

Understandably, if it were common practice to breach confidentiality, patients/ clients would probably lose their trust and confidence in their attending health care professionals, and would probably 'refrain from divulging critical information to them' (Beauchamp and Childress 1989, p. 4). Worse, they might not seek professional help at all — something which might have the undesirable consequence of individuals, groups and indeed the community at large, suffering a health status inferior to that which might otherwise be enjoyed. This argument is particularly persuasive when considered in relation to the world's current AIDS crisis (see, for example, Kirkman and Bell 1989).

The question remains, however, of whether the principle of confidentiality really is as binding as professionals seem to think it is. Where does it come from? And, as Bok (1980, p. 154) correctly asks: 'Was it ever meant to stretch so far as to require lying?'; 'Why is it so binding that it can protect those who have no right to impose their incompetence, their disease, their malevolence on ignorant and innocent victims?'.

In answering these questions, it is important to understand the nature of the principle of confidentiality. One reason why I think it has been so problematic and has caused so many controversies in health professional practice is that people mistakenly view it as an *absolute* principle — that is, one which cannot be overridden under any circumstance, as the *International Code of Medical Ethics* seems to demand. If we examine its parent principles, that is, the broader moral principles from which it has been derived, we can soon see that this absolutist view is questionable.

Confidentiality as a prima-facie principle

On close analysis it can be seen that, at best, the principle of confidentiality is, and can only ever be, a prima-facie principle. Confidentiality has a special link to a person's *right to privacy*, which may be loosely defined as the right to 'have control over information about ourselves' or 'control over who can sense us' (Parker 1974; McCloskey 1980; Thomson 1975). This in turn is connected with the principle of autonomy, which demands that people should be respected as autonomous choosers, and have the right to act on their choices provided these do not seriously impinge on the moral interests of others. Given this, it seems reasonable to hold that, where the maintenance of confidentiality results in the moral interests of others being violated, the principle can and must be overridden. This conclusion is also partially supported by the principles of non-maleficence and justice. Thus, in instances where keeping a confidence or a secret has the unhappy consequence of causing or failing to prevent an otherwise avoidable harm, and/or indeed results in an unequal distribution of harms over benefits, there is a very strong case supporting disclosure of the information being kept secret.

When subjected to the scrutiny of broader moral principles, it can be seen, first, that there are serious limits to the duty of secrecy and of maintaining confidentiality. Second, it is clear that, while in some instances the norm of confidentiality might justifiably extend to include lying, this does not hold unconditionally in all cases. (Given a consequentialist analysis, lying can only ever be justified on the grounds that it is necessary to prevent an otherwise avoidable harm from occurring, and that there is no other alternative action which can be taken to prevent the foreseen harm in question.) Third, it can be seen, given the competing demands of the moral principles of non-maleficence and justice, that the principle of confidentiality can never be used morally to protect those who would impose their incompetence, their diseases and their malevolence on to innocent and ignorant victims.

Unfortunately, the moral principle of confidentiality has sometimes been (ab)used to prevent the disclosure of unscrupulous practices. A poignant example of this can be found in the Chelmsford case referred to in Chapter 7. Of particular relevance to this discussion is the point that, after the '60 Minutes' program in 1977, when some advice was sought by medical authorities on how to deal with the Chelmsford case, the principle of confidentiality was used to impose a duty of silence on the matter, or at least to delay its exposure. When, for example, an eminent professor of psychiatry at Cambridge University was approached about the matter, he advised:

> The inhumanity and cruelty to which the patients appear to have been subjected is quite unique in my experience, and the Scientologists and other organisations will have obtained ammunition for decades to come. There is therefore a pressing need for maintaining strict confidentiality at this stage until one can set these unique barbarities in the context of contemporary practice in psychiatry in a carefully prepared statement that comes from colleges and other bodies concerned.
>
> (Sir Martin Roth, cited in Bromberger and Fife-Yeomans 1991, p. 143)

This appeal to the principle of confidentiality is questionable, and stands as an example of how conventional ethical principles of conduct can be (ab)used to maintain and reinforce the status quo rather than to challenge it. Further, when more parochial interpretations and applications of the principle of confidentiality are considered, what emerges is not a respect for ethical conduct, but rather what Bok (1980) describes as 'primeval tribal emotions: the loyalty to self, kin, clansmen, guild members as against ... the unrelated, the outsiders, the barbarians' (p. 149). Bok (1980, p. 149) concludes by warning that the principle of confidentiality can sometimes serve little more than the drive for 'self-preservation' and 'collective survival in an hostile environment'. The Chelmsford case is an example of this.

It is not being argued here that the principle of confidentiality ought not to be respected. On the contrary: confidentiality is an important moral requirement of any health care professional–patient/client relationship, and one that is crucial to ensuring the protection of a patient's/client's wellbeing and moral interests. Indiscriminate breaches of confidentiality can have morally undesirable and catastrophic consequences for patients/clients. For example, careless breaches of confidentiality concerning persons who are HIV positive can result — and have resulted — in people being dismissed from their jobs, being evicted from their rented accommodation, and being subjected generally to a wide range of negative discrimination and abuse. Similarly, careless breaches of confidentiality concerning a person's mental health status (including mild depression and grieving states) can also result — and have resulted — in harmful consequences, including persons losing their jobs or having their career prospects hampered. It is crucial, therefore, that every effort is made to ensure that information disclosed in the professional–client relationship is kept secret. This is not to say, however, that there is not a need for the principle of confidentiality to be interpreted better and applied more justly than it has been in the past. Points of clarification which need to be particularly addressed are summarised as follows:

- confidentiality is at best only a prima-facie principle, not an absolute one, and thus is one which may be overridden by stronger moral considerations;
- confidentiality should not be upheld in instances where doing so would result in otherwise avoidable harms occurring to innocent others; and
- while patients/clients as a general rule have an entitlement to have certain information about themselves kept secret, the entitlement is forfeited where it stands seriously to impinge on the moral interests of innocent others.

If these points of clarification are accepted, it must also be accepted that patients (or anybody else, for that matter) might not always be entitled to have certain information about themselves kept secret; and that disclosure, in some instances, might even be an overriding moral duty, particularly in cases where non-disclosure entails the probability of innocent others suffering unnecessary and avoidable harms (for example, children as in the case of child abuse). This second demand is also enshrined in legal law, which requires health professionals to report certain infectious diseases (commonly referred to as 'notifiable diseases'), suspected cases of child abuse (to be examined in depth in Chapter 10 of this text), and other activities 'which [are] potentially or actually dangerous to the health of others' (Wallace 1991, p. 303).

Whatever the situation at hand, nurses' decisions to keep secret or to disclose certain information gained in a professional–client or other type of relationship (for example, an employee–employer relationship) must always be based firmly on sound moral justifications and moral decision-making procedures. Nurses also need to remember that arbitrary disclosure is just as morally capricious as arbitrary non-disclosure, and may have just as many devastating consequences. As in any morally troubling situation, dilemmas posed by a controversial application of the principle of confidentiality must be resolved in a way which ensures the realisation of morally just outcomes.

4. The right to dignity and dying with dignity[2]

The right to the maintenance of dignity, and, in particular, *the right to die with dignity*, have both been widely considered in the bioethics and nursing literature (too voluminous to list here).

The terms dignity and dying with dignity have gained popular usage in contemporary debates concerning the invasive and sometimes encroaching nature of technological scientific medical care. They have also featured as key words in debates concerning the moral rights and wrongs of euthanasia. Yet, while the terms 'dignity' and 'dying with dignity' have been and are freely used, there is room seriously to question whether those who use them have a clear understanding of what exactly they mean.

---

2. Section 4, 'The right to dignity and dying with dignity', is revised from M.-J. Johnstone, 'Dying with dignity', *New Zealand Nursing Journal* 81(12), 1989, pp. 34, 37.

Another concern is that these terms have come to be used in a rather clichéd sense, and thus could have the undesirable consequence of a blanket definition of dignity being applied uncritically in all situations, regardless of their ethically significant differences, and in a way which could result in a serious distraction from (rather than a focus on) the moral issues at stake. For example, some speak of the removal of a life-support system, or the withdrawal of some other orthodox medical therapies, as tantamount to 'letting a person die with dignity' (Social Development Committee, Victoria 1986, 1987). What such views dangerously presume, however, is that the terms 'dignity' and 'dying with dignity' in these contexts have a clear-cut, commonsense meaning and use, and, furthermore, implicitly justify the acts or omissions in relation to which they have been expressed.

Two central questions invariably arise here: How should the notions 'dignity' and 'dying with dignity' be defined? What might be the implications of given definitions of these terms for nursing practice?

Can dignity be defined?

The word dignity comes from the Latin *dignitas*, meaning 'merit', and *dignus*, meaning 'worthy'. Needless to say, there are as many definitions of 'dignity' as there are dictionaries. *Collins English dictionary*, for example, defines dignity as:

> [1]. a formal, stately, or grave bearing ... [2]. the state or quality of being worthy of honour ... [3]. relative importance; rank ... [4]. sense of self importance ...

According to the *Oxford English dictionary*, dignity is:

> [1]. the quality of being worthy or honourable; worthiness, worth, nobleness, excellence ... [2]. Honourable or high estate, position, or estimation ... [4]. Nobility or befitting elevation of aspect, manner, or style ...

Webster's dictionary says dignity is:

> [1]: the quality or state of being worthy: intrinsic worth: EXCELLENCE ...

> [2]: the quality or state of being honoured or esteemed: degree of esteem ...

> [5]: formal reserve of manner, appearance, behaviour, or language: behaviour that accords with self-respect or with regard for the seriousness of occasion or purpose ...

Interestingly, the unabridged international edition of *Webster's dictionary* also gives consideration of the word 'decent' (i.e. of the mind and character) as a definition of dignity. It is perhaps worth noting here that the term 'decent' comes from the Latin *decens*, meaning 'suitable', and from *decere*, meaning 'to be fitting'.

Significantly, the question of dignity has also been a topic of philosophical debate. For example, in 1651 the English philosopher Thomas Hobbes defined it as:

> (T)he publique worth of a man [sic], which is the Value set on him [sic] by the Common-Wealth ... And this Value of him [sic] by the commonwealth, is understood, by offices of Command, Judicature, public Employment; or by Names and Titles, introduced for distinction of such Value.
>
> (Hobbes 1968, p. 152)

241

Later philosophers, however, rejected this 'social worth' view and sought to define dignity in more sophisticated moral terms. The German philosopher Immanuel Kant, for instance, defines dignity in quite different terms as 'an intrinsic, unconditioned, incomparable worth or worthiness' (1972, p. 35). Rejecting the 'market value' or 'social worth' interpretations of dignity, he goes on to assert that:

> Morality or virtue — and humanity so far as it is capable of morality — alone has dignity. In this respect it cannot be compared with things that have economic value (a market price) or even with things that have an aesthetic value (a fancy price). The incomparable worth of a good man [sic] springs from his [sic] being a [moral] law making member in a kingdom of ends.
>
> (Kant 1972, p. 35)

More recent definitions and interpretations have tended to capture the essence of Kant's views. One modern philosopher, for example, argues that dignity is akin to 'justified happiness' (a happiness which is 'interpenetrated with a sense of meaning, reason, and worth') and the attainment of 'just goals'; that is, morally valuable ends (Swenson, 1981). The behaviourist B. F. Skinner (1973, pp. 48–62) sees dignity and what he calls the 'struggle for dignity' as having many features in common with freedom and the 'struggle for freedom'.

Some of the most revealing and instructive definitions of dignity and dying with dignity might, however, come from a group of students from the Phillip Institute of Technology (now RMIT University), first-year Diploma of Applied Science (Nursing) course in Victoria. Comments were sought from the students after their clinical placement at a residential care home for the elderly. The results are summarised as follows.

- 'Dying with dignity is dying the way you want to die.'
- 'Dignity is a feeling of pride ... of feeling good about yourself.'
- 'Dignity and dying with dignity is maintaining self-value, self-respect, and self-image ...'
- 'I don't know, but I think, as it is used today, it all boils down to having to look good for other people.'
- 'Dignity is having pride without shame.'
- 'Dignity and dying with dignity is being happy with oneself, and what one has achieved in life.'
- 'Dying with dignity is having no pain, no fear. Feeling valued, and having your opinions valued. Yes. That's it! It involves having control and being valued.'
- 'Dying with dignity is putting yourself above whatever is going on around you.'
- 'Dignity is concerned with self-respect, and how this is related to society — your social worth.'
- 'Dignity is being accepting of one's self, and of what's to come ... the problem is, however, that a lot of people base their self-worth on what other people think of them.'

As the last student voiced her comments, another student interjected with frustration, exclaiming: 'Oh! How can you die with dignity if you have no say about it?'.

In considering all these definitions, it soon becomes apparent that the notions 'dignity', and 'dying with dignity', essentially defy precise definition. What this inevitably warns, of course, is that nurses — and indeed health care professionals generally — must never take the notion of dignity (and its usage) for granted. They must also be cautious in treating these terms as if they had clear-cut, commonsense interpretations. What one person might consider 'dignity', another person might equally reject —and this has important implications for nursing care delivery in particular, and health care management generally.

How, then, should dignity be defined? And what might be the implications of a given definition for nursing practice?

Despite the variety of definitions and interpretations of the notions 'dignity' and 'dying with dignity', there are a number of common elements. In summary, these include:

- that persons have intrinsic moral worth, and thus ought to be treated with respect (see below);
- that persons should be respected as autonomous choosers, and thus as beings capable of exercising self-determining choice;
- that persons should be facilitated and supported in the course of exercising their autonomous choices;
- that persons should be facilitated and supported in their attempts to maintain their self-respect and self-esteem.

Implications for nurses

Whatever nurses or allied health workers take dignity and/or dying with dignity to mean, it is important that they do not unfairly impose their interpretations on their patients. It is a moral imperative of the first order that patients' preferences (which might include them abdicating their autonomy to chosen and trusted lay carers) are respected, even if others do not agree with these. This means that, where possible, and in a manner that is culturally appropriate, patients are morally entitled to participate in decision-making concerning their care, and are morally entitled to give a fully informed consent to the use and withdrawal of recommended medical or other therapies. If patients are not able to participate in decision-making concerning their care and treatment, every effort must be made to establish what their considered preferences might be. Either way, in the final analysis, what is to count as dignity and dying with dignity must be decided from the patients' (or their advocates') point of view, not that of the health professionals.

Given this, nurses should not be asking 'What is dignity?' or 'What does it mean to die with dignity?'; rather, they should be asking: 'What is dignity for *this* or *that* person?' and 'What is dying with dignity *for them*?'. If nurses want valid answers to these questions, they need to ask these questions in the first place.

The challenge to nursing is not just to allow patients the right to the maintenance of dignity, but actually to find out what the patient considers as being dignity and/or a dignified death, and ensuring that this is permitted and upheld on terms of what the patient wants, and not on what the *nurse thinks* the patient wants.

5. The right to be treated with respect

People (regardless of their age, sexuality, cultural backgrounds and social position) have a special interest in being treated with respect. Furthermore, there are significant moral reasons why this interest ought to be protected. Thus, the claim that people have a *right* to be treated with respect is a meaningful one.

Underpinning most moral claims (rights claims included) is the principle that *people ought to be treated with respect*. Otherwise referred to in moral philosophy as 'respect for persons', this principle is generally regarded as being of paramount importance to the establishment, development and maintenance of moral relationships between people, and to moral practice generally (Tadd 1998, pp. 1–3).

The notion of 'respect for persons' is widely used, often without qualification, in the bioethics literature (its meaning more or less taken for granted), and, of significance to this discussion, it is widely used in codes of professional ethics. For instance, common to most nursing codes of ethics is a prescribed demand to 'respect patients' in the provision of nursing care. This demand tends to be interpreted in varying ways as including an obligation to treat with respect a patient's needs, values, beliefs, and culture. As well, nursing codes of ethics prescribe respect for patients' rights. Consider the following examples.

The International Council of Nurses (1973) *Code for Nurses* states:

> Inherent in nursing is respect for life, dignity and rights of man [sic]. [...]
> The nurse, in providing care, promotes an environment in which the values,
> customs and spiritual beliefs of the individual are respected.

The Australian Nursing Council's (1993) *Code of Ethics for Nurses in Australia* takes a similar position. It states:

- Nurses respect persons' individual needs, values and culture in the provision of nursing care (Value statement 1);
- Nurses respect the rights of persons to make informed choices in relation to their care (Value statement 2).

The New Zealand Nurses' Association's (1988) *Code of Ethics* also carries strong statements prescribing 'respect'. Significantly, five of its twelve underpinning core ethical values pertain explicitly to respect:

1. Respect for clients' individual needs and values;
2. Respect for clients' right of choice;
3. Respect for the right of clients to control their own care;
4. Respect for the confidentiality of client related information;
5. Respect for the dignity of clients.

Despite its popular usage in the ethics literature and in codes of ethics, however, just what constitutes 'respect' and 'respect for persons' has received surprisingly little attention by authors. In the remainder of this chapter an attempt will be made to remedy this oversight. Specifically, brief attention will be given to exploring the nature and moral implications of 'respect' and 'respect for persons' — particularly as these pertain to the ethical practice of nursing and the promotion of patients' rights generally.

Every culture has its own conception of respect and 'its own norms of behaviour and ways of being that are considered respectful' (Sugirtharjah 1994). Asian cultures, for example, tend to treat respect as a moral *duty* expressed through such concepts (tautologically) as: *duty, respect* and *honour* (Sugirtharjah 1994). Western cultures, however, tend to give greater primacy to respect as an individual moral *right* (Sugirtharjah 1994, p. 740).

Western conceptions of *respect* and, specifically, the *principle of respect for persons* has borrowed heavily from the work of the 18th Century German philosopher, Immanuel Kant. In his celebrated work the *Fundamental principles of the metaphysics of ethics*, Kant (1959, p. 56) prescribes the (now famous) practical imperative: 'So act as to treat humanity, whether in thine own person or in that of any other, in every case as an end withal, never as means only'. This practical imperative has been variously translated to mean that *people should always be treated as ends in themselves, and never as mere means (for instance, as objects) to the ends of others*. Although commonly accepted, this conception of 'respect for persons' is, however, miserably inadequate and requires expansion to enhance its usefulness as a guiding principle in health care domains. There is, for instance, considerable scope to suggest that respecting persons entails something far more than fulfilling the negative duty of not treating individuals as 'mere means' to the ends of others. It also involves the positive duty of treating people in a manner that is affirming of their *personal identity* as dignified human beings, that is, affirming of *who they are*.

In clarifying the nature and moral implications of rights claims involving respect in health care contexts, it is important first to draw a distinction between respecting *persons* per se, and respecting *the rights* of persons. While the latter is obviously a critical ingredient of the former, the two are nevertheless distinct. In regard to the latter, respecting *the rights* of persons means honouring a range of special interests (moral entitlements) that people might have, say, upon entering a health care domain; for example, the right to health care, to make informed choices, to have information about themselves treated as confidential, to be treated with dignity, and to be treated with respect itself. Moral demands to treat *persons* with respect, in contrast, is fundamentally tied to enhancing the self-identity of persons and involves, in complex ways, acknowledging persons for *who* they are and responding to them in a manner that *prima facie* preserves the integrity of their self-identity and the promotion of moral goods that this preservation will facilitate. Let us explore this claim further.

Respect (from the Latin *respicere*, meaning 'to look back, pay attention to', from *specere*, meaning 'to look') is essentially a moral attitude that when translated into action is manifest as the showing of admiration, regard, esteem, and/or kindly consideration for another. In short, *respect* manifests as the 'good' treatment of people, and invariably results in their being 'humanised' (that is, enabled to experience their 'beingness' both as human persons and as moral entities, and/or characterised as having moral worth). Disrespect, in contrast, manifests as the 'bad' (or ill) treatment of people, and invariably results in them being 'dehumanised' (deprived of qualities that otherwise enables them — and others — to feel they are 'human beings' of moral worth). Or, to borrow from Asian thought, disrespecting another is to 'take away' that other's 'face'; to 'lose face', in turn, is to diminish that person's very identity and dignity, and consequently to 'pollute the web of relationship' (Rivers 1996, pp. 54–5). Respect, in contrast, keeps the door of relationship' open (Rivers 1996, p. 55).

An important example of the manifestation of disrespect in health care can be found in the case of the stigmatisation, prejudicial treatment of, marginalisation and (negative) discrimination of certain groups of people (for instance: the mentally ill; people of different cultural backgrounds and whose first language is not English; the aged; the disabled; people living with blood borne pathogens [for example, HIV]; the homeless and the poor; gay men, lesbians, transgendered and intergendered [viz. hermaphrodite] people). Consider the following.

Stigma (from Latin via Greek meaning 'brand' or 'bodily sign') is literally a distinguishing mark of social disgrace. It presupposes the acquisition of an attribute or attributes that others (usually those who are dominant members of a mainstream culture) find or regard as deeply discrediting (personally, socially and morally) (Goffman 1963). What is regarded as a 'distinguishing mark of social disgrace' will, however, depend on the culture from which it has originated.

The process of stigmatisation evolves into a situation in which an individual is disqualified from full social and cultural acceptance on the basis of his or her carrying a given 'distinguishing mark of social disgrace' (for example, being old, immigrant, disabled, homosexual, mentally ill etc.) (Goffman 1963). Inevitably this means that stigma almost always carries with it commensurate processes of discrimination; that is, the unfair treatment of persons on the basis of their 'distinguishing mark(s)'. This treatment is unfair since judgments are made on the somewhat arbitrary basis of morally irrelevant *distinguishing marks*, rather than on *moral considerations per se*; hence the notion that stigma and stigmatisation are unjustly discriminatory. This outcome is unethical since, by focusing on one (or more) arbitrary characteristic(s) of a person (that is, the marks that may 'distinguish them'), stigma and discrimination undermine the moral worth of a person (results in them 'losing face', if you will) and thus dehumanises them. The stigmatising and (negative) discriminatory treatment of persons thus stands in contradistinction to the respectful treatment of persons. In the case of respectful treatment, responses to persons are guided by profoundly moral considerations, not merely arbitrary ones.

What then are the ingredients of respectful health-professional (nurse–patient) interactions? In conclusion to this discussion on the right to be treated with respect, I would like to suggest that minimally a nurse's respectful interactions with patients, chosen carers and significant others must contain the following:

- acknowledgment of the moral worth and dignity of human beings;
- an unconditional positive regard and valuing of persons for *who they are* as moral beings;
- focused attention on persons (that is, being 'fully present' and being *fully alert to another's presence*, viz. not treating persons in a dismissive, belittling or marginalising manner);
- empathically attuned listening (taking seriously what another says and knows);
- supportive actions aimed at promoting another's moral interests and wellbeing; and
- strategies aimed at 'saving face' and preserving the web of relationship.

Conclusion

The issue of patients' rights to and in health care is an important one for members of the nursing profession. Although a patients' rights approach to ethics in health care is not free of difficulties (as the following chapters of this text will show), it nevertheless serves a number of important functions. Among other things, discourse on patients' rights helps to remind both health professionals and the laity alike: firstly, that upon entering health care domains for care and treatment, people have special interests and entitlements which ought to be recognised and protected; secondly, and related to this first claim, people (patients) are not — and never have been — obliged to be the passive recipients of unnegotiated care. Thirdly, patients' rights discourse helps to remind health professionals (nurses included) that their relationships with patients and their chosen carers are constrained by relevant moral considerations. Fourthly, patients' rights discourse highlights the vulnerability of people in health care contexts and the 'special' actions that are required by others (including nurses) to help reduce this vulnerability and to promote generally the significant moral interests of patients and their chosen carers. Finally, patients rights' discourse helps to remind us that moral decision-making in health care is not just a matter of 'working through normative hierarchies of values', but is also 'a matter of personal extension into the lives and values of other human beings' which deserve respect (Thomasma 1990, p. 250).

Despite the enormous progress that has been made in recent years in regard to the whole issue of patients' rights to and in health care, it is nevertheless evident that serious abuses of patients' rights routinely and unacceptably occur across the continuum of care (as examples given throughout this text make plain). In light of this, it is evident that the nursing profession has a fundamental role to play in advocating the promotion and protection of patients' rights — not just 'at the bedside', but in the broader socio-political sphere as well. Specifically, the nursing profession has an important and justifiable role to play in actively lobbying for such things as:

- the formulation and global recognition of a comprehensive list of principles, together with a set of interpretive statements, which can be appealed to for both identifying patients' rights and guiding their protection (in short, a universal declaration of patients' rights);
- the establishment and maintenance of accessible, just, reliable and enforceable health complaints mechanisms;
- the improvement of health professional education programs aimed at preparing health professionals better to recognise and respond appropriately to patients' rights claims;
- the introduction of broadly-based community information programs aimed at better informing its community members of their rights to, in and against health care; and
- the staging of regular state, national and international multidisciplinary and transcultural symposiums on patients' rights, with a commitment by all concerned (including health care professional groups and governments) to act upon these symposiums' findings.

If such aims can be achieved, the prospect for patients' rights will be considerably brighter than is suggested by present social, political and legal indicators.

Chapter 9

Human rights and the mentally ill

Introduction

Discussions on patients' rights to and in health care have tended to have as their focus persons with 'physical health' problems. While important, this focus has nevertheless been at the expense of attention being given to the moral entitlements of people with 'mental health' problems. Indeed, the subject of moral rights and the mentally ill has been relatively neglected in mainstream bioethics discourse (Johnstone 1995). In light of the past neglect of mental health care ethics in both the mainstream bioethics and nursing literature, 'special' attention to the moral plight of the mentally ill is warranted. In this chapter, a brief overview will be provided of some of the disproportionate and hence unjust burdens that the mentally ill have to carry in the cultural context of Australia. While drawing on the Australian experience, however, this discussion has relevance for other countries.

Discrimination against the mentally ill

In 1993, an Australian national inquiry into the human rights of people with mental illness concluded, unequivocally, that people affected by mental illness continue to 'suffer from widespread, systematic discrimination and are consistently denied the rights and services to which they are entitled (Burdekin et al. 1993, p. 870). The inquiry found that discrimination was particularly widespread in mainstream society, with the mentally ill experiencing 'stigma and discrimination in almost every aspect of their lives' ranging from restrictions on eligibility for insurance and superannuation schemes, to employment, education and training (Burdekin et al. 1993, p. 925). Equally disturbing was the inquiry's additional finding that underpinning this discrimination were deeply ingrained (and often structurally reinforced) societal attitudes of fear, ignorance and intolerance of mental illness and mental health disorders.

It is widely known that people suffering from mental health disorders, mental illness and other mental health-related problems are among the most stigmatised, discriminated against, marginalised, disadvantaged and hence vulnerable individuals in our society (Health Care Committee Expert Panel on Mental Health, 1991; Burdekin et al. 1993; South East Centre Against Sexual Assault, 1994; Tippett et al. 1994; Australian Health Ministers, 1995; Mental Health Consumer Outcomes Task Force, 1995; Senate Community Affairs References

Committee, 1995).[1] And, although human rights violations have occurred repeatedly in the mental health care sector since the inception of contemporary bioethics, the issue of the human rights of people with mental health problems has received relatively little attention in the mainstream bioethics and related literature. Just why this is so, is a matter for speculation. One explanation might be that the issue of human rights in mental health care simply lacks the kudos that, say, other more popular bioethical issues (such as euthanasia, abortion, reproductive technology, organ transplantation, and the like) have. Or, it might be that, the issue itself carries some degree of stigma from which authors writing in the field of health care ethics (bioethics) would prefer to obtain some distance.

In recent years significant efforts have been made in Australia to redress the problem of human rights violations in mental health care settings, and to provide a framework for assuring the protection of the moral entitlements of people suffering from mental health problems (see, in particular, the *National Mental Health Policy* [Australian Health Ministers 1995] and the *Mental Health Statement of Rights and Responsibilities* [Mental Health Consumer Outcomes Task Force 1995]). However, it is evident that a great deal more needs to be done to improve the status quo. Certainly, initiatives aimed at educating the public, promoting mental health through mainstream health promotion activities, establishing preventative mental health programs as an essential component of care provision to people at risk of mental health problems, and promoting research, are all essential to promoting better 'mental health outcomes'. If, however, there is to be a genuine promotion and realisation of 'social justice, equity, access and a compassionate society with mental health as a primary goal' (Raphael 1995), what is also required is the development, promotion and practice of a substantive mental health care ethic which recognises, among other things, that mental health is a 'multi-dimensional, dynamic and interactive phenomenon' (Tippett et al. 1994, p. xii).

The moral responsibilities of nurses in mental health care

The *Code of Ethics for Nurses in Australia* (Australian Nursing Council 1993) makes explicit the moral responsibility of nurses to care for human beings 'regardless of race, religion, status, age, gender, diagnosis or any other ground'. Underpinning this stated moral responsibility of nurses is a recognition of nursing care as being a profoundly moral activity that 'is based on the development of a helping relationship and the implementation and evaluation of therapeutic

---

1. The notions, 'mental disorders', 'mental illness', 'psychiatric disorders' and 'mental health problem' are not synonymous, and thus it would be misleading to use them interchangeably. For instance, a person can have a mental health problem yet not be 'mentally disordered'.

  In Australia, 'mental disorder' is a term used to 'describe individuals suffering from some form of psychiatric condition which impairs their functioning' (Tomison 1996, p. 2). Although the terms 'mental disorder' and 'mental illness' are often used synonymously, 'mental illness' is a form of *legalese* used in legal contexts to refer to persons considered 'patients' under various State and Territory Mental Health Acts. In contrast, persons suffering from a 'psychiatric condition' are defined as 'those who have a mental disorder that has had a disabling effect on them' (Tomison 1996, p. 2). Controversially, a mental health problem, in turn, could be distinguished as a 'problem' of a psychogenic sort which causes discomfort — and even a certain degree of distress, but does not interfere with the sufferer's functioning and performance of social responsibilities.

processes'. Therapeutic processes, in this instance, are interpreted to include 'health promotion and education, counselling, nursing interventions and empowerment of individuals, families or groups to exercise maximum choice in relation to their health care' (Australian Nursing Council 1993). The moral imperatives arising from this interpretation have an obvious significance and poignancy for those working in the area of mental health care.

It has been acknowledged that nurses are at the forefront of providing care to people suffering from mental illness, mental health disorders and other mental health-related problems (Burdekin et al. 1993, pp. 175–8). By virtue of this primary position in mental health care, nurses have a fundamental role to play in promoting social justice, equity, access, compassion and destigmatisation in mental health domains. While many nurses may already be well intentioned in this regard, much more than 'good intention' is required. Specifically, nurses need to be well informed about the ethical issues confronting them, and the kinds of strategies required in order to address these issues in ways that are responsive to and reflective of the lived experiences of the people for whose mental health care they share responsibility. Many of the topics covered in this text will assist nurses to develop a requisite understanding of the ethical issues they face when caring for people with mental health problems. However, it is also important that they have a 'special' understanding of the now widely accepted 'human rights' approach to and in mental health, a brief overview of which will now be given.

A human rights approach to and in mental health care domains

In Australia, as in other countries, it has become increasingly recognised at a social, cultural and political level that people suffering from mental illnesses, mental health disorders and other mental health-related problems need to be protected from abuse and neglect, something which for a variety of reasons they are especially vulnerable to experiencing. This need of protection has also been recognised at an international level as evident by the United Nations General Assembly's adoption in 1991 of the principles for 'The Protection of Persons with Mental Illness and for the Improvement of Mental Health Care'. Although these principles have not yet been incorporated into Australian legislation, they have nevertheless been formally endorsed in the National Mental Health Policy 'which sets 1998 as a target date for ensuring full compliance by Australian mental health legislation with the standards set out in the Principles' (Burdekin et al. 1993, p. 31).

In attempting to secure protection of the mentally ill and disordered from abuse and neglect, a human rights model of mental health care ethics has been adopted. Underpinning the selection of this model is the view that 'all people have fundamental human rights' and that people with mental health problems or disorders should not be precluded from having or exercising these rights *just because* of their mental health difficulties. As the Mental Health Consumer Outcomes Task Force puts it:

> The diagnosis of mental health problems or mental disorder is not an excuse for inappropriately limiting their [people with mental health problems or disorders] rights.
>
> (Mental Health Consumer Outcomes Task Force 1995, p. ix)

In March 1991, the Australian Health Ministers acknowledged and accepted the above viewpoint, and adopted, as part of Australia's national mental health strategy, the final report of the Mental Health Consumer Outcomes Task Force, titled *Mental Health Statement of Rights and Responsibilities*. This report has been reprinted twice since its initial publication (latest edition1995), and stands as an influential guiding force behind other public policy initiatives and statements such as the *National Mental Health Policy* (Australian Health Ministers 1995) as well as health care professional practice in mental health care settings.

The *Mental Health Statement of Rights and Responsibilities* makes explicit and seeks to inform a range of stakeholders of a number of key rights (in fact, a mixture of moral, civil and legal rights) affecting 'individuals seeking promotion or enhancement of mental health or care and protection when suffering mental health problems or mental disorders' (Mental Health Consumer Outcomes Task Force 1995, p. 1). Included in its list are consumers' rights to:

- access adequate, high quality and culturally appropriate mental health care services;
- make informed choices about care and treatment;
- privacy, dignity and respect;
- be treated fairly;
- mechanisms of complaint and redress;
- advocacy;
- have legislation affirm their fundamental rights;
- have mental health legislation reviewed and updated as necessary;
- have access to relatives and friends;
- rehabilitation; and
- 'the right equal to other citizens to health care, income maintenance, education, employment, housing, transport, legal services, equitable health and other insurance and leisure appropriate to one's age' (Mental Health Consumer Outcomes Task Force 1995, p. 1).

As well as specifying a number of key rights, the statement also lists key responsibilities; included here are mental health consumers' responsibilities to 'respect the human worth and dignity of other people; and to participate as far as possible in reasonable treatment and rehabilitation processes' (Mental Health Consumer Outcomes Task Force 1995, p. 2). The rights and responsibilities of service providers, carers and advocates are also listed.

At first glance, the content and intent of the *Mental Health Statement of Rights and Responsibilities* seems to provide an important step forward toward the protection of the human rights of people made vulnerable by mental health problems. On closer examination, however, there is room to suggest that the statement may, in reality, offer those working in the field little guidance on what to do when faced with morally problematic situations involving people who are mentally ill, mentally unwell, mentally disordered or whatever other description may be appropriate of someone experiencing a mental health problem. It also risks raising more questions than it answers and possibly even contributing to an exacerbation of moral problems in mental health care settings rather than remedying them. There are a number of reasons for this, not least the problematic nature of a human rights approach to ethics itself (discussed earlier in Chapter 4 of this text).

Human rights claims entail a range of 'special interests' deserving protection for a variety of reasons. Human rights include moral rights, legal rights, civil rights and so forth, and thus do not exclusively concern moral rights. Of pertinence to this discussion is the *moral rights* aspect of human rights.

As previously explained, a moral right can be defined as a special interest or entitlement which a person has and which ought to be protected for moral reasons. Having a moral right usually entails that another has a corresponding duty to respect that right. Fulfilling a corresponding duty can involve either doing something 'positive' to benefit a person claiming a particular right or, alternatively, refraining from doing something 'negative' which could harm a person claiming a particular right. For example, if a patient claims the right to make an informed choice concerning prescribed psychotropic medication or electroconvulsive therapy (ECT), this imposes on an attending health care professional a corresponding duty to ensure that the patient is fully informed about the therapeutic effects and the adverse side effects of the treatments in question *as well as* to respect the patient's choice to either accept or refuse the treatment, even where the health professional may not agree with the ultimate choice made. The moral force of the right's claim in this instance is such that if an attending health care professional does not uphold or violates the patient's choice in regard to the treatment options considered, that patient would probably feel wronged or that a serious injustice had been done. The health care professional in turn could be judged, criticised and possibly even censured on grounds of having infringed the patient's rights (Johnstone 1998).

As already explained in this text, a human rights approach to ethics is widely used. It is not, however, without difficulties. For example, the *Mental Health Statement of Rights and Responsibilities* (cited throughout this discussion) itself acknowledges that the freedom of people to exercise their human rights (and responsibilities) is 'inherently linked to the mental health functioning of individuals and communities' (Mental Health Consumer Outcomes Task Force 1995, p. ix). Here serious questions arise concerning the status and usefulness of a human rights approach for people who are so mentally ill that they are unable to exercise their own rights. While it might be responded that in such instances an advocate could and indeed should (that is, has a *duty* to) act on behalf of the person in question, this merely begs the question of who can and should undertake this role, as well as when, where and how?

For example, should the role of, and the duty to act as, an advocate fall to an attending health care professional (who may or may not have intimate knowledge of the mentally ill person)? Or a family member (who, while having intimate knowledge of the mentally ill person, may for some reason be estranged from him or her)? Or a friend (who has no legal relationship with the person, but nevertheless has the person's best interests at heart). Or a lawyer or some other legal representative (who, despite having the legal authority to act on behalf of the person, may be a complete stranger and not really be in a position to advocate the person's 'best interests' at all)? How is a matter of this nature to be decided and by whom? There may be no easy answers to the questions posed. An additional problem concerns the philosophical issue of whether human rights are of a nature that allows another to validly act as a 'surrogate decision-maker' and make rights claims 'by proxy' on behalf of another. To put this another way, is the freedom to exercise a human right something that can be 'abdicated' to another? Or does this defeat the whole purpose of having individual human rights in the first place?

Another difficulty is that rights can conflict and compete with one another. For example, the patient's stated right to have 'access to family and friends' could seriously conflict with the family's and friend's moral interests and entitlements to be spared the certain harms that might flow from contact; for example, in the case of a patient who is physically violent and has demonstrable homicidal tendencies. In a case such as this, the patient's right to privacy and confidentiality might also stand in serious conflict with the moral interests of family and friends to be warned of a possible threat to their safety and wellbeing; for example, in instances where the client has disclosed a serious intention to kill a given person, as tragically happened in the 1974 American legal case *Tarasoff v Regents of the University of California* (discussed in Chapter 8; see also Daley 1983). While a human rights approach to ethics may tell us what rights people have, it offers very little guidance in regard to what should be done when stated rights conflict and compete with one another.

Related to the above is the additional difficulty of establishing the extent to which a patient's rights claim entails a correlative duty. Consider, for example, a person's right to access appropriate and quality mental health care services. Consider also that such a claim may be extremely difficult to uphold in instances where services are either seriously under-resourced or simply do not exist (such as in remote areas). Here difficult questions arise concerning who or what has a corresponding duty to respond to a mentally ill person's rights in this instance? Is it an individual nurse? another mental health worker? a mental health service? a general hospital? family? friends? the state? a philanthropist? or some other entity? Compounding this difficulty is the problem of competing rights claims. For example, a number of persons might make equally deserving claims to mental health care services (as they do) but, because of a shortage of resources, it is genuinely difficult to satisfy the rights claims of all persons equally. Compounding these difficulties still further is the additional question of whether it makes sense to even claim a right to something that does not exist, in this instance, a particular type of health care service in a particular region? Further, is it reasonable to condemn someone for not providing a service where no such service exists or where existing services have been totally exhausted? There may be no satisfactory answers to these questions.

Finally there is the paradoxical problem of a human rights approach to mental health care ethics being abused to advance dominant political interests. For instance, recent trends favouring the deinstitutionalisation of the mentally ill might be cynically appraised as having been motivated not by humane concern for people with mental health problems confined to institutional care, but by blatant political interest in reducing the cost (both financial and political) of institutionalised mental health care services around the country — some of which has been shown to be seriously substandard (see, for example, the publicly documented cases of the *Chelmsford Hospital in New South Wales* [Bromberger and Fife-Yeomans 1991], *Ward 10B of Townsville Hospital in Queensland* [Carter 1991], and the *Lakeside Hospital in Victoria* [Burdekin et al. 1993, p. 870]). Consider the following.

In his controversial text *Nowhere to go*, Torrey (1988), an American psychiatrist, persuasively argues that sometimes rights (for example, civil and legal rights) designed to protect the mentally ill often protect their 'right' to *remain* mentally ill. In illustrating this, Torrey (1988) cites an American case of a man suffering from schizophrenia and who was the subject of a committal hearing. The man had been refusing food, but was said to have been ingesting his own faeces. Although in a state of neglect and in need of institutional care and treatment, the man could not be institutionalised against his will without a court order. Significantly, while the court acknowledged that the man was eating his own faeces, it did not regard this as constituting a 'danger to self' (or to others, for that matter). The court subsequently upheld the man's 'civil liberty' not to be institutionalised against his will. An important point to be drawn from this case is that while that man's civil liberties (rights) were protected by the court in this instance, his genuine human welfare and wellbeing was not. As one observer cited by Torrey (1988, p. 31) phrased it, 'we are protecting the civil liberties [of the mentally ill] much more adequately than we are protecting their minds and their lives'.

Problems associated with a human rights approach to mental health care ethics

From the brief discussion above, it can be seen that a human rights approach to mental health care ethics can be very problematic. One reason for this can be found in the nature of a rights approach to ethics itself and the difficulties which can be experienced in determining who has rights, who has corresponding duties to these rights, and how best to try and satisfy all valid rights claims of all people equally. Another difficulty is that what are sometimes put forward as moral rights are not, technically speaking, moral rights at all, but rather a mixture of civil rights (special interests and entitlements people have by virtue of being civilians), legal rights (special interests or entitlements bestowed by law and which ought to be protected for legal reasons) or institutional rights (special interests or entitlements bestowed by an institution in which one is participating in some way) — all of which have differing moral force. This mixture can confuse judgments on what is a morally correct course of action to take and can compound many of the problems outlined above.

An important question to arise here is: If statements on human rights and responsibilities in mental health care are so problematic, is there any point in having them? The short answer to this question is, yes. Whatever the faults, weaknesses and difficulties of such statements, they nevertheless achieve a number of important things:

- they help to remind patients, service providers, caregivers and the general community that people with mental health problems (including mental illness and mental health disorders) do have special interests and entitlements which ought to be respected and protected;
- they help to inform stakeholders (patients, service providers, caregivers and the community) of what these special entitlements are and thereby provide a basis upon which respect for and protection of these can be demanded;
- they help to delineate the special responsibilities that stakeholders (patients, service providers, caregivers and the community) all have in ensuring the promotion and protection of people's special interests and entitlements in mental health care and in promoting mental health generally;
- they help to remind all stakeholders (patients, service providers, caregivers and the community at large) that their relationships with each other are ethically constrained and are bound by certain correlative duties.

What a consideration of the difficulties outlined above warn, however, is that if a human rights approach to mental health care ethics is to be taken, nurses need to be well informed about the pitfalls of this approach and be cognisant of the reality that it may not always be helpful in guiding ethical professional conduct.

Practical ethics in mental health

It is to be expected that in the course of caring for people with mental health problems, nurses will encounter a variety of practical ethical issues. In addition, it is important to understand that these issues will vary both in kind and complexity, depending on:

- who the patient is (for example, whether the patient is an individual, a family, a group or an entire community);
- where the patient is located (for example, whether in a community or institutional setting, a private or public place, whether free or constrained physically, legally or otherwise); and
- what resources are available to assist the patient in whatever form these resources might be required (for example, a patient might be in need of legal aid and accommodation, not merely health care; a patient might also just be in need of 'a friend' — someone who will just sit and listen and reassure them that 'everything will be OK').

These considerations will, in turn, have a bearing on determining the nature of a nurse's given moral responsibilities and the extent to which he or she is obligated to fulfil these.

For instance, it is quite probable that a nurse's responsibilities do not just begin and end with an individual patient. If the whole notion of moral obligation is taken seriously from a professional point of view, then there is considerable room to suggest that the moral responsibilities of nurses extend far beyond their immediate one-to-one professional–client relationships to include other things such as professional and political activism aimed at improving the plight of those who suffer from mental health problems. Activism of this kind could be aimed at securing such things as: the demystification and destigmatisation of mental health disorders, mental illness and other mental health problems, better mental health care services (to be distinguished here from psychiatric services) for the community, and other general mechanisms which will assist those with mental health problems to be spared the devastating consequences of stigma and discrimination which many continue to suffer.

Given the above, it can be seen that practical ethical issues for mental health nurses can and do involve much more than the commonly discussed moral problems of the right to health care, informed consent and competency to decide, privacy and confidentiality, the political abuse of psychiatry and psychiatric research — all of which have been discussed in the bioethics, nursing ethics, psychotherapy ethics and psychiatric ethics literature (see, for example, Engelhardt 1995; Rave and Larsen 1995; Beauchamp and Childress 1994; Bloch and Chodoff 1991; Weinstein 1990; Buchanan and Brock 1989; Gorovitz et al. 1983). Other important practical issues concern the moral imperatives of the professional–client relationship (including mutuality, therapeutic alliance, safety, security, trust, compassion and empathy); the moral dimensions and unacceptable consequences of stigma and discrimination; and the moral imperatives of transcultural mental health nursing, to name some. Unfortunately, due to the limited scope of this discussion, it is not possible to explore all these issues in a manner that would do justice to them or which would provide nurses working in the mental health care sector with the in-depth understanding they need in order to be able to deal with these issues effectively. Nevertheless, they are identified here to alert nurses to the possible range of ethical issues they need to be informed about and which will, at some stage, have a bearing on their practice.

Future directions in mental health care ethics

This discussion on mental health care ethics would be incomplete without some consideration being given to the future directions in which the field of mental health care ethics should take.

It is of some considerable significance that many of the respondents to the National Inquiry into the Human Rights of People with Mental Illness felt that 'one of the most debilitating aspects of being mentally ill was not the illness itself, but the social stigma it attracts' (Burdekin et al. 1993, p. 443). As one respondent disclosed: 'The horrendous consequences of my illness have been [a result of] public attitudes of ignorance, fear, discrimination and neglect and professional indifference (Gillespie — cited in Burdekin et al. 1993, p. 443). Equally significant is the Inquiry's overall finding that what clients of mental health services were largely affected by were not the 'big' ethical issues constructed as being 'paramount' by mainstream bioethics (for example, informed consent, confidentiality, and so forth). Rather, clients were affected by much more 'basic' day-to-day relationship and existential issues which, while perhaps lacking the intrigue of other exotic bioethical issues, nevertheless have a profound moral dimension and warrant just as much attention as do the 'big' ethical issues which have tended to preoccupy contemporary mainstream bioethics discourse. The key issues identified by people with mental health problems were:

- the desperate need for understanding;
- the need to be able to speak openly and to be heard;
- the longing for acceptance by others of the mystery and the unpredictability of their illness, without constantly having to defend and explain to those who have little interest in understanding; and
- the desire to be equal with others and to have basic human rights respected.

(adapted from Burdekin et al. 1993, pp. 439–40)

Similar findings were made by another, although less known provincial report examining the experiences of women survivors of sexual assault who had been seriously misunderstood and mistreated by mainstream psychiatric services (South East Centre Against Sexual Assault 1994).

What, then, are some of the lessons to be gained from these findings and what are their implications for the future development of mental health care ethics?

In the introductory comments to this discussion, it was claimed that: If there is to be a genuine promotion and realisation of 'social justice, equity, access and a compassionate society with mental health as a primary goal' (Raphael 1995), what is also required is the development, promotion and practice of a substantive mental health care ethic. Such an ethic must, by its very nature, be one which is responsive to and reflective of the lived experiences of clients with mental health problems, as well as their carers. To achieve this, it is clear that the very first place the development of such an ethic must begin is not the abstract theories and principles of traditional Western moral philosophy. Rather, such an ethic must take as its methodological starting point the lived realities and experiences of those who suffer as a result of their mental health problems as well as the lived realities and experiences of the people who share the primary responsibility of caring for them. Such an approach will also empower those whose lives have been affected by mental health problems to 'speak for themselves' and in so doing to challenge the status quo by virtue of engaging in the positive political act of 'making visible' their experiences and naming their own reality. 'Speaking for themselves' will also enable survivors of mental health problems to provide the foundations needed for achieving the understanding and respect they are so desperately seeking. Finally, such an approach will facilitate the development of our moral thinking generally and will enable a very 'life-rich' contribution to be made to mainstream bioethics discourse which remains largely incomplete because of the many 'moral voices and moral selves' (adapted from Hekman, 1995) that have not yet been heard.

Conclusion

Over the years there has been a scandalous neglect of mental health care ethics in and by the mainstream bioethics movement as well as by the health professions. The reasons for this are varied and complicated and, in many respects, reflect the very stigma and discrimination that has become so characteristic of the whole field of mental health care in general. Nevertheless, there is increasing evidence that if the field of mental health care ethics has been the most neglected (and it has), it is also the most promising. New and important work is being undertaken which heralds a whole new understanding, acceptance, commitment and approach to mental health care ethics and to the people with mental health problems who stand most in need of the benefits of this work. Whether this work will succeed, however, will depend not on either bioethics or law or government policy. Rather, it will depend on the 'right attitude', and how successful stakeholders in the discourses on mental health care are in demystifying mental health disorders, mental illness and other mental health-related problems, and stripping the stigmatisation from these issues that historically has seen them relegated to the 'too hard basket', not just in mainstream ethics discourse, but in the minds of us all.

Chapter 10

Ethical issues associated with the reporting of child abuse[1]

Introduction

Historically, responses to child abuse and neglect in common law countries have been seriously wanting. Even though the modern problem of cruelty to children was formally recognised in the early 1800s (and, it might be added, even popularised through the fictional writings of the English author Charles Dickens), processes and procedures for protecting children at risk were either: (1) lacking, (2) existed but never enforced systematically, or (3) were themselves abusive or neglectful, thereby compounding further the harm caused to children by their initial maltreatment. Today, the problem of child abuse and protection remains one which is fraught with difficulties and invites controversy at a variety of levels (public, political, professional, legal and moral being key among them). Of particular interest to this discussion is the moral controversy surrounding child abuse and the question it begs of what constitutes a morally just response to child maltreatment and protection — something which remains a moot point and raises many provocative questions. For instance:

- is it the case, as tends to be assumed, that concerned citizens, professionals or public officials ought morally to intervene to protect children from known or suspected instances of abuse and neglect?
- is it unethical for those who hold suspicions about or know that a child is being abused, *not* to intervene in some way?
- are the harms of child maltreatment sufficient to justify overriding a health professional's moral duty to maintain confidentiality in the professional–client relationship?
- are the harms of child neglect and abuse morally significant enough to justify the removal of children from the 'care' of an abusive parent/ guardian or dysfunctional family?
- to what extent, if any, ought the state intervene in the private matters of its citizens (in this instance, parents/guardians who have lawful authority over their children and who have an interest in maintaining their autonomy in deciding how best to raise their children)?

---

1. An earlier version of this chapter was presented under the title *Ethical issues associated with the mandatory and voluntary reporting of child abuse: implications for health professionals in Victoria*, at the Wyeth Health and Nutrition Conference, Hotel Sofitel, Melbourne, 2 August 1997. It has been revised for inclusion in this text.

- is it immoral for the state *not* to intervene to protect children from known or suspected abuse and neglect?
- and so on.

At first glance, answers to these and similar questions might seem manifestly self evident and amenable to consensus. Upon reflection, however, it becomes clear that possible answers to these and related questions are not 'clear-cut', are sometimes hopelessly inadequate and are rarely free of controversy. One reason for this can be found in what appears to be a general reticence in treating the problem of child abuse, neglect and protection as a bona fide moral problem. For instance, while literature abounds on the clinical, legal, sociological and political dimensions of child maltreatment, and some notable discourses on the civil and legal rights of children generally have been advanced (see, for example, Archard 1993; Schrag 1995), relatively little has been written on the *moral* dimensions of child abuse, neglect and protection. Curiously (and significantly) the issue of child abuse has been poorly addressed in the mainstream bioethics literature, which has tended to be preoccupied with addressing the more 'glamorous' ethical issues of abortion, euthanasia, organ transplantation, reproductive technology, and the like. References to child abuse are either conspicuously missing from both the tables of contents and indexes of popular bioethics texts, including those written by feminist moral philosophers, or are included only cursorily (see, for example, Jecker et al. 1997; LaFollette 1997; Engelhardt 1996; Callahan 1995; Reich 1995; Beauchamp and Childress 1994; Macklin 1993; Singer 1993; Holmes and Purdy 1992; Sherwin 1992; Gorovitz et al. 1983). When references and/or discussions are included in these texts, they are often problematic insofar as they tend to be either:

- *minimal and tokenistic in nature* (that is, with only a small number of pages making reference to or containing discussion on the subject; sometimes references to child abuse are contained in endnotes only (see, for example, Jecker et al. 1997; LaFollette 1997; Engelhardt 1996, 1986; Daniels 1996; Callahan 1995; Reich 1995; Macklin 1993; Holmes and Purdy 1992);
- *excusatory and apologist* (for example, advancing arguments defending why it is 'understandable' that professionals feel reticent in intervening in suspected or known cases of child abuse, with little or no attention given to showing why this reticence maybe — and arguably is — morally indefensible and unacceptable [see, for example, Lantos 1995; MacNair 1992]); or
- *elitist*, focussing on the 'philosophically exotic' issues of:
  - *prenatal harm and neglect* termed 'fetal abuse' (such as that caused by smoking and drug and alcohol ingestion by pregnant women; includes debate about the use of contraceptives as a means of 'preventing' child abuse by preventing the existence of the child [Bowman 1995, p. 982; Gallagher 1995, p. 354; Levine 1995, pp. 4–21; Tanne 1991, p. 873]);
  - *'reproductive abuse'* (for example, surrogacy [Oliver 1989, pp. 270–2]);
  - *'religious parental neglect'* (such as in the case of parents declining consent to medical treatment on religious grounds; for example, Jehovah's Witnesses refusing consent for blood transfusions and Christian Scientist parents refusing orthodox medical treatment for their children [Drane 1995, pp. 137–8; Lantos 1995, p. 43);
  - *cultural abuse'* (such as in the case of female genital mutilation [Bond 1996, p. 22]); and

- *'medical abuse and neglect'* (such as in the case of withholding medically indicated treatment from severely disabled newborns and infants [Engelhardt 1996, p. 267]; and the use of children as research subjects [Grodin and Glantz 1994]).

Adding to the above problematic, unlike in the cases of abortion, euthanasia and other popular ethical issues in health care and society, bioethicists themselves rarely (if ever) make public comment on the problem of child maltreatment — and rarely agitate for public policy reform — despite this problem being of at least comparable importance to other more popular bioethical issues deemed to be in the 'public interest' and despite it deserving sustained attention at a public policy level.

In this chapter, an attempt will be made to redress the past neglect of child maltreatment as a substantive moral problem deserving of consideration. Particular attention will be given to briefly examining why child maltreatment stands as a significant moral problem in its own right and why its intervention (such as by mandatory and voluntary notification) is morally compelling. Brief attention will also be given to examining some of the criticism raised against the key interventionist strategies of mandatory and voluntary notification of child abuse and neglect. It will be the ultimate conclusion of this discussion that, given the demonstrable harms caused by child abuse and neglect, everyone (lay and professional alike) has both an individual and a collective moral responsibility to intervene and prevent it. Before commencing this critical examination, however, it would be helpful to first consider some of the historical influences on the development of the child protection movement as we know it today.

The development of the child protection movement in North America: a brief historical overview

In the United States of America, reported cases of child abuse date back to the seventeenth century. In 1655, for example, a master was convicted in a Massachusetts' court and punished for the death of his 12 year old apprentice (Watkins 1990, p. 500). Almost 200 years later, in *Johnson v State* (1840), 'a Tennessee parent was charged with excessive punishment of a child' (Watkins 1990, p. 500). In this case, the court held:

> A parent has the right to chastise a disobedient child, but if he [sic] exceeds the bounds of moderation, and inflicts cruel punishment, he [sic] is a trespasser, and liable to indictment therefor[sic], the excess which constitutes the offence being, not a conclusion of law, but a question of fact for the determination of the jury.
>
> (Johnson v State (1840) — cited in Watkins 1990, p. 500)

It is also known that in the early 1820's, public authorities in New York recognised their duty to intervene in cases of child abuse (including parental cruelty and gross neglect). This, however, often resulted in children being indentured (that is, placed into service or an apprenticeship) in conditions as bad or worse than those from which they had originally been removed (Folks 1902 — cited in Watkins 1990, p. 500). The practice of indenture did not fade out until about 1875 following the passage of the 13th Amendment in 1867 which ended not only slavery but 'involuntary servitude within the United States or any place subject to its jurisdiction' (Watkins 1990, p. 500).

Significantly, laws which could be used to protect children from cruelty existed long before the date of the 13th Amendment being passed. As an early commentator on the care of destitute, neglected and delinquent children noted, during the 1800s, 'laws for the prevention of cruelty to children were considered ample, but *it was nobody's business to enforce the laws*' (Folks 1902 — cited in Watkins 1990, p. 501, emphasis added). Although American 'state statutes were adopted after 1825 that established a public duty to intervene in cases of cruelty or neglect of children', these were rarely enforced (Folks 1902; Thomas 1972 — cited in Watkins 1990, p. 501). Further, these statutes stopped short of mandating 'a responsibility to search out children at risk' (Watkins 1990, p. 500). Significantly, it was not until after the landmark (and now legendary) Mary Ellen child abuse case of 1874 (described below) that this situation began to change, largely due to the establishment and development of a formal movement for the protection of children which was initiated as a result of the widespread publicity given to this case. A key feature of this movement was to make it 'somebody's business' to enforce child protection laws.

The Mary Ellen case

The Mary Ellen case involved a small child (of approximately 10 years of age) who had been severely abused by her guardians since the time of her indenture in 1866. A visitor among the poor, Mrs Wheeler, received complaints about the child's maltreatment and, when unable to get assistance from either the police, benevolent societies or charitable gentlemen, approached the president of the society for the Protection of Animals for assistance in gaining protection for the child against further cruelty by her guardians [Lewin 1994, p. 15; Watkins 1990, p. 501]). The president of the society ultimately agreed to help and, with his assistance, the case was brought before the New York State Supreme Court. Mary Ellen is reported to have appeared in court 'wrapped in a carriage blanket and wearing ragged garments. Her body was bruised, and she had a gash above her left eye and cheek where she had been struck with scissors' (Lewin 1994, p. 15).

The court case was successful, the outcome of which resulted in Mary Ellen being placed in the protective care of Mrs Wheeler; Mary Ellen's abusive female guardian, meanwhile, was convicted of criminal assault and sentenced to 'one year in the Penitentiary at hard labour' (Watkins 1990, p. 502). Following the publicity given to this case, the New York Society for the Prevention of Cruelty to Children (NYSPCC) was formed in 1874 and 'became the child protection and rescue model for several US states and foreign countries' (Watkins 1990, p. 501; see also Lewin 1994, p. 15; Goddard 1996, p. 96). A century later, in 1976, the first international conference on child abuse was held in Geneva. Among other things, this conference increased the world's understanding that the problem of child maltreatment was not just a local or a national one, but was unequivocally international in its scope (Fogarty and Sargeant 1989, p. 149).

Development of the child protection movement in England and Australia

The North American experience was to be influential in the development of the child protection movement in the United Kingdom, with the first Society for the Prevention of Cruelty to Children in England being established in 1883 and ultimately receiving Queen Victoria's patronage in 1889 (Fogarty and Sargeant 1989, p. 17). Like its North American counterparts, this society aimed, among other things, to achieve specific child protection and rescue law reforms, which up until then had failed to be passed. For example, in the 1870's, attempts to introduce anti-cruelty legislation into the English parliament were 'entirely rebuffed' with the prime minister of the day, Lord Shaftesbury, defending:

> the evils you state are enormous and indisputable, but they are so private, internal and domestic in character as to be beyond the reach of legislation, and the subject would not, I think, be entertained in either House of Parliament.
>
> (cited in Fogarty and Sargeant 1989, p. 17)

Australia, as a colony of England, was very much influenced by British attitudes and political antipathy in dealing formally with the issue of cruelty to children (Renvoize 1993, p. 31; Fogarty and Sargeant 1989, pp. 16–17). Of particular interest to this discussion is the situation in the Australian State of Victoria which was not exempt from the problem of child abuse. For example, in 1863, inquests into the deaths of children under 3 years of age found that approximately one-quarter had died as a result of causes 'denoting neglect, ignorance or maltreatment' (Gandevia 1978 — cited by Goddard 1996, p. 10). Although child-specific welfare legislation was passed as early as 1864 (the *Neglected and Criminal Children's Act*) and a Society for Prevention of Cruelty to Children (modelled on the British society) established in 1897, as Fogarty and Sargeant comment:

> Throughout the 19th century the State displayed a deliberate reticence to intervene in family matters. Whereas factory legislation and educational developments increasingly took cognisance of the particular needs of children and there was legislation protecting animals against cruelty, there was a marked antipathy to protect children against maltreatment by their parents or custodians.
>
> (Fogarty and Sargeant 1989, p. 16)

A notable example of this antipathy can be found in an argument that was advanced against a proposed Bill introduced into the Victorian parliament in 1891 and which was aimed at 'making incest a criminal offence' (Renvoize 1993, p. 31). In rejecting the passage of the Bill (which was later passed), it was argued 'that it would be better that a few persons should escape than that such a monstrous clause as this should be placed upon the statute book in this colony' (Renvoize 1993, p. 31). Later examples show that this antipathy persisted well into the twentieth century. For example, between 1966 and 1968, concern about child maltreatment and protection in Victoria was again highlighted when two medical researchers, publishing in the *Australian Medical Journal*, recommended the introduction of mandatory reporting laws (Birrell and Birrell 1966, 1968). The government of the day, however, rejected this recommendation on grounds that it would 'run counter to "welfare ideology" and could lead to hysteria and an urge to punish cruel parents' (Hiskey 1980 — cited in Mendes 1996, p. 27). In its stead, a system of voluntary reporting was recommended. A decade later, in 1986, a recommendation for mandatory reporting was again opposed by the government of the day, this time on grounds that 'it was punitive rather than preventive and likely to lead to a large increase in false reports' (Colyer 1986 — cited in Mendes 1996, p. 27).

Today, the issue of child maltreatment and the need for effective child protection services remains problematic in countries around the world, including Australia.

Over the past few years, there has been a sharp increase in reported incidents of child abuse and neglect Australia wide. 'The system' of child protection has not, however, been able to cope with the increase in demands placed upon it. Despite a rise in the reporting of child abuse, significant numbers of children are still maimed and killed each year as a result of abuse received at the hands of their primary carers (Australian Institute of Health and Welfare 1998; Strang 1996). A troubling aspect of this scenario is that in Australia, as has been shown to be the case overseas, very often 'the circumstances leading to the most serious cases of child abuse almost always were known to the authorities, but there was no intervention because *no-one would take responsibility*' (*Monash Review* 1986, p. 11, emphasis added). In 1996 these failures of the Australian child protection system were described by one critic as a 'national tragedy', and prompted calls by the then Chief Justice of the Family Court, Justice Alastair Nicholson, for the system to be investigated by a royal commission of inquiry (Milburn 1996, p. 3). This call has been largely ignored at both a social and political level (Johnstone, in press). Arguably, what lies at the basis of this social and political inertia is an even more insidious moral inertia and a culpable lack of moral will to challenge and change the status quo. What will shift this moral inertia remains an open question. What is certain, however, is that this moral malaise will continue until it is recognised and understood that child maltreatment is most profoundly a moral problem and, as such, deserves a sustained and comprehensive moral response.

What makes child abuse a bona fide and significant moral issue?

Child abuse constitutes a bona fide and significant moral problem in its own right and, as such, demands a substantive moral response. Reasons for this are outlined below.

As previously considered in Chapter 4 of this text, it is generally accepted that something involves a (human) moral/ethical problem where it has as its central concern:

- the promotion and protection of people's genuine wellbeing and welfare (including their interests in not suffering unnecessarily);
- responding justly to the genuine needs and significant interests of different people; and
- determining and justifying what constitutes right and wrong conduct in a given situation (Frankena 1973; Blum 1980, 1994; Amato 1990; McNaughton 1988; Singer 1993; Beauchamp and Childress 1994; Bond 1996).

Adjunct to these concerns is an additional consideration, namely, that people have a moral responsibility to not cause unnecessary harm to others and, where able, ought to come to the aid of those who are suffering and in distress. As Amato (1990) notes in his *Victims and values: a history and a theory of suffering* (p. 175):

> There is an elemental moral requirement to respond to innocent suffering. If we were not to respond to it and its claims upon us, we would be without conscience and, in some basic sense, not completely human. And without compassion for others and passion for the causes on behalf of human wellbeing, what is best in our world would be missing.

These considerations all apply in the case of child abuse. As can be readily demonstrated, the problem of child abuse fundamentally concerns:

- promoting and protecting the wellbeing and welfare of children at risk of harm because of the abuse and neglect by more powerful others;
- protecting children from this harm requires a careful calculation and balancing of the needs and interests of 'different people'; for example, the children themselves, their primary caregivers (who are often, although not always, the abusers), others (such as family, friends) who may also have an important relationship with the child, prospective notifiers (who may themselves sometimes experience negative outcomes — including violence and abuse — as a result of their interventions aimed at protecting children at risk), society as a whole and, not least, future generations (who may find themselves unwitting participants in the sequelae of intergenerational abuse); and
- determining and justifying the 'rightness' and 'wrongness' of intervening or not intervening in a case of known or suspected child abuse.

Adjunct to these concerns is an additional consideration involving the moral responsibility people have to not cause unnecessary harm to children and, where able, to come to the aid of children who are suffering and in distress as a result of being maltreated and/or neglected by others.

Underscoring child abuse as a moral problem are a number of other important considerations revolving around the extraordinary vulnerability of children generally. Children are among the most vulnerable members of our community. For the most part, they are unable to protect themselves from the harms imposed on them by people more powerful than themselves. Invariably children have to rely on others for help if their wellbeing and welfare is to be safeguarded. Without intervention and help offered by others, the abuse and neglect of children rarely stops (Child Protection Victoria 1993, p. 9; Goddard 1996). Historically, however, children have not always been able to rely on others (including benevolent citizens, health professionals and public officials) to intervene and help them. Nor have they been able to rely on legal law and its processes. As has been pointed out elsewhere, children have long been considered 'different' under law and stand as the 'paradigmatic group excluded from traditional liberal rights' otherwise accorded to and protective of autonomous adults (Minow 1990, p. 283). Equally troubling, neither have children been able to rely on ethics/morality to protect them. Historically, as in the case of law, ethics has also treated children as 'different'; specifically, as not deserving the moral respect otherwise accorded to rationally competent adults (usually men) and which, if accorded to children, could have resulted in 'substantial [and unwanted] intrusion' into the lives of parents (especially fathers) and guardians (male benefactors) (adapted from Schrag 1995, p. 357; see also Archard 1993; Radi 1979; Johnstone, in press). Because of not being able to rely on others, law or ethics for help, children historically have remained at risk of and have experienced otherwise avoidable harms which, if experienced by adults, would have been (and would be) universally condemned, even by the most rudimentary of moral calculations, as being morally unacceptable.

In light of these and other considerations, it is manifestly evident not only that child abuse is a significant moral problem, but that it warrants a substantive moral response. To be effective this response must include moral initiative and action at an individual, group, community and state level aimed at providing genuine *presence* ('being there') for the children who require the assistance of others in order to get the protection they need from a situation of potential or actual abuse and/or neglect.

The problem of ambivalence toward the moral entitlements of children

In an attempt to redress the historical and legitimated vulnerability of children in the case of child abuse and neglect, governments have responded by enacting either mandatory or voluntary reporting laws obligating certain people (on either legal or moral grounds) to intervene by reporting known or suspected cases of child abuse to child protection services. This response has not been without controversy, however. Pivotal to the controversy have been variant moral beliefs, values and attitudes concerning what constitutes the morally most appropriate response to child abuse given the complex of overlapping relationships, responsibilities and variant moral calculations that are inherent in any potential or actual child abuse situation. So intense has been this controversy that, in some instances, it has resulted in a significant and serious 'backlash' against child protection (see, for example, Myers 1994).

While there is little disagreement among stakeholders in the child abuse debate that it is morally wrong for children to be harmed unnecessarily and that children *should* be protected from the harmful behaviours of others, there is considerable disagreement about the kinds of things that can and should be considered *bona fide* 'harmful' to children, the kinds of acknowledged harms that children ought to be formally protected from, and how best to protect children from the harms deemed both *bona fide* and unacceptable. Thus, while there may appear to be a social consensus about the moral unacceptability of child abuse, quite the reverse may be true. As Lantos (1995, p. 45) points out, an apparent consensus about child abuse may, paradoxically, 'mask profound disagreements' about the nature of child abuse and the apparent responsibilities of various parties (including parents/guardians, health professionals and government authorities) to intervene. An example of this can be found in the tragic Australian child abuse case of Daniel Valerio.

The case of Daniel Valerio

On 8 September 1990, Daniel Valerio, a 2-year-old boy living in the state of Victoria, was bashed to death by his stepfather. During the inquest that followed, it was revealed that twenty-one professionals (including three general medical practitioners, a paediatrician, nurses, social workers, a psychologist, a community health worker, teachers and police) as well as neighbours and family friends had all observed bruising on Daniel Valerio's body in the months leading up to his death (Farouque 1993a, p. 3; Garner 1993, p. 24; Goddard 1996, pp. 174–5). Despite making these observations, no action was taken and, as a result, the child remained in an abusive situation. In July, before his death, Daniel Valerio was admitted to a local hospital for assessment and treatment of a large haematoma on his forehead and other bruises observed on his body, head and limbs. Despite suspicions about the nature of the boy's injuries, the attending paediatrician, in consultation with a psychologist acting as a social worker at the hospital, 'decided that there were not sufficient grounds to refer to protective services but that Daniel should be monitored' (Goddard 1996, pp. 174–75). Later it was also revealed that a family doctor had suspected the child was being abused a week before he died 'but left it to the boy's mother — a key suspect — to seek specialist medical advice' (Farouque 1993b, p. 3). Upon autopsy, it was found that Daniel Valerio had sustained 104 external injuries, predominantly bruises, on his body (Farouque 1993a, p. 3; Garner 1993).

The Daniel Valerio case received widespread media attention around Australia and sparked public outrage. A burning question on many people's lips was: How could this have happened? One commentator has since suggested that a possible reason for why the case 'happened' is because the professionals concerned were simply 'not convinced of the need to act' (Goddard 1996, p. 180). He has further contended that had a stranger (rather than a primary caregiver) been suspected of beating the child, 'the responses of all the systems would have been entirely different'; quite probably the child would have received 'immediate medical examination and treatment' and the media would have reported the attack 'and provided descriptions of the attacker' (Goddard 1996, pp. 180–1). Instead, Daniel Valerio's case was met initially with silence and disbelief until it was too late.

Is the 'failure of the system' to blame?

It has been suggested that the failure of 'the system' to be convinced of the seriousness of a child's situation and the need to take protective action rests, in complicated ways, on a prevailing social–cultural ambivalence about violence towards children (Goddard 1996). In support of this claim, it is contended that violence towards children is often viewed, controversially, as being merely 'discipline' (and hence socially acceptable) when carried out at the hands of parents/guardians. (Indeed, this point is underscored everyday in supermarkets around the country where children are physically 'disciplined' [read physically abused] into submission by their adult custodians; were adults treated in this abusive way by other adults, it is likely that local security officers or the police or both would be called, and charges of criminal assault possibly laid against an offending adult.) This explanation is, however, incomplete. The 'failure of the system' to intervene appropriately to protect children rests on something far deeper and more complex than an ambivalence about violence per se towards children. There are other underpinning ambivalences at play, including (and perhaps especially) an extraordinary social–cultural ambivalence about the *moral status, moral interests* and *related moral entitlements of children* and the *correlative moral responsibilities* these entitlements impose on others who come into contact with children. This 'moral ambivalence' has contributed to the 'failure of the system', by undermining the confidence of people in taking what Hoff (1982) calls 'private moral initiative' and 'private benevolence' (read individual moral action) needed to genuinely assist and protect children who are at risk.

If children were genuinely regarded as having moral status and significant moral interests deserving of protection (at least comparable to that otherwise enjoyed by adults), the world's historical response to child maltreatment and protection may well have been very different. For instance, there may have been less of a tendency both privately and publicly to regard the moral interests of children as being subordinate to the interests of adults (in particular, parents). This, in turn, might have resulted in individuals (including professionals), groups, communities and governments responding more effectively to the problem of child maltreatment and protection than has historically been the case. And it might also have resulted in individuals, groups and communities positioning themselves better to break the cycle of intergenerational violence that has become so characteristic of contemporary societies everywhere. Instead, the problem of child abuse has foundered on a bedrock of moral malaise that, arguably, will not shift until there is a concerted effort at both an individual and collective level to challenge and change the status quo.

The ethical implications of child abuse

Whether driven by legal obligation or moral commitment, or both, a health care professional's decision to report child abuse (or not report it, as the case may be) never occurs in a moral vacuum and is never free of moral risk. Even in the face of clinical certainty (insofar as this is possible) and the threat of legal and professional censure for noncompliance with mandatory reporting requirements (insofar as this is probable), there is always room to question: Should I report this particular case of known or suspected child abuse and/or neglect? Underpinning this question are the additional questions of: What are the possible consequences to the child of me reporting or not reporting this case? What are the possible consequences to the child's family/caregivers of me reporting or not reporting this case? and What are the possible consequences to me of reporting or not reporting this case? Possible answers to these questions will depend, in varying degrees, on an effective harm/benefit analysis of the situation.

The moral demand to report child abuse

Child abuse (often used as 'an "umbrella" term that covers a wide range of activities that harm children in some way' [Goddard 1996, p. 28]), can take a number of forms, including physical, sexual, emotional and spiritual. It can also involve neglect, defined here as 'the failure to provide the child with the basic necessities of life, such as food, clothing, shelter and supervision, to the extent that the child's health and development are placed at risk' (Child Protection Victoria 1993, p. 3). In some instances, all forms of abuse may overlap; for example, a child who is sexually abused is *ipso facto* abused physically, emotionally and spiritually as well (Renvoize 1993, p. 36).

Although there is some disagreement about how child abuse can and should be defined (Goddard 1996, pp. 27–40; O'Hagan 1993), this is not sufficient to threaten strong moral arguments against child abuse and its intervention, as some have suggested (see, for example, Lantos 1995, p. 43). Child abuse can be defined in ways that unequivocally distinguishes it from other 'acceptable' behaviours directed at children (for example, play, discipline, 'character building', education) and it is spurious to suggest otherwise. A key feature of child abuse (not carried by other behaviours directed at children) concerns the risk of non-accidental and culpable harm that it poses to a child's genuine welfare and wellbeing. These risks are not merely speculative or imaginary, but substantive and known through the supportive findings of rigorous research, an increasing body of professional literature on the subject, and, not least, by the survivors of child abuse themselves who are increasingly coming forward to share their experiences by making their 'stories' public.

In all its forms, child abuse can cause significant and lasting harm to children and, ultimately, the adults they become. Borrowing from Archard (1993, p. 150): 'A child may be harmed both as a child *and* as a prospective adult. The adult of the future can be harmed by what is now done to the child'. It is this consequence of harm that makes child abuse and neglect morally objectionable. Understanding this, however, requires at least a rudimentary understanding of the notion of 'harm', the way it is linked to human welfare and wellbeing, and why it is morally compelling both *not to cause harm* and *to prevent harm* to others.

The notion of harm and its link with the moral duty to prevent child abuse

As previously considered in Chapter 4 of this text, harm may be taken as involving the invasion, violation, thwarting, or 'setting back' of a person's significant welfare interests to the detriment of that person's wellbeing (Feinberg 1984, p. 34; Beauchamp and Childress 1994, p. 193). Wellbeing, in turn, can include interests in:

> continuance for a foreseeable interval of one's life, and the interests in one's own physical health and vigour, the integrity and normal functioning of one's body, the absence of absorbing pain and suffering or grotesque disfigurement, minimal intellectual acuity, emotional stability, the absence of groundless anxieties and resentments, the capacity to engage normally in social intercourse and to enjoy and maintain friendships, at least minimal income and financial security, a tolerable social and physical environment, and a certain amount of freedom from interference and coercion.
>
> (Feinberg 1984, p. 37)

The test for whether a person's interests and wellbeing have been violated or thwarted rests on 'whether that interest is in a worse condition than it would otherwise have been in had the invasion not occurred at all' (Feinberg 1984, p. 34). For instance, if a person (for example, a child, a young person or an adult survivor of child abuse) is left psychogenically distressed (for example, emotionally unstable, anxious, depressed and/or suicidal) as a result of his/her abusive childhood experiences, our reflective commonsense tells us that this person's interests have been violated and the person him/herself 'harmed'. As the American philosopher Joel Feinberg (1984) explains, the violation of a person's welfare interests renders that person 'very seriously harmed indeed' since 'their ultimate aspirations are defeated too'.

Protecting the interests of children as *children* and as *prospective adults*

It is generally recognised in contemporary bioethical thought that people ought not to cause harm to or to impose risks of harm onto others. It is also accepted that people have a moral obligation to prevent harm to others if this can be done without sacrificing other important moral interests (Beauchamp and Childress 1994). By this view, acts which violate the interests of others, or fail to prevent the interests of others being violated, are prima facie morally wrong. The abuse of children — and the failure to prevent it — clearly violates the interests of children (both as *children* and as *prospective adults*) and renders them seriously harmed. It is the profound risk of the harmful consequences of child abuse (at all stages of life), and the utter preventability of these consequences, that makes intervention in child abuse at all levels morally compelling. Failure to prevent this harm is morally wrong. Further, the moral unacceptability of child abuse is underscored when it is remembered that the harmful consequences of child abuse do not remain quarantined in a 'lost and forgotten' childhood which a person can leave behind upon entering adulthood. As Briere (1992, p. xvi) points out 'in the absence of appropriate intervention, hurt children often grow to become distressed and symptomatic adolescents and adults' — a morally significant and harmful outcome.

What is not always understood in this debate is that the negative effects of child abuse can be long term and sometimes devastating, affecting, in morally significant ways, not only the individuals who survive their traumatic childhoods, but those with whom they share relationships including family, friends, partners, co-workers, service providers and the community at large (see, for example, Mullinar and Hunt 1997; van der Kolk et al. 1996; Phillips and Frederick 1995; Vicki 1995; Loring 1994; Terr 1994; Valent 1993; Elliott 1993; Porterfield 1993; Renvoize 1993; Wilson and Raphael 1993; Briere 1992; Herman 1992; Sanford 1990). This is so, even for those who receive professional help in dealing with their child abuse issues. As one commentator notes:

> Day to day, moment to moment, our feelings and perceptions of the world can change. No matter how long you have been 'working' on your abuse, or how you may feel that at last you can live your life rather than just exist, there are times when you can be overwhelmed quite unexpectedly with painful feelings and memories of your abuse. The 'trigger' can be a smell, a sound, a memory apparently from nowhere. Of this, one survivor says: 'One day, one moment, you can believe that you are all right, that the world and the people in it are all right, and the next be right back down there in the pit of despair'.

> (Longdon 1993, p. 59)

This 'reality' is exemplified by one adult survivor of child abuse, who writes:

> The last seven years have been very difficult for me. For nearly two years I was unable to work, simply being traumatised by the memories that kept bombarding me. My ensuing depression put me in a psychiatric hospital for about eight months in total, and during that time I tried to end my life three times by taking overdoses, and continued to self-abuse by slashing myself. It took me eight years to complete a three-year university degree, as I had to keep dropping out when I had breakdowns.

> (Mono 1997, p. 40)

These examples (which stand as just two among many [see others included in Mullinar and Hunt 1997]) show that adult survivors of child abuse can be seriously harmed (have their welfare interests and wellbeing violated) by their traumatic childhood experiences. The survivors quoted in these examples are plagued by painful feelings and memories of their past childhood abuse and, as a result, are thwarted in realising their ultimate aspirations, not least to be free of the 'absorbing pain and suffering' and 'emotional instability' that has come to characterise and burden their lives. This outcome is morally wrong and ought to have been prevented.

It might be objected here that many survivors of child abuse do not emerge from their traumatic childhood pasts as 'damaged goods' (Sanford 1990), do go on to live productive and satisfying lives (which indeed they do [see, for example, Higgins 1994]), and therefore are no longer 'harmed' by their childhood abuse.

While many survivors of child abuse do go on to live productive and satisfying lives, this is not sufficient to negate or to override the moral obligation to intervene and prevent child maltreatment. There are at least two reasons for this. Firstly, maltreated children are still harmed *as children* by their traumatic experiences irrespective of their survival into adulthood. To deny the suffering of children — or at least to render this suffering as irrelevant — is to discriminate against them in morally unjust ways; it seems to be saying that the suffering of children does not count (or, at least, does not count as much as the suffering of adults) just because it is *children* who are suffering. This 'adultist' view is morally indefensible. Secondly, even though adults who have survived child abuse do go on to live productive and satisfying lives, this is not to say that they do not also suffer in unjustly burdensome ways as a result of their traumatic childhood pasts.

Considerations against the mandatory and voluntary notification of child abuse

Public policy requirements to report child abuse have historically been criticised and even rejected by a range of people including members of the medical profession, community support groups and, not least, members of the judiciary (for example, Family Court judges) (Fogarty and Sargeant 1989; Fogarty 1993; MacNair 1992; Chandler 1993; Magazanik 1993, p. 18; Myers 1994; Goddard 1996; Mendes 1996). The grounds for this criticism and rejection have mostly been utilitarian in nature, involving a calculation of harms and benefits to the: (1) professional–client relationship, (2) parents and families of allegedly abused and neglected children, and lastly (3) allegedly abused and neglected children themselves. Requirements to report child abuse and neglect have also been criticised, controversially, on civil libertarian grounds. Here arguments are advanced to the effect that requirements to report child abuse stands as a fundamental violation of parental rights to be free of state interference and to decide how best to raise their children (Archard 1993). As one commentator observes in relation to the alleged 'dangers' of children's rights discourse, 'taken literally, respect for children's rights may permit substantial intrusion into parents' lives' (Schrag 1995, p. 356). These considerations are not unproblematic, however, and are themselves vulnerable to criticism. Consider the following.

The professional–client relationship

Legitimised requirements to report child abuse and neglect have been viewed as being problematic primarily on grounds that they threaten the sanctity of the professional–client relationship by eroding professional discretion about: (1) duties of confidentiality, and (2) how best to deal with child abuse cases (for example, by discretional and confidential counselling) (Goddard 1996, p. 98; Lantos 1995, p. 44; Winslade 1995, p. 455; Lewin 1994, p. 15; MacNair 1992, pp. 128–9; Quinn 1992, pp. 86–96). A related concern has been that legitimised reporting requirements can also shift and extend the boundaries of responsibility of the professional–client relationship, namely, to include not just the *adult*-client but the *child*-client as well. This is seen as potentially creating an intolerable tension between the possibly competing and conflicting interests of all stakeholders in question. For example, it could create for an attending health professional the moral dilemma of how best to uphold the interests of an abused child-client without also violating the interests of an abusing adult-client, and vice versa. It may well be that, in the end, it is not possible for the health professional to uphold the interests of both clients equally, prompting the question: *What should I do?*

Consequential to the shift in boundaries of responsibility, there is also a commensurate change in role for the health professional, namely, from that of clinician-healer/therapist to that of 'statutory protector'. For some, this assumed role of 'statutory protector' could further threaten the therapeutic sanctity of the professional–client relationship, begging the question of the moral acceptability of health care professionals functioning as the 'eyes of the state'; that is, as agents of a 'state surveillance' system.

Parents and families

Legitimised requirements to report child mistreatment have also been criticised and rejected on grounds that these stand to seriously threaten the 'liberal rights' (to privacy and self-determination), welfare interests and wellbeing of parents and families (Archard 1993, pp. 122–32). The risk of this happening is seen to be especially high in the case of false allegations being made, or where health care professionals are either 'overly zealous' or incompetent or impaired in performing their assessments of allegedly abused children and reporting their findings to child protection services. For example, health care professionals may be lacking in the necessary skills or may make the wrong judgments or, because of their own unresolved personal issues, are just not able 'to come to terms fully with any abuse' (Renvoize 1993, p. 152; see also Goddard 1996; Lantos 1995; Tilden et al. 1994; Miller and Weinstock 1987; Giovannoni 1982). Some critics contend that, in the ultimate analysis, the legitimated reporting of child abuse could result in parents and families being left stigmatised, embarrassment and even irreparably damaged — particularly if the family is 'totally dismembered through termination of parental rights' (Giovannoni 1982, p. 108; Lantos 1995, p. 44). Parents and families could, therefore, be harmed as a result of interventions by child protection services. This, in turn, could seriously harm the welfare interests and wellbeing of the children suspected of being mistreated by their parents and families, but who nevertheless remain dependent on them for care. In short, harmed parents/families could *ipso facto* result in harmed children.

Abused and neglected children

Perhaps among the most serious and troubling criticisms of all is the view that legitimated requirements to report child abuse may, paradoxically, cause further harm to abused children themselves (Goddard 1996; Lantos 1995; Lewin 1994; Miller and Weinstock 1987; Giovannoni 1982). The 'harmfulness' of the intervention, in this instance, is thought to derive from and be compounded by a number of processes.

- Through children being separated (sometimes prematurely) from their parents/primary caregivers and surrendered to 'ambiguous substitute family arrangements' (Giovannoni 1982, p. 108; Miller and Weinstock 1987, p. 162).
- Where separation and removal damages the child–parent/guardian relationship, not least through 'interfering with the ability of abusing parents to deal with their problems and reintegrate their families' (Miller

272

and Weinstock 1987, p. 162). Further, if protective processes (for example, court action) are unsuccessful, this could result in an abused child being returned 'unprotected to an unbelieving family which might scapegoat them and blame them for all the disruption' (Renvoize 1993, p. 152).

- Where protective services simply fail mistreated children, for example:
  - where referrals and protective interventions are handled poorly (for instance, investigations may be delayed or be ineffective; children may be returned to violent and abusive homes and thus committed to a life of re-abuse, crime and death [Fogarty 1993, p. 8; MacNair 1992, p. 129; Pegler 1996, p. 4; Pegler and Farouque 1996, p. 1; Coffey 1996, pp. 1, 4; Daly et al. 1996, p. 1; Hawes and Honeysett 1996, p. 3; Kissane 1993, pp. 24–5, 1995, p. 13; Chandler 1993, p. 28]);
  - where mechanisms for securing child protection may themselves be traumatic and 'abusive' (legal processes [including police involvement and court proceedings] are, for example, characteristically intrusive and 'adversarial' in nature; media coverage is characteristically intrusive and can be harmfully 'exposing' and adversarial in nature) (Lewin 1994); and
  - where protective services are inadequate to meet the needs of mistreated children, resulting in increasing numbers of children being drawn into a child protection system that is 'incapable of caring for them properly' (for example, as can occur in the case of a protective system plagued by budgetary constraints) (Fogarty 1993, p. 7).

Thus, in the final analysis, rather than promoting and protecting the welfare interests and wellbeing of abused and neglected children, mandatory and voluntary reporting requirements might block, thwart, intrude upon, set back, invade and violate these moral entitlements. In short, reporting requirements used as a child protection intervention may ultimately prove to be more harmful than the abuse itself.

Responding to the criticisms

The question remains, however, of whether legitimated demands to report known and suspected cases of child abuse and neglect do stand to 'adversely' affect the nature and boundaries of the professional–client relationship, the 'deserving' interests of parents and families (and, it should be added, other abusing adults) and, not least, the interests of mistreated children. And, if so, what the moral implications of this might be. It is to briefly considering these questions that the remainder of this chapter will now turn.

The problem of maintaining confidentiality

Reporting child abuse, unless consented to by both the abuser and the child (given the child is capable of giving consent), almost always involves a breach of confidentiality and privacy. A key reason health care professionals are reluctant to breach confidentiality concerns a fear that, if abusers cannot rely on or trust professional caregivers to keep secret abuse-related information disclosed in the professional–client relationship, then they (the abusers) may be discouraged from seeking help to remedy their abusive behaviours. In effect, legitimised reporting laws could 'drive people underground' (Goddard 1996, p. 98; Magazanik 1993,

p. 18; MacNair 1992, p. 129). It is not clear, however, that this fear is sufficient to justify maintaining confidentiality in favour of an abusing adult. There are a number of reasons for this. The first of these concerns the very nature of the moral demand to maintain confidentiality itself.

Traditionally, as discussed in Chapter 8 of this text, the rule of confidentiality has demanded that information gained in the professional–client relationship ought to be kept secret even when its disclosure might serve a greater public good. Over time, however, real-life examples and moral theorising have repeatedly shown that treating the rule of confidentiality as being *absolute* is morally unjust, indefensible and unreasonable (Bok 1978, 1983). At best, maintaining confidentiality should be treated as only a *prima facie* obligation. What this means is that while, as a general rule, confidentiality ought to be maintained in the professional–client relationship, there may sometimes be stronger moral reasons for overriding this obligation. An example here would be where an abusing adult discloses to an attending health care professional his or her intention to deliberately injure a child. A decision to disclose this information in order to warn and protect the intended child-victim would be justified on grounds that it could help to prevent an otherwise avoidable harm from occurring.

Superficially, the disclosure of privileged information in the above example might appear to be in breach of a disclosing client's 'rights' to confidentiality. However, confidentiality was never meant to stretch so far as to compel an attending health care professional to lie or to protect those who have no right to impose their malevolence on innocent victims — in this instance an innocent child (Bok 1978, p. 148). Borrowing from Bok (1978, p. 155), 'only an overwhelming blindness to the suffering of those beyond one's immediate sphere' could justify the maintenance of absolute confidentiality in the case where innocent others are at risk of being harmed. Further, a client's moral entitlements to have certain information about themselves kept secret are forfeited where the maintenance of confidentiality about their case stands to seriously impinge on the moral interests and wellbeing of innocent others. In this instance, morally constrained discretionary breaches of confidentiality are morally justified.

In the case of child abuse, there exists strong moral grounds for justifiably overriding an obligation of confidentiality that might otherwise be due to an abusing adult, and for discretionary disclosures to be made to appropriate people. In regard to the 'possible harm' that discretionary disclosures may cause to abusers (for example, driving abusers 'underground' and discouraging them from seeking help; causing them to feel hurt, embarrassed and stigmatised; dismembering families; and so forth), this is not sufficient to justify the maintenance of *absolute* confidentiality. One reason for this is: it is not clear that discretionary disclosures will necessarily harm the welfare interests of abusers. The aim of protective interventions (of which the legitimated reporting of child abuse is a form) is to 'protect children, not to punish abusers' and to be 'curative and remedial rather than punitive' (Lewin 1994, p. 16; Fogarty 1993, pp. 86–8; Miller and Weinstock 1987, p. 167; see also Scott and O'Neil 1996). Thus disclosures that are made to appropriate people stand to not only benefit an abused child, but also set in motion a process that could potentially assist the abuser as well. If the abuser is genuinely accepting of responsibility for his or her abusive behaviour toward children and is committed to rehabilitation, then the problem of competing demands to maintain confidentiality can be overcome by the health care provider negotiating the discretionary disclosure of privileged information gained in the professional–client relationship. If, however, an abuser is unwilling to accept responsibility for his or her abusive behaviour and is unwilling to give permission for a discretionary breach of confidentiality to the relevant authorities, the health care professional has an overriding moral obligation to take the action necessary to protect the interests of an at-risk child or children. Discretionary breaches of confidentiality are morally justified in these instances.

The problem of statutory surveillance

Some claim that legitimised reporting requirements could exacerbate the problem of child abuse in another way; namely, by facilitating its 'over-reporting' (including a proliferation of false allegations being made about its incidence) (Goddard 1996, p. 98; Renvoize 1993; Miller and Weinstock 1987). This, it is contended, might result in 'more children and families being drawn into a system which does not have the capacity to provide the necessary services to them' (Fogarty 1993, p. 12). Furthermore, were health care professionals seen to be spearheading this 'over-reporting' through their surveillance role, this could result in a loss of community trust in service providers and, ultimately, 'the system' which, in turn, could work against an effective overall societal response to child abuse and neglect.

It is not clear, however, whether community trust in health care professionals would be eroded by a proliferation in the reporting of child abuse. For one thing, a proliferation in the reporting of child abuse may not necessarily be spurious. An increase in reporting could be directly linked to a genuine increase in the actual incidence of abuse which, in turn, can be further linked to increased professional and community awareness of what constitutes child abuse and its unacceptability (Fogarty 1993; Goddard 1996). Thus, while being perplexed by an increase in the reporting of child abuse, the community might nevertheless be reassured that 'the system' is working and that children are being protected from unnecessary harm. Contrary to the claims made above, it might be a *failure* by health care professionals to report child abuse that risks undermining community confidence in their services, not the reverse. The Daniel Valerio case (cited earlier in this chapter) is an example of this.

Preserving the integrity of the professional–client relationship

Legitimated requirements to report child abuse do not necessarily threaten the sanctity or integrity of the professional–client relationship. If disclosures are handled in a morally, legally and clinically informed, competent and sensitive manner, this need not involve a collapse of the boundaries between matters of clinical competence and legal and moral prescription/proscription, as some have suggested (Giovannoni 1982, p. 108). To the contrary. Legal and moral prescriptions/proscriptions in the case of child abuse can strengthen the bases and boundaries of clinical competence by reminding health care professionals to always consider carefully the precise impact that their acts and omissions can have on the lives of others (especially children both as children and as prospective adults), and to remain vigilant in regard to their capacity to harm as well as benefit those in their care.

Upholding the interests of parents, families and abused children

It is fully acknowledged that the act of reporting child mistreatment is one which is fraught with difficulties. It is further acknowledged, there are no guarantees that mistakes will not occur. But the risks of *failing* to intervene are equally if not more onerous. By not reporting instances of child mistreatment, there is a risk that abused and neglected children will be 'left forgotten and invisible' (Mullinar and Hunt 1997) and, without help, will go on to be symptomatic adults. There is an additional risk that, without intervention (whatever the risks), the sequelae of child mistreatment could 'continue to wreak havoc generation after generation' (Lord 1997). Appropriate intervention to prevent child abuse (of which reporting may be the first step) can make a significant contribution to breaking the cycle of intergenerational violence.

As suggested earlier, it is not necessarily the case that protective interventions (of which the legitimated reporting of child abuse is a form) will harm the deserving welfare interests of abusing parents and families. It needs to be remembered that a key aim of interventionist strategies is 'to protect children, not to punish the abusers', and, where able, to offer dysfunctional adults and families remediation. Thus appropriate interventions stand to not only benefit an abused child, but also to set in motion a process that could potentially assist and benefit abusers as well.

In the case of children, there is no denying that separation from a primary caregiver can be an extremely traumatic experience for a child — even when the primary caregiver is the abuser. While it might be assumed that an abused child would be 'happy' to get away from an abusive parent, this is not necessarily so. (There are many complex reasons for this which, regrettably, are beyond the scope of this present work to consider [see, for example, van der Kolk 1996, p. 200].) And there is no denying that children can be — and have been — seriously harmed when protective interventions have 'gone wrong'. It is acknowledged that children can be — and are — seriously harmed when the system fails them. What this instructs, however, is not the abandonment of protective services or components of it (for example, reporting requirements). Rather, it highlights the need for protective processes to be improved. In summary, attention ought to be focussed on improving — not removing — the systematic processes that have been put in place to help protect children from the harms of abuse and neglect.

The importance of a supportive socio-cultural environment in child abuse prevention

In her influential text *Trauma and recovery: the aftermath of violence — from domestic abuse to political terror*, the American psychiatrist Judith Herman persuasively argues that:

> In the absence of strong political movements for human rights, the active process of bearing witness inevitably gives way to the process of forgetting. Repression, dissociation, and denial are phenomena of social as well as individual consciousness.
>
> (Herman 1992, p. 9)

Applied in the context of child abuse, there is room to suggest that without a strong political movement for children's right, the process of bearing witness (to child mistreatment) will likewise give way to a communal forgetting. The risk of forgetting is particularly great in an environment which is not supportive of or encourages personal moral initiative and individual acts of benevolence (moral action) aimed at genuinely assisting and protecting children who are at risk.

Herman (1992, p. 8) contends that 'without a supportive environment, the bystander usually succumbs to the temptation to look the other way'. Currently, the social and cultural environment in Australia (as well as overseas) is not generally supportive of child abuse prevention and, to some extent, even supports the position of the 'morally passive bystander' (consider, for example, the positive regard generally given to people who 'mind their own business' and the disparagement made of those who do not). For many health care professionals located in this unsupportive environment, looking the other way may seem a preferable option to 'becoming involved' (Goddard 1996). This 'not becoming involved' might even be seen, controversially, as being a morally preferable option on grounds that it could help to avoid the otherwise unpredictable harmful consequences that can (and do sometimes) flow from intervening or becoming involved in a given child abuse/neglect case. What might not be appreciated, however, is that succumbing to the temptation to look the other way and to avoid involvement is not a morally neutral response. Just because health professionals may have done nothing actively to abuse a child (that is, they may have merely witnessed evidence of possible abuse), this does not mean that they have avoided complicity in the harms to the child caused by his or her initial mistreatment. Borrowing from Joseph Fletcher (1973, p. 675) writing in another context, 'Not doing anything is doing something; it is a decision to act every bit as much as deciding for any other deed'. Thus, a decision to do nothing to intervene in the prevention of child abuse is every bit a decision nevertheless, and still stands as a link in the causal chain of events between an actual instance of abuse and the harm to the child that can and does follow from this abuse.

In their report on protective services for children in Victoria, Fogarty and Sargeant conclude that:

> basically, the issue [of child abuse] is a public one and one in respect of which each section of the community can and should make a contribution. It would we feel be a fundamental mistake to believe that this community problem can be eliminated by a total concentration upon what the government can do for the community. The issue also is — what can the community and individual members of the community do for the state and the children within it? There is too great a tendency both generally and in relation to this particular matter to sit back and demand that the government do this or that but without appreciation of the wider responsibilities which are involved.
>
> (Fogarty and Sargeant 1989, p. 152)

There are not, of course, any 'quick fix' solutions to the problem of child abuse and protection. But there is considerable scope to suggest that a lot more could be done at an individual, familial, group, community and state level to improve the status quo. Health care professionals have a particularly important role to play on account of them being in a prime position to discern and provide evidence of instances of child abuse and neglect, and to legitimately intervene to prevent these instances from continuing. Through their informed and morally judicious interventions, health care professionals could, in turn, make a significant difference to the lives and welfare interests of both abused children and abusing adults. Legitimated reporting requirements should, therefore, not be seen as an intrusion or a violation of the professional–client relationship, but as an opportunity to provide support and care to injured and distressed human beings (both children and adults alike).

A system of child protection is only as good as the people who are charged with the responsibilities of upholding it. All health care professionals have an obligation to become sufficiently informed about the clinical, legal and ethical dimensions of child abuse to enable them to competently participate in child protection processes. And there is small doubt that improving the education of health care professionals about child abuse and protection issues will prepare them to deal better with known or suspected child abuse cases. But, as Judith Herman (cited above) makes plain, commitment and education may not be enough; there also needs to be a supportive social environment and a deeply ingrained cultural commitment to preventing the harms of child abuse and neglect across the board. There are a number of points at which initiatives to improve the socio-cultural environment could begin, two examples of which are given below.

One starting point can be found in the nomenclature commonly used to refer to the child protection intervention of 'reporting'. Rather than speak of 'reporting' child abuse, perhaps it would be less punitive to use the notion of 'making notifications'. The term 'reporting', for example, carries a range of negative connotations, including that of 'making a complaint', 'to lay a charge against a person', 'to present oneself to a person in authority' and variations thereof, something which seems to go against the stated aims of reporting; namely, 'to protect the child, not to punish the abuser' (*The Macquarie Concise Dictionary* 1997). The term 'notification' (meaning 'to tell'), in contrast, does not seem to have the same moralistic loading attached to it. A health care professional could 'notify' a case of child abuse to a relevant authority in much the same way that he or she would notify other 'notifiable' conditions such as an infectious disease or other medical condition.

Another starting point may be the electronic and print media. For instance, television advertisements around Australia remind viewers daily that 'If you drink drive, you are a bloody idiot', 'Every cigarette is doing you harm', and 'Work safety: think it, talk it, work it — some injuries never heal'. The financial costs of running these advertisements are seen to be justified even though the advertisements themselves are only a small (be it so important) part of an overall strategy aimed at changing the health risk behaviours in question. This is because the costs of drink driving accidents, smoking and of work-related injuries have all been deemed unacceptable to our community. It is time that the incalculable costs of child abuse and neglect are similarly deemed unacceptable to our community. Comparable initiatives (to those above) need to be taken to help change community attitudes towards the health-risking behaviours of child abuse generally and towards its own deep responsibility to protect children at risk of abuse. On this note, it is worth speculating what community attitudes might be like today if there had been a concerted advertisement campaign (comparable to the anti-drink driving, anti-smoking and work safety campaigns) along the lines of: 'If you abuse a child, you're a bloody coward' or 'Every act of abuse is doing your child harm' or 'Child protection/safety: think it, talk it, work it — some injuries never heal ...'.

Conclusion

This chapter has attempted to show that the issue of child maltreatment not only raises a number of important ethical issues, but is itself an important and discrete ethical issue. It has also attempted to show that health care professionals have a moral obligation to intervene in the prevention of child abuse and neglect and that this obligation rests on considerations of the welfare interests and wellbeing of children. And while it is acknowledged that the act of reporting child abuse and neglect is one which is fraught with difficulties, the risks of *not* reporting are equally if not more onerous — not just to abused children but to the community as a whole. In the ultimate analysis, and in support of Fogarty and Sargeant (1989) cited above, 'each section of the community [including and perhaps especially health care professionals] can and should make a contribution'.

Children should not have to bear 'silent and unacknowledged witness to their own suffering in many ways throughout their lives' (Valent 1993, p. 4). Everyone has a moral responsibility (irrespective of legal law) to break the culture of silence that surrounds child abuse and which has been so effective in invalidating, marginalising and rendering as invisible its untoward effects. Unless this responsibility is accepted and acted upon at an individual and private level, children will remain at risk of the otherwise avoidable harms caused by child abuse and neglect. To fail in this responsibility is not only to fail the most vulnerable members of our society (children), but to fail ourselves and the community as a whole in which we share membership.

Child abuse does not only affect children, it affects us all. It is, therefore, up to each and every one of us (as co-participating members of a moral community) to do what we can in order to prevent it and the harms that flow insidiously from it. Preventing the harms of child abuse is not merely a charitable cause which people can choose to either support or not support. Rather it is an obligation supported by the deepest of ethical considerations and which is binding on all of us. The ultimate question, then, is not one of *whether we ought to intervene* in the prevention of child abuse, but *how we may best intervene* and achieve the desired moral outcomes of this intervention.

Chapter 11

Abortion and the nursing profession

Introduction

There are perhaps no contemporary ethical issues so emotionally charged and so inviting of public, political, legal and moral controversy as those involving matters of life and death. Abortion is one such ethical issue and, as demonstrated in the opening chapter to this text, one that has the capacity not only to cause extreme and damaging divisions among people, but violence as well. Indeed, few (if any) other mainstream bioethical issues have the distinction that the abortion issue has today; namely, of having literally drawn thousands upon thousands of people out onto the streets, in countries around the world, in public protest (either for or against abortion) and demanding a decisive political response to settle, once and for all, what in the eyes of many stands as an irreconcilable disagreement about the morality of abortion.

The nursing profession is not, of course, immune from the protests associated with the abortion issue. More than this, the demonstrable controversy surrounding the abortion issue has placed the nursing profession globally in an extremely difficult position, and one that raises a number of crucial questions for nurses. Such questions include the following six.

1. What is abortion?
2. Is abortion morally right or wrong? How is this matter to be decided?
3. If abortion is morally wrong, can members of the nursing profession be decently expected to assist with abortion work and/or care for the women who have had them?
4. If abortion is not morally wrong, can nurses justifiably refuse to assist with abortion work and/or care for the women who have had them?
5. If participating in abortion work, what are the obligations (if any) of nurses toward fathers of a pregnancy who are opposed to their fetus being aborted?
6. In the event of no substantive agreement being reached on whether abortion is morally right or wrong, what, if any, public position should the nursing profession take on the issue?

It is to addressing these and related questions that this chapter will now turn.

Nurses' experiences of abortion work: a brief historical overview

In January 1988, Canada shredded its 19-year-old abortion law. An article in the *Leader Post* signed the 'Canadian Press' (1988) reported that everyone was scrambling to gauge what this legislative reform would mean — 'particularly [to] *politicians* and *doctors*' (emphasis added). It went on to report:

> Most authorities agree the ruling will not mean abortion on demand — at least not immediately and not ever in the sense that *doctors have the right to refuse* to perform the procedure.

> (Canadian Press 1988, emphasis added)

In the 1200-word article reporting on this reform, not once is the term 'nurse' mentioned, nor is any thought given to the impact that the new liberal abortion laws might have had on nurse practitioners generally. The Canadian Medical Association is reported as having 'advised its 45 000 members to honour the law until lawyers have studied the ruling', but no mention is made of any response from the Canadian Nurses' Association. Pro-abortionist and anti-abortionist groups are widely quoted, as are eminent theologians and legal authorities — but no nurses.

In the United Kingdom, midwives and nurses have long been expected to participate actively in abortion work — even to the point of coming perilously close to engaging in the illegal practice of medicine on account of their being left without direct medical supervision to manage the actual process of a fetus being aborted following medical intervention. In the United Kingdom, while doctors would prescribe an abortion for a given woman, prescribe the necessary pharmaceutical substances to induce an abortion, and would insert an intravenous and/or an intrauterine line for the purposes of administering abortive substances (for example, intrauterine hypotonic saline), it was left to the midwives to *alone* manage the intravenous/intrauterine lines, to administer and regulate the medically prescribed abortive substances, to manage the actual expulsion of the fetus, and to manage the care of the woman after the fetus had been expelled. This situation emerged because, once prescribing and initiating the abortion procedures, the doctors would leave the vicinity — enabling them to gain some 'moral distance' from the physical act of procuring the abortions they had prescribed.

The position of midwives and nurses in regard to these abortion practices became a very serious professional concern. So much so that, in the early 1980s, the Royal College of Nursing (RCN) in the United Kingdom (UK) attempted to have midwife-assisted abortions stopped by taking the matter to court. The RCN (UK) lost its case, however. In the noted House of Lords case *Royal College of Nursing v DHSS [CA]* (1981), it was held that so long as a 'registered medical practitioner decided on and initiated the procedure', and 'remained throughout responsible for its overall conduct and control in the sense that the acts needed to bring it to its conclusion were done by appropriately skilled staff acting on his [sic] specific instructions', it was not necessary for a registered medical practitioner to be present throughout an abortion procedure (see also Rea 1981). The court also held that while the 'finger of the nurse' was on the button, it was merely performing a mechanical, not a medical, act. Midwives and nurses performing abortion work were thus not seen by the court as engaging in the illegal practice of medicine.

Abortion work in the United Kingdom was problematic on yet another front. Up until the late 1980s midwives were expected to manage the abortion of fetuses of 24–28 weeks gestation. As a result of the 28-week limit (permitted by abortion laws), abortions were resulting in viable births. In 1985, one midwife is reported to have confirmed that her unit had 'one [live] baby born under 28 weeks every three weeks' (*Nursing Times*, 24 July 1985, p. 5). Another midwife confirmed that viable births resulting from abortions were posing serious problems, not least that of forcing midwives and medical staff to 'decide how to dispose of live babies' (*Nursing Times*, 24 July 1985, p. 5). This intolerable situation prompted the question of whether nurses should be asked to participate in abortions of fetuses that might be capable of independent existence (Holmes 1988, p. 19). The problem was partially 'resolved' by the legislative reforms restricting the time limit for 'social' abortions to 18 weeks — where fetal viability is low (*Nursing Times*, 17 February 1988, p. 8).

In Australia, nurses have also faced political and legal difficulties in relation to their abortion-assisting work. For example, in early 1998, nurses involved in abortion work in Western Australia were advised by the Australian Nursing Federation that they risked criminal prosecution if they directly or indirectly engaged in the termination of pregnancies (see previous discussion on this matter in Chapter 2, p. 17). Significantly, the legal advice received contradicted earlier advice received from the State's Health Department to the effect that 'nurses who assist in terminations might be fulfilling their contract of employment' (Reeves 1998, p. 11). The legal advice was given to nurses after two Perth doctors were charged with attempting to procure an abortion, throwing Western Australia into a state of panic and political upheaval (O'Brien and Price 1998, p. 5). Subsequently, the editor of the *Newsletter of the Legal Issues Society* (Royal College of Nursing, Australia) criticised the whole affair, and the highly questionable misinterpretation and misrepresentation of existing abortion laws that underpinned it (Wallace 1998, pp. 2–3). She concluded that the matter highlighted the need for abortion laws to be clarified in all jurisdictions, pointing out that it was 'not satisfactory that nurses must rely on interpretations of cases in the 1970s and 1980s to determine whether an abortion is legal or not', and to have to face the kind of confusion and anguish that Western Australian women and nurses had just endured (Wallace 1998, p. 3).

On a more individual (and personal) level, the abortion issue has, on the whole, proved to be both a complex and an unhappy one for members of the nursing profession. In the past, nurses have been systematically discriminated against and have lost their jobs for refusing conscientiously to participate in abortion procedures (Thompson and Thompson 1981, p. 84; Muyskens 1982, p. 59; Davis and Aroskar 1983, p. 129). Some states in the United States of America have since enacted legislation aimed at protecting individuals who conscientiously refuse to participate in abortion work by making it a felony for employers to dismiss employees (such as nurses) on grounds of conscientious objection (Davis and Aroskar 1983, p. 129). In the United Kingdom, abortion laws now permit nurses, by way of a 'conscience clause', conscientiously to refuse, in non-emergency situations, to participate in abortion work (Tschudin 1986; Rumbold 1986). In Australia, the banning of religious discrimination in public hospitals ensures that *believers*, at least, are not placed in 'situations of moral dilemma'. The situation for *non-believers* is not clear, although most nurses

I have spoken to have indicated that, on the whole, conscientious objection in cases involving abortion is reasonably well accepted in Australian hospitals, despite not being supported legally.

Despite these protective provisions and this general tolerance, however, nurses have a history of and continue to suffer from unfair discrimination, stereotyping and harassment if they have a moral objection to participating in abortion work. The International Council of Nurses (ICN) (1977), for example, cites the case of a midwifery student who had 'problems on ethical grounds' in assisting with abortion and sterilisation procedures. When the student approached the teaching hospital's director of nursing to discuss the matter, she was asked by the director of nursing why she had 'bothered' to come to the hospital to do her midwifery training at all. The student unsuccessfully tried to explain that, for her, midwifery did not entail assisting with abortions or sterilisations. Commenting on her eventual decision to withdraw from the midwifery course, the student wrote: 'Rather than continue in these sad circumstances I packed my bags and returned home the next day. I was a disappointed midwifery student but happy that I had taken the correct action' (International Council of Nurses 1977, p. 13).

In February 1988, a similar case occurred in Australia. The case involved a registered nurse and midwife who was allegedly refused employment at a large New South Wales rural hospital because she was conscientiously opposed to participating in abortion and sterilisation work (Broekhuijse 1988). The nurse had apparently been offered a position at the hospital concerned, and had written back accepting the offer. In her letter of acceptance, however, she pointed out that she was conscientiously opposed to abortion and sterilisation procedures, and that if she was asked to participate in such procedures she would exercise her right to refuse. To this, the director of nursing is reported to have replied: 'It would be quite impractical for you to be excluded from any involvement in the care of these patients' (Broekhuijse 1988, p. 13).

After several more letters had passed between the nurse and the director of nursing, and after the nurse had declined the offer of an alternative position, the original offer of employment was withdrawn. Interestingly, a New South Wales Health Department document is reported as stating that: 'In the case of junior *medical staff* reasonable steps must be taken to reorganise work so as not to place individuals in situations of moral dilemma' (Broekhuijse 1988, emphasis added). Whether this provision also applies to *nursing staff* is a point in question.

More recently, in 1994, nurses in South Australia were the subject of a particularly vitriolic attack in both the lay media and the bioethics literature for their refusal to assist with second trimester abortions (Debelle 1991; Cannold 1994). This stance by nurses, taken for a variety of reasons (including difficulties in clinical practice and a lack of support for nurses assisting with abortions) allegedly resulted in abortion services in South Australia being disrupted for almost two years, with women requiring second trimester abortions having to travel interstate for abortion services (Cannold 1994, p. 86).

One of the most extraordinary examples of negative attitudes toward nurses who are opposed conscientiously to abortion is to be found in a 1972 article published in the *American Journal of Psychiatry*. The article in question, written by two psychiatrists, Walter Char and John McDermott, also provides a classic example of 'an ethical issue being translated into a technical problem which has a clinical solution'. Since this article provides such an important and compelling example of so many things, I make no apology for discussing and quoting from it at length.

On 11 March 1970, Hawaii became the first of the United States of America to liberalise its abortion laws, paving the way for abortion to be available virtually on demand. Psychiatrists applauded the reformed legislation, since it meant that society no longer required them 'to conjure up psychiatric reasons to justify abortion' (Char and McDermott 1972, p. 952). Within a month of the passage of the new abortion bill, however, many nurses began to conscientiously refuse to participate in abortion work, and some threatened resignation. This led to a chief of staff of a major hospital contacting the consulting psychiatrists, Walter Char and John McDermott, and requesting them to help 'deal with the acute psychological reactions of many of their nurses who were so upset by their abortion work' (some were in fact assisting with up to ten abortions a day) (Char and McDermott 1972, p. 952). Soon after, a second hospital also sought the assistance of these two psychiatrists. Char and McDermott (1972) later dubbed the crisis an 'acute *psychiatric* problem' (emphasis added) and one which 'no-one foresaw' would occur as a result of Hawaii legalising abortion.

It is perhaps not surprising that the psychiatrists in this case should perceive the nurses' *moral distress* as a *psychiatric problem*. Nevertheless, their overall analysis of the nurses' reaction deserves to be described as misguided and wrong.

Significantly, Char and McDermott 'found' that all of the nurses 'suffered from strong emotional reactions to their abortion work and welcomed the opportunity to talk about them' (p. 953). In support of this finding, they write:

> The nurses' strong reactions were a surprise to even some of them since many of them, including some of the Catholic nurses, appreciated the problem of unwanted pregnancies and had approved of the new abortion law before it went into operation. But once the nurses became *personally, intimately, and constantly involved* with abortions, their *intellectual* and *professional objective* attitudes favouring legalised abortions were replaced by deeply *personal emotional reactions* so strong that many of them were *even* questioning the wisdom of the new law.
>
> (Char and McDermott 1972, p. 953, emphasis added)[1]

Char and McDermott further stated that all the nurses showed symptoms of anxiety and depression:

> They [the nurses] complained about being tired and being unhappy about their work; they cried *too easily* and got angry *too quickly*; they had difficulty sleeping and had bad dreams; during the day they found themselves preoccupied with disturbing thoughts about their abortion work; and they were *overly sensitive* when their friends teased them about working in a 'slaughter house'. One nurse *even* worried about what her mother would think of her if she found out that she was working in an 'abortion mill'.
>
> (Char and McDermott 1972, p. 953, emphasis added)[2]

---

1. From W. F. Char and J. F. McDermott (1972), Abortions and acute identity crisis in nurses, *American Journal of Psychiatry* 128.(8), pp. 952–7. © 1972, The American Psychiatric Association. Reprinted by permission.
2. From W. F. Char and J. F. McDermott (1972), Abortions and acute identity crisis in nurses, *American Journal of Psychiatry* 128.(8), pp. 952–7. © 1972, The American Psychiatric Association. Reprinted by permission.

The psychiatrists concluded that the nurses' 'symptomatology' fell into the category of 'a transient reactive disorder'. They pointed out, however, that only one nurse appeared to have a more 'severe psychiatric disability', manifested by her going about 'blessing dead fetuses' (a problem which they judged was caused by a pre-existing 'deep-seated emotional difficulty').

One of the disturbing features about this psychiatric assessment is that it assumes that the nurses' reaction to their abortion work was abnormal, and even pathological. Also disturbing is its overt rejection of emotion as a professional behaviour guide. The psychiatrists' labelling of the nurses' reactions as being over-sensitive is also disturbing: it would be interesting to know just what standard they used to measure this 'oversensitivity'. What is particularly noteworthy, however, is the case of the nurse 'compulsively blessing dead fetuses'. This nurse's cultural and religious background is not given. Placed in the context of strong cultural and religious beliefs, her actions might not seem so obviously the manifestation of psychiatric illness. As we saw in Chapter 3, in the case of the young Maori woman who spontaneously aborted her twenty-week fetus, practices of 'compulsively blessing' dead or dying fetuses can have a sound and reasonable explanation.

Char and McDermott also 'found' that many of the nurses 'over-identified with the aborted fetus'. This, they reasoned, largely came about because in the wards fetuses of twelve to twenty weeks were mostly aborted. Abortions in these cases were procured by injecting saline into the uterus, causing labour and the subsequent expulsion of the fetus twelve to twenty-four hours later. Nurses working with patients having this type of abortion found it most disturbing 'to hold a well-formed aborted fetus with movement and with its eyes "still alive"' (Char and McDermott 1972, p. 953). Nurses involved in abortions procured by the dilation and curettage method were also deeply disturbed by seeing 'formed fetal parts such as hair and bits of limbs being sucked out or scraped out'. The psychiatrists concluded that this distress was quite unnecessary, and was largely the product of nurses 'over-identifying' with the fetus and projecting 'into the protoplasmic masses real, live, grown-up individuals' (p. 953). The psychiatrists also concluded that the nurses who over-identified the most with the aborted fetuses were themselves adopted, or had adopted children, or had had difficulty conceiving.

Char and McDermott's assessments must not go unchallenged here. Holding a fetus, feeling it move, hearing it trying to 'cry' (something which usually only happens with older fetuses, those of around twenty weeks' gestation or more), seeing it trying to open its eyes (again, usually with the older fetuses), smelling its death, and the like, are not trivial experiences; nor are they pleasant ones. The psychiatrists' report on nurses' comments do not in fact suggest that the nurses perceived the fetuses as 'grown-up individuals'; live, yes, but not 'grown up'. What they saw was a tiny and uniquely human form of life made vulnerable by medical intervention. This sight — as any delicate sight has the power to do — caused in the nurses feelings of emotion in exactly the same way that nurses observing other medical procedures (for example, the removal of 'beating hearts' from cadavers) experience strong feelings of emotion. This feeling of emotion is understandable, and is in this case hardly a basis for making a sound psychiatric diagnosis. Yet a diagnosis was made, and the process effectively medicalised the nurses' emotions — something which warrants concern given its potential to undermine moral sensibility, and the authority and credibility of the 'moral emotions'.

A third diagnosis formulated by Char and McDermott was that 'the nurses felt hostile toward most of the abortion patients' (1972, pp. 953–4). This, they suggested, was largely influenced by the nurses 'own sexual problems', as well as by the nurses' difficulty in identifying positively with the abortion patients.

The 'catch-22' should be obvious here: on the one hand the nurses were accused of *over-identifying* with the aborted fetuses, and on the other of *under-identifying* with the aborting/aborted mothers. These nurses were thus placed in a 'no-win' situation. It is doubtful whether any degree of identification with the aborting mothers would lessen the emotion provoked by the sight of a tiny moving fetus. Further, the assessment that the nurses' problems stemmed from their own sexual difficulties seems hardly a suggestion to be taken seriously. For instance, it is not difficult to imagine a nurse who has no sexual problems still being overwhelmingly distressed by the sights likely to be witnessed during abortion work (including the sights of distressed and grieving mothers).

Char and McDermott make one further controversial assessment of the nurses, notably that they 'suffered from an acute identity crisis regarding their nursing role and function' (pp. 954–5). This, the psychiatrists reasoned, occurred predominantly as a result of role conflict: on the one hand nurses were trained to save life; now they were being asked to assist in terminating life. This role conflict was exacerbated by the fact that the nurses, unlike doctors (including junior residents), did not have the option of refusing. The reasons given for nurses not having this option were solely practical ones; that is, 'whether she [sic] was in the operating room or on the floor, the nurse *had* to cover whatever case came on her [sic] service' (p. 954, emphasis added). Further to this, the nurses claimed that 'many of the physicians were not as readily available to help in the care of abortion patients as with other patients' (p. 954).

The psychiatrists' diagnosis of identity crisis and role conflict is, in my view, simplistic and open to serious question. The judgment of 'role conflict' in this instance erroneously presumes that the nurse is torn between two bona fide roles. If it can be shown, however, that one of the roles is not in fact a bona fide nursing role, the psychiatrists' diagnosis of role conflict and related identity crisis is immediately without basis. In this instance, it is open to serious question whether *assisting with an actual abortion procedure* (to be distinguished here from *caring for women who have had or are about to have an abortion*) is a bona fide nursing role. Nurses may well be able to fulfil a *technical* and *practical role* in assisting with an actual abortion procedure, but this in no way implies that the role is a bona fide *professional nursing one*. This argument becomes persuasive when we consider the very concept and definition of nursing itself. *Nursing* is typically defined in terms of *caring* and *fulfilling a caring role* (see, for example, Watson 1985; Benner and Wrubel 1989). It is difficult to see, on the basis of this definition, how handing over a set of surgical instruments to a doctor performing an abortion, and/or counting a set of swabs after the procedure has been completed, is the fulfilment of a caring (viz. nursing) role. If, for example, we analyse the tasks performed by assisting nurses during a surgical abortion procedure, we soon see that their role reduces to being little more than *technical assistance* and, what is more, of a kind that does not particularly draw upon *nursing* skills. While nurses may well use their learned skills during the pre-operative and post-operative/recovery stages, it is open to serious question whether they do so in an operating theatre situation. Against Char and McDermott, then, I would suggest that, at least in the case of surgical abortions performed in the operating theatre, it is not a nurse's role to assist. Even if it is

287

conceded that nurses do have a role in assisting with abortion procedures, this still does not rescue Char and McDermott's diagnosis. For what the Hawaiian nurses were clearly suffering from in this case was not *role conflict* but *moral conflict*, complete with all the psychological and moral distress associated with it.

Char and McDermott's solution to the abortion crisis came in the form of psychiatric therapy, notably abreaction, the use of psychiatrists as positive therapeutic figures, assisting nurses to establish a more positive identification with their patients, helping the nurse to 'regain objectivity' about abortions, and calling for the role, philosophy and ethics of nursing and medicine guiding abortion practices to be redefined.

The psychiatrists both felt they had been successful in resolving the crisis. They felt that they had been particularly effective in helping to 'bridge the gap that was separating the nurses from administrators and the medical staff and brought the hospital "family" closer together again' (p. 955). They also felt they had been successful in helping the nurses regain their 'objectivity', and to see 'again that what is aborted is a protoplasmic mass and not a real, live, grown-up individual' (p. 956). Char and McDermott conceded, however, that where nurses continue to 'react poorly' they should be transferred to another type of duty.

The treatment of this moral issue as a psychiatric problem to be solved by a clinical solution has parallels to the 'doubling' described by Robert Jay Lifton (1986) in his analysis of the Nazi doctors and their psychology of evil. It is not being suggested here that the psychiatrists in this case were behaving like Nazis. However, what is disturbing about this case is that the psychiatrists in question had the power to 'condition' a group of others (nurses) to 'double' — to see abortion not as a moral issue but as *good medicine*, and to see the fetus not as a *human form* but as a *protoplasmic mass*. It should be of some concern that psychiatrists have the legitimated authority to function in this way (see also Wikler and Barondess 1993).

It could be argued against the use of this example that the article was after all written a generation ago, and thus is somewhat outdated for the purposes of discussing present-day issues. Significantly, however, the attitudes expressed in Char and McDermott's article are still current. On the basis of informal comments received from nurses involved in organ retrieval work, autopsies and abortion work, or who work with patients who refuse care or for whom decisions have been made to withhold or withdraw medical treatment, I have good reason to believe that these attitudes are far from outdated, and remain relevant to present-day concerns. I have been told, for instance, that psychiatrists are playing an increasing role in 'debriefing' nurses in situations where patients have refused care and treatment, but where these patients' wishes have been overridden on the basis of recommendations made by a consulting psychiatrist.

For example, in one notable case (occurring as recently as 1988) a severely debilitated patient expressed a wish to be allowed to die. When her wishes were refused, she proceeded to decline offers of food and fluids. A consulting psychiatrist was called in and subsequently declared the patient 'rationally incompetent'. Nursing staff who were distressed by the fact that this woman's wishes were not being respected (and they had no reason to believe that her wishes were not rational) were later 'counselled' by the psychiatrist, and assisted to regain their 'objectivity' about the 'medical facts' of the case. When it became evident that the nursing staff could not cope with the woman being force-fed against her will, she was discharged by the hospital into the care of her husband.

As can be seen by the brief historical overview that has just been given of nurses' experiences of abortion work, the abortion question is an important ethical issue for nurses and one that warrants in-depth examination. It is to providing this examination that the remainder of this chapter will now turn.

What is abortion?

As with any moral debate, it is important first to clarify the terms of reference being used. Not surprisingly, abortion is defined differently by those who do support it and those who do not. This is interesting and significant, in that it again raises questions concerning the supposed value neutrality of so-called 'objective' moral definitions and concepts, and the extent to which these can be ethically loaded.

In its 1986 report, *Human embryo experimentation in Australia*, the Senate Select Committee on the Human Embryo Experimentation Bill defines 'abortion' as a 'spontaneous or induced termination of pregnancy' (p. xix), and 'miscarriage' as the 'the spontaneous loss of an early pregnancy at any stage before the twentieth week after conception' (p. xxi). Pro-abortionists use similar language when discussing abortion, tending typically to define it in terms such as 'terminating pregnancy' or 'ridding the products of unwanted conception'. The language in this instance is regarded by proponents of abortion as 'objective' and aims to focus attention away from the emotional aspect of the issue. It also seems to imply the conclusion that abortion is morally permissible. Anti-abortionists, by contrast, tend typically to define abortion in such terms as 'artificially causing the miscarriage of an unborn child', or of 'killing an innocent human being' (Fisher and Buckingham 1985). The language used in these and similar definitions is 'emotive', and aims to focus attention on the emotional aspect of abortion. It also seems to imply the conclusion that abortion is morally wrong.

In light of the ongoing radical disagreement between pro- and anti-abortionist groups, it is unlikely that a consensus on the definition of abortion will ever be achieved. This serves as a timely warning that it is unlikely that the abortion debate itself will ever be resolved to everybody's satisfaction. The question of whether abortion is *moral* (to be distinguished here from it being *legal*) is, however, not one to be answered by a popular vote on what is to count as an acceptable definition. Rather, it is something which can only be decided by rigorous moral analysis and deliberation.

Is abortion morally permissible?

Abortion has an interesting history. Anthropological studies suggest that abortion has been widely practised across cultures and throughout human history, and probably dates back even to prehistoric times (Thomas 1986, p. 77). Abortion techniques have been described in early Chinese, Egyptian and Greek texts, and continue to be widely practised in non-industrialised societies and other Third World countries. Muslim traditions permit abortion, so long as it is procured while 'the embryo is unformed in human shape' (Thomas 1986, p. 79). Japan did not introduce anti-abortion laws until the Meiji Restoration (1869–1912).

Contrary to what many Christian fundamentalists believe, opposition to abortion is not justified by appealing to either the Bible — it simply 'does not discuss it' (Badham 1987) — to church traditions or to Christian reasoning. The early religious fathers, including St Augustine, St Jerome and St Thomas Aquinas, did not believe that the embryo was a human being from the moment of conception, and 'all insisted that early abortion could not be classed as homicide' (Badham 1987, p. 11). They also drew a firm distinction between early and late abortions. As far as the personhood of the fetus is concerned, this too 'has virtually no significant support' in the Christian tradition until the teachings of Pope Pius IX (1846–78). And in the Hebrew version of Exodus 21, accidental abortion is seen as an offence (and one punishable by death) 'only if the woman dies' (Thomas 1986, p. 78).

Where then has contemporary anti-abortion sentiment arisen from? There is much to suggest that it is largely the product of Catholic dogma dating back to the 1854 proclamation of the *Dogma of the Immaculate Conception* and the subsequent series of papal decrees (for example, in 1884, 1889 and 1908), 'which forbade direct termination of a pregnancy even in circumstances where, as in ectopic pregnancies, the result of non-intervention was the certain death of both mother and child' (Badham 1987, p. 12). Given this, it is difficult to avoid the impression that the ongoing abortion debate is as much a matter of disagreement of religious dogma as it is of moral values.

Abortion is usually viewed as both a moral and a legal problem (see in particular Pojman and Beckwith 1994; Dworkin 1993). In this instance, morality and legal law have vitally interdependent roles to play in ensuring the realisation of just outcomes. Common questions which both law and morality attempt to answer include: Who, if anyone, ought to be permitted to have an abortion? Under what circumstances or conditions might abortion be allowed?

Generally speaking, there are roughly three positions that can be taken on abortion: a conservative position, a moderate position and a liberal position.

The conservative position

According to the conservative position (see, for example, Brody 1982; Noonan 1983), abortion is an absolute moral wrong, and thus something which should never be permitted under any circumstances — not even in self-defence, such as cases where a continued pregnancy would almost certainly result in the mother's death. A common concern among conservative anti-abortionists is that, if abortion is permitted, then respect for the sanctity of human life will be diminished, making it easier for human life to be taken in other circumstances. Arguments typically raised against abortion here are almost always based on the sanctity-of-life doctrine. One example of the kind of reasoning which might be employed to argue against abortion is as follows:

> It is wrong to kill innocent human beings; fetuses are innocent human beings; therefore it is wrong to kill fetuses.

> (Warren 1973, p. 53)

Or, to use another example:

> Human beings have a natural right to life; fetuses are human beings; therefore fetuses have a right to life and killing them is wrong.

Whether human beings do in fact have a natural right to life, and whether fetuses are in fact human beings, are matters of on-going philosophical controversy.

The moderate position

According to the moderate position (see, for example, Werner 1979; Bolton 1983) abortion is only a prima facie moral wrong, and thus prohibitions against it may be overridden by stronger moral considerations. Werner (1979), for example, argues that abortion is permissible provided that it is procured during pre-sentience (i.e. before the fetus has the capacity to feel). Since a pre-sentient fetus cannot feel, it cannot be meaningfully harmed or benefited. Thus, as with other non-sentient or pre-sentient entities, it makes no sense to say a fetus has rights, much less a right to life. In the case of post-sentience, Werner argues that abortion may still be justified on carefully defined grounds, namely: *self-defence* (for example, where the life or health of the mother would be at risk if the pregnancy was allowed to continue); or *unavoidability* (for example, where abortion cannot be avoided, such as in the case of ectopic pregnancy or accidental injury). Abortions performed on lesser grounds are, according to Werner, unjustified.

Bolton (1983) takes a slightly different line of reasoning. She argues that, since fetuses are not undisputed persons, they do not have the same rights not to be killed as do actual undisputed persons. Thus, in the case of life-threatening pregnancy, at least, a woman's right to life overrides that of the fetus. Bolton (1983) also argues, controversially, that if women are not permitted to have abortions, the community might find itself deprived of the beneficial contributions that a woman freed of the burdens of child rearing would otherwise be free to make (p. 335). She concedes, however, that there are also cases 'in which others stand to benefit from the pregnant woman's bearing a child' (Bolton 1983, p. 337), and that this too might contribute to the community's benefit. The bottom line of Bolton's position is that abortion is morally permitted in some situations, and might even be 'morally required' in others, and it is not morally permitted in some other types of situations. Either way, the facts of the matter need to be carefully assessed and analysed before an abortion decision is made.

Another popular argument raised in defence of abortion under a moderate's banner is that a woman is under no moral obligation to bring a pregnancy to term, particularly in instances where the pregnancy has been forced upon her (as in the case of rape), or where the pregnancy has not resulted from a voluntary and informed choice (as in cases involving the intellectually impaired, the ignorant and uneducated, or, quite simply, contraceptive failure). In her celebrated article 'A defence of abortion', Judith Jarvis Thomson (1971) contends, for example, that even if it is conceded, for the sake of argument, that a fetus is a person, this still does not place an obligation on a woman to carry it to full term. Her reasoning is simply that morality does not generally require individuals to make large sacrifices to keep another alive. Thus, if pregnancy requires a woman to make a large sacrifice — and one which she is not willing to make — it is morally permissible for her to terminate the pregnancy.

It could, of course, be objected that the kinds of sacrifices a woman might ultimately be required to make by giving birth could be avoided by her allowing the unwanted child to be adopted. And, indeed, many view the *adoption option* as a respectable way out of the abortion dilemma — even in cases involving severely disabled fetuses or severely disabled newborns (see, for example, Rothenberg 1987). Thomson, however, rejects the adoption option, arguing that it can be utterly devastating on relinquishing mothers — a claim which finds considerable support in research studies on the subject (see in particular Howe et al. 1992; Lancaster 1983; Harper 1983; Winkler and van Keppel 1983). It can also be utterly devastating on adopted children, who may grow up 'wondering who they are' and spending a lifetime searching for their unknown biological parents (Lifton 1994; Health and Community Services 1992). In some countries, babies born out of wedlock (especially 'rape babies') can face a life of shame and rejection (see in particular Doder 1993, p. 8). 'Rape babies' can even be prevented by law from being adopted. In Bosnia, for example, it is reported that the government has prohibited adoption of the children of rape victims, in the hope that their natural mothers will one day accept them (Williams 1993, p. 8). The American feminist Barbara Ehrenreich (1985) also strongly rejects the adoption option. She writes:

> Anyone who thinks for a moment about a woman's role in reproductive biology could never blithely recommend 'adoption, not abortion' because women have to go through something unknown to fetuses or men, and that is pregnancy. We are talking about a nine-month bout of symptoms of varying severity, often including nausea, skin discolouration, extreme bloating and swelling, insomnia, narcolepsy, hair loss, varicose veins, haemorrhoids, indigestion and irreversible weight gain, and culminating in a physiological crisis, which is occasionally fatal and almost always excruciatingly painful.

> (Ehrenreich 1985, p. 7)

The adoption option thus is not as 'simple' as its advocates would have people believe.

The liberal position

The third stance on abortion, the liberal position (see in particular Tooley 1972; Warren 1973; Thomson 1971), holds that abortion is morally permissible on demand. Michael Tooley (1972) argues, for example, that since fetuses are not persons, they cannot meaningfully claim a right to life. He points out that the notion 'person', in this instance, is a purely moral concept, and that the unfortunate tendency by some to use it as if it were synonymous with the notions of 'human being' and 'human life' is grossly misleading. Warren (1973) argues along similar lines. She contends that a fetus is not a *human being* and to claim that it is only begs the question. She points out that it is one thing to use *human* to refer 'exclusively to members of the species *Homo sapiens*', but quite another to use it in the sense of being 'a full-fledged member of the moral community' (p. 53). In other words, it is one thing to be human in the *genetic* sense, but it is quite another to be human in the *moral* sense. These two senses are quite distinct, and care must be taken to distinguish between them. She concludes:

> In the absence of any argument showing that whatever is genetically human is also morally human ... nothing more than genetic humanity can be demonstrated by the presence of the genetic human code.

> (Warren 1973, p. 53)[3]

---

3. Copyright © 1973, *The Monist*, La Salle, Il 61301. All quotations from this work are reprinted by permission.

The consequence of this is unavoidable. It has yet to be demonstrated that the genetic humanity of fetuses alone qualifies them to have fully-fledged membership of the moral community.

Judith Jarvis Thomson (1971) also argues that a fetus is not a person. She contends that it is nothing more than a 'newly implanted clump of cells'. In defence of this claim, she argues that a fetus is 'no more a person than an acorn is an oak tree'. The analogy can be extended further to show that, just as stepping on an acorn is significantly different from cutting down an oak tree, so too is aborting a fetus significantly different from killing an actual person.

The conclusion of these and similar views is that, once it is admitted that a fetus is nothing more than a clump of genetically human cells (or a 'protoplasmic mass', as it was called by the psychiatrists cited earlier), the abortion issue is immediately rendered a non-issue. It would make no more sense to speak of the right of a fetus to life than it would be to speak of some other piece of genetically human tissue's right to life, say, a strand of human hair or a piece of human toenail (both of which are genetically human).

A 1987 Saulwick poll conducted by *The Age* suggested that 66 per cent of Australians approved of abortion in some circumstances, and another 19 per cent approved of abortion generally. Only a minority of 14 per cent disapproved entirely (Stephens 1987, p. 5). On the basis of our discussion so far, these findings may be displayed as a diagram, shown here in Figure 11.1.

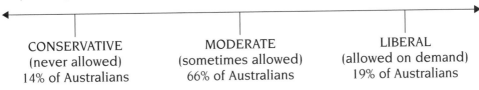

CONSERVATIVE	MODERATE	LIBERAL
(never allowed)	(sometimes allowed)	(allowed on demand)
14% of Australians	66% of Australians	19% of Australians

Figure 11.1 Australian attitudes to abortion

Abortion and the moral rights of women, fetuses and fathers

In the 1990s, public opinion polls in common law countries continue to reflect majority support (of approximately 75%) for women's abortion rights (both legal and moral) (Cannold 1998, pp. 2–4).

The abortion issue essentially turns on two key points: (1) the moral status of the fetus, and (2) the moral rights of pregnant women to control their bodies and their lives. To recap, anti-abortionists argue that the human fetus is a human being, and therefore has a right to life at least equal to that of the mother's. Pro-abortionists, however, reject this view, arguing that, while a human fetus is genetically human, this in no way implies that it is morally a human being with a full set of rights claims.

Pro-abortionists also argue that fetuses are not *persons*; the moral criteria of *personhood*, they contend, are quite different from the criteria of *fetalhood*. Let us consider this claim further.

In 1973 the reputed North American philosopher, Mary Anne Warren, argued controversially that, for an entity to be a person, it must satisfy a number of criteria, namely:

1. consciousness (of objects and events external and/or internal to the being), and in particular the capacity to feel pain;
2. reasoning (the developed capacity to solve new and relatively complex problems);
3. self-motivated activity (activity which is relatively independent of either genetic or direct external control);
4. the capacity to communicate, by whatever means, messages of an indefinite variety of types, that is, not just with an indefinite number of possible contents, but on indefinitely many possible topics;
5. the presence of self-concepts, and self-awareness, either individual or racial, or both.

(Warren 1973, p. 55)

Warren admitted that there were numerous difficulties involved in formulating and applying precise criteria of personhood. Even so, it could be done. Commenting on the criteria she had formulated, Warren argues that an entity does not need to have all five attributes described, and that it is possible that attributes given in criteria 1 and 2 alone are sufficient for personhood, and might even qualify as necessary criteria for personhood. Given these criteria, all that needs to be claimed to demonstrate that an entity (including a fetus) is not a person is that any entity which fails to satisfy all of the five criteria listed is not a person. She concluded that if opponents of abortion deny the appropriateness of the criteria she has identified, she knows of no other arguments which would convince them. She concludes: 'We would probably have to admit that our conceptual schemes were indeed irreconcilably different, and that our dispute could not be settled objectively' (p. 56).

Michael Tooley (1972), like Warren, also interpreted 'person' in rationalistic terms. He argued that in order for something to be a person it must have a serious moral right to life. And in order to have a serious moral right to life, it must possess 'the concept of self as a continuing subject of experience and other mental states, and believe that it is itself such a continuing entity' (Tooley 1972, p. 44). Since fetuses do not satisfy this basic 'self-consciousness requirement', as Tooley called it, they are not persons — they do not have a serious moral right to life, and therefore to kill them is not wrong.

More recently, in a revised version of her earlier work, Mary Anne Warren (1997) expands on and refines the characteristics which she believes are central to the concept of personhood, namely:

1. *sentience* — the capacity to have conscious experiences, usually including the capacity to experience pain and pleasure;
2. *emotionality* — the capacity to feel happy, sad, angry, loving, etc.;
3. *reason* — the capacity to solve new and relatively complex problems;
4. *the capacity to communicate,* by whatever means, messages of an indefinite variety of types; that is, not just with an indefinite number of possible contents, but on indefinitely many possible topics;
5. *self-awareness* — having a concept of oneself, as an individual and/or as a member of a social group; and finally
6. *moral agency* — the capacity to regulate one's own actions through moral principles or ideals.

(Warren 1997, p. 84)

Although conceding that it is difficult to define these traits precisely, or to specify 'universally valid behavioural indications that these traits are present',

Warren (1997, p. 84) nevertheless holds that these criteria of personhood are functional — pointing out that an entity 'need not have *all* of these attributes to be a person'. She explains:

> It should not surprise us that many people do not meet all the criteria of personhood. Criteria for the applicability of complex concepts are often like this: none may be logically necessary, but the more criteria that are satisfied, the more confident we are that the concept is applicable. Conversely, the fewer criteria are satisfied, the less plausible it is to hold that the concept applies. And if none of the relevant criteria are met, then we may be confident that it does not [apply].
>
> (Warren 1997, p. 84)

Warren (1997) suggests that in order to demonstrate that a fetus is not a person, all that is required is to claim that a fetus has *none* of the above six characteristics of personhood.

For some, the personhood argument does little to settle the abortion question. For example, it might be claimed that, even if it is true that a fetus is not a person, it nevertheless has the potential to become one, and therefore it has rights (see also Warren 1977). Thus abortion is still wrong on grounds of the potentiality of the fetus (Glover 1977, p. 122). Or, to borrow from Warren's analogy cited earlier: even though an acorn is not an oak tree, it nevertheless has the potential to become one; therefore crushing an acorn is tantamount to chopping down an oak tree.

There are a number of obvious difficulties with this view. First, the argument tends to presume that what is potential will in fact become actual. In the case of zygotes, however, this is quite improbable. As Engelhardt points out, only '40–50% of zygotes survive to be persons (i.e. adult, competent human beings)' (1986, p. 111). It might then be better, suggests Engelhardt, to speak of human zygotes as being only '0.4 probable persons'.

Second, the argument strongly suggests that it is not the fetus per se that is valued, but rather *what it will become* (Glover 1977, p. 122). It is difficult to interpret just what kind of moral demand this creates. As Glover points out:

> It is hard to see how this potential argument can come to any more than saying that abortion is wrong because a person who would have existed in the future will not exist if an abortion is performed.
>
> (Glover 1977, p. 122)

If we take the *potentiality argument* to its logical extreme, we are committed to accepting, absurdly, that contraception, the wasteful ejaculation of sperm, menstruation and celibacy are also morally wrong, since these too will result in future persons being prevented from existing (Warren 1977, p. 277).

The main unresolved question, however, is: Can a *potential* person be meaningfully said to have *actual* rights and, if so, can these rights meaningfully override the existing rights of actual persons? Or, to put this another way: Can a fetus (a potential person) have actual rights and, if so, can these meaningfully override the existing rights of its mother (an actual person)? The crux of the dilemma posed here is whether the more immediate and actual rights of the pregnant woman should be recognised before the more remote and potential needs of the fetus, or vice versa.

One answer is that, given our understanding of the nature of moral rights and correlative duties, there is something logically and linguistically odd in ascribing rights to fetuses (non-persons), particularly during the pre-sentient stage. If we were to accept that non-sentient fetuses have moral rights, we would be committed, absurdly, to accepting that all sorts of other non-sentient things have moral rights — including human toenails, strands of hair, or pieces of skin. For argument's sake, however, let us accept that the fetus does have moral rights and, further, that these can meaningfully conflict with the mother's moral rights. The question which arises here is which fetal/maternal rights are likely to conflict?

The most obvious is the fetus' and the mother's common claim to a right to life. This is particularly so in cases where the mother's life would almost certainly be lost if the pregnancy were allowed to continue. In such situations it seems reasonable to claim that the mother's right to life must at least be as strong as the fetus' right to life. And, further, since both stand to die unless the pregnancy is terminated, then surely it is better, morally speaking, that only one life is lost instead of two? It is difficult to see how anyone could reasonably and conscientiously choose an outcome which would see both the mother and the fetus die. Furthermore, as has already been discussed elsewhere in this text, morality does not generally require us to make large personal sacrifices on behalf of another, and thus it would be morally incorrect to suggest that the mother has a duty to sacrifice her life in defence of the fetus. In the case of life-threatening pregnancies, then, it seems reasonable to conclude that the pregnant woman's right to life has the weightier claim.

A second set of rights which may conflict is the mother's *right to have control over her body and life's circumstances* versus the fetus' *right to life*. It might be claimed, for example, that a woman's right to choose her lifestyle, career, economic circumstances, standard of health, and similar, override any claims the fetus might have to be 'kept alive'. The mother may then withdraw her 'life support' even if this means the fetus will die in the process (an unfortunate, but nevertheless unavoidable, consequence). Against this, however, it might still be claimed that the inconveniences and other psychological, physical or social ills caused by an unwanted pregnancy are still not enough to justify killing the fetus and violating its right to life (Brody 1982; Noonan 1983). The demand not to kill the fetus becomes even more persuasive when it is considered that there are alternatives available for helping to prevent or alleviate the ills of unwanted pregnancies, such as child welfare and other social security benefits, adoption, counselling, medication, or, as some have suggested controversially, even extracting the fetus and placing it in a surrogate or an artificial uterus (Glover 1977, p. 135). (It should be noted that this latter suggestion is not as far-fetched as it seems. Work is already being carried out overseas on 'maintaining uteri extracted from women outside of a woman's body', and implanting embryos into these wombs [Rowland 1992, pp. 288–9]. Aborted fetuses have been 'kept alive for up to forty-eight hours' in these research projects [Rowland 1992, p. 289].) In cases where alternatives are available, it seems difficult to sustain a claim that the mother's rights ought to be given overriding consideration over those of the fetus.

A third set of rights which might conflict is the mother's *right to health* (and to a quality of life) versus the fetus' *right to life*. In this instance, the mother's health and quality of life are threatened not by her pregnancy but by a progressive debilitating disease, such as Alzheimer's, Parkinson's or diabetes. The mother might, for example, contemplate getting pregnant for the sole purpose of growing tissue which can be harvested and transplanted into her brain or pancreas in an attempt to restore her health. The issue of fetal tissue transplantation is already the subject of intensive debate (see in particular Mandel 1985; *Bioethics News* 1988, p. 10; Griffiths 1988; Gillam 1989; Engelhardt 1989). Although governments are striving hard to prevent this type of scenario from occurring, it is not difficult to imagine cases of women getting pregnant and having abortions for the sole purpose of supplying fetal tissue for transplantation — if not for themselves, for other people. It is rumoured that poor women are already being given financial incentives to supply fetal tissue, in much the same way as the poor are being encouraged to sell their kidneys. Meanwhile, there are already documented cases of women getting pregnant and giving birth for the sole purpose of providing life-saving tissue (such as bone marrow) for transplantation into a newborn's sibling (see Gibbs 1990; Morrow 1991). In the light of this, it is difficult to imagine that women will not become — and are not already becoming — pregnant and undergoing 'altruistic abortions' in order to supply fetal tissue for therapeutic transplantations for a loved one, a needy stranger, or, indeed, themselves.

A fourth set of rights which may cause conflict, and one which is beginning to be given increasing publicity, involves not only the competing claims of a fetus and its mother, but also those of the father (Teo 1975; Purdy 1996, pp. 161–7). Media reports suggest that around the world there is an increasing trend of fathers undertaking legal action in an attempt to stop their (ex)wives and (ex)girlfriends from having abortions (PA 1987; Lowther 1988; AFP 1989; Beyer 1989; Leo 1983). In 1987, for example, a 23-year-old father is reported to have taken court action in an English court of appeal to try and stop his 21-year-old girlfriend, an Oxford University student, from having an abortion (PA 1987, p. 6). The court is reported to have rejected the father's appeal — significantly, not on the grounds of the woman's right to choose, but on the grounds that the fetus was:

> so underdeveloped that, if separated from its mother, it would be unable to breathe either naturally or through a ventilator, was not capable of being 'born alive'.
>
> (PA 1987, p. 8)

Upon learning of the court's decision, the 21-year-old Oxford University student is reported to have taken the position that:

> It is her decision what she does now, but it is a point of principle that she is now able to control her own body.
>
> (PA 1987, p. 8)

The 23-year-old man responsible for her pregnancy is reported to have been 'disappointed and very surprised at the result' (PA 1987, p. 8).

A year later, a similar case occurred in the United States of America. It involved a 24-year-old man who is reported to have 'lost a lower-court appeal for the right to force his estranged [19-year-old] wife to have their baby' (Lowther 1988, p. 8). The court is reported to have ruled against the father, on the grounds that the abortion concerned only the estranged wife (Lowther 1988, p. 8). Rejecting the court's decision, the man decided to 'fight to seek a legal precedent' in favour of fathers — even though his estranged wife had gone ahead and had an abortion after the court's findings. In explaining his decision to take further legal action, the man is reported to have said:

> I was willing to take full responsibility and raise the baby and take care of it; there's nothing for me to do now but let the wounds heal. Maybe the next guy will have it easier.
>
> (Lowther 1988, p. 8)

Critics of his stance, and advocates of a woman's right to choose, argued, however, that 'it is nothing short of involuntary servitude to order a woman to carry a child she does not want' (Lowther 1988, p. 8). Against this, an Indiana lawyer argued in support of the man's actions that what they were asking the court to do was merely:

> to find that there should be a balancing of the interests of the father against those of the mother on a case-by-case basis.
>
> (Lowther 1988, p. 8)

In 1989, one year later again, a similar case was reported in Canada. This time it involved a 25-year-old man who took court action to stop his 21-year-old ex-girlfriend from having an abortion (Beyer 1989). The case took a dramatic twist, however, when, with considerable embarrassment, the woman's lawyer announced, before the court case had concluded and all arguments completed, that his client, 'worried that it might be too late for an abortion even if she won the case, had decided not to wait' (Beyer 1989). Commenting on the case, Beyer writes:

> Defying a lower-court injunction, she had gone ahead with the operation. The court was stunned. But it went on nonetheless to rule unanimously that the injunction barring the abortion was invalid. The court thus seemed to be ending a recent spate of injunctions against abortion sought by angry ex-boyfriends.
>
> (Beyer 1989, p. 60)

Not surprisingly, this upsurge in paternal interest has met with little sympathy from women who historically have been left alone with the burden and hardships of child-rearing after the fathers of their children have long abandoned them. Further, some even worry that, if the paternity rights debate is allowed to progress to its logical extreme, it could pave the way for even rapists to prevent their victims from having abortions, and to press for access rights after the baby has been born. It has also been suggested that recognition of paternal rights may see the courts inviting rapists 'to be present at the birth' (Rogers 1992).

Women's history (or rather *her*story) is, however, unlikely to settle the debate on paternity rights. Given the tenuous relationship women historically have had with the law, it is possible that men may well eventually succeed in obtaining the legal remedies they seek in regard to protecting their paternity, viz. 'property rights over the fetus' (Petchesky 1986, p. 328). It is also possible that they will win their patriarchal fight against 'female-controlled' abortion and the rights of women to control their own bodies and lives (Chesler 1987, pp. 241–5). Just what the ultimate outcome of the 'mothers' rights versus fathers' rights' debate will be, however, remains an open question, and to a very large extent probably will not depend on the genuine moral rights of individuals, or even on substantive ethical arguments. Rather, the outcome will probably depend on the power of the courts — and, more specifically, the men who preside over them — and the extent to which they wish to ensure the 'continual subordination of women to men through the exploitation of pregnancy' (Tribe, cited in Graycar and Morgan 1990, p. 209; see also Luker 1984; Petchesky 1986; Eisenstein 1988; Keown 1988; Messer and May 1988; Rhode 1989; Graycar and Morgan 1990; Chesler 1987; Smart 1992; Shanley 1995; Purdy 1996).

Abortion, politics and the broader community

The abortion issue is enormous and complex; it is also extremely political, as some spectacular overseas incidents have shown. For example, in 1990, Belgium was thrown into a constitutional crisis after King Baudouin, Belgium's reigning monarch, stepped down from his throne temporarily 'because his conscience would not let him sign a law legalising abortion' (Reuter 1990a, p. 7). As a result, the government had to take over the King's powers and pass the abortion law. It is reported that once the abortion law was passed the King's inability to reign ceased, and he resumed his position on the throne (Reuter 1990a, p. 7).

In the same year, it was reported that disagreement over abortion law threatened to 'derail a treaty on German unity' (Reuter 1990b, p. 7). The disagreement was primarily over whether 'West German women may take advantage of East Germany's liberal abortion laws after unification' (Reuter 1990b, p. 7).

In 1992, Ireland (where abortion is illegal) witnessed political uproar and large public demonstrations after the High Court banned a 14-year-old rape victim from travelling to Britain for an abortion (the girl had been raped repeatedly by a friend's father over a one-year period) (Barrett 1992c, 1992d; Holden 1994). It was reported that many European constitutional lawyers considered the ban a breach of the Treaty of Rome, which had brought the European Community (EC) into being almost four decades earlier, and, among other things, 'permitted the right to free movement within the EC' (Barrett 1992c). The situation reached crisis point when it was evident that the ban threatened the European Community's Maastricht Treaty on European political union, which Irish voters were due to vote on a few months later (*Independent* 1992, p. 6; Barrett 1992a, 1992b, 1992f).

The case is reported to have aroused the concerns of a number of influential groups, including Irish legislators and lawyers and members of human rights and women's groups, and to have raised serious questions about how far the state and its officials should interfere in the fundamental rights of its citizens (*Independent, New York Times* 1992, p. 9). The travelling ban was eventually lifted by the Supreme Court in Dublin, and the girl was able to travel to Britain for an abortion (*Independent* 1992 p. 6). Later in the year, two Dublin counselling clinics appealed successfully to the European Court of Human Rights against the Irish Government's prohibition on women gaining access to information about abortion services overseas (Barrett 1992e, p. 8; Holden 1994). The judges who heard the case are reported to have decided that the Irish Government was 'violating fundamental human rights by preventing women from gaining access to information about having abortions abroad' (Barrett 1992e, p. 8). The counselling clinics were also reported to have been awarded costs and damages of more than $400 000 (Barrett 1992e, p. 8).

Abortion was also a major issue in the American presidential election of 1992, with the then presidential contenders Bill Clinton and Ross Perot both trying 'to lure pro-choice voters to their side' (Barrett, L. I. 1992, p. 54). During the campaign, the Bush camp (whose law reforms saw the loss of civil rights protection for United States abortion clinics [*Baltimore Sun* 1993] and the banning of abortion counselling at federally-funded clinics [Toner 1993]) admitted publicly that anything raising the profile of the abortion issue was 'a problem for us' (Barrett, L. I. 1992, p. 54). Initially, the Clinton camp also wanted to avoid too much attention being paid to the abortion issue. It was reported that basically 'he wanted to avoid the appearance of catering to "special interests", including feminists' (Barrett, L. I. 1992, p. 55).

The abortion debate in the United States took a dramatic and historic turn in 1993, when an anti-abortion protester shot and killed a doctor during a pro-life demonstration outside a lawful abortion clinic (Rohter 1993, p. 7) (referred to earlier in Chapter 1 of this text). Abortion rights groups took the shooting of the doctor as a 'symbol of the increasing harassment' of health workers involved in abortion work, which has seen abortion clinics increasingly vandalised and destroyed by arsonists. In one case, a clinic was even firebombed and razed (Rohter 1993, p. 7).

The politics of abortion in the United States took another turn, however, as President Clinton moved to 'reverse a decade of Republican edicts on abortion and other issues, including a repeal on the ban on abortion counselling at federally-funded clinics' (Toner 1993, p. 6). The Clinton administration was also reported to be planning a repeal of the 1977 *Hyde Amendment* (see Eisenstein 1988, p. 188), which effectively:

> barred Medicaid federal funding for poor women to obtain abortions, even when pregnancies arise from incest and rape or when they are deemed medically necessary.
>
> (Cornwell 1993, p. 8)

Despite severe criticism of these plans by proponents of anti-abortion legislation, the White House was reported to be 'determined to fulfil a promise made repeatedly by Mr Clinton during the campaign' (Cornwell 1993, p. 8).

Closer to home, Australia has also experienced the politicisation of abortion, with a small number of politicians attempting, unsuccessfully, to introduce legislation aimed at restricting abortion services for women. In 1988, for example, the Reverend Fred Nile, a New South Wales independent MP, attempted unsuccessfully to introduce his *Unborn Child Protection Bill*, which could have seen doctors performing abortions jailed for up to fourteen years and fined $100 000 (Ansell 1988, p. 21). The Reverend Nile was reported to have said that the Bill would allow abortion only if the mother's life was in danger, and that 'no exceptions would be made for any threat to the mental health of the mother' (Ansell 1988, p. 21). The medical director of the Family Planning Association of New South Wales is reported at the time to have condemned the Bill on the grounds that it would 'not stop women having abortions — it would just drive them underground' (Ansell 1988, p. 21).

Alistair Webster (a Liberal politician in New South Wales) has also made several attempts over the years to introduce legislation aimed at eliminating Medicare rebates for abortion services. An attempt in 1990 was condemned by the Women's Electoral Lobby, who reminded politicians supporting the move that 'no legislation has ever prevented desperate women from terminating unwanted pregnancies' (Schnookal 1990, p. 2). Further, as one ALP member responded during parliamentary debate on the matter:

> Medicare benefits do not cause abortion. It will not go away if we remove the benefit, just as unemployed people will not disappear if we remove the unemployment benefit ... The best way to reduce abortion numbers is better sex education, family planning and support for pregnant women — from their partners and from the government.
>
> (Dr Ric Charlesworth, cited by Wainer 1990, p. 8)

In 1998, however, the abortion debate reached a new dimension in Australia when Western Australian politicians voted in favour of legislation regarded as creating Australia's 'most liberal abortion laws' (Reardon 1998, p. 7). The legislation (introduced by Labor MLC Cheryl Davenport, and ratified by the upper house of parliament within weeks of passing through the lower house) repealed 'criminal sanctions against women for procuring an abortion' (Le Grand 1998, p. 1; Reardon 1998, p. 7; Ewing 1998, p. 3). The legislation was reported as leaving a woman's *informed consent* as the 'minimum requirement for doctors to perform lawful abortion' — literally, *abortion on demand* (Le Grand 1998, p. 11). It is anticipated that these abortion law reforms in Western Australia will 'trigger a review of abortion laws' in other Australian states (Ewing 1998, p. 3).

At a broader international level perhaps one of the most controversial examples of an attack on abortion comes from the Pope. In February 1993, the Pope is reported to have told Bosnian women pregnant as a result of wartime rape that 'they should not seek abortions, but give birth to the children' (*Bioethics News* 1993, p. 3). It is estimated that between 20 000 and 70 000 women have been raped — the majority of violated women being Muslims (Corlett 1993, p. 4). It is reported that the Pope addressed the women in a letter as follows: 'Do not abort. Your children are not responsible for the ignoble violence you have undergone'. He asked the women to 'accept the enemy' into them, and make him the 'flesh of their own flesh' (*Bioethics News* 1993, p. 3).

The Pope's comments have since been the subject of much criticism by Muslims and Catholic theologians alike. One outspoken German Catholic theologian (a woman) is reported to have said that the Pope 'had no right to get involved in matters of which he can have no understanding' and that 'no bachelor ... could decide on matters such as these. A decision can be made only by those who have been raped' (*Bioethics News* 1993, p. 3).

There remains much more to be said on the politics of and the moral controversies surrounding abortion than there is space here to do. For example, we have yet to address the problems of:

- restrictive abortion laws and the real suffering these have caused — and continue to cause — girls and women who find themselves trapped by an unwanted and/or intolerable pregnancy (see, for example, the *Bobigny case* [Henderson 1975], the *Roe v Wade case* [McCorvey 1994], the *Irish 'X' case* [Holden 1994], and Messer and May's [1988] *Back rooms: voices from the illegal abortion era*);
- sex-selected abortions, practised widely in countries where a patriarchal and misogynist preference for sons results in the 'sex-selected' abortions of female fetuses (a form of gendercide) in those countries (see, in particular, Mary Anne Warren's [1985] *Gendercide: the implications of sex selections*);
- homophobic-selected abortions — otherwise referred to as 'gay gene abortions' — proposed in the event of a 'sexuality gene' being discovered (it has been seriously suggested by a leading geneticist and Noble laureate that if a gay gene is discovered, and a fetus is found to be 'gay-gene identified', a mother ought to have the option of aborting a fetus if 'she doesn't want a homosexual child' [Loudon and Wilson 1997; Joyce 1997);
- rape-abortions, and the dilemmas associated with terminating pregnancies resulting from rape and sexual abuse (see also Holden 1994);
- eugenic-abortions, and the dilemmas associated with aborting fetuses with disabilities ranging from the very minor to the extremely severe (for instance, there is anecdotal evidence that fetuses have been aborted for

relatively minor deformities, for example, because of having one leg shorter than the other);

- the role of 'fetal police' (comprised of registered medical practitioners, 'risk managers', legislators, lawyers and judges) who take steps to coerce, detain and even incarcerate women who engage in health-injurious behaviours (such as cigarette smoking, illicit drug taking, alcohol consumption, and the like) during pregnancy (see, in particular, Ruth Macklin's [1993] discussion on 'The fetal police: enemies of pregnant women' included as Chapter 4 of her text *Enemies of patients*; Gallagher 1995);
- the nature and implications of the 'hard choices' women have to make when choosing abortion (Cannold 1998); and, not least,
- the traumatic consequences to women of having abortions, including the terrible complications that abortion procedures themselves can have such as 'sepsis, haemorrhage, uterine perforation, kidney failure and even coma' (Cannold 1998, p. 16; Fisher and Buckingham 1985).

Other problems yet to be examined include the following:

- determining the point at which a fetus actually becomes a person — for example, is it at conception/syngamy, upon achieving viability, or at birth? (see also Buckle and Dawson 1988; Warren 1988; Glover 1977, pp. 123–6);
- 'slippery slope' arguments which reason that, if abortion is permitted, our moral characters and expectations will seriously decline; that is, if we allow abortion today, we will allow infanticide tomorrow and the next day we will allow euthanasia of other 'useless' persons.

Regrettably, consideration of these and similar problems must be left for another time.

Conclusion

Although falling far short of a complete examination of the abortion issue, the discussion is sufficient to clarify the nature of the abortion debate and its implications for nurses. It has been shown that abortion is a highly complex and controversial issue, and one which is unlikely to be satisfactorily resolved. This means that nurses will invariably encounter moral disagreements in abortion contexts — many of which may not be able to be reconciled. The discussion has also warned the nursing profession that it cannot afford to be complacent or indecisive about taking a formal position on policy formulation in relation to abortion practices and procedures and the questions of social justice these raise (see also Bandman and Bandman 1985, p. 136). While nurse leaders and administrators remain indecisive or complacent about reaching a just position on the subject, nurse practitioners will continue to suffer intolerable moral, personal, professional and legal burdens on account of their conscientious opposition to abortion. This in turn could have the unhappy consequence of nursing standards of care being eroded, which could place intolerable and unnecessary burdens on women requiring nursing care before, during and after an abortion procedure. An important question raised by this prospect is: To what extent, if at all, should a nurse's conscientious objection to a given abortion procedure be permitted if, in permitting it, the life, health or wellbeing of the woman seeking the abortion is compromised or violated? It may be that nurses' conscientious objections in such instances should not be permitted, and, if that is the case, the onus falls on nurses not to work in areas where their conscientious objections to morally controversial (although not unequivocally immoral) procedures cannot be accommodated. Since the issue of conscientious objection is important in its own right, it is considered separately in Chapter 15 of this text.

Perhaps most importantly, this discussion demonstrates the need for the abortion issue to be opened up for formal and informed discussion within the ranks of the nursing profession. It can never be assumed that nurses have had a trouble-free path to conscience-free participation in abortion work. If we do not know what experiences nurses have had in this area, we will never be in a position to champion a substantive nursing perspective on the moral permissibility of abortion, much less on the extent to which nurses can be reasonably expected — against their moral conscience — to assist with abortion work. In formulating policies on the abortion issue, however, the nursing profession must be careful not to lose sight of its moral commitment to respecting women's personal choices (no matter how disagreeable these might appear to be). Individual nurse practitioners, meanwhile, must take great care not to fall into the moralising trap of imposing their personal values on others — in this instance, women who have decided, for whatever moral reason, to abort a pregnancy which, if carried to full term, promises intolerable consequences.

Chapter 12

Euthanasia and assisted suicide

Introduction

In 1990, in the United States of America, Janet Adkins, a victim of Alzheimer's disease, died after pushing a red button on a suicide machine — or 'mercitron', as it has been called — designed by a retired pathologist, Dr Jack Kevorkian, whom she had approached for assistance to die (Gibbs 1990, 1993). Adkins, who is reported to have 'feared an excruciating future', soon came to be viewed as a 'symbol of all those patients who confront a horrible disease and vow to maintain some dignity in death' (Gibbs 1990, p. 70). Dr Kevorkian, meanwhile, found himself in the forefront of the pro-euthanasia debate and, as *Time* magazine put it:

> a standard-bearer for all those who fail to see a moral difference between unplugging a respirator and plugging in a poison machine.
>
> (Gibbs 1990, p. 70)

Despite being dubbed 'Dr Death', and 'the devil that doctors deserve' (because of the alleged deceitful, insensitive and neglectful way they often treated dying patients), Dr Kevorkian is continuing his crusade for the legalisation of euthanasia/assisted suicide, or, as he calls it, 'medicide' in the United States of America (Gibbs 1993, p. 52; see also Kevorkian 1991; Brovins and Oehmke 1993). As part of this crusade, in December 1998 it was reported that Dr Kevorkian was successful in getting authorities in the state of Michigan (USA) to charge him with first-degree murder. His trial, which is expected to take place some time in 1999, will represent the fifth time Kevorkian 'has been tried over the deaths of his patients'. This trial, however, will be the first in which Kevorkian 'admitted to having directly administered a fatal injection'. To date, Dr Kevorkian has assisted 130 people to die (Riley 1998, p. 11).

In the Netherlands, meanwhile, a very different scenario was at play. In contrast to the United States of America, euthanasia and assisted suicide was, at the time of Janet Adkins' medically-assisted death, legally tolerated (although still a criminal offence) in the Netherlands. By the time Dr Jack Kevorkian had facilitated his first 'assisted suicide' in 1990, Dutch doctors had already participated in thousands of medically-assisted deaths. In 1986, for example, the Royal Dutch Medical Association reported that there were between 5000 and 6000 cases of voluntary euthanasia each year in Holland (British Medical Association 1986). In 1990, the overall incidence of euthanasia was estimated by formal sources to be between 4000 and 6000 deaths annually (de Wachter 1992, p. 24). However, others contend that the overall incidence of euthanasia is, in reality, unknown and, if informal sources are to be relied upon, could range from between 2000 and 20 000 cases a year (ten Have and Welie 1992; de Wachter 1992; Keown 1992).

Currently, in the Netherlands, under certain clearly defined conditions, euthanasia is not viewed by the courts as a punishable offence (Vervoorn 1987; Browne 1990; Keown 1992). Although euthanasia is still technically illegal, a new law passed in February 1993 clarified and affirmed the strict conditions under which euthanasia is permitted. The passage of this new law is reported as giving the Netherlands the world's most lenient policy on 'mercy killing' (Hirschler 1993, p. 7). It has also given the world a 'laboratory' for 'testing' and 'observing' euthanasia — and one which has attracted many onlookers from both ends of the moral spectrum *apropos* the moral permissibility of euthanasia. Certainly, the Netherlands is currently the only country in the world which is able to offer retrospective studies of substance concerning the practice of euthanasia and any emerging patterns or trends associated with it. Consider the following.

In 1995, in a nationwide study of euthanatic practices in the Netherlands, and which involved a survey of physicians who had attended over 6000 certified deaths, the following statistics were revealed: of the certified deaths evaluated, approximately 43 per cent occurred in persons over the age of 65 years; of these, around 29 per cent were as a direct result of euthanasia, around 31 per cent as a result of physician-assisted suicide, and around 40 per cent as a result of a decision to forego treatment (van der Maas et al. 1996; van der Wal et al. 1996). In contradiction to an earlier 1990 study, van der Maas et al. (1996, p. 1703) found that euthanasia was more common among female patients than males, that decisions to forego treatment tended to be made more often in the case of older females, and that the decisions to forgo treatment were made 'relatively often by nursing home physicians'. Meanwhile, a 1996 study of homosexual men with AIDS found that in the population under study, patients with AIDS experienced death by euthanasia or physician-assisted suicide at a rate twelve times higher than the frequency among all deaths (Bindels et al. 1996). While researchers continue to find no evidence of an increase in euthanasia since laws proscribing it have been relaxed (see, for example, Bindels 1996, p. 503), it is estimated that 59 per cent of euthanatic deaths still go unreported, with cases of physician-assisted death without the patient's explicit request being the most under-reported of all (van der Wal et al. 1996). While there is considerable scope for caution in translating the meaning of these figures for cultural contexts outside of the Netherlands, they nevertheless offer some 'cautionary tales' — not least, that even the best of legal safeguards may still be inadequate (as noted above, 59 per cent of cases of euthanasia still go unreported).

In 1996, Australia became the subject of international attention when it became the first country in the world to fully legalise active voluntary euthanasia. This followed the passage, in May 1995, of the Northern Territory's controversial *Rights of the Terminally Ill Act 1995*, which came into effect on 1 July 1996. Almost one year later, however, the Act was overturned by the Australian Federal Government — although not before five people had sought assistance to die under the Act. Of these people, four were successful in achieving legally-assisted deaths; the only person not successful in achieving his wish was eligible for assistance to die under the Act but was 'unable to find a specialist who was prepared to be one of the three doctors required under the Act' to certify eligibility for an assisted death (Senate Legal and Constitutional Legislation Committee 1997, p. 11). To date, despite the success of the Australian Federal Government in overturning the Northern Territory's euthanasia legislation, proponents of euthanasia speculate that it will only be a matter of time before euthanasia and assisted suicide will be legal in not just one, but possibly all jurisdictions in Australia.

Euthanasia and assisted suicide continues to receive widespread attention both locally and globally, and remains the subject of much controversy. Central to the controversy is the fundamental question of whether a doctor should intentionally and actively assist a patient to die, and, if so, by what means. These same questions can, of course, also be asked of nurses — and that they have not been asked of nurses is curious, particularly when it is considered that nurses play a fundamental role in caring for and promoting the dignity of patients who are incurably ill, suffering intolerably and dying; that these questions *should* be asked of nurses will become self-evident in the discussion to follow.

In this chapter, attention is given to examining the nature and moral implications of the euthanasia/assisted suicide question for nurses. Attention is also given to clarifying what euthanasia is, how it differs from assisted suicide and 'mercy killing', and the kinds of moral arguments that can be raised both for and against the legitimation of euthanatic practices. It is hoped that by examining these and related issues, members of the nursing profession will move a step closer toward answering the following kinds of questions.

- How significant or important is the euthanasia/assisted suicide issue for the nursing profession?
- Should the nursing profession take a formal position either way on the euthanasia/assisted suicide question (for example, should nursing organisations adopt formal position statements advocating a particular view on the moral permissibility or impermissibility of euthanatic practices, or is this a matter that should be left to individual nurses to decide conscientiously)?
- To what extent, if at all, should the broader nursing profession participate in public debate on the euthanasia/assisted suicide question (for example, should nursing organisations actively lobby for the legalisation of euthanasia/assisted suicide)?
- In the event of euthanasia/assisted suicide being decriminalised, what (if any) should be the role of nurses in regard to assisting with or actually performing euthanasia and/or assisted suicide?
- How best can the nursing profession proceed to answer these and related questions (see also Johnstone 1996a)?

Euthanasia and its significance for nurses

Next to abortion, euthanasia is probably one of the most controversial bioethical issues to have captured the world's attention. And, like the abortion issue, it is unlikely to be resolved to everybody's satisfaction.

Euthanasia and the so-called 'right to die' are not new issues for nurses. In Australia, one of the first articles addressing the subject was published as early as 1912 in the *Australasian Nurses Journal*. Reprinted from the *British Medical Journal*, the article contains concerns and viewpoints which remain current — including the agonising question of whether euthanasia should be legalised. Citing an 1873 essay on the subject, the article contends that 'a modified *harikari* should be made lawful in England' (and, one presumes, her colonies, including Australia), and, quoting the essay's author, that: 'on the whole it cannot be doubted that the benefits resulting from a change in the law would be simply enormous' (Lionel Tollemache, cited in the *Australasian Nurses Journal*, 16 September 1912, p. 304).

While euthanasia may not be a new issue for nurses, it has nevertheless become a more substantive, intense and highly significant one. Evidence of this can be found in the increasing attention being given to the experiences of nurses in regard to euthanasia in both the professional and lay press. In 1987, for example, the English nursing periodical *Nursing Times* carried a provocative report on the fate of four Dutch nurses who had been arrested in Amsterdam after it was alleged they had practised euthanasia on three hopelessly ill patients. The report concluded that, if the nurses were found guilty of killing the patients, they could face prison sentences of up to twenty years (*Nursing Times*, 25 March 1987, p. 8).

Almost a decade later, in another (although unrelated) case in 1995 in the Netherlands, a 38-year-old Dutch registered nurse was given a two-month suspended prison sentence for performing active voluntary euthanasia on a patient suffering end-stage AIDS (Staal 1995, p. 7; van de Pasch 1995; van der Arend 1995). What was particularly significant about this case was that the sentence was passed despite the fact that:

- the patient (who was a friend and colleague of the nurse) had specifically requested that the nurse perform the act of assisted death; and
- the procedure fully complied with legal regulations governing euthanatic practices in the Netherlands (for example, the patient had competently requested assistance to die, he was suffering from an end-stage illness, a second medical opinion had been obtained, and the procedure was fully attended to and supervised by a qualified medical practitioner [who, significantly, escaped sentence] (van de Pasch 1995, p. 108).

As I have discussed elsewhere (Johnstone 1996c, pp. 21–2), this case helped to demonstrate the tenuous position of nurses in relation to euthanatic practices — even in countries where euthanasia and assisted suicide are 'legally tolerated'. In this case, the court's decision seemed to hinge on the view that euthanasia and assisted suicide were *medical procedures* of a nature that could not (and should not) be delegated to nurses. More specifically, the court clarified that the deed of 'ultimate care' (the procedure that is the act of euthanasia itself) could only be performed by a doctor and could not be delegated to anyone else (Staal 1995, p. 7).

Nurses in the United Kingdom have also experienced significant problems in relation to the euthanasia issue. For example, in 1991, a UK registered nurse experienced threats of violence and obscene phone calls, was vilified by some sections of the media, and was made a scapegoat in the eyes of the public after reporting to the appropriate authorities that a terminally ill patient had died possibly as a result of being administered 10mmol of potassium chloride by a consultant physician, Dr Nigel Cox (Hart and Snell 1992, p. 19). The incident was discovered after nurses noted the blatant documentation of the drug administration in the patient's case history which 'had been left in the nurses' station for all to see' (Hart and Snell 1992, p. 19). The registered nurse's attempts to contact Dr Cox about the matter were unsuccessful. Not wishing to implicate other staff in the matter and recognising her professional duties as prescribed in the United Kingdom Central Council for Nursing, Midwifery and Health Visiting (UKCC)(1992) *Code of Professional Conduct*, the registered nurse decided that she 'had no choice but to report the incident'. Accordingly she notified the director of nursing services and the unit general manager. One month later, Dr Cox was convicted of attempted murder at Winchester Crown Court. He subsequently received a one-year suspended prison sentence (Hart and Snell 1992, p. 19). He was not deregistered by the General Medical Council (UK), however, and continued to practise medicine. The registered nurse meanwhile carried a disproportionate burden of suffering for her actions.

Besides sometimes finding themselves unwitting witnesses to the illegal euthanatic practices of others, it has been alleged that some British nurses have also practised euthanasia themselves. For example, in 1992, a commentary published in a Voluntary Euthanasia Society publication alleged, controversially, that:

> British nurses are often involved in euthanasia; but that due to the illegality of euthanasia practices, it is difficult to assess the exact extent of the problem — particularly in a culture which prescribes that nurses should not 'tell on colleagues'.
>
> (Turton 1992, pp. 92–3)

At the time of writing, euthanasia and assisted suicide remains a controversial issue for nurses in the United Kingdom (Johnstone 1996c). Significantly, the prestigious Royal College of Nursing (RCN), a leading professional nursing organisation in the United Kingdom, has unequivocally rejected the role of nurses in participating in euthanasia. This position has been made explicit in an issues paper on living wills; in this paper, the RCN takes the following position:

> The RCN believes that this [euthanasia] is contrary to the public interest and to the medical and nursing ethical principles as well as to natural and civil rights.
>
> (Royal College of Nursing 1994)

It further asserts:

> The RCN is opposed to the introduction of any legislation which would place on doctors or nurses a responsibility to respond to a demand for termination of life from any patient or from their relatives.
>
> (Royal College of Nursing 1994)

The euthanasia/assisted suicide question has also proved to be a significant professional issue for Australian nurses. For example, in January 1995, recognising the seriousness of the euthanasia issue for members of the nursing profession, the Royal College of Nursing, Australia (RCNA) took the unprecedented step of releasing for comment a discussion paper entitled *Euthanasia: an issue for nurses* (Hamilton 1995). As I have discussed elsewhere (Johnstone 1996b), the RCNA received over seventy responses to this discussion paper from concerned and interested nursing organisations, groups and individuals from around Australia. The responses received represented nurses working in a variety of clinical areas and fields of nursing (including education) and reflected a great diversity of knowledge, opinion, values and beliefs about euthanasia and assisted suicide. In some cases, the responses also demonstrated a devastating need for information and guidance on how best to respond to the uncertainty, controversy, complexity and perplexity that has become so characteristic of the right to die movement generally. Perhaps most confronting of all, however, was the emerging difficult question of whether the nursing profession should formally and publicly support the legalisation of active voluntary euthanasia. Related to this was the equally confronting question of whether representative nursing organisations should adopt a formal position statement either supporting or rejecting the role of nurses in active voluntary euthanasia and assisted suicide. Not surprisingly, while the responses demonstrated the need to raise and address these troubling questions, they fell far short of offering a definitive answer to them. Recognising the complexity and perplexity of the issue, the RCNA subsequently commissioned, as part of its professional development series, a monograph entitled: *The politics of euthanasia: a nursing response* (Johnstone 1996a). The purpose of this monograph was not to provide nurses with definitive answers to the difficult questions posed by the euthanasia debate. Rather, it was to advance a discussion that would enable nurses 'to formulate their own thinking and viewpoints on the subject and to be able to contribute to broader professional discussion on the whole issue of the right to die' (Johnstone 1996b, p. 22). In July 1996, the RCNA also issued its first position statement on voluntary euthanasia and assisted suicide (Royal College of Nursing, Australia 1996). This position statement primarily focussed on clarifying the illegal status of euthanasia/assisted suicide in Australia, acknowledging that there exists a diversity of moral viewpoints on the euthanasia issue, reminding nurses of their professional responsibility to be reliably informed about the ethical, legal, cultural and clinical implications of euthanasia and assisted suicide, and recognising and supporting the appropriateness of nurses taking a 'conscientious' position on the matter.

The RCNA's initiatives (just outlined above) were to prove extremely timely, coinciding as they did with the enactment of the Northern Territory of Australia's controversial *Rights of the Terminally Ill Act 1995* which came into effect on 1 July, 1996. As already stated in the opening paragraphs of this chapter, the passage of this legislation earned Australia the controversial distinction of being the first country in the world to legalise active voluntary euthanasia. Of significance to nurses (and to this discussion) is that the legislation anticipated and provided for nurse participation in active voluntary euthanasia and assisted suicide (either by way of preparing, or being delegated the task of actually administering, a substance to terminate life [see S16(1)]; see also Trollope 1995 p. 21). What, arguably, was troubling about the legislation's provisions in regard to nurse participation was that they had been enacted even before the broader nursing profession itself had:

- clarified its position on the euthanasia/assisted suicide question (at the time, the issue had not been widely discussed in the Australian nursing literature, and policy statements on the subject were either non-existent, inadequate or only at draft stage); and
- taken the necessary steps to ensure that its membership had been fully informed about and adequately prepared to deal with the complex range of political, social, cultural, moral, legal and clinical issues raised by public policy innovation and legal ratification of active voluntary euthanasia and assisted suicide (Johnstone 1996b).

Significantly, in May 1996, less than two months before the *Rights of the Terminally Ill Act 1995 (NT)* came into effect, the Nurses' Board of the Northern Territory took the unprecedented step of formulating and ratifying a formal position statement on euthanasia (see *Nurses' Board of the Northern Territory Position Statement on the Nurse's Role in Euthanasia*, included in full as Appendix 5 in Johnstone 1996a). This position statement was keyed to the *Rights of the Terminally Ill Act 1995 (NT)* and sought to clarify the role and function of nurses in relation to the Act's provisions. Specifically, the position statement supported:

- the role of nurses assisting in the voluntary euthanasia of competent patients; and
- the rights of nurses to conscientiously refuse to participate in the euthanasia of patients (Johnstone 1996c, p. 36).

The position statement also outlined the obligations of nurses in regard to the ethical and legal aspects of euthanasia, employment policies, professional competence and education (Johnstone 1996c, pp. 36–7).

As stated earlier, the decriminalisation of euthanasia and assisted suicide in the Northern Territory of Australia was short lived. Almost one year after its enactment, intense political pressure resulted in the *Rights of the Terminally Ill Act 1995 (NT)* being overturned by the Australian Federal Government. Currently, euthanasia and assisted suicide is illegal in Australia, and anyone who wilfully assists a person to die would be viewed by the courts as having committed the criminal offence of homicide (Wallace 1991, p. 265, ss. 14–65). As Dix et al. warn:

> It should be made very clear from the outset that the law does not allow mercy killing. Where a person takes steps to end, or hasten the end of another person's life with the intention or the knowledge that this is likely to be the consequence of his or her actions, such a person may be liable for murder or, should death not eventuate, attempted murder. The sentence for murder is imprisonment for life, although in some jurisdictions (NSW, Vic, ACT) there is a discretion in the trial judge to order a sentence of less duration ...
>
> (Dix et al. 1996, p. 339, s. 1223)

Despite the current legal prohibition against euthanasia and assisted suicide in Australia, proponents of euthanasia/assisted suicide speculate that it will only be a matter of time before euthanasia and assisted suicide will be legal in not just one, but possibly all jurisdictions in Australia. Given this prediction, there is ample room to speculate that it will only be a matter of time before Australian nurses will once again have to grapple with the complex and perplexing questions raised by the legalisation of euthanasia/assisted suicide, and, in particular, the possible and actual implications of this for nurses at a personal, professional, and political level (see also Johnstone 1996a).

Public opinion on the euthanasia/assisted suicide issue

In reaching a position on the euthanasia/assisted suicide issue, it might be tempting to appeal to and/or be persuaded by public opinion on the matter. Consider the following.

Over the past fifteen years, public opinion in most common law countries, including Australia, suggests majority support for the legalisation of euthanasia and physician-assisted suicide (Radic 1982; Humphries 1983; Kuhse and Singer 1988; *Australian Dr Weekly*, 10 August 1990, p. 9; Kuhse 1991; Somerville 1996). In Australia, for example, opinion polls conducted by Morgan and Newspoll respectively during 1995 and 1996 showed 75–78 per cent public support for physician-assisted suicide. A Newspoll conducted in July 1996 also found that 39 per cent strongly favoured and 24 per cent partly favoured (making a sub-total of 63 per cent in favour) changes to the law allowing doctors to perform active euthanasia via the administration of a lethal injection (Senate Legal and Constitutional Legislation Committee 1997, pp. 81–3). Just what is to be made of this public opinion, however, is open to question. As discussed earlier in Chapter 3 of this text, public opinion is not a reliable guide to moral conduct; all that it tells us is that a certain group (a majority) of people *hold a particular opinion*, not that the opinion held is 'morally right' all things considered. In short, it tells us nothing about the moral acceptability or the moral authority of the opinion held. We must look elsewhere (that is, beyond public opinion) to guide our deliberations on whether a given practice is morally right or wrong. This applies no less to the euthanasia/assisted suicide issue than it does to other ethical issues which are also the subject of public opinion polls. It is to looking 'elsewhere' to guide our deliberations on the euthanasia and assisted suicide issue that the remainder of this chapter will now turn. This exploration will begin firstly by clarifying what euthanasia is, and how, if at all, it differs from other end-of-life practices such as assisted suicide and 'mercy killing'. This, in turn, will be followed by a critical examination of views popularly raised for and against the legitimation of euthanasia and assisted suicide.

Definitions of euthanasia, assisted suicide and 'mercy killing'

Euthanasia

The term euthanasia comes via New Latin from Greek *eu* (meaning 'easy', 'happy' or 'good') and *thanatos* (meaning 'death'); it is translated literally as 'good death' or 'happy death'. Contrary to popular opinion, the Greeks did not use the term euthanasia (or equivalents) to imply either 'a means or method of causing or hastening death' (Carrick 1985, p. 127). Rather, it was used in a broader and somewhat metaphorical sense 'to describe the *spiritual state* of the dying person at the impending approach of death' (Carrick 1985, p. 127). Historical evidence also suggests that euthanasia, as we understand it today, was in fact prohibited in ancient medical circles (Carrick 1985, p. 81). Plato, for one, even went so far as to suggest that physicians who attempt to poison another 'must be punished by death', whereas the lay person who attempted such a thing should only be fined — indicating that physicians were regarded as having the greater burden of responsibility to refrain from causing death (Carrick 1985, p. 83). Carrick comments that 'if someone's life was terminated without his (sic) consent, normally this was prima facie a case of homicide' (p. 128).

Contemporary English definitions of euthanasia vary. The *Oxford English dictionary*, for example, defines it as 'the action of inducing a quiet and easy death', and the *Collins English dictionary* as 'the act of killing someone painlessly, especially to relieve suffering from an incurable illness'. *Webster's dictionary*, similarly, defines euthanasia as 'an act or practice of painlessly putting to death people suffering from incurable conditions or disease'.

Whether euthanasia *is* any of these things, however, is a matter of some controversy. For example, we can imagine a case of 'inducing a quiet and easy death' which is a case not of euthanasia but of cold-blooded murder. I could, for example, slip a calming and sleep-inducing sedative into my fit grandmother's nightcap, and the moment she starts blissfully sleeping in her armchair administer to her a lethal dose of intravenous morphine. My sole intention might be nothing more than to secure her premature death so that I may receive the large inheritance I know she has left me in her will. There is something about this example which, to borrow from Beauchamp and Davidson (1979, p. 295) 'omits all the subtle aspects of our notion of euthanasia'. Likewise, we can imagine cases involving patients with incurable diseases or conditions who would nevertheless not be candidates for euthanasia. Diabetes, for example, is an incurable disease, and colour blindness an incurable condition. Yet, we would not, I think, regard either of these incurable states as grounds for euthanasia.

The notion of 'painlessly' inducing death is also unhelpful. We can, for example, imagine a *painless means* of causing death (for example, injecting a lethal substance through the side arm of an intravenous line, or removing someone from a life-support system or withholding food and fluids) but where the *death itself* is nevertheless painful and/or distressing (for example, where a patient is acutely aware of the sensations of suffocation after being taken off a respirator or after being given a large dose of narcotics, or is aware of both hunger and thirst sensations when food and fluids have been withheld). Just because the *means* of death was 'pain-free', it does not always follow that the *death itself* was a 'good death'.

All three dictionary definitions are also inadequate in that they say nothing about the kinds of reasons which should be considered for killing another person, leaving it wide open for motivations of self-interest to be admitted (Beauchamp and Davidson 1979, p. 295). The questions remain: How should euthanasia be defined? How can we be sure that a given act is an act of euthanasia rather than some other kind of act, such as murder or unassisted suicide?

Beauchamp and Davidson (1979) argue that for an act to be an instance of euthanasia, it must satisfy at least five conditions.

1. *Intentionality.* Death must be intended and not be merely accidental, and further must be intended by at least one other human being.
2. *Suffering and evidence of suffering.* Here suffering may be in the form of conscious pain, mental anguish, and/or serious self-burdensomeness (as may occur in cases of high quadriplegia, or tetraplegia, or the like). This interpretation of suffering fully upholds the view that ending a person's pain is not always tantamount to ending that person's suffering (see also Cassell 1982, 1991; Kuhse 1982; Hill 1992; Starck and McGovern 1992). In assessing a person's level of suffering, every effort must be made to gain 'sufficient current evidence' (Beauchamp and Davidson 1979, p. 301); in this instance, it is simply not enough to rely on mere guesswork or on supposition based on ignorance.
3. *Reasons for death and the means of death.* Beauchamp and Davidson contend that death-causing acts must be motivated by beneficence or other humanitarian considerations (such as the demand to end suffering). Killing acts which are not motivated by these things are not acts of euthanasia, but murder. Further to this, any means of death chosen must also be of a nature that does not cause more suffering than is already being experienced (Beauchamp and Davidson 1979, p. 302).
4. *Painlessness.* This condition is related to the previous one and demands, quite simply, that any death act performed must be as painless and as merciful as possible. Beauchamp and Davidson (1979, p. 303) explain that if the means of bringing about death causes more suffering than if

that particular means was not used, then the individual will be effectively deprived of a 'good death'.

5. *Non-fetal humanity.* Beauchamp and Davidson (1979, p. 303) contend that if this simple qualification is not included then we would not be able to distinguish acts of abortion from acts of euthanasia.

Beauchamp and Davidson maintain that the five conditions they have formulated supply a 'non-prescriptive definition' of euthanasia, and thus one which avoids dictating a particular moral conclusion. Whether they have totally succeeded, however, is another matter. The definition still seems ethically loaded, and therefore carries prescriptive properties. Nevertheless, the five conditions given supply an important step towards the formulation of a substantive concept and definition of euthanasia, and one which can be meaningfully applied in the euthanasia debate.

Having defined euthanasia, there now remains the task of distinguishing between the different types of euthanasia that can be practised. The bioethics literature typically distinguishes between six different types of euthanasia: (1) voluntary active euthanasia, (2) voluntary passive euthanasia, (3) involuntary active euthanasia, (4) involuntary passive euthanasia, (5) non-voluntary active euthanasia, and (6) non-voluntary passive euthanasia. In the case of *voluntary euthanasia*, a fully competent patient makes an informed and voluntary choice to have a medically-assisted death, asks for assistance to die, and gives an informed consent for the actual procedure of euthanasia to be performed. In short, the patient explicitly requests a doctor or a nurse to administer a lethal injection to hasten his/her (the patient's) death. The Dutch case cited earlier, involving a registered nurse who was prosecuted for performing euthanasia on a patient, is an example of this. *Involuntary euthanasia*, in contrast, involves the exact opposite, namely, killing a patient without the patient's informed consent and/or contrary to that patient's expressed wishes (where these are known or could be known) (Lewins 1996, p. 114). The involuntary killing of patients as part of the Nazi medicalised killing programs (discussed in Chapter 2 of this text) is an important example of this. *Non-voluntary euthanasia* stands in contrast again and involves the act of killing a patient whose wishes cannot be known either because of immaturity, incompetency or both. The killing of severely disabled newborns (albeit with parental consent) would be an example of this. As McGuire (1987) explains, whereas the term 'involuntary' implies an action which is carried out against the wishes of the patient, unlike 'non-voluntary' which simply implies that there is *no* voluntariness — in the sense that the patient is not capable of either denying or giving consent (as in the case of the permanently comatose or brain-injured patient). In the case of the permanently comatose, McGuire contends, euthanasia would be 'neither voluntary nor involuntary, but is simply non-voluntary'.

Active euthanasia, meanwhile, typically involves a deliberate act (or commission) which results in the patient's death. The deliberate act of administering a lethal injection or a lethal dose of pills is an example of active euthanasia. This type of euthanasia is sometimes referred to as positive euthanasia. *Passive euthanasia*, on the other hand, involves a deliberate omission or the withholding of certain life-supporting cares and treatments. Withholding antibiotics, nutrition and fluids, mechanical life supports, or other life-supporting measures from terminally or chronically ill patients are examples of *passive euthanasia*. This type of euthanasia is sometimes referred to as negative euthanasia (Glaser 1975).

The six types of euthanasia just outlined can be expressed diagrammatically, as shown in Figure 12.1.

	PASSIVE	ACTIVE
VOLUNTARY	Voluntary passive euthanasia	Voluntary active euthanasia
INVOLUNTARY	Involuntary passive euthanasia	Involuntary active euthanasia
NON-VOLUNTARY	Non-voluntary passive euthanasia	Non-voluntary active euthanasia

Figure 12.1 Six categories of euthanasia

Assisted suicide

The term 'euthanasia' (and, more specifically, voluntary active euthanasia) is sometimes used interchangeably with the term 'assisted suicide'. As I have explained elsewhere (Johnstone 1996c), this interchanging usage is not, however, strictly correct. While it is acknowledged that there may be no morally significant difference between voluntary active euthanasia and assisted suicide (see Brock 1993, p. 204; Parker 1994, pp. 34–42), there is nevertheless a qualitative (experiential) difference between them. With assisted suicide, a qualified medical practitioner supplies the patient/client with the means (for example, a prescription for a lethal dose of drugs) of taking his or her own life but, unlike in the case of voluntary active euthanasia, it is the *patient/client* (not the doctor) 'who acts last' (Brock 1993, p. 204; Campbell 1992, p. 276). To put this another way, in the case of active euthanasia it is the *qualified medical practitioner who kills the patient/client*; whereas in the case of assisted suicide, the *patient/client kills him or herself*. Interestingly, while there may indeed be no morally significant difference between voluntary active euthanasia and assisted suicide (in both instances the ultimate choice rests with the patient/client, both involve assistance from a qualified medical practitioner [or his or her proxy, for example, a nurse] and both result in the foreseeable and intended death of the patient/client suffering from an irreversible medical condition), the law, public policy and public opinion have all distinguished between them (Glick 1992; Brock 1993). A notable example here involves the recently proclaimed (world first) legislation in the United States of America, the *Oregon Death with Dignity Act*, which has legalised physician-assisted suicide (in the form of prescribing a lethal dose of medication), but not active voluntary euthanasia (see also Kuhse 1995).

'Mercy killing'

A third terminology which has found usage in discussions on euthanasia is that of 'mercy killing'. Although this term is also sometimes used interchangeably with the term 'euthanasia' it can nevertheless be distinguished from euthanasia on a contextual basis. Specifically, as Glick explains:

> Mercy killing is not the same as voluntary active euthanasia since many killings are committed without patient request or consent — typically an

315

elderly husband shoots his terminally ill and unconscious or Alzheimer's disease-stricken wife. But the cases almost always exhibit wrenching long-term personal suffering and sacrifice and financial ruin ... They evoke sympathy for both killer and victim and perpetuate interest in the legalisation [sic] of voluntary active euthanasia, which some believe might eliminate the compelling need that desperate people feel for killing their hopelessly ill spouses.

(Glick 1992, pp. 81–2)

Views for and against euthanasia/assisted suicide

Like other controversial bioethical issues, euthanasia and assisted suicide have proponents and opponents. Attitudes towards them range from liberal and moderate acceptance to absolutist conservative prohibition. It is to examining some of the various viewpoints for and against euthanasia and assisted suicide that this discussion will now turn.

Views in support of euthanasia

Those who support euthanasia typically take the view that it is morally wrong to allow people to suffer unnecessarily. As one author writes:

the most horrible thing in the world for us, living and sentient beings, is inexorable suffering pain, without any possible compensation when it has reached this degree of intensity; and one must be barbarous, or stupid, or both at once, not to use the sure and easy means now at our disposal to bring it to an end.

(Reiser 1975, p. 28)

Popular views advanced in support of euthanasia (and, in particular, in support of legalising it) fall roughly under four main augmentative categories:

1. arguments from individual autonomy and the right to choose;
2. arguments from the loss of dignity and the right to the maintenance of dignity;
3. arguments from the reduction of suffering;
4. arguments from justice and the demand to be treated fairly.

(adapted from Beauchamp and Perlin 1978, p. 217)

A fifth more recent and controversial category of argument raised in support of euthanasia is that, in some instances, patients have a 'duty to die' (Beloff 1992, pp. 52–6).

1. Arguments from individual autonomy and the right to choose

We generally accept that people have a right to choose. And, as we have already seen in Chapter 4, the moral principle of autonomy demands that we respect other people's choices, even if we consider them to be mistaken or foolish. The only grounds upon which a person's autonomous choices can be justly interfered with is if they stand to impinge seriously on the significant moral interests of others. Proponents of voluntary euthanasia argue that the right to choose includes the right to choose death (abbreviated as 'the right to die'). Given the right to die, this means that others (including the state) should not interfere with a person's decision to die, and in some instances may even entail a positive duty to assist a person to die — as in cases where a person desires death but is physically unable to end his or her own life (Johnstone 1988). Voluntary euthanasia is thought to be justified here on grounds of autonomy and the demand to respect a person's autonomous wishes.

An important example of this can be found in the comments of Baume (1996, p. 17) who writes that voluntary euthanasia is justified because 'it is a self-regarding victimless action from an individual decision in a matter which affects individuals alone'.

2. Arguments from the loss of dignity and the right to the maintenance of dignity

Related to the demand to respect a person's autonomous choices is the further demand to respect and maintain a person's dignity. Advances in medical technology have increased medicine's capacity to prolong a person's life. Its methods, however, are not always humane, and can seriously erode a person's self-concept, character, sense of self-worth and self-esteem, and the like. As Beauchamp and Perlin (1978) point out, some patients 'are not only subjected to intense and abiding pain, they are often aware of their own deterioration, as well as of the burden they have become to others' (p. 217). They conclude that under these conditions 'it seems uncivilised and uncompassionate' not to allow patients to choose their own death. Euthanasia in some pain states as well as in some chronic disease states may well be the most dignified option.

3. Arguments from reduction of suffering

Suffering is generally regarded as morally unacceptable and, as we have already seen in Chapter 4, morality demands that, where possible, persons should be spared or prevented from suffering unnecessarily. In cases where patients' suffering is intense, protracted, unendurable and intractable, it seems cruel to deny them the choice of death as a means of release from their suffering. Euthanasia in these kinds of cases is said to be justified on grounds of 'prevention of cruelty' or 'mercy' (Beauchamp and Perlin 1978, p. 217). It is also thought to be justified on the grounds that people have the indisputable right to judge their suffering as unbearable, and the concomitant right to request euthanasia to end their unbearable suffering (see, for example, Admiraal 1991, p. 11). This, in turn, is grounded in the fact that, despite the achievements of modern medicine, doctors still cannot relieve all suffering (Admiraal 1991, p. 16; see also Cassell 1991).

4. Arguments from justice and the demand to be treated fairly

It is argued that everybody is entitled to be treated fairly and to share equally the benefits and burdens of life. To deny patients the option of being spared intolerable and intractable suffering is to treat them unfairly, and to make them carry a burden which others do not have to carry. Furthermore, to deny patients the right to die (that is, in a manner and time of their choosing) is to impose unfairly on them the values of others. Only patients, or those intimately involved with them (for example, family and friends), can judge what is in their own best interests. For others to deny patients the right to choose death is therefore to violate unfairly these patients' autonomy, dignity and entitlement to be spared the harms that will flow from suffering intolerable and intractable pain. Where euthanasia is the only thing that can end patients' intolerable and intractable pain, it stands as a morally just alternative.

5. Arguments from altruism and the 'duty to die'

It is argued that in certain circumstances (such as in the case of old age, chronic illness, or when medical treatment is futile) it may be a person's duty to volunteer for euthanasia (Kilner 1990; Beloff 1992; Schwartz 1993). Beloff, for example, apparently finds it quite plausible that:

> the mere thought of becoming a burden to others, not to mention a drain upon society, would suffice to make [some] choose voluntary euthanasia as the only honourable course of action still open to them.
>
> (Beloff 1992, p. 53)

In situations where a person's primary caregivers are burdened to the point where they cannot live their lives fully and are themselves beginning to suffer as a result of their burden of care, euthanasia, argues Beloff, is not only permissible, but required and deserving of moral praise. Beloff explains that this is because:

> If there *is* a duty to die it is one that arises from our basic human predicament, the fact that we are dependent on others, and it is a duty we owe to those we cherish.
>
> (Beloff 1992, p. 54)

Counter-arguments to views supporting euthanasia

Not surprisingly, those who are against euthanasia are not moved by these kinds of arguments. The anti-euthanasia response typically entails three main approaches: (1) to assert a number of counter-claims and counter-arguments against the views put forward in support of euthanasia; (2) to assert a number of distinctive arguments against euthanasia; and (3) to reject altogether the notion of passive euthanasia (killing by omission) on the grounds that there is a morally significant difference between directly killing a person and merely letting a person die (referred to in the bioethics literature as the 'killing/letting die distinction').

1. Autonomy and the right to choose death

While the moral principle of autonomy is well established in Western moral thinking, it nevertheless has limits. Whether 'autonomy' was ever meant to stretch so far as to impose a moral duty on a doctor or a nurse to comply with a patient's request for euthanasia — to intentionally and actively assist that patient to die — is an open question. If complying with a patient's request for euthanasia has the foreseeable consequence of harming or affecting prejudicially the significant moral interests of others (for example, the doctor[s] or nurse[s] receiving the request, or the patient's family and friends), there is considerable scope for arguing that the doctor(s) and nurse(s) in question have no duty to perform euthanasia, no matter how autonomous the patient's request for it. Further, given the complex nature of the morality of euthanasia, it is rather simplistic to hold that euthanasia can be justified on the grounds of patient autonomy *alone* without consideration being given to other important moral considerations which might also have a significant bearing on a patient's choosing active or passive euthanasia, and on a doctor's, a nurse's, a family member's or a friend's providing it.

(Adjunct to this view, it is important to note here that autonomy discourse is extremely powerful, making challenges to it difficult. So successful has been the promotion of autonomy, and the assumed sovereign rights of individuals to exercise self-determining choices, as mentioned earlier, that the imperatives of these things — especially in the case of euthanasia/assisted suicide — have come to seem 'so self-evident to all "right thinking people" that to question them seems almost perverse' (Moody 1992, p. 50). Those who do question them risk being publicly ridiculed and dismissed by opponents as ill-informed and 'illogical', or worse as being 'insulting' to vulnerable and oppressed groups [see, for example, the reported comments in the Senate Legal and Constitutional Legislation Committee 1997 at pp. 71, 176].)

2. *Dignity and the right to die with dignity*

Dignity and dying with dignity does not necessarily entail choosing death over the artificial prolongation of life. The demand to respect and maintain a person's dignity might equally entail respect for a person's autonomous wish that 'everything possible be done' to prolong or sustain her or his life — and to sustain a sense of hope that is fundamental to living that life meaningfully, even though (and when) dying. Here, it is important to understand that the ethical controversies surrounding the care of dying patients are not just about management at a technological, medical or institutional level. As Campbell (1992, p. 255) points out, they should also be seen 'as a sign of a deeper crisis of meaning in our culture', and as an indication of how impoverished our society has become in 'assessing the significance of suffering, dying and death as part of a whole human life'. Given this, as Campbell goes on to explain:

> The emergence of the individual asserting inviolable rights to self-determination becomes intelligible in this void as a way to create meaning through a freely-chosen style of life and an authentic manner of death.
>
> (Campbell 1992, p. 255)

One way to respond to this crisis of meaning is to 'provide compassionate presence to the sufferer', not to 'end the suffering by killing the sufferer' (Campbell 1992, pp. 269, 276). Another is to deny altogether the philosophical bases for a 'right to die' (see, for example, Kass 1993).

3. *Suffering and the demand to end it*

Suffering is not just a medical problem; it is also an existential problem involving profound questions concerning the meaning and purpose of human life and destiny (Campbell 1992; Starck and McGovern 1992; Amato 1990; Klemke 1981). To 'end suffering by killing the sufferer' is, to borrow from Campbell (1992, p. 276), to misunderstand 'both suffering and ourselves in a way that threatens [infinitely] our moral integrity'.

4. *Justice and the demand to be treated fairly*

To deny patients the right to *choose treatment* — including the artificial prolongation of 'hopeless life' — is as unjust as to deny patients the right to choose death. Denying patients' requests for 'everything possible to be done', where this conforms with their notions of dignity, meaning, value and quality of life, is to impose unfairly on them the values of others. As in the case *for* euthanasia, only patients (or those close to them) can judge what is in their best interests, and they must be permitted to make these judgments.

5. Altruism and the 'duty to die'

In some circumstances, people may have a 'duty to live' in order to spare the pain of their grieving loved ones, who desire their ill loved one to live 'as long as possible'. Being dependent on others is not necessarily being a burden on them (see, for example, Kanitsaki 1993, 1994). Even if dependency does become burdensome — either for the dependent person or her or his carers — it is not clear how, if at all, this gives rise to a so-called 'duty to die'. At best, it may only substantiate 'our basic human predicament' that:

> the very experience of illness, and more fundamentally the process of aging that inevitably culminates in death, not only reveals our shared vulnerability and dependency, but also that we are all subject to some kind of ultimate powers beyond our control. Through our knowledge and technology we may aspire to a mastery of nature and the immortality of the gods, but we continually receive reminders of our dependency and finitude. From this it follows that any control we assert over our dying is already limited, and that dependency and dignity are not mutually exclusive.
>
> (Campbell 1992, p. 270)

At worst, to embrace a 'duty to die' may be to embrace an all-pervasive sense of pessimism and hopelessness which would blind people to understanding that 'the lives of even the terminally ill are precious and matter, right up to the last second of breath' (Mirin, reported by Gibbs 1993, p. 53). And it may risk blinding people to the fundamental insight which has been articulated so well by the late French philosopher and feminist, Simone de Beauvoir (1987, p. 92), that, while all people must die, death is still an accident, and that, even if people know this, and consent to it, death remains 'an unjustifiable violation' (de Beauvoir 1987, p. 92). By this view, therefore, to embrace a duty to die emerges as an embracement of the unjustifiable violation of human life and all that it stands for. It also risks the perversion of morality — and of its ultimate aim, notably, how best to *live* the 'good life'. Finally, if currency is given to the notion of people having a 'duty to die', this might have the undesirable effect of adding 'to the distress and guilt of those who wondered whether they were too great a burden on others' (Muirden 1993, p. 14).

Specific arguments against euthanasia

Specific arguments commonly raised against euthanasia (and the need to legalise it) include:

1. arguments from the sanctity-of-life doctrine;
2. arguments from misdiagnosis and possible recovery;
3. arguments from the risk of abuse;
4. arguments from non-necessity;
5. arguments from discrimination;
6. arguments from irrational or mistaken or imprudent choice;
7. the 'slippery slope' argument.

1. Arguments from the sanctity-of-life doctrine

A popular argument raised against euthanasia draws heavily on the sanctity-of-life doctrine and contends that, since life is sacred and inviolable, *nothing* (not even intolerable and intractable suffering) can justify taking it. Sanctity-of-life arguments against euthanasia run something like this:

1. human life is sacred, and taking it is wrong;
2. euthanasia is an instance of taking human life; therefore
3. euthanasia is wrong.

Whether human life is sacred, and whether taking it is always wrong is, however, a matter of philosophical controversy (see, for example, Kuhse 1987).

2. Arguments from misdiagnosis and possible recovery

An argument often used against euthanasia is that which speaks to the risk of misdiagnosis and the possibility of recovery. Doctors themselves argue that they are fallible and can make mistakes (see in particular the comments of Dr John Mathew, President of the Victorian Branch of the Australian Medical Association [AMA], reported in *The Age*, 4 August 1986a, p. 5). Furthermore, patients can sometimes recover spontaneously (see, for example, Chopra 1989; Dossey 1991), or a new cure might be found. For example, it was reported recently that scientists have shown that the 'human spinal cord may have the capacity to reconnect and regenerate, and that treatment for spinal injuries may be tested on humans within a couple of years' (Ewing 1994, p. 1). If a cure for spinal injuries were found, quadriplegics, for example, might not request assistance to die as they are now doing. What is of concern about the euthanasia option is that once euthanasia is performed it cannot be reversed. Once done, it is done. The risk of error is unacceptable, and overrides any other considerations which might favour euthanasia in a particular case (see also Kamisar 1978; Muirden 1993).

3. Arguments from the risk of abuse

The possibility of euthanasia being abused is an argument frequently raised against euthanasia. For example, Dr Nell Muirden, of the Peter MacCallum Cancer Institute in Melbourne, has emphasised the danger of euthanasia being abused by unscrupulous relatives (Athersmith 1986; Muirden 1993). Further to this, Dr John Mathew is reportedly concerned about legislation giving one group the power to terminate life. The fear that 'the giving of power to terminate life to any one group can easily be misused' is, according to the AMA, by no means 'trivial' (*The Age*, 4 August 1986a, p. 5).

For the anti-euthanasiasts, the risk of abuse is unacceptable and underscores the need to reject the moral permissibility of euthanasia.

4. Arguments from non-necessity

Some contend that it is simply 'not necessary' to legislate or to support euthanasia. The reason commonly offered (mostly by conservative doctors) is that 'the medical profession has been successful over the years in allowing patients to die with dignity' (see in particular Dr Ken Sleeman's reported comments in Harari and Clarke 1987). Since patients are 'dying well' or are having 'good deaths' anyway, why take the matter any further?

5. Arguments from discrimination

It is sometimes suggested that euthanasia entails blatant discrimination, notably by treating some lives as less worthy than others. Margaret Tighe, president of the Victorian Right to Life, for example, repeatedly argues that euthanasia is detrimental to terminally ill, sick and incompetent people. She maintains that euthanasia 'reinforces the concept that there are some lives not worthy to be lived' (Maslen 1986; Harari 1987). By this view, just as any other act of discrimination is morally offensive, so too is euthanasia.

6. *Arguments from irrational, mistaken or imprudent choice*

It is sometimes argued that any person requesting euthanasia is not really exercising a rational or prudent choice, and that, for this reason, among others, an individual's request for euthanasia should not be taken seriously. One of the staunchest supporters of this view is the Vatican. In its 1980 *Declaration on euthanasia*, it states:

> The pleas of gravely ill people who sometimes ask for death are not to be understood as implying a true desire for euthanasia; in fact it is almost always a case of an anguished plea for help and love.

> (Vatican 1980, p. 7)

(Whether a death wish is always the product of irrational or imprudent choice is however a matter of philosophical controversy.)

7. *'Slippery slope' argument*

Also popular in the anti-euthanasia debate, as it is in the anti-abortion debate, is the 'slippery slope' contention. It will be recalled that the slippery slope argument holds that we risk a decline in our moral standards once we permit the taking of human life. For example, if we permit abortion today, we will permit infanticide the next day, and euthanasia the next. In the case of euthanasia, a slippery slope argument might run as follows: once we allow euthanasia for consenting persons, we will permit euthanasia for unconsenting and non-consenting persons, such as infants, the intellectually impaired and the severely brain-injured. Once we compromise the standards for protecting human life, we compromise all other standards pertaining to human life and wellbeing. Euthanasia, then, should never be justified.

An important example of the risk of 'slippery slope' action in the context of euthanasia being practised can be found in the little-known 1991 Dutch case involving a psychiatrist who medically-assisted the suicide of a female patient who was suffering emotionally but who was otherwise physically healthy viz. had no somatic illness (Ogilvie and Potts 1994; Klotzko 1995). Although deemed by her psychiatrist not to be suffering from a psychiatric illness, the patient was nevertheless regarded as being clinically depressed. The social history of this woman is as follows and worth quoting at length:

> She was a 50-year-old social worker. She was also a painter in her spare time. She was divorced. She had been physically abused by her former husband for many years. She had two sons. One son, Peter, died by suicide in 1986, at the age of 20. She then underwent psychiatric treatment for a marriage crisis following his suicide. At the time, she strongly wished to commit suicide, but decided that her second son, Robbie, age 15, needed her as a mother.

> Her son, Robbie, died of cancer in 1991, at the age of 20. Before his death, she decided that she did not want to continue living after he died. She

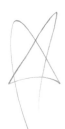

attempted suicide, but did not succeed. On July 13, 1991, she wrote to a social worker at the academic hospital where her second son died of cancer; she asked for a contact and for pills, so that she could kill herself. She had bought a cemetery plot for her sons, her former husband, and herself; her only wish was to die and lie between the two graves of her sons.

(Klotzko 1995, pp. 240–41)

Subsequently, the patient wrote to Dr Boudewijn Chabot, a psychiatrist, requesting assistance to die. On 28 September 1991, Dr Boudewijn Chabot, after assessing the patient, provided her with a lethal dose of medication and remained with her while she swallowed the medication and died (Klotzko 1995, p. 239). He subsequently reported the death to the relevant authorities following which he was prosecuted by the Supreme Court of the Netherlands. On June 21, 1994, in what has been described as a 'historic ruling', the Supreme Court of the Netherlands found Dr Chabot guilty, but declined to punish him. Significantly, in reaching its verdict, the court rejected the contention that 'help in assistance with suicide to a patient where there is no physical suffering and who is not dying can never be justified' (Ogilvie and Potts 1994, p. 492). To the contrary. As Ogilvie and Potts report, the court:

> explicitly accepted that euthanasia and assisted suicide might be justified for a patient with severe psychic suffering due to a depressive illness and in the absence of a physical disorder or terminal condition.
>
> (Ogilvie and Potts 1994, p. 492)

Significantly, the court found that Chabot's guilt lay not in his providing a medically-assisted death to his patient, but in his failure to obtain a second psychiatric opinion on the woman, and his failure to secure independent expert evidence that an 'emergency situation existed' — regarded as providing 'the normal mitigating defence in such cases' (Ogilvie and Potts 1994, p. 492).

Responses to the Chabot case have been mixed. Some have cited the case to underpin their sympathy for the view that:

> in severe and persistent depressive illness, when all appropriate physical treatments, including polypharmacy, electroconvulsive therapy, and psychosurgery, have apparently been exhausted, voluntary euthanasia may sometimes seem to be as justifiable an option as it does in intractable physical illness.
>
> (Ogilvie and Potts 1994, p. 493)

Others, however, take the Chabot case as underscoring the fears of those advancing the slippery slope argument. As Ogilvie and Potts (1994, p. 493) point out, the Chabot case of 'psychiatric euthanasia' has demonstrated that the 'slippery slope' exists. They conclude:

> However well any legislation is hedged about with guidelines and protections against abuse, the slippery slope predicts an inevitable extension of those practices to other, more vulnerable, groups, such as those who are demented, mentally ill, chronically disabled, frail, dependent, and elderly — and perhaps even simply unhappy.
>
> (Ogilvie and Potts 1994, p. 493)

The arguments for and against euthanasia given here are not the only arguments raised in bioethics literature, but they are nevertheless common, and nurses need to become familiar with them. It should be pointed out that none of these arguments is uncontroversial, and that much more remains to be said about them than there is space here to do. Nevertheless, the discussion so far succeeds in supplying a starting point from which nurses can begin to address the question of the moral permissibility of euthanasia.

The killing/letting die distinction

Another response to the euthanasia debate is to argue that there is a morally significant difference between 'killing' and merely 'letting die'. Opponents of euthanasia claim that so-called *passive euthanasia* is merely 'letting die'; it is not euthanasia at all, and is therefore morally permissible. Let us explore this view further.

It is sometimes suggested that where medical treatment is relatively 'expensive, unusual, difficult, painful or dangerous' (sometimes referred to as 'extraordinary' treatment), no moral obligation exists to use it in order to prolong a person's life (Glover 1977, pp. 195–6; Vatican 1980, pp. 10–11). Furthermore, where a given life-prolonging treatment is unduly 'burdensome' to the patient, or even costly, it may, in conscience, be withdrawn (Vatican 1980, pp. 10–11). Even though the withdrawal of life-restoring or life-prolonging therapy may causally result in a patient's death, this need not be regarded as an intentional termination of a life, and therefore an act of passive euthanasia, but rather as merely 'letting nature take its course'. To put this another way, it is merely 'letting die', not direct and intentional killing. Withholding or withdrawing burdensome life-saving or life-prolonging treatment is therefore not, strictly speaking, euthanasia.

Bonnie Steinbock (1983) argues that withdrawing or withholding burdensome life-prolonging treatment should not be viewed as the intentional termination of life, but as 'the avoidance of painful and pointless treatment' (p. 293). Where decisions are made to withdraw treatments, these are really decisions about 'the most appropriate treatment for a given patient', not about killing that patient. She further contends that if a case of ceasing treatment is to hold as a case of euthanasia, it must first be shown that a particular treatment has been withdrawn with the *intention of causing death*. Where this cannot be shown, a claim of killing simply does not hold.

There are cases in which a doctor is simply 'not at liberty', argues Steinbock, to continue treatment — such as where a competent patient has explicitly refused a recommended life-saving therapy. In such cases it seems odd to hold the doctor culpable for failing to provide treatment or for causing the patient's death. Similarly, in cases involving hopelessly ill patients, where 'nothing more can be done', it seems implausible to hold that the discontinuation of a given treatment directly *caused* a patient's ultimate death (Steinbock 1983, p. 294). Here it is *disease* which has provided the causal link to a patient's death, not some act or omission on the part of a doctor or a nurse.

The ultimate conclusion of Steinbock's argument is that the discontinuation of life-prolonging treatment cannot be considered the intentional killing of another — viz. an act of euthanasia. At best, it is merely 'allowing nature to take its course' or allowing the 'natural flow of events to continue'.

The case for 'letting die' fails to consider, however, that deliberately *not acting* in life-threatening situations is itself a kind of *act* (see also Weinryb 1980). In this respect, a conscious decision to withdraw or withhold life-saving therapy still amounts to a 'deliberate inducement of death' (Trammell 1978). As Fletcher points out:

It is naive and superficial to suppose that because we don't 'do anything positively' to hasten a patient's death we have thereby avoided complicity in his [sic] death. Not doing anything is doing something; it is a decision to act every bit as much as deciding for any other deed.

(Fletcher 1973, p. 675)

By this view, it can be seen that withdrawing or withholding life-saving treatment still involves deliberate choice, just as positively administering treatment does, and as such still has 'a place among events' (Green 1980, p. 204). In this respect discontinuing or withholding burdensome life-saving treatment may hold as at least one way of intentional killing.

The view that withholding or withdrawing life-saving treatment is tantamount to intentional killing becomes even more compelling when considering the very nature of medical/health care contexts, which generally have the facilities to restore and/or prolong life. As Gruzalski (1981) points out, failing to treat in a medical setting is one way of killing *precisely because* in such settings there are the means to prolong life; where these means are not used, then a *failure to treat* can be differentiated from *disease* as a causal factor in a patient's death. A good example of this is the celebrated Clarence Herbert case (cited in Veatch and Fry 1987, p. 175). Mr Herbert, a 55-year-old security guard, suffered a respiratory arrest following an uneventful closure of an ileostomy. He was subsequently intubated and transferred to intensive care for treatment. There was, however, some controversy about whether Mr Herbert should be maintained on a ventilator. Nevertheless, the decision was made to discontinue his respiratory support. Although unconscious, Mr Herbert continued to breathe spontaneously and his vital signs stabilised. Despite this stabilisation, a second decision was made to withdraw all intravenous and nasogastric fluids, and to transfer Mr Herbert from the intensive care unit to a room in the hospital's surgical unit. Six days after his respiratory arrest, Mr Herbert died. An autopsy listed 'anoxia and dehydration as two of the causes of death' (Veatch and Fry 1987, p. 175). Here then is one case in which a failure to treat (namely the withdrawal of respiratory support and hydration) contributed causally to a patient's death; in this case a *failure to treat* was clearly distinguishable from mere *disease*.

The killing/letting die distinction is vulnerable to criticism on other grounds as well. Tooley (1980), for example, argues that there is no morally significant difference between *intentionally* killing and *intentionally* letting die, and that it is therefore just as wrong to 'intentionally refrain from interfering with a causal process as it is to initiate it' (p. 58). One of the consequences of this view is that, if there is no significant distinction between intentionally killing and intentionally letting die, it is probably the case that there is also no real distinction between active and passive euthanasia, since, like killing and letting die, these share the same intention — that of bringing about or hastening a patient's death. This, suggests Tooley, forces us to conclude that either euthanasia is somehow justified and therefore not morally wrong, or that we are morally confused or insincere in our thinking about it being wrong.

Arguing along similar lines, James Rachels (1975) contends that not only is there no distinction between killing and letting die, but that letting die 'has no defence' (p. 496), particularly where the period of letting die entails a period of prolonged and intolerable suffering. Cases involving the withdrawal or withholding of fluids and nourishment from severely disabled newborns and severe stroke patients are examples of this (Battin 1983). Rachels further argues (p. 495) that where letting die is allowed for so-called 'humane reasons', it amounts to much the same thing as killing; that is, the *cessation of treatment* amounts to *intentionally terminating another's life*. Consider, for example, the common practice of withholding nourishing fluids from severely disabled newborns. As a result of this practice, the severely disabled newborn almost always dies (mostly as a result of dehydration and starvation). The decision to withhold fluids from a severely disabled infant is usually considered a 'humane' course of action, since if the infant were to live it could only look forward to a burdensome life. In these kinds of cases, withholding fluids from a severely disabled newborn amounts to exactly the same thing as administering lethal injections to it, since both acts have the same intention (and outcome) — that is, of hastening the newborn's death and thereby preventing it from living or having to live a burdensome life.

If we accept these views, against the proponents of the killing/letting die distinction, we are also committed to accepting that there is no morally significant difference between withholding nourishment and fluids and administering a lethal injection. This is particularly so in cases where both have as their intention the hastening of a patient's death, the ending of a patient's suffering, and where both ultimately stand as a causal link to the patient's death when it actually occurs. If we accept this, we are further committed to accepting that in the ultimate analysis there is no intrinsic difference between active and passive euthanasia.

Intentional killing versus alleviating pain

At this point some comment needs to be made on the issue of narcotic administration to chronically and terminally ill patients. Is this, in some cases, tantamount to killing patients? I have spoken to many nurses who feel that their actions in administering prescribed narcotic analgesia to some patients have been tantamount to 'murder'. The question which arises here is: Is the administration of narcotics in some cases the same as intentional killing? If so, is this always morally wrong?

It must be remembered, first, that many cases of medically prescribed narcotic administration are *not* cases of intentional killing, and in fact may prolong life. Second, it is also likely that some cases fall somewhere between prolonging life and intentional killing. Third, it is probably true that some cases of medically prescribed narcotic administration are cases of intentional killing. Let us refer to these three kinds of cases respectively as analgesia without death; analgesia with unintentional death; and analgesia with intentional death.

Analgesia without death

There are some pain states which can only be relieved by the administration of narcotic agents. An effective narcotic regime — even when entailing enormous doses — can, however, control pain without necessarily 'doping' or debilitating the patient. Indeed, many patients receiving large doses of narcotics remain alert, pain-free and as active as their disease will allow. Muirden (1993), for example, cites the case of a 55-year-old man who had cancer and who, at one stage of his illness, was receiving up to 3600 milligrams of morphine by injection (the usual dose is about 10 milligrams every four hours, a total of just 60 milligrams a day). She writes: 'He did not die of an overdose, and did not remain in a drowsy or drugged state' (Muirden 1993, p. 18). In such cases the administration of narcotics is clearly nowhere near tantamount to intentional killing. In fact, it may be quite the reverse. As pain specialists are quick to point out, the correct prescription of narcotic agents (for example, morphine) is more likely to prolong patients' lives than shorten them, because patients are 'able to rest, sleep, eat more and take a renewed interest in life' (Twycross and Lack 1984, p. 183; Muirden 1993).

Analgesia with unintentional death

There are other pain states which can only be relieved by the administration of narcotic analgesia. However, unlike the previous type of case, these pain states require the administration of narcotics at a level which may compromise patients' alertness and physical ability, and may even render them semi-comatose. In these types of cases, death is almost always hastened, even if not directly intended. Fortunately, these types of cases are not the norm, although they do occur frequently enough to be of concern to nurse practitioners.

Analgesia with intentional death

In another type of case, ill or debilitated patients do not have an organic pain state, or have only trivial pain states, but are nevertheless prescribed potentially lethal narcotic regimes. Pat Turton (1987, 1992), for example, cites the case of an elderly stroke patient who was prescribed what one nurse considered an 'unnecessary and dangerous' dose of morphine. The nurse's views were shared by the hospital pharmacy. When the nurse questioned the drug order, however, she was asked by the prescribing doctor 'Is this your first ward?', the implication being that the nurse was naive. Turton comments that the drug was given by another nurse and the woman died within hours. Similar cases occur every day in residential care homes and in some general hospital wards. In other cases, analgesia is given to seriously ill patients who have neuropathogenic pain states which conventional medicine is unable to alleviate. The drug regime given is clearly intended to hasten death, although this intention may be 'disguised' in some way — for example, by stating a rationale to 'alleviate pain', even though it is known that the pain cannot be alleviated. It is difficult to avoid the impression that in all these cases the administration of a given narcotic regime is tantamount to intentional killing or the intentional shortening of life.

Given these three situations, the question remains: Is the administration of potentially lethal doses of narcotics always morally wrong?

The case of *analgesia without death* is morally uncontroversial. Here narcotic regimes enhance not only patients' wellbeing but also patients' lives. Since no moral standards are compromised, the administration of enormous doses of narcotics in this instance is morally permissible.

The case of *analgesia with unintentional death*, however, is not so morally clear-cut. Although a patient may well be spared intolerable suffering by the administration of large and potentially lethal doses of narcotics, this cannot be achieved without compromising the patient's sanctity of life. For some nurses, the conflict between the demand to alleviate a patient's pain and the demand to respect and preserve a patient's life is the most troublesome of all. When caught in such a conflict, these nurses generally find the preservation-of-life principle too compelling to override and, rightly or wrongly, opt for withholding the analgesia. As a point of interest, Donovan et al. (1987), in researching the use of analgesia, found that some nurses administer only one-fourth of prescribed analgesia to their patients, although these patients have significant pain. (The widespread under-treatment of pain is also reported by Hill [1992, p. 76], and Greipp [1992, p. 44].) Donovan et al. do not identify conscientious objection as a possible variable influencing this incredible degree of negligence, but it cannot be altogether dismissed. While 'opting out' might alleviate the nurse's conscience, it does little to alleviate the patient's pain. Thus we are still left with a moral problem on our hands.

Like analgesia with unintentional death, *analgesia with intentional death* is morally controversial. It should also be pointed out that it is illegal and would be viewed by the courts as homicide. This is an issue which requires open and honest intellectual debate, as the entire debate on euthanasia and assisted suicide makes plain.

The doctrine of double effect

Catholic theologians have long recognised the dilemma posed by intolerable pain and the use of potentially lethal doses of narcotics as a means of suppressing pain. Interestingly, although the Vatican totally prohibits euthanasia, it nevertheless permits the use of narcotics as a means of alleviating pain — and, furthermore, permits dosages which might suppress a patient's level of consciousness and even shorten a patient's life (Vatican 1980, p. 9). There are, however, clearly defined conditions which must be met. First, there must be no other means of alleviating the patient's pain; in other words, potentially lethal doses of narcotics must never be prescribed except as a last resort. (This condition has interesting implications for the use of narcotics in cases involving severely disabled newborns and the chronically ill who are given narcotics as a means of suppressing hunger pains.) Second, the intention of using narcotics must be to only *alleviate pain*, not to cause death.

The first condition, that of last resort, is consistent with the general principles governing effective and safe pain management and, as it stands, is relatively uncontroversial. The second condition, however, that of intentionality, takes its force from the controversial 'doctrine of double effect', and thus is vulnerable to the same criticisms as is the doctrine itself.

The doctrine of double effect was developed by Catholic theologians. It states, roughly, that it is always wrong to do a bad act for the sake of good consequences, but that it is sometimes permissible to do a good act even knowing it might have some bad consequences. To illustrate this doctrine, consider the case of a patient suffering intolerable and intractable pain. In this case, ending the patient's life would also result in ending the patient's intolerable and intractable pain. While ending the patient's *pain* would be a 'good thing', ending the patient's *life* would not. Indeed, given the sanctity-of-life doctrine, deliberately ending an innocent patient's life would be a morally evil thing to do. Thus, we could say here, it would always be wrong to end an innocent patient's life (a bad act) in order to alleviate that patient's pain (a good consequence).

Given the 'good' of alleviating pain, however, we are morally permitted to give the patient analgesia — even though this might have the foreseeable and unfortunate consequence of shortening the patient's life. This is permitted since, even though the act of narcotic administration is associated with the foreseen possibility of hastening death, ending the patient's life is not the conscious intention behind the act. In short, the decision and action of giving the narcotics was not done with 'murder in your heart', to borrow from Cattanach (1985). To express the doctrine of double effect another way, we could say: it is always wrong to end patients' lives for the sake of alleviating their pain, but it is sometimes permissible to give potentially lethal doses of narcotics to alleviate pain, even though this might result in the patient's death — *as long as the patient's death is not the intended outcome.*

The doctrine of double effect has been the subject of much philosophical criticism, most notably on account of its over-reliance on what is called the foreseeability/intentionality distinction. This distinction holds roughly that foreseeing that a bad consequence will occur as a result of a given act is not the same thing as intending that bad consequence. For example, foreseeing that a patient will die as a result of being given large doses of narcotics is not the same thing as intending to end that patient's life; therefore the person who administers the narcotic is not morally culpable.

Critics reject this, however, and argue that the distinction drawn here is misleading. They contend that foreseeing a bad consequence of an action is exactly the same as intending it, since the agent knows that a bad consequence is pending but deliberately refrains from preventing it. To some extent, this position is also upheld in legal law. As Kuhse (1984) points out, the law presumes: 'everyone must be taken to intend that which is the natural consequence of his [sic] actions' (p. 26).

Given these criticisms, then, it seems that we cannot rely on the distinction between merely alleviating a patient's pain and intentionally ending a patient's life. Although it might perhaps be psychologically more tolerable to admit this distinction, it is not morally tolerable to do so. Where does this leave us?

The position is clear — nurses must all pursue a path of rigorous moral analysis of their actions. Acts involving narcotic prescription and administration must satisfy the ultimate standards not only of medicine and nursing, but also of ethics.

First and foremost, narcotic administration must accord with patients' considered preferences. This means that every effort must be made to establish what patients' preferences are, and to what extent patients are prepared to tolerate or not tolerate pain. Nurses must be open to the possibility, for example, of some patients preferring to suffer a certain degree of pain rather than compromise their mental alertness and physical ability. While a nurse might not agree with this kind of decision, it is nevertheless the patient's prerogative to make it.

Second, pain management must be guided by moral as well as clinical considerations.

Lastly, those involved in the administration of narcotics must be free conscientiously to refuse to administer drug regimes which they judge to be morally controversial or unacceptable.

Implications for nurses of narcotic administration

Narcotic administration will always remain a controversial issue for some nurses. Nevertheless it is not insurmountable. In most cases, a sound knowledge of the principles of pain management, proper pain assessment, and correct drug administration will help to reduce the likelihood of moral dilemmas occurring. In other cases, a clear articulation of relevant moral standards and values will help to reduce and/or resolve many of the moral problems associated with pain management and drug administration. Either way, the position nurses are morally obliged to take is clear: the patients are always the nurses' primary concern. If nurses have good reason to believe that a patient's safety, dignity, autonomy and wellbeing will be compromised by a given drug order or regime, then they must question it. This is not only a moral requirement, but also a legal requirement. It is far better to question a narcotic order and be wrong than not to question a narcotic order and be wrong — with the former, what is at stake may be only a little self-pride; with the latter, at stake may be a patient's life.

'Nursing care only' directives

A common, although not widely acknowledged, euthanatic practice — and one that has significant implications for nurses — is that of doctors prescribing 'nursing care only' for patients deemed 'medically hopeless'. In many (although, of course, not all) instances, this medical prescription has become a euphemism for non-voluntary and involuntary passive euthanasia since what is in fact being ordered is not *nursing care*, but rather the *withdrawal* of both *competent nursing care* and *life-sustaining medical care*. To illustrate this point, consider the widely discussed Dr Leonard Arthur case (Kuhse 1984), and the Danville case (Robertson 1981). Although these two cases are now somewhat dated, the issues they raise remain current in contemporary nursing care contexts.

The Dr Leonard Arthur case

On 1 July 1980, in a small English city, a Down's syndrome infant named John Pearson died in the arms of a nurse. The case would have escaped public attention had it not been for a member of staff reporting the circumstances of the case to Life, an anti-abortion organisation. On the basis of the information obtained by Life, John Pearson's attending physician, Dr Leonard Arthur, was charged with murder. The charge was based on the prosecution's claims that:

1. Dr Arthur had ordered the administration of the drug DFl18 with the intention of bringing about the baby's death;

2. the fact that Dr Arthur had ordered 'nursing care only' showed that he had intended the infant to die.

(Kuhse 1984, p. 22)

Dr Arthur's 'nursing care only' order in this instance directed the feeding of *water only* to the infant, and the administration of the drug DFl18 '*at the discretion of the nurse in charge* but not more than every four hours' (Kuhse and Singer 1985, p. 2, emphasis added). Since John Pearson had no organic pain syndrome as such, it would seem that the DF118 was prescribed for the purposes of sedating him and suppressing his hunger sensations.

However we look at this case, it is clear that what Dr Arthur ordered was *not* nursing care, or, if it was, it was highly negligent nursing care. For example, feeding water only to an infant who is perfectly able to take and tolerate a full and nourishing fluid regime falls far short of reasonable and acceptable standards of nursing care, as does the administration of a narcotic to an infant who does not have a commonly recognised organic pain syndrome. Let us explore this claim further.

Nurses are formally educated to assess individuals' fundamental health needs, to diagnose needs deficits (viz. health problems) and to plan nursing interventions aimed at helping people to meet their own health needs. Nurses are also formally educated to evaluate the outcomes of their nursing interventions and to modify their plans of care if an individual's health needs and health goals have, for some reason, not been met. Among the ten or so basic health needs which nurses are taught to assess are nutrition (including hydration), comfort (including being pain-free) and safety (including being kept free of injuries which might be caused by the over-prescription or inappropriate prescription of certain drugs). The formal education given to nurses in this area provides the minimal legal standard of reasonable and acceptable nursing care. Any nurse who fails to assess and diagnose correctly a person's health problems and plan nursing interventions to help meet the health needs of a patient is practising below a reasonable and acceptable standard of nursing care, and is thus practising negligently. The line between failing to meet the nutrition, comfort and safety health needs of a severely disabled newborn and professional negligence is, then, a very thin one.

Even if hunger is conceded as a genuine pain syndrome, this still does not justify the administration of large doses of narcotics or sedatives, nor does it rescue nurses administering these from culpability. There are at least two reasons for this. First, it is not normal practice to administer large doses of narcotics or sedatives to alleviate hunger pain. If it were, patients hungry from, say, pre- and post-operative fasting would be routinely administered narcotics or sedatives as part of their care. As we know, this is not done. Nurses should be rightly suspicious of medical prescriptions directing the administration of potentially lethal doses of narcotics or sedatives to infants who do not have a genuine organic pain syndrome and who are suffering hunger only from not being fed adequately.

A second reason why narcotic or sedative administration is not justified in the case of hungry severely disabled newborns is that there is no clinical basis for preferring a narcotic agent or a sedative agent over a bottle of milk for alleviating these infants' so-called 'pain states' and associated distress. As a general rule, narcotics are prescribed only for extreme organic pain states or where other non-narcotic agents are known to be ineffective in alleviating a given type of pain. In less extreme pain states, the tendency is to prescribe non-narcotic agents (such as aspirin or paracetamol), or even to avoid prescribing analgesia altogether, with preference being given to other methods of pain management such as exercise, change of bodily position, massage, physiotherapy, transneuronal stimulation, the administration of antacids, and, in the case of babies and infants, simply nursing them on one's lap and spending time with them. Since hunger is not generally regarded as an extreme pain state (in fact hunger is not even listed as a pain state in general analgesic guidelines and manuals), it is again highly suspect that narcotics should be chosen as a preferred 'treatment' option over the simple administration of a bottle of warm milk. Similarly, sedatives are usually prescribed for children only as a last resort. Where children's distress can be easily resolved by feeding them and/or nursing them on one's lap, there seems little to justify the administration of potentially lethal doses of a given sedative or narcotic analgesic.

It is, I think, fairly obvious that 'nursing care only' orders, as given by doctors in the case of severely disabled newborns, are prescriptions for euthanasia. It is also clear that, by so ordering 'nursing care only', doctors are placing nurses in a position of legal negligence and possibly of even committing homicide. Obvious as these points are, however, they have been conveniently ignored by some courts.

In the case of Dr Leonard Arthur, the suggestion that John Pearson had been killed by the *nursing care only* order was dismissed. Significantly, the defence council's success was largely based on showing that ordering 'nursing care only' was *proper medical practice* (Kuhse and Singer 1985, p. 9). In this case, the judge ignored any thought that the attending nurses had acted negligently by giving 'water only' to a hungry infant otherwise capable of feeding, and had effectively committed homicide by giving potentially lethal doses of narcotics to an infant who did not have a genuine organic pain syndrome (see also Gunn and Smith 1985). Following his trial at Leicester in November 1981, Dr Arthur was acquitted of the criminal charges brought against him. His acquittal is reported to have sparked 'rejoicing' (Kuhse and Singer 1985, p. 10).

The Danville case

On 6 May 1981, Siamese twins were born at a hospital in Danville, Illinois. The babies were joined at the waist with three legs. Upon seeing the deformity, the attending anaesthetist passed the order: 'Don't resuscitate, let's just cover the babies' (Robertson 1981, p. 5; Horan 1982). The father of the twins, also a doctor, gestured support for the anaesthetist's decision. It was later revealed that the decision to let the infants die had been made on little more than a visual impression of the infants' condition. Robertson (1981) writes that in fact no assessment was made to check whether there was any brain damage, whether the twins could be separated, or what their prognosis was. No effort was made to explore either adoption or institutional alternatives for the babies. The decision was made in total ignorance, and furthermore was made at the most stressful point in time — at delivery. Nevertheless, an order was written in the medical notes not to feed the babies, and they were taken to the newborn unit to die.

Nurses involved in caring for the twins, not surprisingly, became increasingly uncomfortable with the decision to withhold feeds from the babies. And it is claimed that at least one of the nurses 'fed the babies several times' (Robertson 1981, p. 5). The case received public attention after an anonymous caller reported it to the Illinois Department of Children and Family Services. Upon receiving the call the department immediately investigated the caller's claim, and the babies were transferred to another hospital for assessment and care. Later, in an unprecedented step, criminal charges were filed against both the parents and the doctors for 'conspiracy to commit murder and endangering the life and health of children' (Robertson 1981, p. 5). In the legal case that followed, nurses described how the twins 'cried in pain because they were hungry; how the cries dwindled down to whimpers as they were starved to death, how the skin started to wrinkle ...' (Robertson 1981, p. 6; Horan 1982).

As in the Dr Arthur case, nurses were once again placed in a legally and morally intolerable position on account of a 'routine' medical order to withhold nourishment. Curiously, because the nurses were unable 'to link the parents and the physicians directly with the orders to withhold food and fluids from the twins', the judge hearing the case dismissed the charges on grounds of lack of evidence (Robertson 1981, p. 5). It seems that either the nurses' expert testimony was not admitted, or, if it was admitted, it was considered insignificant. Either way, the universal euphemism for euthanasia, viz. 'nursing care only', remained intact.

Position statements on euthanasia/assisted suicide and the nursing profession

A pressing question currently facing the nursing profession concerns what, if any, formal position nurses ought to take on the euthanasia/assisted suicide issue? For many, this question remains an open one. For some, the failure by some nursing organisations to formulate a firm position, either way, on the euthanasia/assisted suicide question is untenable and paradoxical — paradoxical since even a 'non-position' is a position (Johnstone 1996a).

Significantly, there is no universally agreed nursing position on the ethics of euthanasia/assisted suicide; different nursing organisations in different countries hold quite distinct and sometimes opposing views on the matter, and on whether it is appropriate for nurses to assist with euthanatic procedures (Johnstone 1996b, pp. 32–43). For example, whereas some nursing organisations (such as the Royal College of Nursing in the United Kingdom, and the American Nurses' Association in the United States of America) have stated positions firmly rejecting the role of the nurse in participating in or assisting with active voluntary euthanasia and/or assisted suicide, others (such as the National Nurses' Association in the Netherlands, and the Nurses' Board of the Northern Territory of Australia) have stated positions supporting the role of the nurse in assisting with euthanasia/assisted suicide (Johnstone 1996b, pp. 32–43). While there does seem to be some agreement among nursing organisations on the matter of patients rights to self-determination, and to die with dignity and peace (Johnstone 1996b, p. 38), this support has stopped short of being translated into a frank pro-euthanasia/assisted suicide position with the matter tending to be left to individual nurses to decide on the basis of conscience.

In several respects it is not surprising that there exists moral uncertainty and disagreement among members of the nursing profession about the 'rightness' and 'wrongness' of euthanasia/assisted suicide; about the kind of position the nursing profession should take, if at all; and, in the event of euthanasia/assisted suicide being decriminalised, about what kind of role nurses should play in the medically-assisted deaths of patients. Many people hold differing views on these and related issues, and there is no reason why nurses should be any exception in this regard. Furthermore, it is important that this moral uncertainty and disagreement exists — a point that is not always understood. Nurses like other members of the community should not fear moral uncertainty. Appropriately felt and placed it imports what I shall call here 'moral vigilance' — a moral 'watchfulness', as it were, that can and does provide an important check against moral complacency. Neither should nurses fear moral disagreement or the diversity of opinion underpinning it (provided, of course, this does not spill over into violence, as has happened with the abortion debate where pro-life supporters have murdered pro-choice supporters in the name of 'upholding their pro-life beliefs' [see Chapter 1 of this text]). As has long been recognised in philosophy (and has been alluded to earlier in this text), disagreement is the beginning of our thinking, not its end. Philosophical disagreement can help to stimulate our moral imagination, and to sharpen and refine our moral thinking. In this respect, moral disagreement can, paradoxically, be creative and protective, not destructive; it can enable us to discover new solutions which might otherwise have alluded us — to see not just new things, but a new way of thinking about the things we have discovered. Moral uncertainty and disagreement, therefore, can both provide important beginning points for developing our moral thinking and finding sustainable and satisfying moral stances from which to view the world and guide our moral conduct. Consider the following case scenario.

A few years ago I was participating in a panel discussion on euthanasia and assisted suicide which had been scheduled during a one day seminar on the topic. During the panel discussion (in which a number of distinguished guests participated) I noticed a young woman (a nurse) crying silently in the audience. Concerned about this young woman's obvious distress, I approached her during the morning tea break to ask if she wished to discuss with me what was troubling her. This she agreed to do. Upon hearing her story, I asked whether she would be willing to share her situation with the rest of the seminar participants once the proceedings recommenced after the morning tea break. This she also agreed to do. When the proceedings of the seminar recommenced, I had the opportunity to call on the young woman to share her feelings about the topic under discussion. She bravely faced her audience and related the following:

> I am sitting here listening to you all. And I am so envious because you all seem so to be so sure about where you stand on the [euthanasia] issue. You are either *for* or *against* it. But I do not have the benefit of such certainty. I simply do not know where I stand and this makes me feel very upset. You see, it is like this: I am a 'good Catholic girl', with a good Catholic education. My church tells me 'euthanasia is wrong' and that I must not support it. But then, I am also a nurse. I believe I am a good nurse and I believe in nursing. And my profession tells me I must support patients' rights — I must be an advocate for my patients' rights. And then there are my patients. Sometimes my patients want to die and ask for assistance to die. And I want to do what is right by them. And then there is me, the human being, torn between what my church tells me I should do, what my profession tells me I should do, and what my patients want me to do. I just feel so torn, because I really feel so uncertain about what *is* the right thing to do. I just don't know. I just don't know which side of the fence I should be on. And I feel that somehow maybe I am stupid or deficient because of this — especially when I listen to all of you here being so sure about the positions you are holding.

With this brave and frank admission came other admissions from other people in the audience: significantly, and contrary to superficial appearances, most of the people attending the seminar felt the way this nurse did, but had been unable to say so publicly. We then spent some time exploring the permissibility of feeling 'uncertain' about new and previously unexplored ethical issues, of taking the time necessary to consider other points of view and to explore possible answers to the difficult questions raised, and to ultimately reach a position on the issues identified that the person in question could 'live with'.

Some time later the nurse in question contacted me. She had reasoned the issue through and had reached a position about which she felt confident at both a personal and professional level. What had helped her most in reaching this position was peer support, and the 'permission' her peers had given her to take the time she needed to 'think through' the issue at hand. She also particularly valued the opportunity the seminar had provided in regard to exposing her not just to the issues raised but to the many different points of view expressed in response to them. But most important of all, she valued being able to share her story, and in this sharing to 'make visible' a problem that she was soon able to discover was not hers alone.

Coming to terms with the complex questions raised by the euthanasia/assisted suicide issue requires a systematic response by both individual nurses and the broader nursing profession. Specifically, it requires of nurses to gain knowledge and understanding of the profound ethical, legal, cultural, clinical and political dimensions of euthanasia/assisted suicide, and the influence these dimensions have on the profession and practice of nursing (Johnstone 1996a). Equally important, it requires peer support and understanding among nurses and a recognition that the euthanasia/assisted suicide question is not — and never has been — simple and clear-cut.

In concluding this section, it is my considered view that in order for a position statement on euthanasia/assisted suicide to be meaningful to members of the nursing profession, it must minimally reflect that euthanasia and assisted suicide are controversial moral issues, that there exists a diversity of opinion on whether euthanasia and assisted suicide are morally justified, and that nurses are likely to encounter this diversity of opinion during the course of their work. Further, such a position statement must also reflect that there exists a diversity of opinion on whether nurses have a legitimate role to play in providing medically-assisted deaths to patients and that all nurses have a responsibility to ensure that they are reliably informed about the ethical, legal, cultural, political and clinical dimensions and implications of euthanasia and assisted suicide as a 'health care' option.

Conclusion

Euthanasia and assisted suicide are issues that have obvious significance for members of the nursing profession. While nurses can choose to accept or reject the findings of public debate on the euthanasia/assisted suicide issue, they cannot ignore them since, to do so, would be to risk not just their own moral interests, but importantly the interests of patients for whose care they share responsibility.

The issues of euthanasia and assisted suicide have not been widely discussed in the nursing literature, and the need to do so is long overdue. If this neglect is not redressed, it will be to the peril of the nursing profession, as the recent respective experiences of nurses in the Northern Territory of Australia and the Netherlands reminds us. It will be recalled, for instance, that in 1996, Northern Territory nurses had to confront the reality of being enabled by law to participate in euthanasia and assisted suicide *before* the broader nursing profession had reached a position on the matter and had determined what it regarded as 'acceptable standards of nursing practice' in relation to the actual practice of euthanasia/assisted suicide. In the Netherlands, meanwhile, nurses had to confront the reality that they could be successfully prosecuted for performing euthanasia even when such an action was in accordance with legally prescribed criteria. Nurses are — and have always been — in a tenuous position in regard to their role in participating in end-of-life practices. It is timely that this tenuous position is addressed in the interests of reducing not just the vulnerability of nurses, but of the patients otherwise reliant on nurses for quality care at the end stages of their lives.

Chapter 13
Suicide and parasuicide

Introduction

For many years, suicide has ranked among the top ten causes of death in Western countries (Suicide Prevention Victorian Task Force 1997, p. 9). It has been estimated by the World Health Organisation (WHO) that 'nearly one million people worldwide will die by suicide each year' (Suicide Prevention Victorian Task Force 1997, p. 9).

In 1992, it was estimated that the overall suicide rate in Australia was approximately eleven per 100 000 of population per year (Davis 1992, p. 93); in 1995 this figure was reported to have increased to thirteen per 100 000 (Suicide Prevention Victorian Task Force 1997, p. 12). These figures do not include attempted suicide rates; while reliable data on the incidence of attempted suicide are difficult to obtain, it has been estimated that for every male suicide there are approximately 30–50 attempts; and for every female suicide there are approximately 150–300 attempts (Suicide Prevention Victorian Task Force 1997, p. 21). It has been further estimated that of those who engage in suicidal behaviour (attempt suicide), 15 per cent will ultimately succeed in ending their own lives (Suicide Prevention Victorian Task Force 1997, p. 21).

Alarmingly, suicide is now the second most common cause of death among young Australians (Davis 1992, p. 90). The reality of this trend was underscored in 1992 with the revelation that twenty young people had suicided over a two-year period in the small Victorian township of Kyneton. The suicides were reported to have left the local community feeling stunned, alarmed, and extremely concerned about the welfare of its youth (Kennedy 1992, pp. 4–5; Deane 1992, p. 81; *The Leader* 1992, p. 8). In the following year, 1993, again in the State of Victoria, suicide deaths were reported to have outnumbered the state's road fatalities (Ryle 1993). The probability that some of these road fatalities were also 'autocides' (deaths as the result of premeditated [suicidal] automobile accidents [Donnelly 1990, p. 8]) exacerbates the significance of these statistics. In 1993, a United Nations study showed that 'Australia had the highest suicide rate in the industrialised world among males aged 16–30' (Middleton 1994, p. 3).

Currently, Australia still has one of the highest rates of suicide among young people aged 15–24 years, with male suicide rates being significantly higher than female suicide rates (Suicide Prevention Victorian Task Force 1997, p. 9). Youth suicide is over-represented in remote and rural areas; it is also over-represented among gay and lesbian youth (especially those living in remote and rural areas), possibly accounting for up to 30 per cent of completed youth suicides each year)(Suicide Prevention Victorian Task Force 1997, pp. 19, 40). Explaining this statistical over-representation, one commentator has written that 'homosexual orientation, cultural homophobia and geographical/social isolation are clearly a lethal mixture' (Christian 1997, p. 9). Other high risk groups include: men over 80 years of age, Aboriginal people, the homeless, people with HIV/AIDS, and people in custody (Suicide Prevention Victorian Task Force 1997, pp. 38–40).

Suicide figures in the United States of America are comparable with those in Australia (Davis 1992, p. 92). In 1987, the incidence of suicide in that country was estimated at 12.7 deaths per 100 000 (Donnelly 1990, p. 9). Youth suicide rates in the United States are also alarmingly high with suicide standing as the third leading killer of young people and accounting for '14 per cent of all deaths in the teenage-range' (Remafedi 1994b, p. 7; Davis 1992, p. 92; Donnelly 1990, p. 9). There is also consistent evidence showing 'unusually high rates of attempted suicide among gay [and lesbian] youth, in the range of 20–30 per cent, regardless of geographic and ethnic variability' (Remafedi 1994b, p. 7). As in Australia, gay and lesbian youth may comprise 'up to 30 per cent of completed youth suicides annually' in the United States of America (Gibson 1994, p. 15). These rates are thought to be causally linked to these youths' traumatic experiences of coming to terms with their sexuality in contexts (such as families, communities, society as a whole) that are for the most part unsupportive, alienating and aggressively homophobic (see in particular Remafedi 1994a).

The magnitude of the suicide problem in the United States was highlighted in 1993 with the reported suicide of a six-year-old girl, believed to be the youngest recorded suicide in the State of Florida (Power 1993, p. 9). The child was killed after she deliberately placed herself in front of an oncoming train. Her death was witnessed by three other children aged six, seven, and eight years old respectively — all of whom 'tried to move her as the train approached' (p. 9). The engineer was unable to stop the train 'until nearly a kilometre after impact' (p. 9). It is believed that the little girl wanted to die so that she could 'become an angel and be with her mother', who was dying of cancer (p. 9).

(As a point of interest, contrary to popular thought, child suicide is not an isolated or new phenomenon. During the late Middle Ages and early modern period, for instance, children under the age of 15 years were regarded as being at increased risk of suicide owing to the violent and abusive ways in which they tended to be treated during this period [Williams 1997, p. 153]. Today, while suicide rates are relatively low in children under 15 years of age, there is some suggestion these may be increasing. In 1995, for example, in the Victorian State of Australia, four deaths by suicide were of children aged between 10 and 14 years [Suicide Prevention Victorian Task Force 1997, p. 16].)

Suicide, by its very nature, is an extremely difficult and complex issue to address. At a personal level, the suicide of a loved one, a friend or an associate can be a devastating experience. Those 'left behind' may find themselves struggling 'to make sense of the suicidal act and the causes of suicidal behaviour' (Davis 1992, p. 90). They may also find themselves overwhelmed by feelings of grief, shame, remorse, anger, despair, and possibly even guilt at the thought that 'perhaps they could have done more' or that 'if only they had been there ... it might never have happened'. It has been estimated that for every suicide, between six and ten people (including family, friends and co-workers) are directly and strongly affected by the event (Suicide Prevention Victorian Task Force 1997, p. 25; Williams 1997, p. 224). Significantly, people bereaved by suicide are themselves ten times more likely than the general population to die from self-inflicted deaths (Suicide Prevention Victorian Task Force 1997, p. 25).

Suicide is also difficult to address at a professional/therapeutic level. Even the very best of psychotherapies may still fail to prevent a person suiciding; and even the very best of medical and nursing care may still fail to restore someone who has attempted suicide to a life that is 'worthwhile' and worth living. Equally if not more problematic are the difficulties of addressing the suicide issue at a moral level. Included among these difficulties is the challenge suicide and attempted suicide pose to fundamental moral notions about the value, sanctity and meaning of life. An important question here is not 'how to achieve a better more fruitful [good] life' — a central question in Western moral philosophy — but, as Heyd and Bloch (1981, p. 185) point out, 'whether to live at all'. More seriously, suicide challenges morality itself, and not least the values, standards and principles comprising it which might otherwise be appealed to for guiding deliberation on such issues as the entitlements and responsibilities of people contemplating suicide; the moral permissibility and impermissibility of suicide prevention; the entitlements and responsibilities of others toward those contemplating or attempting suicide; and other similar issues. Compounding the moral complexity of these issues is the additional consideration that, unlike other causes of death, suicide (or, more specifically, death from suicide) is relatively preventable (Baume 1988, p. 43).

Nurses who have either cared for a person who has attempted suicide, or who have been involved in the care of family members and friends of someone who has attempted suicide or succeeded in suiciding, will be only too familiar with the deep emotional agony that inevitably comes with this kind of situation. They will also be very aware of the complex moral problems that are commonly associated with implementing interventions aimed at preventing suicide, with caring for those who have attempted unsuccessfully to suicide, and with the difficulties of addressing these problems in a satisfying and helpful way.

It is not the purpose of this discussion to examine or present a treatise on the clinical aspects of suicide (its underlying causes, and means of prevention), or, indeed, on the philosophy or sociology or anthropology of suicide. Such a task would require major works in their own right — as has already been undertaken (see, for example, Durkheim 1952; Stengel 1970; Farberow 1975a; Battin and Mayo 1980; Battin 1982; Clemons 1990; Colt 1991; Kaplan and Schwartz 1993). Rather, the task here is to assist nurses to gain an understanding of the moral aspects of suicide and suicide prevention, and the nature of nurses' moral obligations when caring for people who are contemplating or who have attempted suicide. In undertaking this task, attention will be given to examining briefly:

- the history of suicide in different cultures and societies;
- definitions of suicide, and possible criteria which must be met in order for an act to count as suicide; and
- some important moral concerns which are raised by the suicide question, and which have significant implications for the profession and practice of nursing.

Socio-cultural attitudes to suicide: a brief historical overview

Concepts of and attitudes toward suicide have varied enormously across different cultures and throughout time (see in particular Farberow's [1975a] *Suicide in different cultures*). Just what was regarded as an act of suicide and whether suicide was approved or disapproved depended on a range of factors, including cultural norms and mores, religion, law, politics, and personal and social morality (Stengel 1970, pp. 65–73; Farberow 1975b, pp. 1–13; Beauchamp and Perlin 1978, pp. 88–92; Alvarez 1980, pp. 7–32; Battin 1982, pp. 27–75; Amundsen 1989, pp. 77–153; Brody 1989b, pp. 39–75; Beauchamp 1989, pp. 183–219; Cooper 1989, pp. 9–38; Ferngren 1989, pp. 155–81). These factors have seen Western attitudes toward suicide shift dramatically from those of socio-cultural approval through to religious prohibition, criminalisation, and ultimately the medicalisation of suicide (see Figure 13.1).

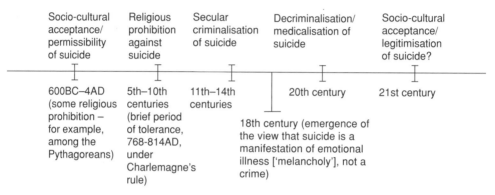

Figure 13.1 The transformation of attitudes to suicide

Socio-cultural acceptance of suicide, 600 BC – 4 AD

In the introduction to *Suicide: the philosophical issues*, Battin and Mayo (1980, p. 1) note that 'suicide has not always been assumed to be tragic or a phenomenon that is always to be prevented'. They go on to point out that, in both the early Greek and the Hebrew cultures, 'suicide was apparently recognised as a reasonable choice in certain kinds of situations', and that for some early North African Christians, 'suicide — like martyrdom — was a mark of religious devotion practised as a way of insuring attainment of immediate salvation' (Battin and Mayo 1980, p. 1).

In Ancient Greece and Rome, suicide was viewed as permissible (at least for the upper classes[1]) if it was chosen for 'the best possible reason' (Alvarez 1980, p. 18). The 'best possible reasons' included to preserve honour; to avoid dishonour or ignominy; as an expression of grief or bereavement; and for high patriotic principle or for a patriotic cause (Farberow 1975b, p. 5; Alvarez 1980, p. 18). There are many famous examples of suicide deaths in the history and mythology of ancient Greece and Rome. Notable among these are the Greek mythological character Jocasta (the mother of Oedipus, King of Thebes), who hanged herself to avoid the grief and shame she felt upon learning of her unwitting complicity in the sins imposed on her by fate (Sophocles 1911, vv. 1213–86); Socrates, the famed ancient Greek philosopher, who killed himself

---

1. Initially, suicide was prohibited on religious grounds. As religious forces weakened, however, attitudes to suicide changed. Farberow (1975b, p. 4) explains: 'while the attitudes of horror and condemnation for suicide were preserved in the lower classes, the upper classes seemed to develop a different religion and different morals, expressing tolerance and acceptance [of suicide]'.

patriotically by drinking hemlock after he was sentenced to death for corrupting the minds of the youth of Athens with his philosophical ideas (see Plato's *Euthyphron, Apology, Crito*, and *Phaedo* in Church's [1903] translation *The trial and death of Socrates*, and in Tredennick's [1969] translation *The last days of Socrates*); and the Roman matron Portia, who, upon learning of the death of Brutus at Philippi, killed herself by swallowing red-hot coals in what French (1985, p. 142) suggests was a kind of *suttee*. Zeno, the founder of Stoic philosophy (who apparently supported Seneca's view that suicide was permissible, but only as a last resort in the case of intractable suffering), also suicided. He apparently hanged himself in disgust at the age of 98 after falling and dislocating a toe! (Farberow 1975b, p. 5). The Roman view of suicide was perhaps among the most liberal during this period. Alvarez comments:

> the Romans looked on suicide with neither fear nor revulsion, but as a carefully considered and chosen validation of the way they had lived and the principles they had lived by ... To live nobly also meant to die nobly and at the right moment. Everything depended on the dominant will and a rational choice.
>
> (Alvarez, 1980, p. 23)

Not all the ancient Greeks and Romans had a permissive attitude to suicide, however. The Pythagoreans, for example, were vehemently opposed to suicide on religious grounds (Wennberg 1989, p. 41). And both the famed ancient Greek philosophers Plato and Aristotle opposed suicide, on religious and secular grounds respectively (Wennberg 1989, p. 42). While Plato was sympathetic to suicide 'when external circumstances became intolerable' (Alvarez 1980, p. 20), Aristotle was opposed even to this, on the grounds that:

> to kill oneself to escape from poverty or love or anything else that is distressing is not courageous but rather the act of a coward, because it shows weakness of character to run away from hardships, and the suicide endures death not because it is a fine thing to do but in order to escape from suffering.
>
> (Aristotle 1976, p. 130 [1116a 12–15])

Aristotle also opposed suicide on the economic grounds that it deprived 'society of one of its productive members' (Wennberg 1989, p. 42). Interestingly, extant taboos against suicide in the city of Athens saw the corpse of the suicide victim 'buried outside the city, its hand cut off and buried separately' (Alvarez 1980, p. 17). Alvarez points out, however, that suicide taboos and the treatment of corpses in these instances were linked not so much as might be thought to religious prohibition or to Aristotelian notions of one's duty to contribute productively to the state. Rather, they were linked 'with the more profound Greek horror of killing one's own kin. By inference, suicide was an extreme case of this, and the language barely distinguishes between self-murder and murder of kindred' (Alvarez 1980, p. 18).

In Rome, on the other hand, while permissive attitudes towards suicide were enshrined in law (Alvarez 1980, p. 22), there were exceptions based on practical and economic grounds. For example, it was a criminal offence for a slave to suicide, since it deprived the master of his capital investment (if this offence was committed within the first six months of a slave being purchased, he could be returned dead or alive to the original master and a refund obtained) (Alvarez 1980, p. 23). Soldiers who suicided were also deemed to have committed a serious offence — 'desertion'. This was because a soldier was 'considered to be the property of the state [a chattel] and his suicide was tantamount to desertion' (Alvarez 1980, p. 23). Finally, it was considered an offence for a criminal to suicide 'in order to avoid trial for a crime for which the punishment would be forfeiture of his estate' (Alvarez 1980, p. 23). Relatives were, however, entitled to defend the accused in his absence. If successful, they would retain property rights to the deceased's estate; if unsuccessful, they would forfeit all property rights, and the deceased's estate would go to the state. Thus, as Alvarez concludes:

> suicide was an offence against neither morality nor religion, only against the capital investments of the slave-owning class or the treasury of the state.
>
> (Alvarez 1980, p. 23)

There are many other examples of old and ancient cultures in which suicide was tolerated, permitted and even esteemed: the Druids, for example, viewed suicide as a passport to paradise, and as a means of accompanying their departed friends (Alvarez 1980, p. 13); in Japan, suicide was ritualised in the form of *seppuku* or *hara kiri* (more commonly known in the variant spelling *harikari*) (Farberow 1975b, p. 3; Smith and Perlin 1978, p. 1622); and in India and China, the ceremonial sacrifice of widows (of which the Hindu custom of *suttee* is an example) was also common (Wennberg 1989, p. 39). (Whether this 'ceremonial sacrifice' should be viewed as *suicide* rather than *homicide* is, however, a contentious point — see, for example, Daly 1978, pp. 114–33.)

Perhaps some of the most poignant examples of the tolerance, if not the permissibility, of suicide can be found in the early Jewish and Christian traditions.

Suicide in the orthodox Jewish tradition has been and continues to be viewed as an abhorrent and heinous sin, and is expressly forbidden (Smith and Perlin 1978, p. 1622; Kaplan and Schwartz 1993). Historically, suicides in Jewish communities have resulted in the people who have suicided being denied full burial honours and other associated rituals, for example, mourning (Farberow 1975b, p. 4; Wennberg 1989, p. 48). There have, however, been some interesting and heart-rending exceptions to this attitude of prohibition. Possibly one of the most famous of these was the mass suicide in 73 AD of 960 Zealots (men, women and children) at Masada, on the western shore of the Dead Sea. In this instance, the Zealots preferred to die at their own hands rather than submit to the Roman legions surrounding their sanctuary (Wennberg 1989, pp. 49–50; Battin 1982, p. 166; Alvarez 1980, p. 17; Farberow 1975b, p. 4). Significantly, the Masada victims are honoured, not condemned in the Jewish tradition (Wennberg 1989, p. 50). In more recent history, in what has been referred to as 'the incident of the ninety-three maidens' (Wennberg 1989, p. 50), ninety-three Jewish female students and teachers (including the head teacher) chose to suicide rather than to submit themselves to the infamous Gestapo for 'immoral purposes'. Describing the incident, Battin writes:

> During the Second World War, the directress of an orthodox Jewish girls' school in a Nazi-occupied city came to understand that her girls, ranging in age from twelve to eighteen, had been kept from extermination in order to provide sexual services for the Gestapo. When the Gestapo announced its intention to avail themselves of these services — ordering the directress to see that the girls were washed and prepared for defloration by 'pure Aryan youth' — she called an assembly and distributed poisons to each of the

students, teachers and herself. The ninety-three maidens, as they came to be called, swallowed the poison, recited a final prayer, and died undefiled.

(Battin 1982, p. 166)

Commenting on this mass suicide, Wennberg (1989, p. 50) explains that, like the suicide of the 400 children facing defilement in the Talmud, rather than this act being viewed as a sin it would be viewed as 'an act of faithfulness to God'; that is, of the victims submitting themselves to God's purpose, rather than to the immoral purposes of the men who would violate them.

The Christian religion, and more specifically its sacred writings, the Bible, also offers some interesting examples of tolerant if not permissible attitudes toward suicide (Wennberg 1989, p. 47; Rauscher 1981, pp. 105–7; Farberow 1975b, p. 4; Smith and Perlin 1978, p. 1622). The first and perhaps most poignant example of all is what Wennberg (1989, p. 45) describes as the Bible's 'curious silence' on the subject of suicide. Indeed, as Smith and Perlin (1978, p. 1622) also observe, 'the Bible contains neither an explicit word for suicide nor an explicit prohibition of the act'.

Despite the apparent omission of an explicit condemnation of suicide, there are a number of significant and famous incidents of suicide mentioned in the Bible:

- Samson, who pleaded 'Let me die with the Philistines' as he toppled the temple filled with God's enemies and was crushed to death (Judges 16: 30);
- Saul, who 'took a sword and fell on it' (1 Samuel 31: 4);
- Saul's armour-bearer, who 'also fell on his sword' (1 Samuel 31: 5);
- Ahithophel, who 'hanged himself, and died' (2 Samuel 17: 3);
- Zimri, who 'burned the King's house down upon himself with fire, and died' (1. Kings 16: 18);
- Judas, who 'went and hanged himself' (Matthew 27: 5).

Another (although less certain) Biblical example of suicide (contrary to popular thought, it may in fact be more an example of euthanasia) is the case of Abimelech (Judges 9: 52), who, in the course of attempting to set fire to a tower in which men and women had locked themselves for protection, was seriously injured after a woman in the tower 'dropped an upper millstone on Abimelech's head and crushed his skull' (Judges 9: 53). Fearing that his manner of death would tarnish his posthumous reputation, he begged his young armour-bearer:

'Draw your sword and kill me, lest men say of me, "A woman killed him."'
So his young man thrust him through, and he died.

(Judges 9: 54)

Some even suggest that the death of Jesus Christ is an example of suicide (Alvarez 1980, p. 12; Rauscher 1981, p. 107). Whether Jesus' death can be regarded as suicide, however, depends entirely on how suicide is defined.

The Bible's apparent failure to prohibit or condemn suicide explicitly, while significant, should not be taken as implying Christian approbation of the act. As Wennberg (1989, p. 46) points out, acts of suicide are — and have long been — incompatible with Christian theology (see also Amundsen 1989, pp. 77–153; Ferngren 1989, pp. 155–81; Beauchamp 1989, pp. 183–219; Boyle 1989, pp. 221–50; Kaplan and Schwartz 1993). The only apparent exception to this prohibition, at least until the teaching of St Augustine, was if suicide was the only option available in order to 'protect one's virginity or to avoid forced apostasy' (Battin 1982, pp. 3, 70–1).

Attitudes of religious prohibition against suicide

Until about 250 AD, attitudes towards suicide were largely permissive, and suicide was common even among the early Christians (Farberow 1975b, p. 6; Alvarez 1980, p. 12; Battin 1982, p. 71). In fact, the rise of Christianity as a persecuted religion brought with it an 'almost epidemic rate of self-destruction', justified as martyrdom (Heyd and Bloch 1981, p. 191). The reasons for this martyrdom are said to have included:

> pessimism, longing for a better life, a struggle for redemption, and a desire to come before God and live there forever.
>
> (Farberow 1975b, p. 6)

The religious fathers of the day were, however, appalled by the 'squandering of human life', and sought to halt it immediately by making it the subject of explicit and absolute religious prohibition (Wennberg 1989, p. 54). Thus, writes Farberow:

> As the 4th century began, changes appeared, with the Church adopting a hostile attitude that progressed from tentative disapproval to severe denunciation and punishment. Antagonism toward suicide developed. Suicide became proof that the individual had despaired of God's grace, or that he [sic] lacked faith and was rejecting God by rejecting life, God's gift to man [sic].
>
> (Farberow 1975b, p. 6)

The Church's emphatic and official prohibition saw a marked decline in the incidence of suicide, with one writer commenting that, by the twelfth century, 'while the Catholic Church held sway in Europe, suicide became practically unknown' (Farberow 1975b, p. 6).

Two highly influential figures in the fight against suicide/martyrdom were the Christian theologians St Augustine (354–430 AD) and St Thomas Aquinas (1225–74). St Augustine's principal theological argument against suicide rested on his interpreting the sixth commandment ('thou shalt not kill') as applying not only to *homicide* (the killing of another), but to *suicide* (the killing of the self) (Heyd and Bloch 1981, p. 191). Rejecting the popular view at the time that suicide was a way of avoiding sin and gaining a passport to eternal paradise, St Augustine countered that 'suicide is itself the gravest sin' (Heyd and Bloch 1981, p. 191). Thus St Augustine denounced suicide 'as a crime under all circumstances' — a view that was quickly ratified as the official view of the Church (Stengel 1970, p. 68). In 452 AD, for example, the Council of Arles declared the act of suicide to be 'an act inspired by diabolical possession'; one century later, the Church set another disincentive to suicide, this time by ordaining that 'the body of the suicide be refused a Christian burial' (Stengel 1970, p. 69).

St Thomas Aquinas' views against suicide were as absolute and as uncompromising as were St Augustine's (Wennberg 1989, p. 65). His arguments were, however, more systematic (Heyd and Bloch 1981, p. 191) and less vulnerable to criticism (Wennberg 1989, p. 66). Central to Aquinas' position were the arguments that suicide constituted an offence to and a violation of one's duty to oneself, the community, and God; he also regarded suicide as 'contrary to the natural law and to charity', and hence wrong (St Thomas Aquinas 1978, pp. 103–4). Whether suicide is, in fact, any of these things has been and remains the subject of much controversy, which will not be settled here (see, for example, Szasz 1988; Beauchamp 1978a, 1978b; Brandt 1978, 1980; Margolis 1978; Battin and Mayo 1980; Battin 1982; Barrington 1983; Hume 1983; Kant 1983; Brody 1989a; Wennberg 1989; Donnelly 1990).

As Christian religious prohibition against suicide spread across Europe, so too did 'the acts of violence and indignity perpetrated against the dead body' — partially, at least, because of 'fears of evil spirits released by the suicide' (Stengel 1970, p. 69). In some countries, for example, 'a stake was driven through the body and it was buried at the crossroads' (Stengel 1970, p. 69; Farberow 1975b, p. 7); an alternative to skewering the body with a stake was to place a stone on the face of the corpse, which would have the same effect as a stake — namely, it would prevent the victim from 'rising as a ghost to haunt the living' (Alvarez 1980, p. 8). The last degradation of the corpse of a person who had suicided occurred as recently as 1823 in England, when a Mr Griffiths was buried at the crossroads of Grosvenor Place and King's Road, Chelsea (Stengel 1970, p. 69; Alvarez 1980, p. 8). For fifty years after this, however, the bodies of suicide victims were still not treated with full respect, and, if unclaimed, were donated legitimately to schools of anatomy for dissection (Alvarez 1980, p. 8).

In France, as in England, it was also common practice to treat the corpse of a suicide victim in a violent and undignified way. Alvarez writes, for example, that:

> varying with local ground rules, the corpse was hanged by the feet, dragged through the streets on a hurdle, burned, thrown on the public garbage.
>
> (Alvarez 1980, p. 9)

As well as this, as in other European countries, the property of suicide victims was legally confiscated, and their memories legitimately defamed (Alvarez 1980, p. 9; Stengel 1970, p. 69). Perhaps worst of all, especially for followers of the Christian faith, was the punishment of being denied a proper Christian burial within the consecrated grounds of the church — a punishment which existed around the world right up until the 1960s and 1970s, and which may still exist in some countries even today. In 1968, for example, a United States study of Roman Catholic and Greek Orthodox priests in Los Angeles found that suicide victims were still sometimes — albeit rarely — denied Christian burial (Demopolous 1968, cited in Farberow 1975b, p. 12). Apparently the many sympathetic priests who were burying suicide victims essentially overcame canonical prohibitions against providing Christian burials to suicide victims by accepting that the deaths in question were either 'accidental', 'natural', or the 'irresponsible act of an unsound mind', and hence not a culpable sin (Farberow 1975b, pp. 12–13; Donnelly 1990, p. 9). In the mid-1970s, a similar situation existed in Catholic Italy. In an article examining the psycho-cultural variables in Italian suicide, Farber noted:

> Suicide is more severely disapproved and regarded with more horror than in many other countries. A suicide cannot be buried in sacred ground; the family is grievously shamed. On a practical level, for example, an applicant will be rejected by the police force if there has been a suicide in the family. It is understandable, therefore, that a sympathetic doctor, priest, or police official will collaborate in having a suicide reported as a death from some other cause. Such behaviour is widely accepted in the Italian culture, in which family loyalty outweighs the value of civic responsibility.
>
> (Farber 1975, p. 179)

Significantly, this collaboration has resulted in what Farber describes as a 'severe distortion of official statistics on suicide and the reasons for suicide', with 'mental illness' being cited as the main reason (p. 179). This is because:

> in the eyes of the Church, only suicide by a sane person, who is responsible for his [sic] decision, is a sin. The label of mental illness allows for normal, religious burial and provides a shield for the family.
>
> (Farber 1975, p. 180)

The criminalisation of suicide

Prohibitions against and punishments for suicide were not only enshrined in and made a part of canon law. Under the influence of religious views, sanctions against suicide were also enshrined in (secular) common law (Stengel 1970, p. 70). Opinion varies on when suicide was first deemed a crime in England; some suggest that it could have been as early as the tenth century, while others contend that it was not until as late as 1485 (Stengel 1970, p. 70). By around 1554, however, suicide was definitely 'equated with murder as a criminal offence (*felo de se*) and attempted suicide a misdemeanour' (Stengel 1970, p. 71). Legislation in other European countries also viewed suicide as a crime equivalent to murder, and worse. In 1670, for instance, pressure from the Church saw secular legislation enacted making suicide 'not merely murder but high treason and heresy' (Farberow 1975b, p. 9).

Anti-suicide legislation, like its counterpart in canon law, brought with it inordinate prejudice and penalties against suicide. This resulted in bizarre treatment of those unfortunate enough to be caught surviving a suicide attempt. An example of the gross inhumanity that anti-suicide legislation could both prescribe and enforce can be found in what was probably a public execution held some time during the 1860s in London and reported in the contemporary press. (Note: executions in England were public until 1868 [Carr 1961, p. 336].) Nicholas Ogarev, a Russian exile staying in London at the time, described the incident in a letter to his beloved, Mary Sutherland:

> A man was hanged who had cut his throat, but who had been brought back to life. They hanged him for suicide. The doctor had warned them that it was impossible to hang him as the throat would burst open and he would breathe through the aperture. They did not listen to his advice and hanged their man. The wound in the neck immediately opened and the man came to life again although he was hanged. It took time to convoke the aldermen to decide the question what was to be done. At length the aldermen assembled and bound up the neck below the wound *until he died*. Oh my Mary, what a crazy society and what a stupid civilisation.
>
> (quoted in Carr 1961, p. 336)

This example of gross inhumanity and absurdity — and the 'weird vindictiveness [of] condemning a man to death for the crime of having condemned himself to death' (Alvarez 1980, p. 8) — was sanctioned by both the church and the state. Further, this 'weird vindictiveness', as Alvarez (1980, p. 8) describes it, did not end until almost 100 years after this incident occurred. Stengel (1970, p. 71) comments, for example, that even as late as 1946–55 in England and Wales, 5794 people were brought to trial for attempting suicide. Of these, 5447 were found guilty; and of these, 5138 were fined or put on probation, and 308 were sentenced to prison without the option of a fine or probation

(Stengel 1970, p. 71). The capricious way in which the law was implemented is exemplified by a 1955 English case in which a 'sentence of two years' imprisonment was imposed on a man for trying to commit suicide in prison' (Stengel 1970, p. 71).

As religious and social opponents of suicide began to lose their influence, the old, cruel, prejudicial, religiously-based superstitious attitudes against suicide and attempted suicide gradually changed. Medical dogma replaced religious dogma, and suicide came to be viewed as the act of a 'diseased mind', rather than a diseased ('diabolically possessed') soul. Laws prescribing the desecration of corpses and the confiscation of property were abolished (Farberow 1975b, p. 12). In 1961, England decriminalised suicide (Stengel 1970, p. 71; Glover 1977, p. 170; Browne 1990, p. 10). In Canada, suicide was decriminalised in 1972; and in the United States, while attempted suicide continues to be illegal in some States, suicide itself 'is not illegal in any state' (Browne 1990, p. 10).

Just over 200 years ago, in 1790, France emerged as the first country to repeal its anti-suicide legislation (Stengel 1970, p. 71). Two centuries later, 'both suicide and attempted suicide are not criminal events in any civilised society' (Browne 1990, p. 10).

The medicalisation of suicide

The pressure to reform anti-suicide legislation came mainly from doctors, followed by sympathetic magistrates, and lastly members of the clergy (Stengel 1970, p. 71). However, the medical profession's political lobbying in this instance achieved considerably more than mere legislative reform; it also achieved legitimation of the medicalisation of suicide. In England, for example, soon after the 1961 *Suicide Act* was passed, the Ministry of Health in London advised all doctors and relevant health authorities that:

> attempted suicide was to be regarded as a medical and social problem and that every such case ought to be seen by a psychiatrist.
>
> (Stengel 1970, p. 72)

Whether this 'reform' has been, as Stengel (1970, p. 72) claims, a less 'moralistic and punitive reaction' than that expressed in former legislation remains to be seen. Those who attempt suicide are still frequently the subject of 'negative attitudes', even on the part of attending health care professionals (Baume 1988, p. 44; Donnelly 1990, p. 10; Lindars 1991, p. 30; Knight 1992, p. 260; Bailey 1998); further, they can still find themselves incapacitated involuntarily by the law. As Beauchamp and Childress (1989) point out:

> Although the act of suicide has been decriminalised, a suicide attempt, irrespective of motive, almost universally gives a legal basis for intervention by public officers and for involuntary hospitalisation. In most jurisdictions involuntary hospitalisation is permitted to establish whether a person is mentally ill and a threat to his or her own person or to others.
>
> (Beauchamp and Childress 1989, p. 225)

As well, social and religious taboos still necessitate a degree of secrecy about the circumstances of a person's 'unexpected illness' or 'accidental death'. Donnelly (1990, p. 9) claims that the legacy of past taboos concerning suicide still sees doctors and coroners pressured into using euphemisms when officially certifying or describing the cause of death of a suicide victim. In one notable example, a British report described as 'accidental' the death of a man 'who just happened to shoot himself while cleaning the muzzle of his gun with his tongue!' (Donnelly 1990, p. 9).

The 'medical gaze' of Foucault's (1973) *la clinique* ('the clinic') may well prove ultimately to be a more humane alternative than the punitive gaze proposed by Jeremy Bentham's penitentiary panopticon, thought to be justified as a system of 'moral accounting' (Foucault 1977, p. 250). There is, however, no way of predicting this with certainty — or even agreeing about its possibility or probability (see also Heyd and Bloch 1981, p. 193).

When I think of the many people — young and old, vulnerable and desperate — who have been admitted to hospital following a failed suicide attempt, and in whose care I have been involved (mostly in accident and emergency departments or intensive care units), I am inclined to think that the anti-suicide law reforms we have inherited in the twentieth century have not really changed the status quo. These law reforms have resulted not so much in the *decriminalisation of suicide* as in the *medicalisation of the law*: where once suicide victims and their families were made to account to the law, now they must account to medicine (psychiatry); where once suicide victims were made to prove their innocence before the law, now they must prove their competence; and where once those who attempted suicide were imprisoned for the crime of stealing the gift of life from God, now they are hospitalised involuntarily for violating the gift of civil liberty from society. As Alvarez observes:

> modern suicide has been removed from the vulnerable, volatile world of human beings and hidden safely away in the isolation wards of science. I doubt if Ogarev [the Russian exile] and his ... mistress would have found much in the change to be grateful for.
>
> (Alvarez 1980, p. 31)

Over the past few decades there has been a renewed interest in the moral aspects of suicide, prompted largely by the euthanasia/euthanatic suicide (assisted suicide) debate (discussed in Chapter 12 of this text), and increasing public demand for the 'right to die' to be enshrined in law. This renewed interest has, arguably, marked the beginning of a trend back (rightly or wrongly) to permissive attitudes toward suicide and, more specifically, the socio-cultural normalisation of suicide — particularly in cases of intolerable and intractable suffering (see Figure 13.1). It is no small irony, however, that whereas in the ancient world economic considerations provided the grounds for the legal prohibition of suicide (particularly among the poor and working classes) and for the just punishment of those who attempted suicide, in the modern world economic considerations will probably provide many of the grounds for legalising suicide (and more particularly, euthanasia/ assisted suicide), and for abandoning legal punishments against those who assist people to die before they become — or even *because* they have already become — a financial and material burden, not just on their primary caregivers but on the state (see also Battin 1982, pp. 96–106).

Defining suicide

Before examining some of the moral issues raised by the suicide question, it is necessary first to establish at least a working definition of *suicide* — a term which, incidentally, entered the English language only in 1651 (Wennberg 1989 p. 17; Battin 1982, pp. 22–58).

The word *suicide* comes from the Latinate *sui*, 'of oneself' and *cidium*, 'a slaying' (from *caedere*, 'to kill'). Like many other terms used in moral discourse, *suicide* is not easy to define; indeed, there is no universally agreed definition of what suicide is, or of what criteria should be met in order for an act to count as an instance of suicide. As Margolis (1978, reprinted in Beauchamp and Perlin 1978, pp. 92–3) explains, the 'culturally variable character of suicide' has given rise to many competing views on what it is, with the unhelpful consequence that some acts have been included as suicide and others firmly excluded. This, in turn, has had some important practical consequences, including the difficulty of ascertaining accurate and comparable statistics on the incidence and causes of suicide (Beauchamp 1980, pp. 68–9).

For Wennberg (1989, p. 17), wrestling with the problem of defining *suicide* is to be taught a lesson in 'linguistic humility'. Nevertheless, our commonsense notions of what suicide is, our ability to recognise instances of suicide and to distinguish these from other kinds of death (for example, homicide, patricide, matricide, fratricide, sororicide, infanticide, regicide and euthanasia or euthanatic suicide [Battin 1982, p. 20]), and the very existence of terms in our language which make it possible to speak of suicide as a distinctive kind of death, all provide considerable grounds for optimism about our ability to achieve at least a working — if not a universal — definition of suicide.

According to Stengel, a commonsense notion of suicide can be expressed in the following terms:

> A person, having decided to end his [or her] life, or acting on a sudden impulse to do so, kills himself [or herself], having chosen the most effective methods available and having made sure that nobody interferes. When he [or she] survives he [or she] is said to have failed and the act is called an unsuccessful suicide attempt. Death is the only purpose of this act and therefore the only criterion of success. Failure may be due to any of the following causes: the sense of purpose may not have been strong enough, or the act may have been undertaken half-heartedly because it was not quite genuine; the subject was ignorant of the limitations of the method; or he [or she] was lacking in judgment and determination through mental illness.
>
> (Stengel 1970, p. 77)

This definition is not, of course, without controversy. For example: what constitutes a 'genuine' suicide attempt? and when is a suicide attempt to be regarded as 'half-hearted' as opposed to 'whole-hearted'? (see also Knight 1992). Further, as Stengel himself points out, the definition may not do justice to what has become 'a very common and varied behaviour pattern' (1970, p. 77). Nevertheless, it provides an important insight into the kinds of criteria that should be met in order for an act to count as suicide. One such criterion is that of *intention* — specifically, the *intention to end one's life* (Margolis 1975, reprinted in Beauchamp and Perlin 1978, p. 95). As Beauchamp points out (1980, p. 70), central to what is called the 'prevailing definition' of suicide is the following premise: 'Suicide occurs if and only if there is an intentional termination of one's own life'.

Beauchamp (1980, pp. 73–9) suggests that other criteria should be met in order for an act to count as suicide, including the following:

1. death is chosen voluntarily (that is, is free of coercive or manipulative influences);
2. an active means of death is chosen;

3. death is caused by the person desiring death (one dies by 'one's own hand', as it were);
4. death is *self-regarding* (rather than altruistic or *other-regarding*); and
5. the person seeking death does not have a fatal or terminal illness.

Windt suggests similar criteria of suicide (all of which have been mentioned in the suicide literature). These are:

1. death [must be] caused by the actions or behaviour of the deceased;
2. the deceased wanted, desired, or wished death;
3. the deceased intended, chose, decided or willed to die;
4. the deceased knew that death would result from his [or her] behaviour; and that
5. the deceased was responsible for his [or her] own death.

(Windt 1980, p. 41, tabulations added)

At first glance, these and similar criteria of suicide appear helpful. On closer analysis, however, a number of problems quickly become apparent — not least the problem of so-called 'exceptional cases', and whether the criteria listed are relevant to or can be applied appropriately and meaningfully to these cases. Consider, for example, the cases of people engaging in dangerous and potentially life-threatening ('suicidal') sports (for instance, bungee jumping, mountain climbing, racing car driving, hang gliding); dangerous work activities (being a member of a bomb disposal squad or a combat soldier are paradigm examples here); or other life-threatening activities such as cigarette smoking, eating and drinking excessively, illicit drug taking, and so on (see also Glover 1977, p. 173; Beauchamp and Perlin 1978, p. 88; Beauchamp 1980, p. 72). In all these cases, it is probably true that the people concerned chose the activities in question; were aware of the potential threats the activities posed to their lives and wellbeing; voluntarily engaged in the activities chosen; and, were they to die as a result of engaging in these activities, were 'responsible for their own deaths', insofar as they were witting accomplices to the activities and the associated risks. Further, while the people concerned might not have *intended* their own (accidental) deaths, they nevertheless foresaw their deaths as a possibility associated with the risky activities they had engaged in, and thereby, ipso facto, can be said to have intended their own demise. Given the criteria for suicide outlined above, it seems we are committed to accepting that people who die as a result of their deliberately engaging in dangerous sporting activities, work activities or lifestyles have, in essence, suicided. Yet, this does not seem to accord with our intuitions on the matter — nor does it sit comfortably with what we would perhaps ordinarily regard as suicide. Let us examine another example to see if this will clarify the matter.

In 1982, Barney Clark, aged 62, became the first human being to receive an artificial (mechanical) heart (Beauchamp and Childress 1989, p. 222). Recognising that this medical experiment had the potential to make Barney Clark's life burdensome, his doctor, Willem Kolf, gave him a key that could be used to turn off the compressor sustaining the artificial heart's action. Defending his decision to supply this key, Dr Kolff argued that if Barney Clark:

> suffers and feels it isn't worth it any more, he has a key that he can apply ... I think it is entirely legitimate that this man whose life has been extended should have the right to cut it off if he doesn't want it, if life ceases to be enjoyable.

(cited in Beauchamp and Childress 1989, p. 223)

The conceptual dilemma which arises here is this: if Barney Clark had chosen to use the key he had been given, and had turned off the compressor driving his artificial heart, which of the following statements would have been the most accurate description of his action and the cause of his death:

1. forgoing extraordinary means of life-sustaining treatment;
2. withdrawing from an experiment;
3. letting nature take its course;
4. natural death;
5. euthanasia;
6. suicide?

To complicate the issue, as Beauchamp and Childress point out:

> If Clark had refused to accept the artificial heart in the first place, few would have characterised his act as one of suicide, because of his overall condition and the experimental nature of the artificial heart, but if he had shot himself while on the artificial heart, it would have been difficult to avoid characterising the act as one of suicide.
>
> (Beauchamp and Childress 1989, p. 223)

And, to complicate the issue still further, what if Barney Clark had consented to receiving the heart in the belief that the risks associated with the experiment were so great that a hastened death would be assured? Could this be classified as a kind of suicide?

Part of the difficulty in sorting out the conceptual confusion surrounding the development of an adequate definition of and criteria for suicide can be linked to the lingering legacy of varying socio-cultural historical and religious taboos against suicide. Beauchamp and Childress (1989, p. 223) suggest, for example, that we often shield acts of which we approve (or at least acts of which we do not disapprove) from the stigmatising label of 'suicide' — preferring instead to use terms that are more socially acceptable, such as 'euthanasia' or 'withdrawing extraordinary life-saving treatment', and similar notions. If this is correct, it is ironic, considering that the term 'suicide' was first adopted in the seventeenth century as a more 'acceptable' alternative to the then contemporary usages 'self-murder' and 'self-slaughter', which were regarded by more liberal-minded people of the day as having unacceptably negative connotations (Battin 1982, pp. 22, 58).

In the light of these considerations, perhaps an important first step in developing a workable definition of and criteria for suicide is to demystify suicide, and to strip it of the taboos and stigmatisations which still seem to linger around it — and which may encourage people to be less than intellectually honest when speaking of its incidence and cause. A second and related step is to modify the negatively connoted language that tends to be used in referring to and discussing suicide. In this instance, the problem of language is highly significant, and should not be underestimated. As Wennberg explains:

> 'suicide' is not a neutrally descriptive term like 'cat', 'car', or 'flower'. Rather, it carries with it a strong negative connotation, especially when it is part of the phrase 'commit suicide'. For one typically does not *commit* X where X is either something approved or something of neutral standing (cf. 'commit murder', 'commit a felony', 'commit a crime', 'commit adultery', 'commit a sin', 'commit treason', 'commit a *faux pas*', etc.).
>
> (Wennberg 1989, p. 17)

The lesson here is important and obvious: the use of the phrase 'committed suicide' (as opposed to using the term *suicided*) is misleading and unhelpful — not least because it seems to imply the commission of a crime, or even a sin, when clearly there has been none.

A third and final step toward developing a working definition of and criteria for suicide is to reinstate the authority of our own ordinary commonsense experience of the world, and our collective experience-based knowledge of what is and is not an act of suicide or attempted suicide. One reason for this is that, in the ultimate analysis, the distinction between suicide and other types of death (for example, euthanasia) may rest not on sophisticated philosophical criteria, but on our fine intuitions informed by life-experience. I suspect, however, that in the main, conceptual clarity in regard to what is and is not an act of suicide will rest on something far more substantial than abstract criteria or even well informed intuition. Rather, the matter will be decided by appealing to:

1. the known intentions and motivations of the person who has died (for instance, whether the death was pursued as 'an alleged solution for the ills of dying' [euthanasia], or pursued as an 'alleged' cure for the ills of living [suicide] [Donnelly 1990, p. 9]);
2. the context in which the person died;
3. whether the person who died genuinely believed there was no other alternative besides death in order to alleviate his or her suffering, or to transcend the life circumstances which for him or her had become unbearable.

The problem remains, however, that ascertaining these things may be just as difficult as establishing reliable criteria for suicide. Nevertheless, it is important that suicide be defined. One reason for this is that without an adequate definition of suicide it will remain extremely difficult to assess accurately the incidence, cause and appropriate means of preventing suicide. It will also be difficult to eradicate the spurious distinction which is sometimes drawn between 'genuine' and 'non-genuine' suicide attempts, with the tragic consequence that some who are suffering and needing help will be dismissed as malingerers, and worse, as not suffering or needing help at all.

(To advance understanding on the raw suffering and despair that suicidal people experience, see in particular: Williams [1997] *Cry of pain: understanding suicide and self-harm*; Heckler [1994] *Waking up alive: the descent to suicide and return to life*; and Knight's [1992] discussion on the suffering of suicide.)

Finally, without an adequate definition of suicide it will make it difficult to engage in substantive moral debate on the ethical aspects of suicide, and to respond effectively and appropriately to the many moral problems raised by the suicide question, some of which are considered below.

Before continuing, however, a brief clarification is required on the working definitions of the terms 'suicide' and 'parasuicide' to be used in the remainder of this chapter, and on the distinction which might otherwise be drawn between 'suicide' (as presently being considered in this chapter) and 'euthanasia' (as considered in the previous chapter).

Although there is no universally agreed definition of suicide, and, as shown, the term itself is difficult to define (see also Soubrier 1993), suicide is generally recognised as being one of the five medical-legal classifications of modes of death, which are taken to include (in addition to suicidal death): accidental, natural, homicidal, and undetermined death (Colt 1991, pp. 263–4). Furthermore, while acknowledging the many difficulties associated with formulating a precise and universally agreed definition of suicide, there is a strong sense in which suicide (at least in the Western world) can be meaningfully understood as:

> a conscious act of self-induced annihilation, best understood as a multidimensional malaise in a needful individual who defines an issue for which the suicide is perceived as the best solution.
>
> (Shneidman 1985, p. 203)

A more elaborate explication of this view is as follows (advanced by Edwin Shneidman, popularly regarded as the 'father' of contemporary suicidology [Leenaars 1993, p. xi]):

> My principal assertion about suicide has two branches. The first is that suicide is a multifaceted event and that biological, cultural, sociological, interpersonal, intrapsychic, logical, conscious and unconscious, and philosophical elements are present, in various degrees, in each suicide event.
>
> The second branch of my assertion is that, in the distillation of each suicide event, its essential element is a *psychological* one; that is to say, each suicidal drama occurs in the *mind* of a unique individual. Suicide is purposive. Its purpose is to respond to or redress certain psychological needs. There are many pointless deaths but there are no needless suicides. Suicide is a concatenated, complicated, multidimensional, conscious and unconscious 'choice' of the best possible practical solution to a perceived problem, dilemma, impasse, crisis, or desperation.
>
> (Shneidman 1993, p. 3)

Parasuicide (a term which came into usage in the late 1960s in an attempt to overcome the confusion associated with using the term 'attempted suicide [see Kreitman 1969; Williams 1997, p. 68]) can, in turn, be defined as:

> An act with non-fatal outcome, in which an individual deliberately initiates a non-habitual behaviour that, without intervention from others, will cause self-harm, or deliberately ingests a substance in excess of the prescribed or generally recognised therapeutic dosage, and which is aimed at realising changes which the subject desired via the actual or expected physical consequences.
>
> (Williams 1997, p. 69)

For the purposes of this discussion, both suicide and parasuicide are taken here as being the 'unequivocal expression of raw suffering' (and it might be added 'psychache' [Shneidman 1993]) of individuals — a suffering from which, for a variety of reasons (not always known or understood by others), these individuals have not been able to secure relief (Heckler 1994, p. xxiv). Suicide ideation (suicidal thoughts) and suicidal behaviour are also taken here as being 'the result of extreme and unusual human predicaments' which require our deepest and most empathetic understanding (Heckler 1994, p. xxv), not our derision as has so frequently been the case (see Bailey 1994, 1998).

Suicide, as being considered in this chapter, is taken here as referring to a different kind of death that might otherwise be brought about by voluntary active euthanasia or physician-assisted suicide. While euthanasia, physician-assisted suicide and 'unassisted' suicide (the topic of this chapter) share many features in common, as we will go on to see, there are also some significant differences between them. One such difference was captured recently by the following insightful comments made in class by an on-site overseas student undertaking a Bachelor of Nursing (Conversion) degree at RMIT University in Melbourne, Australia:

> As I see it, in the case of euthanasia/assisted suicide, the person wants to live, but *cannot* (and it is too hard to die); whereas in the case of 'suicide proper', the person can live, yet *does not* want to (it is too hard to live).
>
> (Su Chia Hsian, personal communication)

Other differences will become more apparent as the discussion in this chapter is advanced. One key difference, however, warrants mention here: whereas euthanasia and physician-assisted suicide tends to be conducted in the context of a breakdown in physical health and wellbeing, suicide (as being considered here) tends to occur in the context of a breakdown in mental health and wellbeing viz. is linked in important ways to a lethal combination of the psychogenic distress states of depression, hopelessness, despair, and apathy (Williams 1997; Heckler 1994; Lester and Tallmer 1994; Remafedi 1994a; Shneidman 1993; Leenaars 1993; Colt 1991).

Suicide: some moral considerations

As discussed earlier under the subheading 'Socio-cultural attitudes to suicide: a brief historical overview', the Judaeo-Christian traditions have, for the most part, regarded suicide as the gravest sin imaginable, and as constituting the most serious violation of one's duties to oneself, to others and to God. These views have been extremely influential and, not surprisingly, the subject of much philosophical debate. Today, however, as Knight (1992, p. 262) correctly points out, 'religiously speaking, the notion of suicide as an unforgivable sin has few, if any, defenders in contemporary moral philosophy'. Further, unlike the days when religious prohibition saw suicide condemned as a grossly immoral act, it is difficult today to find tenable moral arguments against the suicide of people who are able to choose autonomously to end their own lives (Knight 1992, p. 262). Nevertheless, a number of troubling questions remain about the ethics or morality of suicide, such as: Is there a right to suicide? If so, what conditions must be satisfied before this right can be claimed? What are the obligations of others in regard to those contemplating or attempting suicide? Is there a duty to prevent suicide? If so, under what conditions should a suicide be prevented? It is to briefly answering these questions that the remainder of this discussion now turns.

Autonomy and the right to suicide

Fundamental to Western moral thinking is the principle of autonomy. As discussed in Chapter 4 of this text, the moral principle of autonomy prescribes that a person's considered choices should be respected — even if others disagree with them or regard them as foolish — provided they do not interfere with or harm the significant moral interests of others. If we accept this principle, we must also accept that people who choose autonomously to suicide are entitled to have their choices respected, and further, that it would be morally indefensible to prevent these people from exercising their choices. By this view, as Beauchamp explains:

If people are autonomous, then they have the right to be left alone and to do with their lives as they wish, so long as they are sufficiently free of responsibilities to others. From this perspective, the intervention in the life of a suicide is simply an unjust deprivation of liberty.

(Beauchamp 1980, p. 100)

Jonathan Glover argues along similar lines, explaining that once it is admitted that suicide need not always be regarded as an 'irrational symptom of mental disturbance' (see also Wennberg 1989, p. 39), then:

[it] is a matter for each person's free choice: other people should have nothing to say about it, and the question for someone contemplating it is simply one of whether his [or her] future life will be worth living.

(Glover 1977, p. 171)

It is far from certain, however, that people contemplating or attempting suicide are, in fact, entitled to be 'left alone and to do with their lives as they wish' (Beauchamp 1980, p. 100), or that 'other people should have nothing to say about it' (Glover 1977, p. 171). There are a number of reasons for this. First, an act of suicide is never without moral consequences: not only does it have an impact on the significant moral interests of the person suiciding, but it can significantly affect the important moral interests of others (as stated earlier, between six and ten people can be directly and significantly affected by the suicide of another). As experience tells us, suicide can shatter, injure and destroy the lives of other people; it can also cause substantial loss to society (see also Battin 1982). Where suicides do affect the significant moral interests of others, there are at least prima facie grounds for justifying paternalistic intervention to prevent those suicides occurring. As well as this, where other people's significant moral interests are at stake, there may even be an obligation on the part of people contemplating suicide not to proceed with planned actions aimed at ending their own lives (Brandt 1978, p. 128) — although it is an open question just how realistic this demand is in the case of people suffering severe psychological distress.

In the light of these circumstances, it is evident that claims to autonomy *alone* are not sufficient to justify an unequivocal acceptance of a person's decision to suicide, or to justify non-intervention or 'non-postvention' (counselling and therapy after a suicide attempt [Battin 1982, p. 16]) in the case of contemplated or attempted suicide. Of course, there is always the possibility that the concerns or interests of others may not be strong enough to override a person's autonomous choice to suicide. This, however, is something which must be determined by careful evaluation and a 'balancing of considerations' of all the moral interests involved (Beauchamp and Perlin 1978, p. 91), not just by an uncritical deontological acceptance of the moral principle of autonomy. Such a calculation might even show that a contemplated suicide, once carried out, should indeed be permitted in the interests of others. For example, the suicide of a long-term abusing spouse might be shown to be more permissible morally than the homicide of his abused wife and children. Whether this would really be a morally desirable outcome, however, is a contentious point and unfortunately one which is beyond the scope of this work to address.

A second reason why it is not clear that people contemplating or attempting suicide should not have their choices interfered with is that the *quality* of the autonomy behind the choice may not be optimal. As discussed in Chapter 4 of this text, as a *concept* (to be distinguished here from a *principle*), autonomy refers to a person's independent and self-contained ability to decide. At issue in the case of suicide is the question of whether a person contemplating suicide is really capable of making the evaluative, deliberative and reflective choices that are fundamental to a 'rational' and autonomous decision to suicide. While it is true that even so-called 'incompetent' people are still capable of making self-interested choices (see, for example, the discussion on competency in Chapter 8 of this text), the extent to which the choices of these people should be respected is not something that can be decided solely on the basis of the demands prescribed by the moral principle of autonomy; there are other moral considerations that need to be taken into account — including the moral demand to prevent otherwise avoidable harm to people, which a suicide-death could cause.

The issue of the quality of a suicidal person's autonomous choice to kill himself or herself is an important one and, even when considered from a clinical as opposed to a philosophical perspective, has an important bearing on deciding the ethical acceptability of paternalistic interventions aimed at preventing people from suiciding.

It has been suggested that depression 'is a substantial part of the picture of at least 50 per cent of suicides' (Knight 1992, pp. 249–50). Research in the United Kingdom, however, has shown that *70 per cent* of suicides involve people suffering from major depression (Williams 1997, p. 51). While depression alone may not result in suicide, when it is coupled with abiding and intolerable feelings of hopelessness about the future, despair and apathy, the risk of suicide is extremely high (Knight 1992, p. 250, Heckler 1994; Williams 1997). Of importance to the discussion at this point is the consideration that feelings of depression, hopelessness, apathy and despair can have a significant and far-reaching impact on a person's ability to make 'truly' autonomous choices. As has long been recognised in the bioethics literature, these feelings can:

- restrict people's abilities to evaluate and calculate correctly the range of possibilities and probabilities available when planning and making judgments about their lives and future prospects (Brandt 1978, p. 131; Beauchamp 1980, p. 101);
- skew calculations of the probable harms and benefits that may flow from suicide (as Beauchamp [1980, p. 101] points out, 'without depression, persons might make quite different calculations even when their situation is dire');
- result in suicidal people overestimating the magnitude and insolubility of their problems (Knight 1992, p. 266);
- result in impulsive and imprudent choices which might otherwise not have been made (Heyd and Bloch 1981, p. 187).

In short, feelings of depression, hopelessness, apathy and despair can undermine in very significant ways a person's ability to make sound autonomous choices. The question remains, however, of whether these feelings and a possible associated diminution in the ability to make sound autonomous choices are of a nature that justifies paternalistic intervention to prevent a person suiciding — including using invasive procedures to resuscitate someone who has attempted suicide. Or would such intervention — no matter how benevolent — still constitute an unacceptable violation of the moral principle of autonomy?

The short answer to these questions is that intervention may not only be justified, but may even be required, in the interests of both promoting a person's autonomy and saving a worthwhile life. On this point, Jonathan Glover explains:

> Where we think someone bent on suicide has a life worth living, it is always legitimate to reason with him [or her] and to try and persuade him [or her] to stand back and think again. There is no case against reasoning, as it in no way encroaches on the person's autonomy. There is a strong case in its favour, as where it succeeds it will prevent the loss of a worthwhile life. (If the person's life turns out not be worthwhile, he [or she] can always change his [or her] mind again.) And if persuasion fails, the outcome is no worse than it would otherwise have been.
>
> (Glover 1977, pp. 176–7)

Glover goes on to contend that where suicidal tendencies are the product of temporary depressive mood-swings — for instance, where the person 'alternates between very much wanting to go on living and moods of suicidal depression' — then intervention aimed at overriding a decision to suicide 'is less disrespectful of autonomy than overriding a preference that plays a stable role in a person's outlook' (p. 178). If, for example, a person repeatedly and persistently attempts suicide, and the underlying preference (that is, to die) informing these attempts remains constant, then the onus is on would-be 'rescuers' or interveners to reconsider their own judgments about whether the life of the person attempting suicide is, in fact, worthwhile and worth living, or whether they have been mistaken in their views. Unpleasant as it may be, the demand in the latter instance may be an overriding one in favour of *not* intervening to save the person's life (Glover 1977, p. 178). Before this position is accepted, however, there are at least prima facie grounds for asserting that the following five conditions must be met:

1. that the decision to suicide is based on a realistic assessment of the life-circumstances or situation at hand (Motto 1983, pp. 443–6; Knight 1992, p. 254);
2. that the person contemplating suicide has made an 'exhaustive examination' of all available options and has taken into account the 'various possible "errors" and [made] appropriate rectifications of his [or her] initial evaluation' (Brandt 1978, p. 132);
3. that the thought processes used in reaching the decision to suicide have not been impaired by severe emotional distress, feelings of hopelessness and despair, mental illness or the adverse side-effects of drugs (Knight 1992, p. 254);
4. that the degree of ambivalence between wanting to live and wanting to die is minimal (Motto 1983, pp. 443–6; Glover 1977, p. 178; Donnelly 1990, p.8); and
5. that the desire and motivation to suicide is of a nature that 'uninvolved observers from their community or social group [would find] understandable' (Knight 1992, p. 254).

While the satisfaction of these criteria may not always result in the prevention of morally undesirable consequences in situations involving people wanting to suicide, it may nevertheless result in more appropriate assessments of when it is right and when it is not right to paternalistically override a person's autonomous choice to suicide.

One problem which emerges here, however, is that, even if these criteria are not satisfied, does that necessarily justify paternalistic intervention to prevent a person suiciding? What if the suicidal person in question is in a state of intolerable suffering as in the *Chabot case* discussed in the previous chapter (see

Knight 1992; Slater 1980)? Here the additional question arises: Can those who are suffering intolerably and intractably (whether on account of physical or mental illness or some other state of physical or psychogenic distress) be expected decently to go on living? Or should people in these situations be released from the 'obligation to live' — if, indeed, it is an obligation — irrespective of their ability to decide autonomously what is in their own best interests? Are others entitled morally to force a person to go on living a life characterised by excruciating feelings of depression, hopelessness, apathy, despair and a sense that life has lost all meaning and purpose?

It is not unreasonable to hold that a person in this state would prefer death to life. As Glover points out:

> Most of us prefer to be anaesthetised for a painful operation. If most of my life were to be on that level, I might opt for a permanent anaesthesia, or death.

> (Glover 1977, p. 174)

Margolis (1978, p. 96) argues, however, that while prolonged anaesthesia may indeed be 'prudentially preferable to enduring pain', the desire to reduce pain in itself 'cannot justify suicide to end pain as a decision of a prudential sort'. One reason for this is that enduring even intolerable pain may, in the ultimate analysis, still be preferable to no life at all (Margolis 1978, p. 96; see also Glover 1977, p. 174). Another reason is that to allow suicide as a means of alleviating suffering is to compound the hopelessness underpinning the suffering of suicide; it is also to abandon as hopeless those who have abandoned themselves as hopeless, and thereby to violate a fundamental professional ethic of care and responsibility to aid the distressed (see also Murphy 1983, p. 442).

If suicide is viewed as a 'violent statement about human connections, broken and maintained' (Lifton 1979, p. 239), and not simply as a matter of exercising an autonomous choice (as Hauerwas [1986, p. 107] reminds us, 'life has a purpose beyond simply being autonomous'), perhaps our moral obligations toward those contemplating or attempting suicide will become clearer. In particular, as Knight's (1992) discussion on the suffering of suicide clarifies, there needs to be a much greater understanding of the excruciating sense of hopelessness and despair that underlies and motivates many a decision to suicide. Drawing on the remarkable work by Heckler (1994), there also needs to be a much greater appreciation by others that behind every suicide and parasuicide is a life story of 'overwhelming circumstances'. As Stubbs (1994, p. xii) reminds us, in the Foreword to Heckler's insightful study *Waking up alive: the descent to suicide and return to life*:

> Suicide is caused by feelings not by facts — a similar event may be borne by one person and may lead another to suicide or attempted suicide. Events, feelings and experiences add strands to a net that can drag you under. The final straw can be the weight of gossamer but the combined effect can be devastating. Or the final straw can weigh like an iron girder ... Unless we have stood on the edge of the precipice of our own life, we can only begin to grasp how it feels.

Once these and related considerations are understood, it may become clearer that the way to remedy the suffering underlying a decision to suicide is not to do away with the sufferer, but to do away with the sense of hopelessness and despair fuelling the suffering. This, however, requires great compassion, empathy and commitment on the part of those intervening and preventing people suiciding. As Knight puts it:

> Intervention in suicide involves walking down that 'dark road' and immersing oneself into that world in which the suicidal person is living. One soon discovers that most suicidal persons have a predisposition to overestimate the magnitude and insolubility of their problems. Coupled with this, as has been emphasised by those 'who have been there', is an exaggerated negative view of the outside world, of themselves, and of the future. An awareness of what and how a suicidal person is thinking and feeling may lead those intervening to see quickly that the suicidal person's plight has a way out, and soon hope begins to dawn.
>
> (Knight 1992, p. 266)

Suicide prevention: some further considerations

It is probably true that most health care professionals feel obliged to:

- try and persuade people contemplating suicide to change their minds;
- counsel those who have lost their sense of hope, purpose and meaning in life, in order to modify their perceptions and regain a more optimistic outlook on the future;
- resuscitate people who have attempted suicide and who are on the brink of death; and
- treat the injuries of people whose suicide attempts have failed.

Whether health care professionals do, in fact, have these obligations may, in the end, be a matter to be decided not by moral theory, or even by law, but by empathy, compassion, kindness and wisdom, informed by a profound understanding of human vulnerability and suffering, together with a commitment to take each case on its own unique and individual merit (see, in particular, the life stories presented in Heckler [1994]). Either way, it is important not to forget that our obligation to render aid to a person contemplating or attempting suicide is as strong as it would be to aid any person in distress (Brandt 1980, pp. 129–31), and that this may require more than merely protecting a person's autonomy; it may require the more substantive task of protecting a person's genuine human welfare, and restoring in them a sense of hope that, often due to circumstances quite beyond their control, has abandoned them.

Conclusion

Some may find it attractive to view suicide as the manifestation of a mental illness, and hence something that is 'irrational' and 'irresponsible' and ipso facto quite beyond the realms of moral inquiry (see, for example, Stengel 1970, p. 58; Margolis 1978, p. 96; Heyd and Bloch 1981, pp. 193–4; Beauchamp and Childress 1989, p. 224; Wennberg 1989, p. 18). This discussion has shown, however, that even if suicide is the product of mental illness or extreme emotional distress, depression, or other psychogenic pain states, it still has a profound moral dimension, and still requires those involved in suicide prevention and intervention to justify their views and actions, and not to merely assume that these are in themselves morally correct just because they have as their end the preservation of life or the maximisation of autonomy.

Suicide and parasuicide is an issue of importance and concern to *all* nurses, not just to those working in the area of mental health. How well nurses and others respond to the moral issues raised depends, however, on a variety of factors — including the success with which suicide is stripped of the taboos which still surround it, and the degree to which suicide is demystified as a desperate act aimed at transcending a situation which a distressed person has come to perceive as hopeless (Knight 1992; Heckler 1994; Williams 1997).

Some years ago I was involved in the care of a woman who had attempted suicide by pouring a can of petrol over herself and setting fire to it. She arrived in casualty with 100 per cent burns to her body. Incredibly, despite the horrendous injuries her body had sustained, her eyes were unharmed. The extent of her burns made it impossible to insert an intravenous line in the usual way, and a cut-down (which involves a surgical incision to expose a deeply situated vein) had to be performed. I remember the doctor looking at me while he was performing the cut-down, and gasping in horror as the woman's burnt flesh parted in his hands. Nevertheless, this compassionate man succeeded in inserting the intravenous line, and consoled the woman as he did so. As we all worked diligently to retrieve this injured life, the woman looked on smiling, and reassuring us all with the words, 'Don't worry dears, I will be all right'. I remember looking up at this woman and, on observing her terrible injuries, thinking how desperate she must have been to have engaged in such an act. She, however, looked back at me with eyes that were clear and shining, and, bizarre as this whole scene was, I could see that she had found incredible peace within herself. The image of her burnt and tortured body did not sit well with the peace expressed in her eyes, but I knew that she had achieved her goal, and that it would be only a matter of time before she would be released from the suffering that had motivated her to undertake such a desperate act. Her death a day or two later was no surprise. Yet I still cannot help thinking that this woman paid a terrible price for the peace she eventually found in death, and could not find in life.

During the same year, I was involved in the care of a man who had also attempted suicide, in this instance by placing the muzzle of a gun in his mouth and shooting himself. He failed in his attempt to kill himself, however, and succeeded only in destroying one side of his face. After receiving plastic surgery to repair the serious gunshot wound sustained, he was admitted to intensive care. Unlike the woman who had set fire to herself, however, he was not at peace within himself. As he lay corpse-like on his bed, I remember noting that his eyes were like the eyes of a dead man — fully dilated, dull, and unresponsive to light. It was as though his soul had died, and nothing mattered any more. Once, when his plastic surgeon visited to check his wounds, the man handed the doctor a note. Written on the note were the words: 'Dear Dr X — did you do this [the surgical repair] for your sake or mine?'. Understandably, this very compassionate and gentle surgeon was devastated. Shortly after being transferred out of the intensive care unit to a general ward, the man climbed out through a toilet window and plunged to his death several storeys below. Many of the staff were left feeling that they had failed this man. The circumstances motivating his initial suicidal attempt had not seemed insurmountable to them, and they sincerely believed he was 'better'. But he was not getting better, and eventually he too achieved his goal of death. As I recall the case of this desperate and hopeless man, I cannot forget the costly suffering and distress of those he left behind — especially his wife and young children. How different things would have been if he, like the people caring for and about him, could have perceived that his problems were not as overwhelming as he thought, and that it was not necessary to take the desperate action that he ultimately took. To this day, I am reminded by this case of the importance of never underestimating the capacity of human beings to feel deeply and to suffer profoundly on account of things which seem (though they may not necessarily be) insurmountable, and of how feelings of desperation and hopelessness associated with problems perceived as insurmountable can so easily override the desire to go on living.[2]

In June of 1993, a Victorian coroner's court was reported to have found that the suicide of five severely depressed patients at Larundel Hospital was, among other things, a regrettable consequence of a well intended but nevertheless misguided priority being given to upholding patients' rights to confidentiality (i.e. the 'right' not to be observed too closely) at the expense of patient care. Further, there had been a less than optimal level of commitment to 'patient-centred *continuity of care* rather than changes in treating medical personnel due to patient progress' (Pegler 1993, p. 26, emphasis added). The coroner is reported to have also found that 'the most important issue arising from the inquests was family and carer involvement in treatment', and that 'a policy needed to be developed on the conflict between patient rights and patient care' (Pegler 1993, p. 26).

Whether matters such as these can — or, indeed, should — be the subject of institutional policy is a debatable point. As experience tells us, even the very best of policies may still fail to prevent this kind of situation from occurring. Nevertheless, it is clear that there is room for improvement in the care and treatment of those contemplating or attempting suicide, and, more importantly, in understanding the moral issues involved in caring for those who, for whatever reason, are unable to care about themselves. It is also clear that, in securing these improvements, nurses must ensure that, in attempting to uphold the moral rights of their emotionally distressed, severely depressed and mentally unwell patients, they do not lose sight of the importance of also protecting and promoting their patients' *welfare and wellbeing* — something which may not always be secured by paying homage to abstract moral rights and principles. By doing this, nurses, and others involved in caring for people who are contemplating suicide or who have already attempted suicide, may well succeed in helping to prevent and remedy the terrible sufferings and tragedies that have become so characteristic of the whole phenomenon of suicide in our community and in the world.

---

2. Names and details of times and places have been suppressed, but these are true stories that reflect the experience of all nurses everywhere.

Chapter 14

Quality of life, 'Not For Treatment' and 'Not For Resuscitation' directives

Introduction

Our discussion on matters of life and death would not be complete without some consideration being given to three additional ethical issues which, in recent years, have assumed increasing importance for nurses: quality of life, 'Not For Treatment' (NFT) directives and 'Not For Resuscitation' (NFR) directives. As with abortion, euthanasia and suicide, unless nurses are well informed about the nature and moral implications of the issues of quality of life, Not For Treatment (NFT) directives and Not For Resuscitation (NFR) directives, they will not be in a good position from which to contribute to community and professional debate about them. It is to examining these three issues and their moral implications for nurses and nursing practice that this chapter now turns.

Quality of life[1]

The notion of quality of life is a popular one; many see it as a highly important if not central consideration when making life and death decisions. Like other terms and concepts in the health care repertoire, however, the notion of quality of life is not entirely unproblematic, and is vulnerable to criticism. Part of the difficulty here is that 'quality of life' is not a term that can be easily defined. As Welch-McCaffrey (1985, p. 151) correctly points out: 'Quality of life is not a term that has unequivocal meaning nor is it unambiguously determinable in any given case'.

Despite the difficulties associated with trying to define quality of life, nurses and allied health professionals continue to use the term as if it has an objective and clear-cut commonsense meaning, and, further, they also take it as implying binding prescriptions and proscriptions in relation to how a given individual

---

1. An earlier version of the discussion on 'Quality of life' was included in a paper entitled: 'Ethical issues for the health professional when planning for rehabilitation of patients with advanced cancer', presented at the seminar: *Rehabilitation in patients with advanced cancer — a contradiction in terms?* organised by the College of Nursing, Australia in conjunction with the Victoria Association of Hospice Care Programs, Melbourne, 17 October 1988. This segment has been revised for publication in this text.

human life ought and ought not to be regarded. What is troubling about this is that people (particularly those with significant life-threatening diseases) may find themselves being subjected to a quality of life view which is not only inappropriate for them, but also woefully inadequate in terms of guiding the choices which are critical to both the realisation and the maximisation of their significant moral interests. This raises two very important questions. First, if it is possible to define quality of life, how should it be defined? Second, in what way and to what extent ought a given quality of life view influence decision-making in health care domains?

Defining quality of life

The question of how to define quality of life is complex and difficult, and might never find a wholly satisfactory answer. Nevertheless, the question deserves serious attention by nurses. It is hoped that the comments given in this chapter will help to shed some light on how the issue might be meaningfully approached.

In examining discussions in both nursing and bioethical literature, it quickly becomes evident that there are as many different interpretations of 'quality of life' as there are authors. It also quickly becomes evident that different authors have quite different views on how and the extent to which quality of life considerations should be permitted to influence therapeutic decision-making. Consider the examples which follow. Foltz (1987) argues that an individual's quality of life is interdependent with that individual's self-concept. Describing the influence that cancer and cancer treatment can have on a person's self-concept (taken here as comprising four fundamental components, notably the body self, the interpersonal self, the achievement self and the identification self), Foltz goes on to suggest that, where an individual's self-concept is diminished or undermined, so too is that individual's quality of life. She concludes that one way of enhancing quality of life is to intervene in a way that bolsters or promotes self-concept, whichever aspect (or aspects) of it is warranting attention.

Germino (1987) takes a slightly different view. She argues that quality of life is linked in an important way to symptom distress. She goes on to suggest that improving quality of life thus becomes very much a matter of improving symptom control. Germino also points out that improved symptom control stands to improve not only quality of life but also its quantity or survival (Germino 1987, p. 300). Another important point which Germino makes is that a balance needs to be achieved between what a *health professional* might regard as 'effective and reasonable' in terms of symptom management, and what the *patient* might regard as being so. She gives the example of how a patient and a nurse might agree that comfort is a mutual goal, but that 'the meaning of comfort to each and the cost each is willing to pay may differ' (Germino 1987, p. 300). She writes:

> For instance, decreasing mental alertness or awake time to achieve total freedom from pain may not be agreeable to the patient while the nurse sees it as worthwhile ... Quality of life [thus] becomes a personal decision with choices to be made about the extent to which symptom distress outweighs the actual or potential distress of unmet or frustrated needs.
>
> (Germino 1987, p. 300)

Other authors, however, seek to define quality of life in quite different terms. Fredette and Beattie (1986, p. 315), for example, in researching the need for patient education programs to address the informational and emotional concerns of cancer patients and their families, found 'unexpectedly' that *hope* emerged as an important measure of quality of life. Graham and Longman (1987, p. 339), on the other hand, viewed quality of life more in terms of 'the degree of satisfaction with present life circumstances, as perceived by the patient'.

Still other authors define quality of life in quite different terms again; for example, as 'a combination of minimal anxiety, a purpose in life, and adequate self-esteem' (Germino 1987, p. 299); as a 'complex of physical function, personal attitudes, perceived wellbeing, and support' (Germino 1987, p. 299); as a 'perceived control over one's life' (Graham and Longman 1987, p. 339); or, more simply, as a person's ability to lead an 'independent and minimally satisfying' life (Kuhse 1987, p. 6).

In 1998, a class of students undertaking the Bachelor of Nursing (Conversion) course at RMIT University, Melbourne, identified the following characteristics of what they would regard as constituting a 'quality life':

- enjoyment and being happy, further defined as:
  - feeling contented;
  - having no worries;
  - being stress free;
  - feeling fulfilled;
- being healthy (and not having to suffer in any way);
- being valued and respected;
- having freedom and independence (being self-determining);
- being able to function effectively;
- actual achievement and/or being able to achieve important goals;
- having the love of family and friends.

(In other classes taught over the past five years, it has become immediately apparent that there exist as many conceptualisations and views on what constitutes a 'quality of life' as there are people participating in the discussion.)

There are many more views which could be considered here, but these few examples show the difficulties likely to be encountered in attempting to formulate a universal view on how quality of life should be defined and used to guide important life and death decisions in health care domains. Against this backdrop, it is probably reasonable to conclude that the notion 'quality of life' essentially defies precise definition, or at least a definition which could be regarded as being universally acceptable. Even so, as Downie and Calman (1987) argue:

> Most ... would agree that quality of life relates to the individual person, that it is best perceived by that person, that conceptions of it change with time, and that it must be related to all aspects of life.
>
> (Downie and Calman 1987, p. 190)

The message that quality of life is a concept which lends itself overwhelmingly to subjective interpretation is an important one. However, whether given views are in themselves reliable in terms of their ability to guide important moral choices in health care domains is quite another question, and one which is now briefly addressed.

In reaching a position on how best to interpret and use the term quality of life, it is important first to carefully distinguish the different philosophical senses in which the term might be meaningfully employed. Reich (1978), for example, argues that 'quality of life' may be used in at least three different ways: *descriptively, evaluatively*, and/or *prescriptively* (that is, morally).

Reich (1978, p. 830) explains that where the term quality of life is used as a descriptive statement, an observation is being made merely about the properties or characteristics of a human individual. In other words, quality of life in this sense simply refers to an *observable* and *'objective' description* about certain features or traits a person might have, and thus is morally neutral. An example of a descriptive quality of life statement would be: 'this person has pain', or 'this person has lost her or his functional ability', or 'this person is totally dependent on others for care'. By this view, to say someone has lost quality of life would be to say nothing more than that she or he has lost a particular property or characteristic (or set of characteristics) of life, not the value of life itself.

Quality of life in the evaluative sense, however, is quite different. Here a quality of life statement would express that 'some value or worth is attached to the characteristic of a given individual or to a kind of human life' (Reich 1978, p. 831). For example, an evaluative quality of life statement might assert that 'the pain suffered by this person is bad' and 'the absence of pain in this person is good', or that 'the loss of functional ability experienced by that person is bad' and 'the regaining of function by this person is good', or that 'this person's dependency on others for care is bad' and the 'regaining of independence by this person is good', and so on. To say a person has lost quality of life in this sense would be to assert merely that some property or aspect of her or his life has lost value, not that life itself has lost value — although the attachment of value to certain qualities or characteristics, in this instance, often becomes the very basis upon which an individual human life might be judged worth living or not worth living, as the case may be.

Quality of life in the morally normative or prescriptive sense, on the other hand, is quite different again. Here, a quality of life statement would entail a *moral judgment* on a given (already evaluated) quality or set of qualities of an individual human life. Quality of life expressed as a moral judgment in this instance would seek to prescribe what would be a good or bad, right or wrong way of regarding a given individual human life or, more specifically, on the basis of its qualities, what ought and ought not to be done 'to support and protect' it. An example of a morally prescriptive quality of life statement would be: 'a life marked by intense pain is a life which it is not in an individual's best interests to go on living; ending such a life would thus be a morally just thing to do'; or 'a life free of pain is a minimally decent life, and thus one worth living; to take such a life would be morally objectionable'; or 'a life which cannot be lived independently is a life not worth living; therefore, ending such a life would be a morally decent thing to do'; or 'a life which can be lived independently of others is a minimally decent life and therefore a life worth living; taking such a life would be morally objectionable'. In this instance, a statement concerning the loss of quality of life could most certainly be interpreted as indicating that the life in question no longer has worth and thus is dispensable. Alternatively, a statement concerning an increase in quality of life could most certainly be interpreted as indicating that the life in question has improved worth and thus warrants preservation and protection.

In the light of these three different senses of quality of life, it can be seen that there is enormous potential for making moral errors when deciding quality of life matters in health care domains. This observation raises a number of important points. First, it wisely instructs the need for nurses to distinguish carefully the senses in which they might be using, or rather misusing, quality of life statements. This is particularly important in situations where decisions need to be made about which interventions should be implemented in order to enhance or promote the objective qualities of a person's life, and, further, about which quality or qualities ought to be enhanced or restored over others. For example, once it is identified that a person is in a state of pain which can be observed and described 'objectively' and that the pain in question is evaluated negatively by that person, an attending nurse will be in a relatively strong position to assert that interventions aimed at alleviating pain ought to take priority in that situation. If, however, it is determined that the person in question does not regard the pain as a disvalue, or at least regards its relief as being less valuable than, say, maintaining mental alertness, an attending nurse might be in quite a different position. Chosen interventions aimed at alleviating pain might assume quite a different priority, and indeed might take on quite a different form.

A second important point here is that, by distinguishing the different senses in which the term quality of life can be used, the nurse may become more aware of the logical leap between making a *descriptive* judgment on the quality or qualities of a person's life and then making a *prescriptive* judgment (on the basis of that descriptive judgment) concerning what ought or ought not to be done in relation to that person's life. For example, if we distinguish between the different senses of 'quality of life', it soon becomes apparent that it is one thing to say a given person has lost one or two objective (descriptive) qualities or properties of their life, but it is quite another to say that, on the basis of those lost properties or qualities, the life of the person in question has less moral value or ought to be treated in one particular way rather than another. If such a judgment is to be made, this should be done on the basis of sound critically reflective moral standards, not on the basis of mistaken deductive reasoning.

Lastly, when we examine the fragile connection between the descriptive, evaluative and morally prescriptive senses of quality of life, the fundamental questions emerge of *who should decide* which values ought to be given to certain qualities or properties of life, and, further, on the basis of these ascribed values, of whether an individual human life in a particular context ought to be regarded as having one type or degree of moral value rather than another.

In relation to this last point, there is little doubt, at least from a moral point of view, that only the people whose lives are in question can decide what values to ascribe to their properties or qualities of life and which moral value to ascribe to their lives generally. For example, only those people can know what pain or dependency levels they can tolerate, and accordingly only they can identify the boundaries within which their pain or dependency states will be ascribed either positive or negative value. Only those people can know the point beyond which pain or dependency on others would render their life intolerable, and the point at which they would judge their life as being either morally less or morally more worthwhile. Bear in mind here that, while some might view pain as diminishing life's worth, others might view it as their passport to salvation. Likewise, some might consider dependency on others as diminishing their life's worth, while others might consider it quite irrelevant to either the meaning or value of their life — as Kanitsaki (1988) makes abundantly clear in her informative article 'Cancer and informed consent: a cultural perspective'. What is important to understand is that, no matter how well-intentioned a nurse might be, or how knowledgeable or experienced, this probably will never be enough to enable that nurse to judge correctly either the evaluative or the morally prescriptive aspects of another person's (that is, that patient's) 'quality of life'. Even the descriptive aspect, for that matter, is difficult to judge, given the highly subjective nature of some so-called 'objectively observable' qualities, such as pain or loss of function. Since describing qualities is also very much a matter of interpreting them, there is always room for making judgment errors. It is for this reason that the people whose quality of life is at issue must be respected as the only ones who really are the best judges of what is to count as being in their best interests, and, further, as the only ones who are able to judge correctly what is to count as being their quality of life. In instances where people are unable to judge their own quality of life or best interests, this task should rightly fall to those (for example, close family members and/or friends) who intimately know the person in question and who know thoroughly their world views.

It can be seen that in using the notion of quality of life, nurses must be very careful to distinguish the exact sense in which they are using it. They must also be very aware of how easy it is to leap from a *descriptive statement* concerning a person's qualities of life to a *prescriptive statement* on what should be done for that life — morally, medically, or otherwise. Furthermore, they must take steps to guard against making this leap in judgment, particularly in instances where doing so might result in another not only losing a minimally decent *level* of life, but losing *life* itself.

Not For Treatment (NFT) directives

At the end stage of life (across the life span) or, as in the case of extremely premature newborns, at the beginning of life there invariably comes a point at which decisions have to be made about what cares and treatment are 'appropriate' for persons in this stage. Very often medical decisions are made not to treat a given condition or to withdraw various treatments that are in the process of being administered on grounds that such treatment would be medically 'futile'. In such instances, a medical directive may be given to the effect that the patient in question is 'Not For Treatment' (NFT). Sometimes a patient or his or her surrogate will agree with the NFT decisions that have been made, sometimes they will not. It is when there is disagreement about a treatment choice — that is, where a decision is 'contested' (for example, there is disagreement about the decision to treat or not to treat) — that the matter becomes problematic. Here important questions arise, namely: When is it acceptable, if ever, to provide, withdraw or withhold cares and treatment which may be medically futile or marginally beneficial to people (infants, children, adolescents, adults and the elderly alike)? When, if ever, is it permissible for patients and/or their surrogates to request that everything possible be done even when it is evident that a person's case is 'medically hopeless'?

The problem of treatment in 'medically hopeless' cases

In the past, decisions about what treatments to provide — when, where and by whom — were made paternalistically by consultant/attending doctors. This sometimes lead to a situation in which people were being 'aggressively' treated even when their cases were deemed 'medically hopeless'. In other words, people were treated 'aggressively' even where it was evident to experienced bystanders that such treatment would not make a significant difference to their health or life expectancy. Sometimes treatment of this nature was imposed without the patient's knowledge or consent (for example, those in a persistent vegetative state), and gave rise to varying degrees of suffering by both patients and their chosen carers.

This situation began to change, however, as the public started to become weary of and started to question the wisdom of people being 'hopelessly resuscitated'. This public questioning saw a number of key cases reaching the public's attention. Rosemary Tong (1995) explains:

> As a result of various factors, the withholding and withdrawing cases that captured the imagination of the public in the 1960s and 1970s were ones in which patients or their surrogates resisted the imposition of unwanted medical treatment. The media portrayed dying patients as routinely falling prey to physicians who, out of fear of subsequent litigation ... or out of obedience to some sort of 'technological imperative' ..., insisted on keeping them 'alive' irrespective of the quality of their existence.
>
> (Tong 1995, p. 166)

Tong (1995) suggests that during the 1960s and 1970s, economic resources permitted everything possible to be done. During the 1980s and 1990s, however, it became increasingly evident that neither individuals nor society as a whole could sustain the 'technological imperative' to treat regardless of the outcomes. Thus communities in the Western world entered into a new era that was characteristically 'burdened with new obligations of social justice' in health care (Tong 1995, p. 167). Whereas end of life issues in the 1960s and 1970s were more concerned with *patient autonomy versus medical paternalism*, in the 1980s and 1990s they had become chiefly concerned with *patient autonomy versus distributive justice* (Tong 1995, pp. 166–7). In the 1990s, then, a key question dominating bioethical thought is: Are people at the end stages of their lives (or their surrogates) morally entitled to request 'medically inappropriate' 'non-beneficial' and 'expensive' (futile) medical treatment? Before proceeding, it should be noted here that what is at stake in answering this question is not just the entitlements of dying individuals but, as Tong concludes:

> the future wellbeing of the health care professional–patient–society relationship — a relationship best understood not in terms of competing rights (though that is an aspect of it), but in terms of intersecting responsibilities.
>
> (Tong 1995, p. 167)

Disputes about futile or useful treatments at the end stages of life invariably represent 'disputes about professional, patient and surrogate autonomy, as well as concerns about good communication, informed consent, resource allocation, undertreatment, overtreatment, and paternalism' (Kopleman 1995, p. 109). They also represent dispute about 'how to understand or rank such important values as sustaining a life, providing appropriate treatments, relieving suffering, or being compassionate' and the bearing these values may have on deciding questions of resource allocation (Kopleman 1995, p. 111). It should be noted, however, that even the notion of 'futile' medical treatment (generally taken as referring to medical treatment that 'fails to achieve the goals of medicine' in that it offers no benefit to the patient viz. it fails to overcome the patient's medical problem, or results in the patient surviving, but only to lead a 'useless live' [Jecker 1993]) is itself controversial, and one which appears to be serving a highly questionable function. Brody and Halevy (1995, p. 124–5), for example, suggest that the function of invoking 'futility' (a notion that is subject to a variety of contentious interpretations) 'is to authorise physicians to unilaterally limit life prolonging interventions in certain cases, while preserving the rights of patients and surrogates to decide about the provision of such interventions in other cases'. Nevertheless, the notion of medical futility continues to have currency in biomedical and bioethical discourse.

Who decides?

The question of who and how to decide these matters is a difficult one to answer. Choices include:

- the medical practitioner (unilateral approach);
- the health care team (consensus approach);
- the patient or his/her surrogate (unilateral approach);
- society (consensus).

While all plausible, neither of the above approaches are without difficulties (even in the case of a consensus being reached, this alone is not enough to confer moral authority on the decisions made). For example, while all clearly entail respect for the autonomy of individuals, they nevertheless risk decisions being made that are arbitrary, biased, capricious, self-interested and based on personal preferences. This is unacceptable (especially in contested cases) since, as Kopleman points out:

> If one ought to do the morally defensible action in the contested case, then the final appeal cannot be solely preferences of someone or some group. Preference or agreements may be unworthy because they result from prejudice, self-interest or ignorance. In contrast, moral justification requires giving and defending reasons for preferences, and by doing so relying on methodological ideals of clarity, impartiality, consistency and consideration of all relevant information. Other important, albeit fallible, considerations in making moral decisions include legal, social, and religious traditions, stable views about how to understand and rank important values, and a willingness to be sensitive to the feelings, preferences, perceptions and rights of others. The evolution of contested cases often illustrates the pitfalls of failing to take the time and clarify people's concerns, problems, feelings, beliefs or deeply felt needs or even to consider if people are treating others as they would wish to be treated ... Overtreatments may be burdensome to patient and costly to society, yet undertreatments can compromise the rights or dignity of the people seeking help.
>
> (Kopleman (1995) pp. 117–18,119)

In the case of requests being made for 'everything possible to be done' some have suggested that there is no obligation to acquiesce to such requests in so-called medically hopeless cases. Jecker and Schneiderman (1995, p. 160) clarify, however, that 'saying "no" to futile treatment should not mean saying "no" to caring for the patient'. They conclude:

> [saying 'no'] should be an occasion for transferring aggressive efforts away from life prolongation toward life enhancement. Ideally, 'doing everything' means optimising the potential for a good life, and providing that most important coda to a good life — a 'good death'.
>
> (Jecker and Schneiderman 1995, p. 160)

Decisions about whether or not to initiate or to withhold and/or remove medical treatment on patients deemed 'medically hopeless' will rarely be without controversy (sometimes referred to in the bioethics literature as the 'not starting *versus* stopping' debate [see, for example, Gert et al. 1997, pp. 282–3]). While the medical futility debate has tended to focus on the withdrawal of treatment from patients deemed to be suffering from a 'persistent vegetative state' (PVS), as Mitchell et al. (1993, p. 75) observe there are 'already efforts to extend the notion of futility beyond PVS to cases of severe dementia and organ failure'. Nurses are not immune from the medical futility controversy, and may even find themselves unwitting participants in it. It is essential therefore that nurses are well appraised of the relevant views for and against decisions aimed at limiting the medical treatment of patients deemed (rightly or wrongly) to be 'medically hopeless'.

'Not For Resuscitation' (NFR) directives[2]

At some stage during their careers, nurses will be confronted with the difficult moral choice of whether to follow a 'Not For Resuscitation' (NFR) directive (also referred to as 'Do Not Resuscitate' [DNR], and 'No Code'). This type of directive is usually given by a doctor in an attempt to 'avoid over-treatment and CPR (cardiopulmonary resuscitation) abuses', particularly in cases involving hopelessly ill patients 'who would be otherwise hopelessly revived' (Humphry and Wickett 1986, p. 209). NFR is thus a form of NFT, and probably is the most common NFT directive given in health care contexts. Typically, an NFR directive directs that: 'in the event of a cardiac arrest, neither basic nor advanced life support measures will be instituted by physicians, nurses, or other hospital staff' (Cushing 1981, p. 22; Honan et al. 1991, p. 54).

A decision not to resuscitate a person is popularly thought to flow from a medical judgment concerning the irreversible nature of that person's disease and their probable poor or hopeless prognosis (see, for example, Haines et al. 1990, p. 228). This popular view is, however, a highly controversial one. Yarling and McElmurry (1986), for example, persuasively argue that the NFR decision is not a *medical* decision per se, nor is it a legal or nursing decision. Rather, they contend, the NFR decision is fundamentally a *moral* decision, since it is based primarily on *moral values*, such as those concerning 'the meaning, sanctity, and quality of life' (p. 125).

Despite its serious moral and indeed legal implications, the issue of NFR directives has, on the whole, been poorly addressed by the nursing profession in Australasia — not only in academic terms (as suggested by the surprising paucity of nursing literature on the subject), but also in practical terms (as evidenced by the lack of explicit guidelines and policies governing NFR procedures and practices in many Australasian hospitals; or, where these exist, a lack of compliance with formally adopted guidelines).

Just why this state of affairs has occurred is a matter for speculation. It may be that nurses have come to view the NFR directive as absolutely constituting a lawful and reasonable medical directive, and thus not something warranting

---

2. An earlier version of the discussion on 'Not For Resuscitation' (NFR) directives was originally presented under the title: 'The nature and moral implications of "Not For Resuscitation [NFR]" directives' at the *Nursing law and ethics, First Victorian State Conference. Theme: 'Matters of life and death'*, Monash University, Melbourne, 30 September 1988 (organised by the School of Nursing, Phillip Institute of Technology). The paper has been revised for publication in this text.

any special or particular concern. Or it may be that nurses *are* troubled by current practices in this area but say or do nothing out of fear that their employment or career prospects may be hampered in some way if they speak out. Or it may be that nurses are troubled by current practices and do wish to speak out, but genuinely do not know how to go about articulating their concerns.

Whatever the reasons for the nursing profession's failure to address the NFR issue, the fact remains that nurses can no longer ignore the serious moral, legal and professional questions which current NFR practices raise, much less their implications for clinical nursing practice, nursing education and administration. Neither can the nursing profession ignore the point that, while the practice of prescribing NFR for seriously ill patients is a commonly *accepted* one in most Australasian hospitals and residential care agencies (as it is in many hospitals and residential care agencies worldwide), it is nevertheless open to serious question whether the practice is wholly *acceptable*. A whole range of important moral, legal and professional considerations must be taken into account, as it is hoped the following discussion will show. Two central questions are involved: What is the nature of NFR (DNR/No Code) directives? And what are the implications of NFR (DNR/No Code) directives for members of the nursing profession? Possible answers to these questions are considered now in relation to two cases, those of Mr H and Mr X. These cases both occurred in Australia.

Case 1: Mr H

Mr H[3], 60-years-old, was admitted to the intensive care unit of a major city hospital with a provisional diagnosis of septicaemia. At the time of admission he was pale, markedly short of breath, and had an axillary temperature of 40°C. Mr H's past medical history included severe coronary artery disease and a malignant condition. The malignant condition had, however, been successfully treated with chemotherapy, and Mr H was presently in a state of remission. In the light of his provisional diagnosis, a regime of intravenous antibiotics was commenced.

A few hours after Mr H's admission, the on-coming nursing staff for the afternoon shift gathered for 'hand-over'. During hand-over, the charge nurse informed the nursing staff present that she had just received a telephone call from Mr H's physician confirming that the patient was Not For Resuscitation (NFR). As she proceeded to give the afternoon report, a second consulting physician — also involved in Mr H's medical care — approached the assembled nursing staff and reaffirmed her colleague's initial NFR directive. The physician then wrote up her clinical assessment of Mr H and made other important documentations on his medical history chart. She did not, however, make any attempt to document the NFR directive which she had just given to the nursing staff. This 'oversight' was later dealt with by the nursing staff writing the initials 'NFR', in pencil, on the top left-hand corner of Mr H's nursing care plan, which was held in his medical history chart.

A short time later, a nurse who had been sent to help in the unit became involved in a deep conversation with Mr H. During the conversation, Mr H

---

3. Details of this case have been altered to disguise the identity of the patient, the staff and the hospital concerned. Any resemblance the case of Mr H might have to an actual case is therefore purely coincidental.

spontaneously and emphatically exclaimed: 'Oh, I wish they would operate on me!' (referring to coronary artery bypass surgery, the opportunity for which he had recently been denied). In response to this the nurse gently asked Mr H whether he had discussed the possibility of bypass surgery with his doctor.

To this Mr H replied quite openly: 'Sure I have, many times, but they won't do it because they say there's only a 50–50 chance of success ...'. He went on to say: 'What can you do? You can't hit them over the head with a bottle and make them do it, can you?'. The nurse enquired further: 'So even though you'd only have a 50–50 chance — you'd still want this coronary bypass surgery?'.

Mr H replied, sombrely:

> Oh, yes. I'd do anything to buy some time. You see, my wife's very ill at home. She has cancer which can't be operated on. She's always been totally dependent on me — even more so since she's been sick. She doesn't have very long to live, and all I want is to live long enough for her, because she's so afraid of being left alone. We can't do much, and we each stay in separate rooms at home. But at least we're reasonably independent and together. I can bring her a cup of tea when she wants it and things like that. I don't care about me, but I want to live long enough for her ... she's so afraid of being left alone ...

Smiling, Mr H concluded: 'It's such a comfort knowing that you and the doctors are doing all that you can for me here ...'.

Realising that Mr H clearly had no knowledge of the NFR directive against him, the nurse went immediately to discuss the matter with the other nurses, who were still in the nurses' bay, having not yet moved to care for their respective patients. There, she discreetly asked whether Mr H or his relatives had been involved in making the NFR decision. To this question one nurse replied: 'Oh! Surely that's silly to include the patient or the relatives ...' and, almost simultaneously, another nurse replied: 'No. We don't do that in this hospital. It's the doctors' decision, and we're obliged to obey their orders ...'.

The nurse caring for Mr H then attempted to point out that her patient had indicated that he very definitely wished to risk the odds of active resuscitation. She then asked further whether the doctors were aware of Mr H's desires. To this, the nurse in charge replied sternly: 'Of course the doctors know! It's their decision, and it's the policy of this hospital to follow such orders'.

As the afternoon shift progressed, Mr H experienced a number of bradycardiac episodes, with the cardiac monitor showing his heart rate dropping to as low as 34 in some instances. The arrhythmia could have been treated relatively easily by the attending nurse administering a prescribed bolus dose of intravenous atropine. When the nurse caring for Mr H went to have the drug checked with the nurse in charge (as was required by unit policy), she was told: 'You don't need to worry about that, he's NFR ...'. Despite the attending nurse's protests, the nurse in charge still refused to check the atropine. Fortunately, during the time of intense debate between the attending nurse and the nurse in charge, Mr H's cardiac rhythm reverted spontaneously to a rate of between 80 and 90 beats per minute. Mr H had several more bradycardiac episodes throughout the shift, but each time spontaneously reverted to a safe rate of 80–90 beats per minute.

A few days later, Mr H's temperature dropped significantly to within normal limits. He stated that he felt better and was looking forward to going home. His blood cultures came back negative (negating his provisional diagnosis of septicaemia), his heart rate was more stable, and his breathing continued to improve. Despite this, however, the NFR directive was not rescinded. Mr H's condition dramatically improved even further one afternoon when he was given a stat dose of intravenous lasix (a diuretic). Following this, it was decided that the presenting medical condition had not, in fact, been septicaemia but pulmonary congestion (secondary to his heart disease) and pneumonia.

Just six days after his initial admission into the intensive care unit, Mr H was judged sufficiently well recovered to be discharged home. He left, happy, thanking the nursing staff for all that they had done and expressing his eagerness to leave and be reunited with his dying wife.

Rightly troubled by the incident, the nurse made an appointment to discuss the matter with the then director of nursing. During the conversation, the nurse indicated that in future she would override any nurse in charge and would contact the prescribing doctor to clarify an existing NFR directive. To this the director of nursing replied:

> Well, of course, if you had contacted the doctors involved in this case, you would probably have found that they wouldn't be very forthcoming anyway. In fact, they would probably have told you it was not your concern. You will find here that it is really the doctor's decision in cases like these, since it is *they* who have the contract with the patient, not the nurses ...

After many days' deliberation and discussions with trusted friends and colleagues, the nurse resigned from her position, since she believed this was the only way of avoiding the kinds of dilemmas that would be posed when she had to care for patients who had been deemed 'Not For Resuscitation' without their knowledge or informed consent, or against their express wishes.

Case 2: Mr X

The second case to be considered here is taken from the Victorian State Government Social Development Committee's *Inquiry into options for dying with dignity: second and final report* (1987). It involves the case of Mr X, who was also cared for in a major city hospital.

Mr X, 78-years-old, was admitted to hospital with a provisional diagnosis of 'Transitional Cell Carcinoma, with metastatic spread to the lungs, liver and spinal cord and brain' (Social Development Committee 1987, p. 111). On admission, Mr X was observed to be lethargic, disorientated and suffering a greater degree of pain than on previous admissions. He had lost weight and admitted to having lost his appetite. The nurse relating the case stated that:

> it was apparent to me that Mr X's disease process had insidiously created a decline in his overall wellbeing, to a point where it had now affected his quality of life.

(Social Development Committee 1987, p. 112)

On Friday morning, upon consultation with the ward's resident medical officer, it was stated that Mr X 'had now reached the terminal stage of his illness' and that, apart from keeping him comfortable, nothing more could be done for him, medically speaking. On Friday evening, Mr X's deteriorating condition was discussed with his relatives. It was reported that:

> His relatives were distressed over the deterioration they had observed over the past few weeks in Mr X's condition and wellbeing. At this time they

emphatically expressed their wish that should Mr X arrest while in hospital, they in no way wanted an emergency procedure of resuscitation performed on him, and wished for him to be allowed to die peacefully with a degree of dignity assured.

(Social Development Committee 1987, p. 112)

Later that same evening, Mr X himself requested (via the hospital chaplain) that 'should he die that evening he had no wish to be actively resuscitated and would prefer to die peacefully' (p. 113).

Mr X's condition continued to deteriorate. On Saturday morning, the nurse in charge called the covering resident medical officer to examine Mr X medically so that it could be formally established that Mr X 'would not be for resuscitation' in the event of his suffering a cardiac arrest. The Social Development Committee (1987) further reports:

The doctor examined Mr X, and agreed that he should not be for cardiopulmonary resuscitation. However, he also stated that he could not instigate that decision until Monday morning, until he had consulted the Registrar and Consultants of the unit, thereby allowing his decision to be reached as a team decision. On this note, Mr X was still for resuscitation should he arrest, in spite of his and his relatives' wish to allow him to die with peace and dignity.

(Social Development Committee 1987, p. 113)

Over the next 24-hours, Mr X's condition declined even further, and at 5 pm on Sunday, in the presence of his relatives, he suffered a cardiac arrest. As the covering resident medical officer had requested that Mr X should still be resuscitated — at least until the matter could be discussed with the unit team — an immediate resuscitation code was called. Full resuscitation procedures were instigated and continued for approximately twenty minutes. No positive outcome was achieved, however, and Mr X was declared clinically dead. Understandably, Mr X's relatives were very distraught about the incident and 'even more so', as the report goes on to quote, 'about the fact that Mr X had been resuscitated both against his and their wishes' (p. 113).

Raising the issues

The cases of Mr H and Mr X are just two among many — possibly even thousands — which serve very well to illustrate the moral dangers of permitting misguided (or indeed unguided and/or ethically unconstrained) medico-nursing decision-making in life and death situations in the clinical setting. In short, ethically unconstrained or misguided decision-making in arrest situations could result in the undesirable moral consequence of patients either *not being resuscitated* when they otherwise wish to be (as in the case of Mr H) or, alternatively, of *being resuscitated* when they have clearly indicated a preference to die peacefully and without the undignified intrusion of active resuscitation interventions (as occurred in the case of Mr X).

In most Australasian hospitals and residential care agencies, NFR policies are tacitly assumed rather than clearly stated. Actual practices are, on the whole, covert rather than overt, and may vary from hospital to hospital, agency to agency, or doctor to doctor and nurse to nurse. This is the case in Victoria, as the *Inquiry into options for dying with dignity: second and final report* found just over one decade ago (Social Development Committee 1987, p. 108). The Social

Development Committee was so disturbed by its findings with regard to current practices in Victorian hospitals and related health care agencies that it made the following formal recommendation:

> that the Health Department Victoria as a matter of urgency obtain all relevant health care institutions' 'not-for-resuscitation' (NFR) guidelines in order:
>
> - to review current practices in this area, and that such information be referred to the National Health and Medical Research Council (NH & MRC) by the Minister for Health at the next Health Ministers' Conference; and
> - that the NH & MRC develop a commonly accepted set of standards and practices that can be incorporated into guidelines, and observed.
>
> (Social Development Committee 1987, p. v)

At the time of writing, the Human Services Department (formerly the Health Department Victoria) has still not undertaken any action to improve NFR practices in Victorian hospitals and residential care homes. This non-action compares poorly with the initiative of the New South Wales Health Department, which in 1993 issued guidelines on prescribing and implementing CPR/NFR directives (NSW Health Department 1993, section 5).

For many who have uncritically followed institutional NFR practices, this debate might seem somewhat irrelevant and even unnecessary. After all, they might reason, these practices have worked well for the past thirty years; why worry about them now?

What such a view ignores, however, is that, if there are no carefully formulated and clearly documented guidelines and policies governing NFR procedures and practices, a number of otherwise avoidable harmful consequences might occur — and have already occurred, as literature on the subject painfully reminds us (see for example Macklin's discussion, 'Law as an advocate for patients: a case study of DNR' [1993, pp. 29–51]). The kinds of morally undesirable outcomes that might occur include, among others:

- patients' rights and interests being unjustly violated (particularly in instances where an NFR/CPR decision does not accord with a patient's considered preferences);
- nurses being left to carry a disproportionate burden (in moral, legal, professional and personal terms) with regard to actually carrying out NFR/CPR directives;
- other allied health workers (including less senior doctors) carrying disproportionate legal, moral, professional and personal burdens on account of the dilemmas posed by administering uncertain and ambiguous NFR/CPR procedures and practices.

These and similar considerations, needless to say, raise two further questions: What exactly is wrong with current NFR practices and procedures? And what can and should the nursing profession do in order to ensure that morally just NFR policies and guidelines are formulated and implemented in hospitals and related health care agencies?

The difficulties surrounding current NFR practices can be roughly categorised under three general headings:

1. problems concerning NFR decision-making criteria, guidelines and procedures;
2. problems concerning the documentation and communication of NFR directives; and
3. problems concerning the implementation of NFR directives.

Problems concerning NFR decision-making criteria, guidelines and procedures

Criteria and guidelines used

As already briefly mentioned, most hospitals and related health care agencies lack clear guidelines on how NFR decisions should be made and implemented, or, if they do have guidelines, their practices do not always conform with them (Lipton 1989, p. 112; *Bioethics News* 1992, p. 4). As a result, patients have very often been subjected to arbitrary and at times haphazard and even whimsical decision-making with regard to their being resuscitated or not resuscitated in life-threatening situations. Different doctors and nurses may appeal to different *criteria* (to be distinguished here from *procedures*) for making an NFR/CPR decision (see also Stewart and Rai 1989; Thom 1988). For example, some doctors and nurses might appeal to *quality of life* criteria (such as age, mental competence, pain states, chronicity of disease, poor prognosis, and so forth) when making an NFR/CPR decision. An NFR decision based on such criteria might well be in accordance with a patient's preferences, but it might equally be thoroughly opposed to them, as occurred in the Fred Walker case (Hastings Center 1982). Fred Walker was a previously fit 90-year-old who required admission to hospital for multiple medical problems. While in hospital Mr Walker suffered a cardiac arrest and was not resuscitated, even though both he and his wife had clearly indicated that they wished 'everything possible' to be done to try and preserve his life (Hastings Center 1982, pp. 27–8).

Alternatively, some doctors and nurses might appeal to *sanctity of life* criteria (which essentially demand that life be preserved, whatever the cost) when making an NFR/CPR decision. Doctors' or nurses' decisions in this instance might well accord with patients' expressed wishes, but, as with the previous example, they could also be violatory of them. Annas (in Bandman and Bandman 1985), for example, cites the case of a 70-year-old woman 'who was resuscitated over 70 times within a few days' (p. 236). And Dolan (1988) cites the case of a patient who was resuscitated 52 times before 'family members literally threw themselves across the crash cart to prevent the team from reaching the patient' for the fifty-third time (p. 47).

Still others, however, may appeal to nothing more than a personal sense or 'gut feeling' of right and wrong when making NFR/CPR decisions. What is troubling about this is that, while attending doctors or nurses might 'feel' that a particular NFR or CPR decision is right (or wrong, as the case may be), it does not follow that the decision in question is morally sound. Whether an NFR/CPR decision is morally sound can and should be decided only by critical reflection and appeal to sound moral standards, not, as some might contend, by appealing solely to the dictates of 'gut response', for reasons considered previously in this text.

Even more troubling is the practice of deeming patients NFR on the basis of an NFR decision made during a previous hospital admission. For example, if a patient is made NFR during an admission to hospital in March, is discharged, but comes back into hospital in April, the patient can be made NFR again on the basis of the March hospital admission decision. The rationale behind this is not entirely clear.

Equally disturbing is the over-reliance on *age* as a decisional criterion when making NFR/CPR decisions. Many residential care homes for the aged, for example, have a blanket (unwritten) policy of not resuscitating their residents. Persons entering these homes are asked 'whether they wish to be cremated and where they wish to be buried, but not whether they wish to be resuscitated' if and when they should cardiac arrest (Johnstone 1988, p. 8). This practice is disturbing for two main reasons: first, it totally violates the residents' autonomy; second, it relies on what research has shown to be an unreliable and invalid decisional criterion — notably *age* (see in particular Sage et al. 1987).

As a point of interest, one American study investigating the implementation of a 'Do-Not-Resuscitate' (DNR) policy in a nursing home found that, of the 48 residents (who were of a mean age of 81.7 years) who were deemed capable of deciding whether they wanted CPR/DNR, 30 (62.5 per cent) 'chose to be resuscitated in the event of a cardiopulmonary arrest', compared with only 18 (37.5 per cent) who 'decided in favour of DNR' (Fader et al. 1989, p. 545).

In a later British study involving 100 inpatients (mean age 81.5 years) on an acute hospital elderly care unit, 73 per cent of those patients questioned indicated that they would want cardiopulmonary resuscitation (CPR) in the event of a cardiac arrest; this compared with 18 per cent of those questioned indicating that they would not want CPR in the event of a cardiac arrest, and nine percent who indicating that they were unsure (Mead and Turnbull 1995). However, in another North American study (involving 287 elderly people with a mean age of 77 years), a team of researchers found that, in contradiction to most other studies suggesting that a majority of elderly patients would want to undergo CPR in the event of a cardiac arrest, once respondents were informed about the probabilities of survival following CPR, their preference for CPR declined significantly (that is, almost halved) (Murphy et al. 1994). These two studies were nevertheless unanimous in their conclusions: elderly people are capable of being — and should be — consulted about their CPR status in health care contexts

The exclusion of patients from decision-making

Some doctors and nurses genuinely believe that patients or their relatives should not be included in the process of making NFR decisions (see also Perry et al. 1986; Schade and Muslin 1989; Loewy 1991). Responding to the Fred Walker case (mentioned above), Professor Carson (1982) points out that the admitting hospital in that case had an official policy which effectively took the position 'that entering patients should not be bothered with the details of resuscitation policy but should assume that they will be well cared for and coded if necessary' (p. 28).

Also commenting on the Fred Walker case, Mark Siegler (an associate professor of medicine) goes even further, and argues that where a physician knows ('within limits of uncertainty that characterise all medical knowledge') that CPR would be of no possible benefit to the patient, it should not be initiated — *regardless* of a patient's preferences to the contrary (Siegler 1982, p. 29).

Carson's and Siegler's comments on the Walker case alert us to some of the moral dangers of uncritically following institutional policies, norms, etiquette and the like when making important life and death decisions, as well as to the unnecessary suffering which can be caused by an unthinking and dogmatic application of them. The unnecessary suffering caused in this case is summed up very well by Mrs Walker's comments upon being informed that no attempt had been made to resuscitate her husband. The *Hastings Center Report* (1982) describes her response in the following terms:

> Upon being informed that no emergency measures were taken in her husband's case, Mrs Walker said that that decision was against her wishes. 'Doing everything,' she says, 'is the difference between life and death. The doctor was playing God when he decided he should not try to save my husband. You're not playing God when you've tried everything and exhausted all methods. All I wanted was for them to try. My husband knew how to love and be loved. That was his quality of life. That suited him and it suited me'.
>
> (Hastings Center 1982, p. 28)

Many doctors believe that patients should not be 'burdened' with having to decide whether they should be resuscitated in the event of a cardiac arrest — particularly if the patient's condition is 'medically hopeless' and any further treatment — including CPR — would be 'futile' (Perry et al. 1986; Schade and Muslin 1989; Haines et al. 1990; Tomlinson and Brody 1990; Scofield 1991; Lo 1991; Loewy 1991). This has resulted in patients often not being consulted about an NFR/DNR directive that has been made against them. In one American study, for example, it was revealed that only 22 per cent of patients surveyed had been involved in the DNR decision in their case (Lipton 1989, p. 108). Another study found that, while fewer than 50 per cent of nurses and doctors surveyed agreed that patients should be given information about 'No Codes' on admission to hospital, 75 per cent of lay persons surveyed 'believed this information should be available' (Honan et al. 1991, p. 60). And another study revealed that 68 per cent of respondents surveyed indicated their wish to discuss the use of life-sustaining treatment, yet only 6 *per cent* had been given the opportunity to do so (Lo et al. 1986). More recently, a 1994 study found that 86 per cent of respondents (all elderly inpatients of an acute aged care unit, with a mean age of 81.5 years) were willing to be consulted about their CPR status, and 77 per cent were willing for their relative to be consulted (of these, 45 per cent *wanted* their relative to be consulted); 64 per cent indicated that they would be willing to 'follow their doctor's advice about the appropriateness of CPR' (Mead and Turnbull 1995). While these and other findings (see, for example, Council on Ethical and Judicial Affairs, American Medical Association, 1991) cannot be generalised as applying universally, it is nevertheless possible to speculate that, were these studies to be duplicated in Australia, New Zealand, England and other Western countries, they would probably yield very similar results.

Misinterpretation of directives and questionable outcomes

Another major difficulty associated with current NFR guidelines and procedures is that they are essentially inadequate for ensuring that given NFR directives are interpreted in a precise, reliable and uniform manner. Consider, for example, the case of Mr H, described at the beginning of this discussion. In this case the NFR directive was interpreted, controversially, as also including the non-treatment of a potentially fatal but relatively easily treatable cardiac arrhythmia. This interpretation becomes even more troubling, and the appropriateness of the NFR decision more questionable, when it is considered that the patient was, after all, being cared for in an *intensive care unit*. What clearly needs to be questioned here (particularly in cases involving patients who have been admitted to intensive care units) is that, if a patient's condition is so medically hopeless, and an NFR directive is therefore medically justified, why is that patient being cared for in an intensive care unit, where the imperative 'to treat' is usually considered to be both foremost and overriding? There is surely something seriously questionable — and, indeed, inconsistent and contradictory — in caring for patients in an intensive care situation (or any other ward), having their heartbeat monitored, observing and recording presenting cardiac arrhythmias, having a standing prescription for drugs to treat given arrhythmias, and yet doing absolutely nothing when and if that patient cardiac arrests.

Another disturbing example of the way in which an NFR/DNR directive can be misinterpreted can be found in the case of a dying patient who had pulmonary congestion and pneumonia, and, associated with these two conditions, copious mucus production. In this case, the nurses (mis)interpreted the NFR directive to include withholding oropharyngeal/nasopharyngeal suctioning. As a result, the patient was left, quite literally, to drown in his own secretions — until another nurse detected the error and took immediate action to correct the other nurses' misinterpretation of the directive. The lesson to be learned from this case — and others like it — is that 'No Code' does not mean 'no care' (Saunders and Valente 1986; see also Lo 1991).

'Go slow' codes

Another common but questionable NFR practice which prevails in some institutions is the 'go slow' code or 'slow code' (Social Development Committee 1987, p. 108; Bandman and Bandman 1985, p. 235; Honan et al. 1991, p. 55) — loosely defined here as 'responding to a code slowly or not using every available lifesaving measure' (Humphry and Wickett 1986, pp. 210–11). Humphry and Wickett explain:

> Here attempts are made to revive the patient, but only after a delay, usually long enough to ensure that the patient won't respond. In this way, the patient's wishes — or so the physicians can claim — have been honoured, while the hospital is protected from litigation.
>
> (Humphry and Wickett 1986, p. 211)[4]

Citing the comments of a nurse, these authors go on to point out, however, that:

> resuscitation, even when delayed, is rarely done for the patient's benefit: 'Resuscitation is more for the benefit of the living than helpful to the dead or dying patient. The family can say they tried everything, but [the loved one] was too far gone to bring him [sic] back, and the act of resuscitation makes the professional staff look efficient'.
>
> (Humphry and Wickett 1986, p. 211)[5]

An extraordinary example of 'go slow' codes can be found in the case of residential care homes for the elderly. There is considerable anecdotal evidence (be there a regrettable dearth of formal research on the topic) that many residential care homes for the elderly lack the means (either in terms of functioning resuscitation equipment, or trained staff, or both) to initiate CPR in

---

4. Reprinted with permission of Angus & Robertson/Collins.
5. Reprinted with permission of Angus & Robertson/Collins.

the event of an elderly resident suffering a cardiac arrest (Johnstone 1994a). Thus, in the event of a cardiac arrest occurring, it is common practice for staff to call an ambulance. However, it has been alleged by some nurses working in the field that once the ambulance service realises the emergency call is from a residential care home for the elderly, it takes the attitude 'oh well, there is no point hurrying since there will be little chance of achieving therapeutic success'. Nurses have alleged that, during their years of experience working in the aged care sector, it is not uncommon for an ambulance to take over an hour to attend an emergency call to a residential care home. In essence, this practice amounts to an elaborate 'go slow' code.

The practices of formulating and following 'go slow' codes, while common, are nevertheless vulnerable to a number of criticisms. First, those who uphold 'go slow' codes seem erroneously to presume that a morally valid distinction exists between 'going slow' (as in the case of 'go slow' directives) and 'doing nothing' (as in the case of NFR directives). On closer analysis, it can be seen that in essence there is very little distinction between the two, for the following three reasons.

1. Both entail intentional omission (in this instance, doctors, nurses, and allied health workers deliberately refraining from performing CPR when they have both the ability and opportunity to do so) at a point in time otherwise critical to the achievement of positive therapeutic outcomes — that is, the actual resuscitation or revival of the patient in question. (For further insight into the problem of 'intentional omission', see the discussion on euthanasia (Chapter 12), as well as Kuhse 1987, p. 43.)
2. The intentional omission of CPR or other basic resuscitation measures by doctors, nurses and allied health workers (whether in response to a 'go slow' or an NFR code) results in the same foreseeable and intended outcome — notably, the irreversible death of the patient.
3. Given the intentionality of 'go slow' and NFR directives (notably, the *intention* of bringing about or hastening death by deliberately withholding certain cares and treatments), both of these orders unquestionably stand as acts of passive euthanasia. (See the discussion on euthanasia in Chapter 12.)

A second criticism here relates to the legal aspect of 'go slow' codes. Proponents of 'go slow' codes, for example, seem to assume that such codes are legally permissible and thus preferable. Cushing (1981) writes, however, that it is doubtful 'that a court would legitimise a partial code order' (p. 27), since such a code generally means 'that the procedure is not to be carried out according to acceptable practice standards' (p. 27). In short, those upholding 'go slow' codes or 'partial codes' could be held legally negligent for their outcomes (Cushing 1981).

Problems concerning the documentation and communication of NFR directives

A second major area of concern in the NFR debate involves the means by which NFR directives are documented and communicated to health care providers generally, and to nurses in particular.

Modes of communicating NFR directives are, for the most part, disturbing. Common practices include the following.

- NFR directives are given verbally only (i.e. they are not formally documented in the patient's medical or nursing notes). This practice has come about largely because doctors are 'loathe to indicate in written notes in patient records that a patient is not for resuscitation' (Social Development Committee 1987, p. 108).
- NFR directives are 'confirmed' by sticking coloured dots (usually black ones) or scribbling an asterisk either on the patient's medical history chart and/or by the patient's name on the ward's bed allocation board. As a point of interest, in 1988 the Association of Medical Directors of Victorian Hospitals recommended to the Victorian Hospital Association that 'a round white sticker with "sky" blue border and an oblique "sky" blue stripe be adopted by hospitals to denote Not For Resuscitation'. They advised that the sticker should be 'placed on the front of the patient record, on the bed card and on the patient's wristband' (*Victorian Hospital Association Report* 1988, p. 3). (Whether the colour sky blue is significant or not is anyone's guess!)
- NFR directives are 'confirmed' by pencilling the initials 'DNR' or 'NFR' or some other equivalent in an inconspicuous place on the patient's medical history or nursing care plan, or both.
- NFR directives are written euphemistically as 'routine nursing care only', or 'cares for comfort only' (Cushing 1981, p. 24).

These types of practices may well be commonly *accepted* throughout institutional health care settings, but, as noted earlier, it is far from clear that they are *acceptable*, morally, professionally or legally. As with *any* verbal directives, verbal NFR directives are vulnerable not only to misinterpretation but also to denial, in the sense that doctors could always deny that they ever gave such a directive in the event of an intentional omission in relation to a cardiac arrest being discovered. Michael Adams (1984), for example, cites an instructive example of how very serious errors can be made on account of verbal NFR directives being given and, equally instructive, how easily an attending doctor can deny ever having giving an NFR directive.

The case in question involved a patient, identified as Mrs M, who suffered a cardiac arrest while being cared for in an intensive care unit. A medical student covering the unit was called. After initiating CPR he is alleged to have stopped, saying: 'What am I doing? She's a no-code,' and then stopped performing cardiac massage (Adams 1984, p. 54). The case was eventually brought before a grand jury after a nurse anonymously informed Mrs M's daughter that 'her mother had died "unnecessarily" because "a no-code was sent out"' (Adams 1984, p. 55). As a point of interest, the medical student testified that he never made the comment. When the medical student was later asked in an informal situation why he treated Mrs M as a 'no-code', he replied that the directive to do so had been given to him verbally by a cardiologist (Adams 1984, p. 55).

It is popularly but erroneously presumed that a verbal directive, in the case of either NFR or 'go slow' codes, will 'convey the directive without attaching any legal liability' (Cushing 1981, p. 27). Cushing warns, however, that: 'while many hospitals allow no code orders to be "unofficial", it is difficult to justify a continuation of this practice. Once the medical decision has been made, the order should be written as any other medical directive' (1981, p. 27).

Also commenting on the legalities of verbal no-code orders, Kellmer (1986) writes that legal liability is in no way diminished by not writing NFR directives; if anything, failure to document a no-code or NFR directive adequately would probably increase legal liability (a view shared by Cushing). These two authors are admittedly writing from an American context, but in the Australian State of Victoria, given the Victorian State Government's *Medical Treatment Act 1988*, it is not difficult to imagine that nurses and other health care professionals could be found legally negligent for not initiating full CPR in cases where there is absolutely no written documentation of patients exercising their legal right to refuse orthodox medical treatment. This point was made abundantly clear in the parliamentary debates leading up to the enactment and proclamation of the *Medical Treatment Act 1988*. In the parliamentary session of 3 May 1988, for example, the Hon. D. R. White (the then Minister for Health), citing a hypothetical NFR example, stated that, if a person dies as a result of a doctor (and, it may be presumed, a nurse) failing to initiate CPR in the event of a cardiac arrest, 'a relative can sue the doctor under common law for negligence where there is no evidence that the patient has consented' (Parliament of Victoria, Legislative Council, 3 May 1988, p. 1015). Earlier in the same parliamentary debate, Mr White also commented:

> if a person in a hypothetical circumstance — and I repeat that it is hypothetical — has been resuscitated three times and decides not to seek further treatment, or not to be resuscitated a fourth time, under common law the issue is by no means clear. If a medical practitioner decides, in good faith, that he or she wishes to continue resuscitating that patient, the patient must go to court to get a court to uphold the patient's right to refuse medical treatment. This is a difficult process because there is no effective procedure. Moreover, the outcome of the action before the court is by no means certain.
>
> (Parliament of Victoria, Legislative Council, 3 May 1988, p. 1019)

It is also worth noting here the former Victorian Nursing Council's (1988) position statement, 'Resuscitation by the nurse', which, among other things, warns that:

> Registered Nurses must be aware that acting within a guideline or policy statement of a professional organisation or an employer does not relieve them of responsibility for their own acts and may not provide immunity in case of negligence.
>
> (Victorian Nursing Council 1988, p. 4)

The practice of giving verbal NFR directives has seen the emergence of other questionable methods for communicating given NFR directives, such as the use of coloured dots, asterisks and pencilled initials and abbreviations. Like verbal directives, however, coloured dots, asterisks and pencilled initials and abbreviations are less than adequate in terms of their ability and reliability in guiding sound and defensible practices in arrest or emergency situations. Such methods of communicating NFR directives are, in fact, quite dangerous — not only on account of their *anonymity* (for example, it would be extremely difficult to prove who, in fact, stuck a dot or sketched an asterisk on a patient's chart), but also on account of their being *inarticulate* (they are, after all, merely a symbol of a supposed medical directive, not the carefully worded medical directive itself) (see also Macklin's discussion on the 'Purple dots in Queens' [1993, pp. 34–6]). It seems quite inconceivable that important and competent medical decisions concerning the life and death of a human being could be reduced to something so careless and so vulgar as a simple black dot, an asterisk, or a set of unintelligible initials. It is also almost inconceivable that competent health professionals could rely so readily on nothing more than a set of crude symbols for determining whether or not the interventions needed to aid a seriously ill or dying patient should, in fact, be initiated. The additional dangers of dots are, of course, that they can be bought and placed on charts by almost anybody; they can also become dislodged, stick to the wrong chart, or be placed by the wrong person's name on the bed allocation board, and so on (Adams 1984; Macklin 1993, pp. 34–6). To further complicate the problematic use of dots, recent anecdotal evidence points to the emergence of yet another questionable practice: the use of dots to identify patients who *are* for resuscitation (that is, on wards or in residential care homes where the number of patients/residents deemed NFR outnumber those who are for resuscitation) (confidential source, personal communication). It is not yet known how widespread this practice is. In the light of such difficulties, I am not convinced that the recommendation of the Association of Medical Directors of Victorian Hospitals that the use of a specially designed sticker will improve the situation. It merely replaces one problem with another; it does not resolve it.

The use of initials such as 'NFR' or 'DNR', and variations thereof, is also seriously problematic. In one case, for example, a nurse informed me that a doctor had once ordered her to write the initials 'NFR' on a patient's chart. When she queried this directive, she was politely told: 'Don't worry. If there are any problems, we'll just say it means 'Not for Referral ...'. In another case, the initials 'NFR' were written on a patient's nursing care plan, which was left hanging on the end of his bed. During visiting hours, a family member visiting the patient took the liberty of examining the nursing care plan and noticed the initials 'NFR' on it. She asked a passing nurse what the letters meant. To this question the nurse replied: 'Oh, don't worry about that. It just means 'Nice Fellow Really ...'.

In yet another case, a dietitian writing in a patient's integrated case notes (that is, where all members of the health care team — doctors, nurses, and other allied carers — write up their notes) wrote the initials 'NFR' meaning 'not for referral'. Understandably, the dietitian was very distressed when the significance of what she had written was pointed out to her.

The practice of using *pencilled* abbreviations provokes one more comment. This is done so that the initials can be erased when and if the patient dies or alternatively is discharged; the task almost invariably falls to attending nursing staff.

A last concern to be considered here is the practice of ordering 'nursing care only' or 'cares for comfort only' when it is considered that nothing more can be done medically for the patient. The professional — not to mention the moral — acceptability of using 'nursing care only' as a euphemism for withdrawing life-saving medical treatment warrants questioning, however. Nurses need to realise — and need to make it publicly known — that, contrary to popular medical opinion, writing such orders is not an acceptable medical tactic for refusing to accept responsibility in instances where it is decided on the basis of questionable criteria that 'nothing more can be done (medically)'. For one thing, in situations where all means have not, in fact, been exhausted, there is always room to question whether CPR (or any other life-supporting measure, for that matter) should, in fact, be rightfully withheld from a patient. On this point it is worthwhile to consider Veatch's helpful comments. In his book *Death, dying and the biological revolution*, Veatch writes:

The question should never be, 'When should we stop treating this patient?' as if the patient were an object to be repaired or discarded. Rather the moral question must be, 'When, if ever, should it be morally and/or legally possible for the patient to decide to refuse medical treatment even if that may mean that dying will no longer be prolonged?'

(Veatch 1977, p. 8)

Whatever the reasons for permitting verbal NFR directives, and for using dots, asterisks, abbreviations and initials to communicate these, the provocative question remains:

> *If the practice of ordering NFR is so medically, morally and legally justified, why are doctors so reticent in and so loathe to document their NFR directives formally? Why are nurses so ready to use crude and erasable symbols to communicate such important directives?*

Until satisfactory answers to such questions can be given, the practices in question should rightly be condemned as professionally, ethically and legally unsound.

Nurses who continue to use dots and similar symbols to communicate a doctor's NFR directive must accept that they alone are the ones responsible for documenting the decisions which doctors otherwise refuse to put in writing (Adams 1984, p. 53; Macklin 1993, pp. 34–6). If they do not wish to have this responsibility, clearly they need to stop enforcing and upholding the communication modes currently being employed in this area. They must insist that their medical colleagues take full responsibility for the decisions they make and the directives they give to nursing staff on the basis of those decisions.

Problems concerning the implementation of NFR directives

A third major area of concern in the NFR debate involves following or carrying out the NFR directives. While at first glance this might seem to be a relatively trivial concern, literature on the subject suggests otherwise (see also *The Regan report on hospital law* 1985).

It is probably true to say that many nurses experience no difficulty whatsoever in carrying out NFR directives — indeed, in some instances, they may be largely responsible for encouraging doctors to prescribe them. Humphry and Wickett (1987), for example, cite a 1984 poll surveying nurses' attitudes towards withholding life-sustaining procedures from dying patients (p. 128). The poll suggested that a staggering majority (70–84 per cent) of those nurses surveyed were in favour of withholding life-support procedures and extraordinary means of life-saving treatment in given situations.

Polls such as these should, however, be treated cautiously. I would argue, for instance, that it is also probably true that many nurses suffer significant hardships on account of covert institutional demands to follow NFR/CPR directives (see also Dolan 1988). The case of the nurse involved in caring for Mr H, cited earlier, stands as an important example of the kinds of difficulties nurses can face, particularly in instances where an informed consent has not been obtained before giving an NFR directive. Very often, nurses follow a questionable NFR directive simply to avoid the wrath of a prescribing doctor — or even nurse superiors — both of whom have the power to 'make life difficult' for a dissenting nurse.

385

Conversely, nurses who decide not to initiate resuscitation in the absence of a medical NFR/DNR directive can also face enormous difficulties. In one noted English case, for example, a registered nurse 'who chose to let an elderly man die rather than call in a resuscitation team' was dismissed for gross misconduct (*Nursing Times* 1983, p. 20; see also Johnstone 1994b, pp. 258–9). The fact that the man was 78-years-old, had lung cancer, and essentially died of 'natural causes' apparently had no bearing on the case (Buchanan 1983; Regan 1983).

The issue of carrying out NFR directives is, of course, of particular concern to nurses; quite simply, they are almost invariably left with the ultimate decision whether or not to initiate CPR in an arrest situation. They are also thus invariably left with the burden of having to accept the responsibility for the consequences of both their actions and their omissions in arrest situations — a point which, I believe, is not always fully understood by attending nurses. Given this, it is nothing short of nonsense to suggest that nurses have no separate moral, legal or professional responsibilities in situations where a patient's life and wellbeing are hanging in the balance. What such considerations wisely instruct is that nurses, who carry the legal, moral, professional and indeed personal burdens of implementing NFR directives, must take a much stronger stand on ensuring that sound and reliable guidelines and policies are brought into being — not only to protect their own interests, but equally importantly, if not more so, the interests of their patients.

Improving NFR practices

Until now it has been contended that NFR decision-making has, on the whole, been:

- arbitrary and unsound;
- based on questionable and unreliable criteria — particularly in instances where doctors and nurses have relied on little more than institutional norms for guiding NFR decisions, rather than on critically reflective moral judgment;
- not always respectful of a patient's considered preferences;
- open to serious misinterpretation as a result of inadequate guidelines;
- made in a way that serves the interests of attending health care professionals and the health care agency, rather than those of the patient;
- unfairly left to nurses, who then have to carry an enormous share of the burdens associated with doctors prescribing NFR directives.

As a response to some of the weaknesses in current NFR decision-making practices, I shall briefly outline seven important points which I believe ought to be reflected in NFR guidelines.

1. There needs to be a recognition that NFR decisions have a profound moral dimension, and are not just medical, nursing or legal in nature, and because of this must be made by appealing to sound moral criteria and standards as well as to relevant clinical information.
2. Any NFR decision made ought to reflect the *patient's informed choice* (given informed choice in its most stringent sense here).
3. NFR decisions/directives should be *properly written* on patients' medical and nursing charts, and should include all the relevant information upon which the decisions have been based (including descriptions of the patients' statements relevant to their request that given life-saving

measures be withheld). Alternatively, an 'NFR authorisation form' could be signed; an example is shown in Figure 14.1.

4. Mechanisms must be established to ensure the *correct interpretation* of non-treatment directives.

5. Once an NFR decision has been made, it should be *reviewed and re-affirmed* in writing at intervals which are appropriate to the patient's changing condition (Clinical Ethics Committee 1984).

6. An NFR directive should be *able to be revoked* at 'any time at the request of the competent patient, or in the case of the incompetent patient, by the cited next-of-kin or legal representative', or as is morally appropriate (Clinical Ethics Committee 1984).

7. An NFR decision should be carried out only by those who have freely, and possessing the necessary information, agreed to carry out such directives. Where nurses or doctors have genuine conscientious objection to following an NFR directive, morally they ought to be *permitted to abstain* from being actively involved in caring for the patient in question. (See the discussion on conscientious objection in Chapter 15.)

Directing NFR/DNR on patients is a common and widespread practice in hospitals both in Australia and overseas. In one Australian study, for example, it was found that of the 272 people who had died over a three-month period during 1987 in a major South Australian teaching hospital, 166 (61 per cent) had been the subject of an NFR directive (Stanley and Reid 1989, p. 260). This figure was noted by the investigators to be consistent with the findings of other studies (Stanley and Reid 1989, p. 261). Several studies in the United States, meanwhile, have shown that NFR/DNR occurs in 'approximately 3–14% of [all] hospital admissions' (Lipton 1989, p. 108). In some residential care homes in Australia, however, the percentage of those made NFR is likely to be 100 per cent, because unwritten policies in some homes prescribe that all residents are *automatically* NFR/DNR on admission.

Where, then, does this leave the nursing profession? What can and should the nursing profession do about the NFR/DNR issue? I believe that a number of important activities can and should be carried out. In summary, the nursing profession must actively work to:

- ensure that its members are adequately informed of the issues at stake and are adequately prepared to articulate the important concerns facing them when confronted with NFR decisions and directives during their everyday practice;
- ensure that sound and reliable mechanisms are put in place to protect patients' rights and interests when confronted with a life-threatening or harm-causing situation;
- encourage open and honest public debate on the NFR issue and help to promote the community's awareness of what is at stake for the health-care seeking public;
- promote the community's entitlement and duty to participate in any public debate on the NFR issue;
- fight for the entitlement to participate in the development of criteria for NFR policies, and guard against the likelihood of criteria being formulated and imposed that do not ensure the achievement of morally desirable outcomes in arrest or life-threatening situations (the *patient's preferences or expressed wishes*, regardless of what others might think of these, ought to have primary consideration here);

Heidelberg Repatriation Hospital

Banksia Street
Heidelberg West
Victoria 3081 Australia

Surname	Given names	File number

(Affix patient label if available)

PATIENT MANAGEMENT PLAN

In the event of a cardiac arrest ....

UR No. ...., is not to undergo cardiopulmonary resuscitation (CPR)

Name of consultant in charge of patient's care who has given approval ....

Reason for decision to withhold CPR ....

Specific treatment to be continued other than CPR (eg. antibiotics, blood transfusion)...............

Extent of communication with the patient and next of kin (with names)...............

Staff (medical, nursing, allied health) consulted about the decision to withhold CPR ....

Staff informed about the decision to withhold CPR (especially nursing staff)...............

Other relevant information (eg. Refusal of Medical Treatment certificate, role of patient's guardian, role of Director of Medical Services) ....

Signed ....   Name ....

Position ....   Date ....

Not For Cardio-Pulmonary Resuscitation MR/120

Figure 14.1 An example of a form authorising a 'Not For Resuscitation' directive (reproduced with permission by the former Heidelberg Repatriation Hospital, Heidleberg West, Victoria, now the Austin Repatriation Medical Centre)

(Figure 14.1 continued)

NOT FOR CARDIO-PULMONARY RESUSCITATION GUIDELINES

A decision to withhold CPR should be carefully considered, and only made after investigating all available options.

1.   INDICATIONS

a)   If after being adequately informed about the diagnosis, prognosis and the nature of the procedure, and having had time and adequate counselling to adjust emotionally, a competent patient expresses the seriously considered judgement that he or she not be resuscitated in the event that the current condition results in a cardiac arrest, and there is no reason to believe that the patient is suicidal.

b)   If on medical grounds, the procedure is considered futile.

c)   If the medical team is reasonably certain that in the event of a cardiac arrest, resuscitation being achieved, the patient would be so severely disabled and have such a poor prognosis that the distress caused by the resuscitation procedures would be disproportionate to the result.

d)   The patient may have appointed, whilst competent, an agent with enduring power of attorney (under the Treatment Act 1990) to make decisions regarding treatment in the event that the patient becomes incompetent. An agent may refuse treatment on behalf of the patient.

2.   COMMUNICATION

If CPR is not considered appropriate it should be discussed with the patient if his or her emotional and cognitive state permits. The clinician in charge should fully outline the diagnosis, prognosis and treatment options available, allow the patient time to review and discuss this information, involve the patient in the decision about CPR and ensure that the patient is informed of the final decision. If the patient is not competent or is emotionally incapable of being involved these discussions should take place with the patient's next of kin.

If the patient presents a Refusal of Treatment certificate issued under the Treatment Act 1990, or if the patient has an enduring power of attorney or a legally appointed guardian then the matter should be referred to the Director of Medical Services.

3.   DOCUMENTATION

a)   The names of the person making the Not for Resuscitation Order and the consultant who approved the order. A Not For Resuscitation Order should not be signed without the approval of the consultant in charge of the patient's care.

b)   The reason for the decision.

c)   Specific treatment to be continued other than CPR (eg. antibiotics, blood transfusions).

d)   The extent of communication about the decision with the patient or the patient's next of kin.

e)   The names of other staff consulted about the decision (medical, nursing, allied health).

f)   The names of other staff informed of the decision (medical, nursing, allied health).

g)   Any other relevant information (eg. Refusal of Medical Treatment Certificate, role of patient's guardian, role of Director of Medical Services, names of those to be contacted if the patient dies).

A Not for Resuscitation Order is not irreversible and should be reviewed at regular intervals. In particular it should be reviewed if there is a change in the patient's prognosis or if a new consultant takes on a significant role in the patient's management (eg. during the immediate post-operative period if the patient undergoes surgery). Wherever possible, this should be discussed with the patient or the patient's next of kin.

- ensure that morally sound and reliable policies and guidelines are adopted in the clinical setting for guiding NFR/CPR decisions; and, lastly,
- ensure that provision is made for individual nurses who are otherwise conscientiously opposed to a given NFR/CPR directive and thus wish to be exempted from caring for a patient who is the subject of such directives.

It is not being suggested here that NFR directives have no place among the care/treatment alternatives available to seriously ill patients. To reject the moral acceptability of NFR directives outright — without any regard for the kinds of circumstances under which they might well be justified — would be capricious. What is being suggested here, however, is that, if NFR directives are to be formulated, this must be done on the basis of morally sound criteria and decision-making processes.

Responding to the difficulties posed by the use of life-support systems and the NFR issue, the Clinical Ethics Committee of Physicians and Dentists of the Royal Victoria Hospital, Montreal (1984), argues that guidelines must be directed towards:

> defining important ethical principles and their application, recognition of the autonomy of the competent patient, the role of the family, the importance of good communication at all levels, special mechanisms to deal with persistent disagreement, and circumstances in which judicial opinion must be sought.
>
> (Clinical Ethics Committee, Council of Physicians and Dentists 1984, p. 1)

By incorporating these and the many other similar considerations in NFR policies and guidelines outlined in this chapter and elsewhere (see Hickie 1990), nurses and doctors can rest assured that they truly have done all that is possible to ensure that patients' rights and interests have been properly respected in life-threatening situations, and that they have not overstepped their authority as health care providers. Members of the community at large can also rest assured that their assumptions about being well cared for upon coming into hospital or other related health care agencies are not misplaced, and that they can indeed trust and rely on those people who will most probably care for them during those delicate, life-threatening moments which are all too often characterised by intense personal need and human vulnerability.

Conclusion

In a study on quality of life following spinal cord injury (SCI), a team of researchers found that emergency health care providers' (including nurses') attitudes about quality of life following spinal cord injury were substantially more negative than the attitudes expressed by those who had actually sustained such an injury. For instance, whereas only 18 per cent of emergency health care workers 'imagined they would be glad to be alive with a severe SCI', a substantial 92 per cent of those who had a true spinal cord injury were glad to be alive (Gerhart et al. 1994). And whereas only 17 per cent of emergency health care workers 'anticipated an average or better quality of life' following an imagined spinal cord injury, 86 per cent of those who had a true spinal cord injury had an average or better quality of life (Gerhart et al. 1994). Other studies have yielded similar results (Gerhart et al. 1994).

Many health care providers (nurses among them) assume that people who suffer devastating injuries (or illnesses) have — or will have — a poor quality of life. Further, this belief is sometimes translated into the judgment that 'those who cannot lead normal lives would be better off dead' (Gerhart et al. 1994, citing Dunnum 1990). Not infrequently, these kinds of judgments influence decisions about whether or not to treat (see NFT directives) or to resuscitate (see NFR directives) patients deemed 'medically hopeless'. As the above research has shown, however, those who provide health care and those who receive it may not always share the same view about the conditions under which a quality of life is possible. *Quality of life* judgments can have a significant bearing on *quality* (and *quantity*) *of care/treatment* decisions. The views and attitudes of health care providers may not only significantly affect the care they provide, but may also 'influence patients and families struggling with critical treatment decisions' (Gerhart et al. 1994, p. 807). It is therefore vital that health care providers exercise great care when making quality of life judgments, and act in a morally responsible way when using these judgments to inform clinical decisions. Anything less could result in morally undesirable consequences. For example, a prejudicial judgment about a patient's quality of life could result in needed care and treatment being withheld or withdrawn prematurely, and the patient dying prematurely as a consequence. It is therefore crucial that those making quality of life judgments (including nurses) are fully aware of the nature of their judgments, and the extent to which these might influence decisions about a patient's care and treatment — including whether it should be initiated at all, continued, or be withdrawn. It is also crucial that decision-makers are aware that, inevitably, judgments about quality of life, NFT and NFR involve not merely clinical judgments, but also moral judgments and ones which, once acted upon, will always have a moral consequence. Whether this consequence will be 'good' or 'bad' may, in the end, depend less on professional judgment than on personal integrity.

Chapter 15

Taking a stand: conscientious objection, strike action and institutional ethics committees

Introduction

A time invariably comes when nurses must take a stand on what they consider, after careful and critical reflection, to be morally important. Taking a stand can involve either individual or collective action. Individual action may involve a nurse refusing conscientiously to participate in a controversial medical procedure; reporting a troubling incident to a superior or some other authority (including an external statutory authority); seeking nomination on an institutional ethics committee; or, quite simply, speaking out in either a conference or workshop, or some other type of public forum. On rare occasions, a nurse might decide to 'blow the whistle' or approach the media. Collective action, on the other hand, may involve groups of nurses embarking on an organised lobbying campaign aimed at particular target groups. Or, as is becoming increasingly common around the world, it may involve all-out strike action.

Whatever action is taken, it is never free of moral risk. There are many examples of nurses having suffered both personally and professionally because they took a stand on what they deemed to be an important professional or moral issue. Nurses conscientiously refusing to participate in morally controversial medical procedures have lost their jobs or have been made to resign 'voluntarily'. Some of those undertaking strike action have likewise lost their jobs, and have even been threatened with deregistration and charges of criminal negligence for their actions. (Examples are given in the discussion on strike action later in this chapter.)

Despite the associated hazards and risks, nurses have a moral obligation to take a stand on important ethical issues (see also Johnstone 1998). Nevertheless, there are some misconceptions about the nature of this obligation, the options open to nurses for taking a stand, and even about whether it is right to take a stand at all. Some nurses even fear that some of the options open to them (such as conscientious objection, strike action, appealing to an institutional ethics committee, or lobbying) are incompatible with their broader professional obligations as nurses and are therefore 'unprofessional'. For some nurses this has caused enormous personal conflict, and has served more to exacerbate the moral problems they face in the workplace than to help resolve them.

This chapter attempts to clarify some of the confusion surrounding the options open to nurses for taking a stand, and to show that these options might not only be compatible with professional nursing obligations, but may even be prima facie professional nursing obligations in themselves. It is to discussing the options of conscientious objection, strike action, and institutional ethics committees that this chapter now turns.

Conscientious objection[1]

Nurses have for years been 'conscientiously refusing' in private or informal ways. Their objections have sometimes gone beyond informal 'cafeteria' conversation and gained public attention — but only in extreme situations, such as when a nurse has been dismissed or denied employment, or has been threatened in some way. Those who have had the courage to formally voice their conscientious refusal to participate in certain medical procedures, or to carry out certain directives given by a superior, have sometimes done so at great personal and professional cost. In Chapter 2, for example, we examined the case of Corinne Warthen, a registered nurse who was successfully dismissed from her employing hospital of eleven years for refusing to dialyse a terminally ill unconscious patient on conscientious grounds — i.e. that the procedure was causing him more harm (see also Johnstone 1988, 1994, 1998); and in Chapter 11 we discussed the case of a New South Wales registered nurse who was allegedly denied employment as a midwife because of her conscientious objection to abortion and sterilisation. And we saw the case of a registered nurse who 'voluntarily' resigned because she was conscientiously opposed to her employing hospital's unwritten policy on 'Not For Resuscitation' (NFR) directives (see Chapter 14). (Other examples not included in this text involve nurses who have been dismissed for refusing to assist with electroconvulsive therapy (ECT) or other involuntary psychiatric treatment, such as the forced administration of psychotropic drugs — see, for example, Beardshaw 1982; Parsons 1982; *Nursing Times*, 22 September 1982, p. 1573; Hicks 1982; *Nursing Times*, 20 October 1982, p. 1738; *Nursing Times*, 6 April 1983, p. 17; *Nursing Times*, 10 August 1983, p. 18; *Nursing Mirror*, 20 June 1984, p. 2; Vousden 1985; *Nursing Times*, 31 December 1986, p. 7; Crabbe 1988, p. 18.)

These and similar cases illustrate convincingly that the issue of conscientious objection among nurses is by no means trivial. Nevertheless, despite the threat it poses to the moral integrity of both individual nurses and the nursing profession as a whole, the issue of conscientious objection remains poorly addressed in nursing domains: there is a paucity of nursing literature and nursing research on the subject; professional nursing position statements on conscientious objection are either non-existent or seriously wanting in content; and mechanisms for protecting nurses who claim conscientious objector status are either wholly lacking or grossly inadequate, making it virtually impossible for nurses to conscientiously refuse to participate in certain procedures without fear of censure or of being discriminated against in some other way. One unfortunate consequence of the nursing profession's neglect of this issue is that it makes it easier for policy makers, employers and others to dismiss the problem of conscientious objection among nurses as either a non-issue or at most only a trivial issue, and therefore one not warranting serious attention or concern.

---

1. An earlier version of the discussion of conscientious objection was presented as a paper entitled 'Conscientious objection and professional obligation — a contradiction in terms?' at the Nursing Law and Ethics, 2nd Victorian State Conference, *Dealing with dilemmas*, Monash University, 5 May 1989 (organised by the School of Nursing, Phillip Institute of Technology). The paper has been revised for publication in this text.

The issue of conscientious objection by nurses is, however, far from being a trivial matter, and deserves the attention of all concerned. In particular, attention needs to be given to clarifying the nature and authority of conscience, distinguishing between genuine and bogus claims of conscientious objection, and determining the kinds of policy there should be towards those who conscientiously refuse to perform or to participate in morally controversial medical and/or nursing procedures. As well as this, attention needs to be given to the question of when, if ever, a superior can decently direct nurses to perform tasks which they are conscientiously opposed to performing. An additional question is: Can nurses decently refuse to assist with tasks which others do not regard as morally problematic? These and other key concerns raised by the conscientious objection debate are addressed in the following sections.

The nature of conscience explained

The *Oxford English dictionary* defines 'conscience' as 'the internal acknowledgment or recognition of the moral quality of one's motives and actions; the sense of right and wrong as regards things for which one is responsible; the faculty or principle which pronounces upon the moral quality of one's actions or motives, approving the right and condemning the wrong'. The *Collins English dictionary* defines 'conscience' as a 'sense of right and wrong that governs a person's thoughts and actions'. These definitions, however, are inadequate to answer questions concerning the legitimacy and power of conscience as a bona fide moral authority. In short, while they help to describe what conscience is, these definitions say nothing about whether individuals should always obey their conscientious senses of right and wrong, or whether others can reasonably be expected to respect another's conscientious claims. Once again, we must turn to moral philosophy for some more substantive answers.

Philosophical accounts of conscience fall roughly into three categories: as *moral reasoning*, as *moral feelings*, and as a *combination of moral reasoning and moral feelings* (see also Mill 1962, pp. 281–4; Hume 1888, p. 458; Kant 1930, pp. 129–35; Rawls 1971, pp. 205–11, 368–9; Beauchamp and Childress 1989, pp. 385–94).

Conscience as moral reasoning

A reasonable or rationalistic account of conscience regards rational moral principles and reason as the source of one's moral convictions. Conscientious judgments, by this view, are really critically reflective moral judgments concerning right and wrong (Garnett 1965; Broad 1940). Rational insight can be either religious or non-religious in nature, depending on what a person's world views are. Either way, a rational conscience typically manifests itself as 'a little voice inside one's head saying what one should and should not do'. Or, to put this in moral terms, it tells us what our moral obligations and duties are. Statements of conscientious objection then are, by this view, merely statements of moral duty which individuals recognise and commit themselves to fulfil. Whether the duties or obligations identified impose overriding or absolute demands, or only prima facie demands on the individual is, however, another matter entirely, and one that is considered shortly.

Conscience as moral feelings

There are two possible versions of a 'moral feelings' account of conscience — emotivist and intuitionist. Both consist of a tendency to spontaneously experience either emotions or intuitions 'of a unique sort of approval of the doing of what is believed to be right and a similarly unique sort of disapproval of the doing of what is believed to be wrong' (Garnett 1965, p. 81).

It is generally recognised that these feelings are quite different from the sorts of feelings we might have when, for example, looking at a beautiful painting (aesthetic approval) or an awful painting (aesthetic disapproval), or eating a favourite food (the feelings of mere liking) or smelling an awful smell (feelings of mere disliking), or witnessing an act of remarkable human achievement (feelings of admiration) or an act of extraordinary human failure (feelings of disdain). By contrast, in the case of wicked acts or the violation of duty, conscience may manifest itself in strong and distinguishable feelings of moral loathing, shame, remorse, or even guilt, or, as Beauchamp and Childress (1989) suggest, the unpleasant feelings of 'a loss of integrity, wholeness, peace, and harmony' (p. 387). To borrow from Fletcher (1966), conscience can manifest itself as 'a sharp stone in the breast under the sternum, which turns and hurts when we have done wrong' (p. 54). In the case of virtuous acts, conscience may manifest itself as strong feelings of reassurance or moral goodness (Fletcher 1966, p. 54; Kant 1930, p. 130), or, as Beauchamp and Childress (1989) suggest, as feelings of integrity, wholeness, peace and harmony (p. 387). Either way, moral feelings instruct individuals on what they ought and/or ought not to do. As with the rationalistic account, statements of conscience emerge as statements of obligation and duty.

Conscience as moral reason and moral feelings

The concept of conscience as a combination of reason and feelings basically involves an integrated response to moral triggers in the world. It does not rely on 'blind emotive obedience', as Kordig (1976) calls it, nor on an exclusive and blind devotion to reason. Rather, it relies on the mutually guiding and instructive forces of both *moral sensibilities* and *moral reasoning*. This account of conscience is, in my view, the most plausible of the three given, and is thus the one that underpins this discussion.

How conscience works

Now that we have briefly examined the essential nature of conscience, the next question is: How does conscience function as a moral authority?

It is generally recognised that conscience functions as a *personal* (internal) *sanction* and as a *personal moral authority* (Childress 1979; Beauchamp and Childress 1989, p. 388). Claims of conscience typically identify individual people with their self-chosen or autonomously chosen standards and principles of conduct (Nowell-Smith 1954, p. 268); further, they *commit* individual people to act in accordance with those principles. In other words, claims of conscience commit the individual person to act morally (Timms 1983, p. 41). Thus, when conscience is said to be 'personal' or 'one's own', all that is being claimed is that a particular set of autonomously chosen moral standards has authority over a particular person — not, as is sometimes mistakenly thought, that the person has a unique and different set of moral standards from everybody else, and thus is a kind of 'moral freak'.

Conscience can be appealed to both as a kind of 'reviewer' or 'judge' of past acts, and as an 'authority on' or as a 'guide to' future acts. Whether conscience is appealed to as judge or guide, however, it is important to understand that conscience is not *morality itself*, nor is it the *ultimate standard* (or even *a standard*) of morality. Rather, as Gonsalves explains, it is:

> ... only the intellect itself exercising a special function, the function of judging the rightness or wrongness, the moral value, of our own individual acts according to the set of moral values and principles the person holds with conviction.

(Gonsalves 1985, p. 55)

Or, as Childress explains, it is merely 'the mode of consciousness resulting from the application of standards' (1979, p. 319).

Gonsalves' and Childress' views make it plain that statements of conscience are not statements of a unique moral faculty or of unique moral standards. Rather, they are statements of a *particular application of adopted moral standards*. Conscientious objection, by this view, essentially translates into a case of *moral disagreement* in regard to which moral statements apply and what one's moral duty is in a particular situation. If this is so, the case for respecting a conscientious objector's claims becomes compelling — particularly in instances where there are no clear-cut moral grounds for settling a specific disagreement (as sometimes occurs in the cases of abortion, organ transplantation, assisting with the involuntary administration of ECT or psychotropic medication, administering blood to Jehovah's Witness patients, and similar cases).

It should be noted here that, once it is accepted that claims of conscience translate into claims of duty, it is conceptually incorrect to speak of conscientious objection as a *right* (as some nursing position statements on the subject do). To assert this would be to assert that an individual has a 'right to have a duty', which is conceptually incorrect. It is more correct to speak of others being bound to respect another's claim of conscience, just as they are bound to respect another's claim of moral duty.

The problem remains, however, that consciences are fallible and can make mistakes (Seeskin 1978). As Nowell-Smith (1954, p. 247) points out, some of the worst crimes in human history have been committed by people acting on the firm convictions of conscience. Hitler, for example, believed he was fulfilling a supreme moral duty by purging the German race of its 'Jewish disease' (Kordig 1976). Others also point out that, in some instances, what appears to be a claim of conscience may be nothing more than a claim of prudence or self-interest or convenience. This invariably raises the question: Should I always obey my conscience? Further to this, claims of conscience can be insincere or counterfeit, raising the additional questions of: How can I distinguish between genuine and bogus claims of conscientious objection? Should I always respect another's conscientious claims? It is to answering these questions that this discussion now turns.

Bogus and genuine claims of conscientious objection

For a conscientious objection to be genuine, it must satisfy at least five conditions.

1. It must have as its basis a *distinctively moral motivation*, as opposed to the motivations of mere self-interest, prudence, convenience or prejudice. By this is meant:
   a. that the action has as its aim the maintenance of sound moral standards, and the achievement of a moral end (Garnett 1965);

    b. that the person performing the act sincerely believes in the moral characteristics of the action in question, and sincerely desires to do what is right (Broad 1940, p. 75; Childress 1979, p. 334); and

    c. that the desire to do what is right is sufficient to override considerations of fear, cowardice, self-interest, and prejudice.

2. It must be performed on the basis of *autonomous, informed, and critically reflective choice*. By this is meant:

    a. that the action must be the agent's 'own', so to speak — that is, it is not the product of coercion or manipulation; and

    b. that that action has been carefully considered — that is, that the person has taken into account all the relevant factual as well as ethical information pertaining to the situation at hand, possible alternatives to the action being contemplated, and predicted moral outcomes of the action once it is taken (Broad 1940, p. 75).

3. Conscience should be appealed to only *as a last resort* — that is, in defence of one's moral beliefs. A claim of conscientious objection is a last resort when all other means of achieving a tolerable solution to a given moral problem have failed. Here conscientious objection is justified on grounds analogous to those justifying self-defence, which permit people to use reasonable force in order to preserve their integrity (in this case, their moral integrity) (Machan 1983, pp. 503–5).

4. The conscientious objector must admit that *others might have an equal and opposing claim of objection*. For example, a nurse refusing on conscientious grounds to assist with an abortion procedure must be prepared to accept that the aborting surgeon may feel obliged as a matter of conscience to go ahead with the abortion. To quote from Broad: 'What is sauce for the conscientious goose is sauce for the conscientious ganders who are his [sic] neighbours or his [sic] governors' (Broad 1940, p. 78).

5. *The situation in which it is being claimed must itself be of a nature which is morally uncertain*; that is, there are no clear-cut moral grounds upon which the matter at hand can be readily and satisfactorily resolved, and competing views can be shown to be equally valid.

If we accept these criteria, the task of distinguishing bogus from genuine claims of conscientious objection becomes considerably easier. To illustrate this, consider four types of situations in which nurses commonly claim conscientious objection: the lawful but morally controversial directives of a superior; a conflict of personal values between a nurse and a patient; personal fear of contagion; and unsafe working conditions.

Conscientious objection to the lawful but morally controversial directives of a superior

Nurses as employees are compelled by the principle of employment law to obey the lawful and reasonable directives of an employer or superior. The problem is, however, that nurses might not always agree morally with the lawful directives they have been given, and thus may sometimes find themselves in the uncomfortable position of having to perform acts which violate their reasoned moral judgments (Johnstone 1988, 1994, 1998).

There are many examples of nurses having been caught in both personal and professional dilemmas on account of legal demands to obey the lawful though morally controversial directives of doctors and nurse superiors. Several examples have already been given in this text, typically involving situations in which nurses have been directed, against their will, to assist with morally controversial procedures such as abortion, euthanasia, electroconvulsive therapy (ECT) and organ transplantation. The difficulties nurses have encountered in such situations have been compounded by the fact that they have had little, if any, avenue for officially expressing their conscientious refusal without fear of losing their jobs or facing other threats.

Situations involving nurses' conscientious refusal to follow lawful but morally questionable directives invariably pose the age-old question of whether an individual can, all things considered, be decently expected to follow morally controversial or morally bad, although legally valid, laws — or, in this case, lawful directives.

As I have stated elsewhere (Johnstone 1988), the problem of legal–moral conflict is not new to philosophy. Questions of, for example, what is the proper relationship of morality to law, what is to count as a *good* legal system, or whether individuals ought to be compelled to obey immoral laws, are still matters of great philosophical controversy. Hart, an Oxford scholar and professor of jurisprudence, argues persuasively that existing law must not supplant morality 'as a final test of conduct and so escape criticism' (Hart 1957). He also argues that the demands of law must be submitted to the scrutiny and guidance of sound morality before they can be justly enforced (Hart 1961). Not surprisingly, these kinds of views have sparked enormous debates in both philosophy and law. It is beyond the scope of this text to discuss Hart's views and address the interesting questions concerning the philosophy of law that they raise. Nevertheless, it is assumed for argument's sake here that any law which fails the test of sound moral scrutiny should be either adjusted or rejected; it is also assumed that to punish autonomous moral agents for refusing to obey lawful but morally questionable directives is *morally unjust*.

A number of other important considerations are worthy of attention here. First, there is the persuasive view that forcing nurses to act against their reasoned or conscientious judgments is to not only ignore or diminish their moral autonomy, but also to violate the principles of critical morality itself — not least those of autonomy and reflectivity (Muyskens 1982, p. 61). Perhaps even more troubling is the possibility that violating nurses' consciences would also unjustly violate their integrity as moral agents (Childress 1979).

Second, it is generally recognised that if people are forced constantly to violate their conscience then their conscience will gradually weaken and lose its authority (Kant 1930). This in turn makes it easier for individuals to avoid fulfilling their perceived moral duties and/or acting in accordance with autonomously chosen moral standards. As a result, there is likely to be a general breakdown in compliance with moral rules and principles, and a general erosion of individual moral responsibility and accountability. It takes little to imagine what would happen to the moral fabric of the community at large if all its members were forced, say, by order of the state, constantly to violate their reasoned moral judgments or consciences. No less consideration is due to what may ultimately happen to the moral fabric of the nursing profession if its individual members are constantly forced to abandon their reasoned moral judgments and consciences in favour of preserving the prescriptions and proscriptions of law and convention.

Related to this is a third consideration — that moral duty 'is mainly concerned with the avoidance of intolerable results' (Urmson 1958, p. 72). If fulfilling one's supposed duty does not avoid or prevent intolerable results, it seems reasonable to question whether in fact it was one's duty in the first place. As with the case of supererogatory acts (that is, acts above the call of duty, such as those performed by saints and heroes), care must be taken to distinguish those deeds which can be reasonably expected of 'ordinary' persons (or 'ordinary' nurses) from those which it would merely be nice of 'ordinary' persons (nurses) to perform, but which could never be reasonably *expected* of them (Urmson 1958, p. 68). On this point, Urmson (1958, p. 71) argues: '... a line must be drawn between what we can expect and demand of others and what we can merely hope for and receive with gratitude when we get it'.

Fourth, those who coerce others to act against their conscience erroneously presume that coercion vitiates moral responsibility. This, however, is not so. Just as more sophisticated claims of duty cannot be escaped or deceived, neither can claims of conscience. It is a mistake to hold that, if a person is forced to perform an act to which they are conscientiously opposed, they are less morally culpable for that act, and that they will feel less morally guilty for having performed it. What users of force fail to understand is that an instance of moral violation still stands, regardless of whether it has been caused by an act of coercion or an act of free will.

Fifth, nurses are not automata or robots, but thinking, reasoning, feeling, responsible human beings. Legal law recognises this by the very fact that it can and does hold nurses independently accountable for their actions (Johnstone 1994). Given this, it is a mistake to hold that nurses have an *unqualified* duty to obey the directives of a superior.

Lastly, it is ultimately more desirable than not to have a health care system comprised of conscientious nurses. Nurses comprise 70 per cent of the health care work force. The prospect of 70 per cent of health care providers being morally unconscientious is a bleak one. Since most of us cannot be saints, but can be conscientious, we need to preserve and cultivate conscientiousness (Nowell-Smith 1954, p. 259; Garnett 1965, p. 91). Only by doing this can we be assured of achieving and maintaining some sort of moral order in health care domains. As Seeskin (1978) argues, '... we have no guarantee that our deliberations will be perfect or our moral sensibilities adequate' (p. 299); it is for this reason, among others, that conscience and moral conscientiousness should be given a place among the moral virtues. We might be condemned as fanatics if we hold conscience to be infallible, but if we do not at least acknowledge its ultimateness in the scheme of moral reasoning, we might be guilty of moral negligence and moral irresponsibility (Seeskin 1978; Kordig 1976).

The consequences of such views have interesting implications for policy makers attempting to respond to the conscientious objection problem. These views seem to suggest that, even if nurses' consciences are mistaken, on balance there are moral benefits to be gained by permitting their conscientious objections — not least, the benefits of fostering moral sensitivity and moral responsibility in the workplace. These views also suggest that, if nurses are not permitted conscientiously to object, then health care contexts, not to mention the community at large, will be morally worse off by virtue of being more at risk of suffering moral harms on account of receiving care that is not informed or guided by conscientious ethical beliefs and standards.

It might be objected here that permitting conscientious objection is not conducive to the efficient running of hospitals and other health services. There is, however, little support for this kind of claim. In the case of military service, for example, it has been found that objectors are rarely amenable to threats and usually make unsatisfactory soldiers if coerced, and that in fact there are generally not enough objectors to frustrate the community's purpose (Benn and Peters 1959, p. 193). I would suggest that something similar is probably true of objectors in nursing. As some of the examples in this text have shown, nurses have preferred to resign and risk dismissal than perform acts which they find morally offensive. Further to this, those nurses who have been coerced have not wholly complied with given orders. (For example, I know of nurses who have resuscitated patients in cases of controversial NFR directives, and not resuscitated patients in the case of controversial CPR orders. A more common disobedience, however, involves night nurses who secretly feed severely disabled newborns on whom a medical directive has been given to withhold nourishing fluids with the purpose of hastening death.) It is also unlikely that there are enough objecting nurses to obstruct the efficient running of the hospital system.

Where lawful directives entail a demand to perform morally controversial procedures, there is considerable scope for suggesting that a nurse has a firm moral basis upon which to conscientiously object. Issues such as abortion, organ transplants, electroconvulsive therapy, the enforced and involuntary treatment of psychiatric patients and euthanasia are all morally controversial, and, as yet, no morally clear-cut grounds exist for resolving them. Until these issues can be resolved satisfactorily, it would be morally indefensible and unjust to insist that nurses must, when directed, assist with abortion, organ transplantation, electro-convulsive therapy and euthanasia work — or any other work which is morally controversial. In other words, where a so-called 'standard' or 'reasonable' medical or nursing procedure is morally questionable, nurses cannot decently be forced to perform or participate in that procedure. Further, it is worth noting once again that what we have in a situation of conscientious objection is moral disagreement — something which, as discussed in Chapter 7, may not be resolved. The most amenable solution seems to be to permit conscientious objection.

Conscientious objection and the problem of conflict in personal values between nurse and patient

The International Council of Nurses' (1973) *Code for Nurses* states that 'the nurse's primary responsibility is to those who require nursing care'. It further states that: '... the nurse, in providing care, promotes an environment in which the values, customs and spiritual beliefs of the individual are respected' (International Council of Nurses 1973). Sometimes, however, a nurse may find it difficult to respect a person's values, customs and spiritual beliefs, and for this reason may decline to be involved in caring for that person. Consider the following cases.

Case 1

A registered nurse working in a general medical ward was assigned a male patient who was known to be an orthodox Muslim. Upon learning of the man's religion, the nurse refused to care for him, stating that she could not accept the attitudes of Muslim males towards women, and that if she cared for him she would be as good as condoning his views.

Case 2

A registered nurse working in an infectious diseases unit was assigned a male patient in the end stages of AIDS. Upon learning that the patient was a homosexual, the nurse refused to accept the assignment. He argued that as a Christian he could not condone homosexuality, and therefore it would be against his religious beliefs to care for the patient.

Case 3

A registered nurse working in a country hospital was asked to admit and care for a patient injured in a fight. When she recognised the patient as a member of a family who had been engaged in a feud with her own family for years, she declined to care for him. She stated as her reason that, were she to care for the man, she would be violating the loyalties she owed to her own family.

There is little doubt that all three registered nurses in the cases just given have sincere motivations behind their refusals to care for the patients in question. What is not so clear, however, is whether these motivations have a *moral* basis. For instance, their refusals to care for these patients seem to be based more on, for example, non-moral personal dislike, prejudice, fear, disdain or mere disapproval than on sincere moral motivation and the desire to achieve morally desirable ends. Second, it is not clear whether, by refusing to care for these patients, the nurses will preserve their moral integrity. In fact, it may be quite the reverse, since they have allowed personal interests to override the significant moral interests of their patients. Lastly, the professional demand to care for the patients in question is not *itself* morally controversial — at least, not in the same way that, say, the demand to care for and stabilise a 'brain dead' patient for organ donation is (see Johnstone 1989, pp. 302–18). While it may be imprudent to compel the nurses in these cases to care for the patients assigned to them, it is not immediately apparent that it would be immoral to do so. It might be concluded then that their refusals can, at least from a moral perspective, be justly overridden. Nevertheless, there may still exist pragmatic grounds for permitting their refusals. If they cannot be relied upon to give adequate care, for example, it might be better to allow their refusal. If their prejudices and personal feelings are of such a nature as to seriously cloud their prudential judgments and indeed their ability to *care* and engage in an effective therapeutic relationship, it may be that they should not be allocated the patients in question. This, however, may be more a practical consideration rather than a fully-fledged moral one — although, granted, one which will probably have a significant moral dimension, namely, the patient's wellbeing.

Conscientious objection, the fear of contagion, and homophobia

The question of if, and when, and under what circumstances nurses may refuse to care for certain patients has become a particularly important and challenging one over recent years, largely because of the worldwide HIV/AIDS epidemic.

Questions have been asked, both in Australia and overseas, about whether nurses can rightly refuse to care for HIV/AIDS patients (including infected newborns). Overseas research studies and opinion polls even suggest that some nurses would rather abandon their practices and nursing careers than place themselves at risk by caring for HIV/AIDS patients (Beard et al. 1988; Lester and Beard 1988; Huerta and Oddi, 1992). In one United States opinion poll, published in *Nursing 88*, it was revealed that 73 per cent of nurses surveyed were concerned about their own safety, and 47 per cent believed they had a right to refuse to care for HIV/AIDS patients; interestingly, an overwhelming majority (93 per cent) stated that they had never refused to care for an HIV/AIDS patient, despite their fears (Brennan et al. 1988). The poll also revealed that a staggering

80 per cent of nurses surveyed stated that their own families were concerned about their (the nurses') safety when caring for HIV/AIDS patients.

Other studies have found that nurses caring for HIV/AIDS patients have actually been shunned by family, friends and neighbours, and even by other health care workers, who apparently feared association 'with one who provides direct care' (Huerta and Oddi 1992, p. 221; *Nursing Times*, 29 October 1986, p. 10). This further demonstrates the complexity of the refusal to care issue, and the difficulties associated with answering the question: To what extent should nurses be expected to sacrifice their own important interests for the sake of those for whom they care?

Significantly, two of the most commonly cited reasons for refusing to care for HIV/AIDS patients are fear of contagion, and disapproval of patients' lifestyles (especially those involving either homosexuality or intravenous drug use) (Huerta and Oddi 1992, p. 223). A poignant example of how fear of contagion and disapproval of a patient's lifestyle can affect the ability of nurses to care and, in turn, the patient's overall wellbeing, is given below.

> A client was diagnosed as having AIDS upon his admission to hospital. During his inpatient stay, nurses often cracked open the door and called in to him to learn of his condition, but would not enter the room. The hospital staff would not bathe him, and he was not allowed to shower. Bloody linens were not removed from the room. His emergency bedside signal [call bell] was left unanswered for as long as eight hours. A pamphlet was left at his bedside that described homosexuality as a sinful practice.
>
> (Staff of the National Health Law Program 1991, p. 260)

Although this is an American case, the prejudicial attitudes it demonstrates are not restricted to the national borders of the United States. As recently as 1989 the respected Freemasons Hospital in Melbourne caused a public outcry when it imposed a ban on treating all people who had AIDS or who carried the HIV virus (Miller 1989). The decision to impose the ban was made by the hospital's medical advisory board, and was allegedly supported by both doctors and nurses working at the hospital, as well as by the Victorian Branch of the Australian Medical Association (AMA) (Athersmith 1989a; Price 1989). As a point of interest, it was later revealed that nurses had *not* in fact been consulted about the decision to effect the ban (Curtis 1989). The Freemasons' ban is believed to be the first case of its kind in Australia (Allender and Robinson 1989). Subsequently the Victorian Government took steps to outlaw hospital policies which effectively discriminate unjustly against HIV/AIDS patients.

The right of nurses to refuse to care for HIV/AIDS patients is a tough question, which may never find a wholly satisfactory answer. Nevertheless, a serious attempt must be made to address it.

It is doubtful whether HIV/AIDS (and/or other cases of infectious diseases — for example, hepatitis B and C) presents a situation in which conscientious objection claims would be valid. Certainly, claims in these sorts of cases do not seem to satisfy all the five criteria of genuine conscientious objection listed earlier. For example, it is not clear that claims in these cases are based on a distinctive moral motivation aimed at maintaining sound moral standards or achieving a desired moral end. Nor is it clear that claims in these cases are based on informed and critically reflective choice (many may, in fact, be based on misinformed, fearful and arbitrary self-interested choice). It is also not clear that the claims of conscientious objection in these cases are necessary as a 'last resort' in 'the defence of one's moral integrity'. For one thing, it has yet to be shown how, if at all, caring for someone who is HIV positive threatens the moral integrity or standards of a caregiver (a point to be examined further shortly). Finally, it is far from clear that these cases involve a situation that is characteristically 'morally uncertain'. (It has yet to be shown convincingly that it is unethical to care for someone who is seriously ill with an infectious disease.) While the objector may recognise that others' conscientious claims are equally deserving in these cases, and thereby satisfy at least one of the five criteria listed, this is not enough to uphold a genuine claim of conscientious objection.

It should be noted, however, that, even though a claim of genuine conscientious objection might fail in cases of caring for people with potentially life-threatening infectious diseases, this does not necessarily mean that a given refusal to care by a nurse should not be permitted.

One set of circumstances under which this might be so is where nurses are so distracted and so disturbed by their fear of contagion that they can no longer be relied upon to give safe, appropriate and therapeutically effective care. In such instances, it would obviously be better for the patient who has an infectious disease not to be cared for by such nurses. One reason for this is that the patient's sense of wellbeing and self-worth — not to mention, his/her health outcomes — are not going to be maximised by nurses who are so overwhelmed by their own fear that they would neglect the patient (as happened in the case cited above). It needs to be noted, however, that nurses whose practice is 'impaired' by a personal fear of contagion have an obligation to seek remedial education and counselling to help address the problem of their 'impaired practice' (Johnstone 1998). In some jurisdictions, it might even result in a nurse's deregistration. In 1990, for example, a nurse was deregistered by the United Kingdom Central Council (UKCC) for refusing to care for people who were 'HIV, AIDS and hepatitis B positive' (Young 1994, p. 103).

Another problem which needs to be addressed is that of homophobia (the 'irrational fear of homosexuality'), which, as Huerta and Oddi (1992, p. 223) argue, can further compound the fear of caring for HIV/AIDS patients. Significantly, attitudinal studies have found that some nurses feel uncomfortable with caring for male homosexuals and exhibit avoidance behaviour towards HIV/AIDS patients who belong to this group (Huerta and Oddi 1992, p. 223). Nurses opposed to homosexuality also tend to believe that HIV/AIDS patients are 'responsible' for their disease, and, accordingly, these nurses 'blame the victim' (Viele et al. 1984). Equally significant are research findings which show that nurses who are homophobic manifest 'the greatest fear of HIV/AIDS and the least empathy for AIDS patients' (Huerta and Oddi 1992, p. 224).

While these studies are not conclusive, they nevertheless point to a need for nurses to examine their attitudes towards homosexuality and to explore ways in which prejudicial attitudes towards and fear of HIV/AIDS patients can be overcome. One study has found, for example, that nurses can be helped to gain a more positive attitude towards and less fear of homosexuality by participating in sexuality workshops where opportunities can be provided to explore and share feelings about the issue, and to engage in other learning activities (Young 1988).

One group of people who may not be amenable to this kind of education, however, are those who are fundamentally opposed to homosexuality on religious grounds. I have, for instance, heard some nurses who hold conservative religious beliefs express the view that they 'could not possibly care for a homosexual patient with HIV/AIDS, since to do so would be tantamount to condoning homosexuality, and thereby supporting a sinful practice'. (Similar arguments are used in the case of abortion; some nurses have expressed the view, for example, that caring for women who have had abortions is tantamount to condoning abortion.) The reasoning used here is, however, flawed. It is a fallacy to hold that caring for a particular class of patients is tantamount to condoning the lifestyles or life circumstances of those patients. If we were to accept this line of reasoning, we would be committed to accepting that, for example, caring for poor people is tantamount to condoning poverty, or that caring for unemployed people is tantamount to condoning unemployment, or that caring for homeless people is tantamount to condoning homelessness. We would, I think, reject the view that caring for these latter groups of people is tantamount to condoning their respective lifestyles, or to providing grounds upon which a morally defensible refusal to care for them could be based. Since the acts of caring for HIV/AIDS patients are demonstrably remote from the sexual acts to which some nurses are opposed on religious grounds, and since caring for patients who are homosexual does not entail performing acts proscribed by religious doctrine, it is not clear that a refusal to care for patients who are homosexual can be sustained. (Readers may also find Fitzpatrick's discussion of the Catholic principles of cooperation/ complicity helpful [1988, pp. 128–34].)

It might be objected here, however, that, unlike homosexuality, poverty, unemployment and homelessness are not 'sins' and therefore nurses opposed to sinful practices can care for people in these latter groups without compromising their religious beliefs and moral integrity. In fact, caring for these people might even be construed as 'virtuous'. This, however, is not a satisfactory reply, since it fails to show *why* caring for these groups of people is *not* tantamount to condoning their lifestyles, which, significantly, can be shown to be injurious to these groups of people's wellbeing and moral interests. Let us explore this further.

Why, for instance, is caring for a homosexual patient regarded as tantamount to condoning homosexuality, yet caring for an unemployed person *is not* regarded as tantamount to condoning unemployment? If we take out the descriptive statements referring to these groups whose respective lifestyles are in question, what we end up with is something like this: *caring for members of group X is tantamount to condoning their lifestyles, but caring for members of group Y is not tantamount to condoning their lifestyles*. No reasons are given why this is the case, however, demonstrating that the thinking being used here is at best arbitrary and at worst fallacious. Even if it is conceded that what makes a morally significant difference in this case is the 'sinful' nature of homosexuality, this will not help, since this seems to say that what makes caring for a particular group of people tantamount to condoning their lifestyles is the fact that what they do is 'sinful'. If nurses holding conservative religious beliefs were to accept this, however, they would be committed logically to accepting that caring for a whole range of people would be tantamount to condoning their 'sinful' lifestyles, and thus that there exists a whole range of people for whom they should refuse to care. Nurses holding conservative religious beliefs would, for instance, be obliged to refuse to care for people who work on Sundays, bear false witness, steal, murder, covet their neighbours' goods, fornicate, commit adultery, blaspheme, do not fear God, worship other gods, tell lies (including telling children that Father Christmas is a real person and that tooth fairies bring money in the night), take contraception, have attempted suicide, and have performed a whole range of other acts deemed sins in the Bible or other religious texts. Clearly, if nurses were to accept the view that caring for people who commit sins is tantamount to

405

condoning the sins in question, they would probably have to give up nursing altogether, since many people have committed the 'sinful' acts given above.

While the arguments presented here have had as their focus male homosexuals, they could, of course, be applied equally to the cases of other groups of people whose lifestyles some nurses regard as being problematic or sinful — for example, intravenous drug users and prostitutes.

Conscientious objection and the problem of unsafe work conditions

A final type of situation to be considered here involves the common problem of nurses being expected to work in unsafe working conditions, most notably those caused by severe staff shortages. Typically, nurses might be ordered to work in an area with which they are unfamiliar and/or in which they are not educated to work, such as in an intensive care unit. They might also be expected to work at a staffing level which places patient safety and quality of care at risk. These two situations are inextricably linked. For example, if there was not a shortage of properly educated intensive care nurses, nurse administrators would not have to order an inexperienced nurse to go and 'help out' in the hospital's intensive care unit.

The problem of declining and unsafe working conditions is being increasingly responded to by nurses by all-out strike action, which, in many respects, might also qualify as a type of conscientious objection. Since this topic warrants in-depth attention, it is discussed separately later in this chapter.

Conscientious objection and policy considerations

For a conscientious objection policy to be effective and reliable, it must carry at least two minimal requirements (see Childress 1979). First, conscientious objectors must demonstrate that their claims are sincere. A given proof need not be religious in nature, nor necessarily absolute. As we have seen throughout this text, it is not always inconsistent for nurses (or for anyone) to have a 'moderate' position on the moral permissibility of certain procedures, such as abortion and euthanasia/assisted suicide. Thus, it would not necessarily be inconsistent of nurses to, say, support abortion and to participate in most abortion procedures at their place of employment, yet nevertheless be opposed to a 'particular case' of abortion where the procedure in question fails to satisfy certain autonomously chosen moral standards. The same applies in the case of euthanasia/assisted suicide. Conscientious objection policies, then, must recognise and make provision for the moderate's position, and accept that sometimes conscientious objectors might refuse to assist with a type of procedure they have previously assisted with, such as abortion.

A second minimal requirement is that employers must carry the burden of proof that no alternative is available when not permitting nurses to refuse on conscientious grounds to assist with a given procedure. It is difficult to accept that a claim of conscientious objection cannot be accommodated in cases where nurses have used rightful means in expressing a conscientious refusal — that is, superiors have been given advance notice of an intention to refuse, reasons for refusal have been made explicit, replacement or other attending personnel have not been unduly compromised, other interests of comparable moral worth have not been sacrificed, and patients have not been stranded (Johnstone 1988, p. 153). Where an administrator does not accept a nurse's genuine conscientious objection claims, serious questions need to be asked about whether the administrator has sincerely tried to find viable alternatives which would make it possible for conscientiously objecting nurses to withdraw from situations they deem morally troubling or intolerable.

The key to settling the conscientious objection debate does not lie only in having enforceable mechanisms for protecting genuine conscientious objection claims, but also in having a demonstrable threshold beyond which nurses can base their claims. However, this threshold is one which can only be supplied by sound ethics education and agreed ethical standards within the profession (see Johnstone 1998).

Can superiors decently order nurses to perform tasks to which they are genuinely conscientiously opposed? The answer is 'no'. To compel nurses to act against their conscience is to risk weakening their moral conscientiousness and hence their ability to be moral. To deny moral conscientiousness in health care domains is also to risk the moral interests of those requiring health care. Furthermore, superiors simply do not have the moral authority to dictate to another which moral standards ought and ought not to be appealed to in a given situation.

There is much to support the view that a health care system comprised of morally conscientious and sensitive nurses would be much better than one without such nurses. This seems to support the conclusion that genuine conscientious objection is not only morally permissible, but may even be, in the ultimate analysis, morally required.

The issue of conscientious objection in nursing is at last receiving the attention that is warranted by professional nursing organisations. One notable example of this can be found in the Royal College of Nursing, Australia, which, in February 1998, issued its first position statement on conscientious objection (included as Appendix XII of this text).

Strike action[2]

In 1988, Dr Amelia Mangay-Maglacas, the chief nurse at the World Health Organisation, urged nurses worldwide to engage in an unprecedented two-hour global strike. In defence of this initiative, Dr Mangay-Maglacas is reported to have argued that:

> … a two hour global strike supported by all the world's nurses may be the only way to focus attention on the profession's problems.
>
> (*Nursing Times*, 6 April 1988, p. 5)

Rejecting the view that the nurses were mainly concerned with money, Dr Mangay-Maglacas responded that what nurses wanted was simply:

> … the satisfaction of doing what they believe is right, developing and managing their own service and not being dictated to by others.
>
> (*Nursing Times*, 6 April 1988, p. 5)

In the past, strike action has been popularly viewed as the antithesis of professionalism, of caring, and even of professional responsibility (Kelly 1985, p. 187; Tschudin 1986, p. 15; Williams 1988, p. 6). One Melbourne writer would

---

2. An earlier version of the discussion on strike action was presented as a paper entitled 'Professional responsibility and the dilemma of strike action' at the New Zealand Nurses' Association International Conference, *Challenges–options–choices*, held Rotorua, 5 August 1987, in conjunction with the International Council of Nurses' Representatives meeting, Auckland. The paper has been revised for publication in this text.

have us believe it is also the antithesis of 'feminine behaviour'! (see Women's Electoral Lobby 1987, p. 4). The underlying presumption of this view seems to be that *professionalism* is generally regarded as intrinsically 'other serving' (i.e. its end is the welfare of others, and to serve the public good), unlike *strike action*, which is generally considered to be 'self-serving' (i.e. its end is the welfare of self, sometimes even at the expense of the welfare of others). Nurses, both in Australia and overseas, have, I believe, been persuaded by this view and have, at least until just over a decade ago, resisted taking strike action.

The nursing profession's traditional (and universal) anti-strike position has nevertheless been gradually overturned as representative nursing associations and organisations around the world moved to delete the 'no-strike' clauses from their rule books. However, such moves have not been without a sense of consternation, and have served to raise many serious questions about the professional integrity of nurses — both as individuals and as a group — in terms of their commitment to serving the public good in general, and the welfare of patients in particular.

This discussion attempts to address the questions of whether strike action by nurses is ever justified; and whether strike action by nurses entails a violation of both professional ethics and the interests of the community at large. In answering these questions I shall briefly outline some of the central professional and industrial issues which motivated the fifty-day-long Victorian nurses' strike of 1986; describe some of the extraordinary events which occurred during this strike; and critically examine some central philosophical and ethical arguments which might be raised both in criticism and in support of nurses' strikes in general.

Central issues of strike action

In Australia the 'no-strike' clause (section 31C) was deleted from the rules of the then Royal Australian Nursing Federation (RANF), now the Australian Nursing Federation (ANF), after a national poll in 1984 found that 65 per cent of nurses were in favour of such a move (Gardner and McCoppin 1986, p. 31). As work conditions and standards of patient care continued to decline, and heavy and diverse workloads continued to increase, nurses around Victoria began to 'dig in their industrial toes' in a way they had never done before.

Work bans and short-duration strike action occurred in 1984 in support of a variety of long-standing issues ranging from 'non-nursing duties' to 'tertiary education for nurses'. Tired of the government's tardiness in settling these issues, and becoming increasingly suspicious of the government's overall intentions towards them, nurses decided once and for all to take their working futures firmly into their own hands. At a mass meeting on 11 October 1985, attended by over 5500 of Victoria's nurses, the decision to strike received overwhelming support. Settlement was reached by October 21 and the strike ended (Gardner and McCoppin 1986). Nevertheless, even a year later the issues at stake had still not been satisfactorily resolved. Propelled by the principle of 'last resort', the RANF (now the ANF) organised yet another mass meeting, this time for 30 October 1986, and it was here that the decision to strike 'indefinitely' was finally reached. Thus, less than three years after the removal of the 'no-strike' clause from the RANF's rules, an historic fifty-day-long nurses' strike took place (unprecedented in Victoria, and indeed in the Southern Hemisphere), affecting 70 per cent of Victoria's public and private hospitals.

While the central issues of the strike were longstanding, they were by no means extraordinary. Indeed, they were reminiscent of those for which nursing colleagues worldwide have fought in the past, and for which nurses everywhere are continuing to fight (see, for example, Williams 1988, pp. 6–7, 9–14; Bickley 1988, p. 6; *New Zealand Nursing Journal* 1988, p. 5). In brief, the issues at stake included:

- career structure;
- wage justice;
- better nurse–patient ratios;
- control over admissions and discharges;
- role in decision-making (the Australian Medical Association totally opposed this demand [Gardner and McCoppin 1986, p. 29]); and
- better supervision of student nurses (student nurses were often left in charge of wards during night shifts).

The consensus among nurses seemed to be that unless these issues were satisfactorily settled, the mass exodus of nurses from Victoria's hospitals would continue, as would the decline of patient care standards. It was estimated that as many as 56 per cent of registered nurses had already left active practice (Gardner and McCoppin 1986, p. 31). Given the issues at stake, nurses believed their cause to be just, in both professional and moral terms.

Events of the 1986 Victorian state nurses' strike

As the strike progressed, nurses found themselves just as much victims of the strike as they stood to be its beneficiaries. The government threatened striking members with professional deregistration, dismissal, pay cuts, criminal charges for withdrawing labour (including charges of manslaughter in cases of patient deaths thought to be directly attributable to the strike), police intervention, and invoking the Essential Services Act (RANF 1986a; RANF 1987; Gardner and McCoppin 1986, p. 33). Meanwhile, previously recruited overseas nurses began arriving (Birnbauer 1986), and it was alleged that during the strike some student nurses were 'pushed out of hospital accommodation' in order to provide residence for these incoming recruits (RANF 1986c, p. 2).

As if the recruitment and arrival of the overseas nurses was not enough, the government then added 'insult to injury' by publicly announcing a proposal to extend the range of duties carried out by the state's enrolled nurses (SENs) to include those otherwise carried out by registered nurses, such as drug administration, intravenous therapy maintenance, complex dressings, and the like. In effect, what the government was really saying was 'we can do without you' (the registered nurses). Significantly, this proposal was unanimously supported by the Australian Medical Association (Davis 1986a; Cossar and Evans 1986). The RANF was quick to point out, however, that such an irresponsible move would place SENs in the legally indefensible position of practising outside the level of their skill and training, and thus negligently (RANF 1986e, p. 1; Davis and Menagh 1986b).

Tension between the government and the nurses mounted even further when it was publicly revealed that several hospitals were recruiting 'paid volunteers' to perform essential tasks for their inpatients (RANF 1987, p. 7). Angered by this blatant use of 'scab labour', the RANF agreed to the 'in-principle' support of a variety of non-nursing trade unions — including, among others, the Federated Engine Drivers' and Firemen's Association, the Electrical Trades Union, the Building Workers Industrial Union, and a number of 'blue collar' unions, to name a few (Davis and Menagh 1986a; Davis 1986b). Some nurses feared, however, that the involvement of non-nursing unions would undermine the already seriously tarnished professional image of nursing — a fear which was not unreasonable under the circumstances.

Picket lines, meanwhile, were beginning to have their effect, and hospital supplies were running seriously low. Intent on breaking both the strike and the nurses' morale, the government again threatened police intervention. Initially this angered the police, resulting in a public statement from Victoria's then Chief Commissioner of Police, Mr Miller, to the effect that 'no one had the right to use police as a threat' (Davis and Noble 1986). He went on to point out that the police had traditionally enjoyed an excellent rapport with the nursing profession 'and we propose to keep it that way' (Davis and Noble 1986). This sentiment had evidently changed, however, when senior police took up positions to break the picket lines. Here the peacefulness of the nurses' protest ended.

In one incident, a nurse was removed by police by way of 'pressure being asserted on both carotid arteries in her neck — a technique that the SAS trains its "commandos" to use against enemy forces' (RANF 1987, p. 8). Thus what started as an *orderly protest* was suddenly turned into something ugly and obscene. While many nurses received generous donations of food, money (donated to the RANF 'strike fund') and other items, just as many found themselves being evicted from their flats and subjected to physical, verbal and emotional abuse. Some were stood down by their employers (RANF 1986d, p. 2), while others suffered incredible ostracism by family, friends and colleagues. Grotesque cartoons appeared in the daily newspapers. One depicted a nurse with her entrails spilling out over the floor, following a surgical incision performed by a caricature figure of the minister of health dressed in surgeon's garb (see Figure 15.1). Another blatantly sexist cartoon depicted the RANF Secretary, Irene Bolger, in bed with David White, the then Minister of Health, with each accusing the other of forcing them 'to do it' (see Figure 15.2).

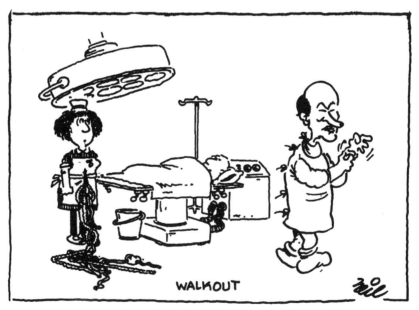

Figure 15.1 Cartoon published during the fifty-day nurses' strike in Victoria in 1986 (cartoon by Neil, reproduced with permission from Neil Matterson. Appeared in the Melbourne *Herald*, 6 November 1986, p. 6)

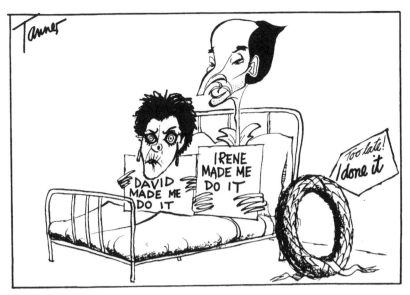

Figure 15.2 During the 1986 nurses' strike, Irene Bolger, Secretary of the Royal Australian Nursing Federation, and David White, Minister of Health, were caricatured in this cartoon by Tanner
(reproduced with permission from *The Age*, 13 November 1986)

The media accused nurses of being 'unprofessional and irresponsible', of abandoning or losing their professional ethics, and even of being inspired by Soviet trade unionism (Davis 1986c; Coster 1986). One particularly scathing editorial argued that nurses had engaged in 'industrial terrorism which, trampling on reason, ethics and compassion, turns the sick, the suffering and the scared into expendable hostages' (Forell 1986, p. 13).

Still other media reports piously asserted that there could be no justification for this kind of strike action by nurses, and repeatedly called upon them to end their strike (*The Herald* 1986; Cole-Adams 1986). As a point of interest, the 1988 spate of nurses' strikes in New Zealand met with similar abuses and accusations. In one reported incident, for example, the President of the Auckland Medical Association, Dr Stuart Ferguson, commented publicly 'that prostitutes were being more professional than striking nurses'. A number of prostitutes were quick to express their opinion in a letter to Dr Ferguson, a copy of which was sent to the *New Zealand Nursing Journal*. It reads:

> Thank you for your favourable comparison of the professionalism of prostitutes to that of nurses. We get very little positive comment in the media. We are aware, however, that throughout history nurses have strived to improve our working conditions.
>
> Nurses get one tenth of our hourly wage and often perform less pleasant duties. We therefore support them in their struggle for better working conditions.
>
> Signed: 14 'working girls of 'K' Road'.
>
> (New Zealand Nursing Journal 1988, p. 5)

Philosophical and ethical questions about nurses' strikes

Strike action by essential service workers such as nurses raises a number of interesting philosophical questions. Notable among these are the following three.

1. Under what conditions, if any, might strike action by nurses be justified?
2. Does strike action by nurses necessarily entail a violation of (their) professional ethics?
3. Is strike action by nurses tantamount to an abdication of the profession's responsibility towards upholding the public good (i.e. the health and welfare interests of both immediate patients and the community at large)?

In attempting to answer these questions, let us examine a number of arguments which might be raised against the view that nurses do, in fact, have a just and morally defensible claim to engage in strike action.

Argument 1: *Patients have a right to receive health care in general, and nursing care in particular.* For nurses to withdraw their services as a mark of industrial dispute is seriously to interfere with patients' rights to receive the care they are otherwise entitled to receive. Since strike action by nurses entails violating other people's rights (in this instance, the patients'), it stands as morally objectionable (Rumbold 1986).

Argument 2: *Nurses have a fundamental moral and professional duty to provide safe care to their patients* (Benjamin and Curtis 1986, p. 156). Strike action undertaken by nurses necessarily entails a violation of the principle of safe nursing care. Unsafe nursing care is in itself a moral harm. Nurses who engage in strike action are, therefore, not only failing to fulfil their broader professional and moral obligations (and thus failing to prevent otherwise avoidable moral harm), but are also wittingly violating their professional ethics, and are guilty of actually *causing* moral harm.

Argument 3: *Nurses are morally bound to fulfil their otherwise immediate duties to provide (safe) nursing care.* The purposes of achieving some 'future good' (such as better future work conditions, patient care and the like) are not sufficient to override these more immediate duties, and thus strike action for these purposes can never be morally justified (Muyskens 1982b, pp. 174–5; 1982c).

Argument 4: *Strike action stands necessarily to cause otherwise avoidable (and in some instances irrevocable) harms* — such as patients suffering intolerable pain, deterioration in medical conditions, and even death. Where strike action does result in such harms, it cannot be justified morally.

Argument 5: *The benefits of strike action by nurses (for example, improved patient care, better work conditions, salary justice) do not always outweigh the harms* (for example, loss of public trust, patient suffering, socioeconomic and political costs). Given this, nurses' strikes are morally unacceptable.

Argument 6: *Strike action by nurses necessarily entails holding patients 'hostage' for the purposes of advancing the nursing profession's interest* (Muyskens 1982b, p. 173). To use patients to further the nursing profession's interests is to treat patients as means to ends of others, or as 'objects', and not as ends in themselves or as entities with intrinsic moral worth. The failure to treat persons (patients) as ends in themselves is to seriously violate the moral principles of autonomy and respect for persons. Strike action which treats persons as means to ends (as objects) constitutes an intrinsic moral wrong.

Argument 7: *It is not the role — much less the duty — of nurses to seek improvements in seriously substandard health care systems.* Improving substandard health care systems is rightfully the domain of doctors, health care administrators and politicians, not nurses. By assuming such a role (or duty), nurses are usurping the moral responsibilities of others.

Argument 8: *Strike action might, in the final analysis, prove thoroughly self-defeating* (Baly 1984, p. 15). Nurses might, for example, find themselves being 'fairly' dismissed from their places of employment, charged with criminal negligence, and becoming the targets of bitter criticism from a mistrustful and unforgiving public. Such 'self-inflicted' harm or professional martyrdom constitutes a significant moral wrong.

Argument 9: *Strike action is not the best possible means of securing better patient care and work conditions for nurses* (Muyskens 1982a, p. 175). Other measures can be taken that might equally secure the benefits that strike action is intent on securing. Given this, strike action is in itself an avoidable harm which nurses are bound, for moral reasons, to reject.

Argument 10: *As professionals, nurses have a duty to serve the public interest and to uphold the 'service ideal'* (Newton 1981; Kelly 1985). To engage in strike action is to break the social contract that the nursing profession has with society, and the tacit promises inherent therein. To break one's contracts or promises (tacit or otherwise) is to commit a moral wrong (Freedman 1978).

Although the arguments raised against the notion of 'just' nurses' strikes are persuasive, they are not entirely unproblematic and are vulnerable to a number of possible counter-arguments. Consider the following.

1. Response to arguments 1 and 10. Since nurses are human beings, they too have fundamental moral interests deserving protection, such as to be respected as persons, to be treated fairly, and to be protected from harm in the workplace. To hold nurses to ransom just because they perform a certain type of work (Stephens 1986), or to deny nurses the right to strike on grounds of the special nature of their work, is to subject nurses to an act of negative discrimination (i.e. unfair treatment on the basis of some distinguishing or differentiating characteristic that dominant others do not share or value). Where nurses' work conditions exploit them, and patient and/or employer expectations stand to cause them otherwise avoidable harms, employers, patients, and, indeed, society at large forfeit their rights to have the terms of the nurses' 'social contract' honoured, and thus to receive the services that nurses might otherwise be expected to give. Where nurses can demonstrate 'just cause', their right to strike is at least, prima facie, as weighty as the right to strike that others in the community enjoy (Rumbold 1986, pp. 145–6).

2. Response to arguments 2, 3 and 7. The ultimate end of nursing is the welfare of others (in this instance, patients). In upholding the welfare of others nurses must strive to prevent harm and promote good; this includes providing safe and ethically defensible nursing care, and alleviating patients' sufferings. In a seriously substandard health care system, nurses can no longer guarantee either the safety of their patients or the alleviation or prevention of patient suffering. Since nurses form a major component of health care systems, they are necessary contributors to the functionings (or dysfunctionings) of such systems. If nurses do nothing to correct a seriously substandard health care system (of which they are a part), they cannot escape culpability for that system's deficiencies and inadequacies; indeed, as Muyskens (1982a) argues, they sit as accomplices to them. It is morally naive to suppose that nurses do not have any real moral duties to correct the imbalance of moral harms and benefits in such instances. Given this, it is morally defensible to assert that, not only do nurses have a prima facie right to strike, but, in certain instances, they may even have a moral duty to do so. In the light of the morally compelling circumstances supplied by seriously substandard health care, not only would it be wrong to claim that strike action entails a violation of the principle of safe nursing care; it would also be wrong to assert that nurses do not have a duty to work towards some 'future good', particularly when this future good stands necessarily to include the realisation of the principle of safe and therapeutically effective nursing practice.

3. **Response to arguments 4 and 5.** Patients and the community do not always suffer on account of strike action undertaken by nurses. Indeed, during the Victorian nurses' strike, some claimed that nurse–patient ratios were better (safer) than they had been before the strike! Further to this, unlike other groups who take strike action, the nurses usually stop short of 'total walkouts' and work diligently to ensure that 'skeleton staff' are left to provide emergency and essential care. (As I overheard one nurse say one day, 'Nurses are the only ones I know who go on strike, but stay on duty'!) Finally, such a view presumes that the suffering which supposedly occurs during an alleged strike action is greater than that which was already occurring before the strike action. Given the length of hospital waiting lists around the country and the declining quality of care in hospitals following the introduction of case-mix management, there is room to seriously question the validity of such a claim. There is also room to question here whether the harms of strike action do, in fact, outweigh the benefits, given the suffering caused by the dysfunctionings of a substandard health care system.

4. **Response to argument 6.** To expect nurses to perform demanding and responsible duties without fair reward, and to expect them to endure legally risky, physically and emotionally harsh, and even health-hazardous, work conditions is to exploit nurses and to treat them as *social and political slaves*. In short, it is to treat them as means to ends (objects), and not as ends in themselves (entities with intrinsic moral worth), which is, as already argued elsewhere, an intrinsic moral wrong. During just strike action it is not the nurses but the government and its hospital administrators who hold patients political 'hostages'.

5. **Response to argument 8.** To decline a morally obligatory act is to be morally negligent. To pay undue regard to one's own self-interests is to risk a very serious kind of moral error; it is to treat one's own interests as more deserving than the interests of others just because they are one's own interests, which is open to moral objection. Where a just nurses' strike stands to correct the otherwise avoidable and harmful inadequacies and deficiencies of a seriously substandard health care system, nurses are morally obliged to take such action — even though at some personal cost and inconvenience to self. Where nurses can act to prevent an otherwise avoidable harm from occurring without sacrificing anything of comparable moral importance, they are bound to perform that act (adapted from Singer 1979).

6. **Response to argument 9.** It is somewhat naively optimistic to suppose that those who are satisfied with a given status quo would be even remotely disposed to settle quickly a table of claims likely to incur significant financial costs. If there were other satisfactory measures for achieving a quick and functional settlement of claims, moral considerations would, of course, oblige people to use them. Where such measures are not readily accessible, the 'last resort' principle (i.e. the principle which sets 'moral deadlines') seems as weighty as any other in the face of potentially harmful odds.

Strike action by nurses can be justified in another way, and that is by appealing to certain criteria. Gonsalves (1985, p. 436), for example, suggests that, in order for strike action to be just, it must satisfy at least four conditions: it must be for a just cause; it must have proper authorisation (i.e. be freely chosen by striking members, and backed by a democratically elected union body); it must be considered only as a last resort (i.e. after all other possible measures have failed); and, lastly, it must be carried out by rightful means (i.e. the property of others must be respected, protests must be conducted peacefully, and sabotage and violence must be avoided). He further argues that, even in cases where certain harms result, a given strike action can still be regarded as just, provided that:

- the strike action was necessary to bring about an equal distribution of harms and benefits (on this point Gonsalves contends [p. 436], 'the more painful and widespread the evil, the greater must be the cause [or action] required to balance it');
- the strikers do not intend to bring about the evil or harmful consequences of their actions; and
- the strikers do not intentionally use the bad effects of their actions to bring about the good effects of their employer assenting to the demands made (here the bad effects must only 'accidentally put added pressure on the employer' to accede to the workers' demands).

There is not space here to discuss these criteria at length. It should be noted, however, that these criteria are not entirely unproblematic (particularly those which obviously derive from the doctrine of double effect), and are vulnerable to a number of objections which might be raised against them (for a more detailed examination of the doctrine of double effect, see Chapter 12). Nevertheless, Gonsalves' framework does, I believe, supply an instructive and useful starting point from which the nursing profession can begin to generate sound and morally defensible policies concerning strike action by its members.

Strike action — some further considerations

The views briefly considered in this discussion succeed, I think, in showing that, contrary to popular anti-strike views, just strikes are not wholly self-interested, and, indeed, can serve very effectively to promote and uphold the interests of others and/or the public good. While striking nurses may well be fighting to have their own interests justly protected, this is not the same as acting purely and simply out of self-interest; these two things are quite distinct and care must be taken to separate them.

In reply, then, to the three questions raised at the beginning of this discussion, there is room to answer, first, that strike action by nurses can be said to be morally justified when it stands, among other things, to prevent an otherwise avoidable harm from occurring or serves to correct a serious imbalance of harms over benefits. Second, given the nursing profession's broader moral responsibilities in terms of preventing harm and promoting good (i.e. alleviating suffering, conducting safe nursing care, upholding the welfare and interests of other human beings), strike action staged as a protest against a seriously substandard and harm-causing health care system does not entail a necessary violation of professional ethics; to the contrary, it upholds such a system of ethics. Third, where nurses succeed in achieving the moral ends of their action, it would be erroneous to hold that a just strike is tantamount to an abdication of the nursing profession's responsibility towards upholding the public good.

Whatever our personal experience or commitments, the decision to either support or refrain from strike action must always be made by way of rigorous and critical moral thinking and the application of sound moral standards. While nurses may well have the courage of their personal convictions, they must not lose sight of their duty as professionals to subscribe to a standard of morality 'more exacting' than that of the ordinary person in the street (Himsworth 1953). If nurses are to assert a supposed common right to strike, it must always and only be done on a sound moral basis and within the boundaries of sound moral considerations.

Institutional ethics committees[3]

In March 1988, the Australian Health Ministers' Conference (AHMC) agreed to the establishment and membership of the National Bioethics Consultative Committee (NBCC). The NBCC was later charged with the responsibility of advising the health ministers on the social, ethical and legal issues arising from a full range of bioethical matters. As well as this, the Committee played an important role in offering guidance to the Commonwealth and state/territory governments in the development of policy — particularly in the area of reproductive technology.

As a point of interest, one of the prime movers in getting the NBCC established and working was a registered general and psychiatric nurse, Marie-Louise Evans. Ms Evans was originally appointed director of the federal government's Bioethics Unit. It was through this appointment that she acted as the NBCC's first executive director, and it was under her directorship that the Committee had its inaugural meeting in August 1988. In 1991, however, the federal government disbanded the NBCC, and its (the NBCC's) responsibility for advising the government on bioethical issues was transferred to the National Health and Medical Research Council (NH & MRC) (*Bioethics News*, July 1991, p. 1).

At its 106th Session, in 1988, the NH & MRC approved and later publicly released a discussion paper, *Ethics of limiting life sustaining treatment*, signalling an expansion of its traditional and previously somewhat parochial role to include stimulating 'further discussion of important ethical issues within the community'. This paper raises the issue of patient care ethics committees and the kinds of roles they should play. The NH & MRC (1988) makes plain its recommendation:

> ... that patient care ethics committees in hospitals should be available to provide information, discussion of options, expert opinions and counsel for both patients and caregivers, but should never determine and direct what is to be done in any situation.

> (National Health and Medical Research Council 1988, p. 14)

In the 1990s, many Australian hospitals, residential care homes and other community-based health care agencies have established ethics committees. The primary function of these ethics committees is to deal with the ethical issues arising from patient/client care, as opposed to the function of the more traditional institutional ethics committee, which has been primarily to approve, monitor, and/ or disapprove *experimental human research projects* (see McNeill et al. 1990).

---

3. The discussion on institutional ethics committees was presented as a paper entitled 'The role of an institutional ethics committee' at the 14th Australian and New Zealand Scientific Meeting on Intensive Care, Conrad International Hotel, Gold Coast, Queensland, 3–6 December 1989.

In most cases the workings of ethics committees remain concealed from the public eye; sometimes, however, their workings are made public, as occurred in the historical 1988 case of Mrs N, involving a 39-year-old woman suffering end-stage motor neurone disease (Wilmoth and Pirrie 1988). Mrs N died after the St Vincent's Hospital medico-moral committee (alias institutional ethics committee) approved her conscious and rationally competent request to have the ventilator supporting her life removed (Cossar 1988). The case was reported as being 'the first time an Australian hospital has removed such a life-support system from a conscious patient to comply with the patient's wishes' (Pirrie 1988, p. 3). It was also probably the first time that an ethics committee had been actively involved in supporting such a request.

The establishment of the 'new' institutional ethics committees in the late 1980s and early 1990s marked the beginning of a new conscientiousness in the Australian health care arena, and a recognition that *the system* (or, rather, those who comprise it) had been ill prepared and inadequate to deal with the many moral complexities and controversies arising from orthodox medical practice and health care delivery. Whether institutional ethics committees will be the panacea for all the moral ills plaguing the health care system, however, remains to be seen. It is difficult to avoid asking the additional question: 'Will institutional ethics committees really help? Or will they emerge as little more than health care's "white elephants", as one writer warns that they might?' (Blake 1992).

Experience in the United States has shown that institutional ethics committees *can* help, and in a significant way. It has also shown, however, that the success of any given institutional ethics committee is conditional on a number of factors, notably its function, composition, authority/power, and accessibility. It is to examining these factors that this discussion now turns.

What is an institutional ethics committee?

In discussing the issue of institutional ethics committees, it is important first to be quite clear about what is being referred to. There is, for example, a common tendency for 'institutional ethics committee' to be used as a generic term for other health care institutional committees that are clinically oriented, such as critical care committees, organ transplant committees, research committees, optimal care committees, and prognosis committees (a tendency which, as a point of caution, can be misleading). As Brodeur (1984, p. 233) correctly points out: 'using the misnomer "ethics committee" to describe a committee whose function is different, muddles the medical decision-making process'. It could be added here that it also 'muddles' the ethical issues at hand and creates the very real risk of ethical issues (as previously explained in Chapter 7 of this text) being translated into technical problems warranting clinical solutions.

Carol Levine defines a institutional/hospital ethics committee as:

> a group established by a hospital or health care institution formally charged with advising, consulting, discussing, or otherwise being involved in ethical decisions and policies that arise in clinical care ... The committee may serve the entire hospital or a special unit, such as a neonatal intensive care nursery or a cardiac intensive care unit.
>
> (Levine 1984, p. 9)

While this is not the only definition of a hospital or institutional ethics committee, it is nevertheless an apt one, and the one which will tentatively be relied upon in this discussion. As a point of clarification, the notion of an 'institutional ethics committee' is to be distinguished from what I shall later refer to as a 'patient care ethics committee'.

Factors influencing the rise of institutional ethics committees

There are many factors which have contributed to the rise of institutional ethics committees. Special institutional ethics committees were formed in the United States as early as the 1920s to review sterilisation decisions, and in the 1950s to review abortion decisions (Levine 1984, p. 9). It was not until the mid-1970s, however, owing to the much publicised Karen Quinlan case (Muir 1978; Hughes 1978; Ross et al. 1986, pp. 5–8), that interest in institutional ethics committees began in earnest. This interest was primarily sparked by the New Jersey Supreme Court's decision in the Quinlan case, which made it clear:

> that the issue at stake was not definition of death, but rather the decision to stop treatment on one who has suffered serious neurological injury.
>
> (Veatch 1977, p. 22)

The next few years saw interest in institutional ethics committees heighten as physicians began to be charged with first degree murder for removing, at the request of the family or patients, life-supporting care and treatment (Cranford and Doudera 1984, p. 13). As doctors increasingly began to recognise their legal vulnerability (La Puma et al. 1988), and as nurses began to feel increasingly frustrated with having 'nowhere to go when confronted by ethical dilemmas' (Cranford and Doudera 1984, p. 15), so too the institutional ethics committee movement gained support, and eventually saw the establishment of working ethics committees in hospitals across the United States (see also Ross et al. 1986).

Factors influencing the rise of institutional ethics committees in Australia are similar to those which have influenced the American scene. With the increasing sophistication of medical technology has come increasing legal and public pressure to meet perceived legal and moral standards of care. The patients' rights movement is witnessing the rise of a public more willing and able to assert its rights to, in and against health care, together with the passage of major legislative reforms to protect these rights (Consumers' Health Forum of Australia 1990). And a more liberally educated health care work force is seeing the rise of a collective attitude demanding that moral/ethical considerations be given at least as much attention, if not more, as scientific considerations when making health care and medical treatment decisions. Inquiries into options for dying with dignity, patients' rights, medical malpractice, psychiatric care, the care of the aged and the disabled, and similar issues, have also created a greater awareness in both the professional and the lay communities of the need for developing reliable mechanisms for ensuring just decision-making in health care contexts, and particularly in cases involving patient/client care.

Institutional ethics committees are a relatively new phenomenon in Australia. Some committees have been functioning for only a few years and, even then, only on an ad hoc basis, and have yet to receive mainstream support from the medical profession and hospital administrators. Doctors fear that the committees will erode their authority (Levine 1977, p. 26; McCormick 1984; Rudd 1992), and personal sources indicate that nurses are continuing to find that their presence on existing ethics committees is not wholly welcomed by the more conservative medical practitioners and hospital administrators. Academics, meanwhile, squabble about the merits and demerits of institutional ethics committees generally, and about what can and should be done to ensure that they achieve desired moral ends (Levine 1977, 1984; Veatch 1977; Noble 1982; Randal 1983; McCormick 1984; Kuhse and Singer 1985; Kuhse 1988; Blake 1992).

Whatever the uncertainties and criticisms generated by the institutional ethics committee movement, the fact remains that Australia's state/territory governments and hospitals are already committing themselves to supporting the establishment of working ethics committees and to taking the activities and findings of these committees seriously. Yet whether this commitment is well placed depends at least partially on what is expected of these committees, and how well they will in fact fulfil their given tasks. This raises the following seven questions.

1. What role or function should an institutional ethics committee have?
2. What authority and power should institutional ethics committees generally have?
3. Who should serve on institutional ethics committees?
4. How should institutional ethics committees approach moral decision-making?
5. Who should have access to them?
6. Do institutional ethics committees really work (i.e. what are their merits and demerits)?
7. Of what significance are institutional ethics committees to the nursing profession?

Each of these issues is discussed below.

The role and function of institutional ethics committees

There has been much debate on what the proper function or role of the institutional ethics committee should be (see, for example Levine 1977, 1984; Veatch 1977; Freedman 1981; Caplan 1982; anonymous 1983; Cranford and Doudera 1984; McCormick 1984; Youngner et al. 1984; Blake 1992). Debate has centred on whether its function should be *decisional* (i.e. deciding morally hard cases); *prognostic* (i.e. establishing prognostic criteria and determining what a patient's actual prognosis is); *monitoring* (i.e. establishing quality assurance programs and evaluating health care practices); *advisory* (i.e. advising and supporting others on how and what to decide); *educational* (i.e. running workshops, seminars and conferences aimed at addressing ethical issues arising in clinical practice and preparing health providers to deal with these better); or a combination of all five.

Interestingly, the response in the philosophical literature has been almost unanimously supportive of the institutional ethics committee having a multi-purpose/multi-faceted role:

- *as a consultative/advisory/supportive mechanism* for assisting individuals (whether caregivers or care receivers) to make their own moral decisions, and to help ensure that the decisions they make are reasonable and fair;
- *as an education and resource facility* aimed at preparing individuals and groups to better deal with moral problems and moral conflict in clinical practice (activities to be undertaken here include grand round discussions,

seminars, workshops, and conferences, with a particular focus on ethical issues arising from clinical practice);

- *as a mechanism for policy formulation, development and review* (i.e. scrutinising past and existing policies for their moral adequacy and acceptability, and identifying areas where policy is lacking or where new policy is required, as in such areas as NFR procedures, the use and withdrawal of life-saving treatment, conscientious objection, and the like);
- *as a forum* where individuals can express their concerns and views without fear of ridicule or repercussions, and where moral disagreements among staff, patients and families can be aired and resolved; and
- *as a reviewer of morally troubling (hard) cases,* offering advice and viewpoints to all those involved.

Whatever the role the institutional ethics committee in fact plays, it should never be viewed as being absolute or static in nature, and should always be subject to review as ethics and experience demand.

The authority and power of institutional ethics committees

As with the question of function, there has also been considerable debate on the kind of power and authority that institutional ethics committees should have. Attention has mainly focused on whether the use of these committees and the demand to follow their findings should be voluntary/optional or compulsory/mandatory.

John Robertson (cited in Levine 1984, p. 11), of the University of Texas Law School, suggests that four possibilities are available to a committee:

1. *optional–optional* (it is optional for individuals to approach the ethics committee for consultation and advice, and optional to follow its recommendations);
2. *optional–mandatory* (it is optional for individuals to approach the ethics committee for consultation and advice, but if they do they must carry out its recommendations);
3. *mandatory–optional* (it is mandatory for individuals to approach the ethics committee for consultation and advice, but optional to follow its recommendations);
4. *mandatory–mandatory* (it is mandatory for individuals to approach the ethics committee for consultation and advice, and mandatory to follow its recommendations).

(Reproduced by permission © The Hastings Centre)

Levine (1984) points out that very few in the United States favour the *mandatory–mandatory* model, and that, in fact, many committees operate on the *optional–optional* model, although not altogether effectively. She also points out that there is mounting political pressure to make some cases the subject of mandatory review — particularly those involving severely disabled newborns, and the chronically and terminally ill from whom doctors wish to withhold life-supporting treatment. In Australia, institutional ethics committees (with the notable exception of research ethics committees) tend to operate on the optional-optional model.

Cases typically brought before institutional ethics committees involve moral dilemmas and moral controversies arising from treating the rationally incompetent, the critically ill and the hopelessly ill (i.e. those with poor prognoses), or in situations where health professionals (most notably treating doctors) are 'uncomfortable' with family demands (Brennan 1988, p. 803). These cases are commonly referred to by health professionals as 'hard cases' — that is, cases which are plagued by moral uncertainty and which are of a nature that defies easy resolution.

Composition of institutional ethics committees

A third major issue to receive considerable attention in the bioethics literature is that pertaining to just who should rightly serve on the institutional ethics committee.

Many have worried that institutional ethics committees would become dominated by those representing the interests of the medical profession and hospital administrators — a fear not without some grounds. For example, a 1984 study in the United States found that 57 per cent of institutional ethics committee members were physicians (Levine 1984, p. 12).

There is general agreement in the philosophical literature that ethics committees should be *interdisciplinary* and should include lay persons independent of the institution. As a point of interest, Australia's National Bioethics Consultative Committee, referred to earlier, took stringent steps to ensure that no *one* professional, gender or age group dominated its membership. Membership was representative of expertise in the areas of science, medicine, health care (other than a doctor), economics, social science, ethics/ philosophy, community/consumer interest, law, and moral theology. An effort was also made to ensure complete geographical representation. The committee was not culturally representative, however, and tended to be dominated by people of Anglo–Celtic Australian backgrounds.

Institutional ethics committees in the United States typically include doctors, nurses, lawyers, social workers, hospital administrators, psychologists, members of the clergy, and at least one non-staff member (Levine 1984; Ross et al. 1986, pp. 37–42). Whether these people are the most appropriate to serve on the committees is a matter of some controversy. First, as Kuhse and Singer point out, the composition tends to give 'too much power to the institution' (1985, p. 183). Thus, even if 'outsiders' are represented on the committee, there is still the risk of the committee deciding in favour of the hospital's or the institution's interests. Second, there is no guarantee that this kind of composition will in fact result in appropriate and effective moral decision-making. While the people represented may well be technically expert, this in no way guarantees their expertise as moral decision-makers. As Veatch has argued in relation to another matter, 'technical competency does not a value judgment expert make' (1972, p. 536). Thus, rather than pooled moral knowledge and competence, such a committee may only yield pooled moral ignorance and incompetence. Third, such a composition may be self-defeating; for example, if all members have radically different views on the matters brought before the committee, they may be quite unable to offer constructive advice and guidance to the people seeking assistance. This is a problem which may be exceedingly difficult to resolve. Fourth, and last, it is not clear why some of these entities should be on an ethics committee at all. While the need for a lawyer can be appreciated (given that some ethical decisions could have serious legal ramifications), and while the need for clinical practitioners (such as doctors, nurses and social workers) can be appreciated (insofar as these people are in a unique position to contribute relevant factual information to the decision-making process), it is far from clear that the presence of a theologian or clergyman is needed. As Dr Swan, producer and presenter of ABC Radio's 'Health Report', is reported as saying:

> I would love to hear a good reason why a Jew should be subjected to an Anglican's view even though he [sic] may try to hide his [sic] dogma behind an objective gloss. Why should a Catholic be subject to a rabbi or a Hindu to the local priest?

(Voumard 1988, p. 17)

Further to this, Kuhse and Singer point out that, while 'some experienced ethicists are also members of the clergy', it is not the case that 'all members of the clergy are knowledgeable about ethics' (1985, p. 182). In light of these and similar comments, it seems that there is no compelling reason for a member of the clergy to be included in the composition of an ethics committee.

Many of the difficulties identified here can be overcome by ensuring that those who are included in the committee's membership are morally sensitive and responsible (Freedman 1981), are respectful of the other committee members' views, have good communication skills, and have at least a working knowledge of bioethics (Levine 1984) and are able to think critically and use a 'problem-solving approach that is primarily reflective' (Ross et al. 1986, p. 37). Humility and a willingness and ability 'to work cooperatively with people who come from different levels within the hospital hierarchy' are also essential attributes (Ross et al. 1986, p. 38). Youngner et al. (1984) argue further that full cooperation between members is essential if 'resentment, political discord, and dysfunction' are to be avoided. However, even if all these things are attended to, there remains the uneasy feeling that the typical composition of institutional ethics committees might still not be *right*, particularly in terms of their role in advising, and possibly even deciding on behalf of a patient, what is to count as an ultimate 'good'.

A study in the mid-1980s of patient attitudes towards institutional ethics committees found, significantly, that while 76 per cent of patients surveyed felt that institutional ethics committees 'could be useful', only 12 per cent felt that an ethics committee should 'make the final decision' (Youngner et al. 1984, p. 23). When asked what they thought the 'ideal purpose' of an institutional ethics committee should be, the overwhelming majority (76 per cent) stated that it should be only to 'provide consultation and advice' (Youngner et al. 1984, p. 27). Meanwhile 43 per cent indicated that the committee should become involved only in cases 'where there is disagreement and uncertainty'. As well, 76 per cent felt that 'all patients and family should be automatically informed about the committee's existence upon admission to the hospital'. Also of interest are the patients' views on who should serve on institutional ethics committees: 96 per cent chose physicians, with nurses ranking a close second at 74 per cent. Only 58 per cent thought clergymen should serve, and only 55 per cent thought social workers should serve (Youngner et al. 1984).

Some argue that, in cases of specific patient care dilemmas, perhaps what is called for is not a committee comprised of *hospital and health care agency* caregivers, but rather one which is comprised of persons belonging to the *patient's own support group*. Levine (1977), for example, suggests that patients' interests might, in the end, be better served by a committee (a true patient care ethics committee) made up of the patient's own family, friends, clergyman, lawyers, and the like. This seems a plausible possibility, as long as conditions are carefully defined, and one which should be seriously considered by policy makers and law reformers. Attending health professionals and hospital administrators need not feel threatened by this suggestion, since there need be nothing stopping them from declaring their concerns and interests and imparting their clinical knowledge and other relevant clinical facts to the patient committee. Indeed, there is room to suggest that the only role that attending health professionals and administrators should play is that of giving the relevant clinical information necessary for the patient committee to make an informed choice.

In some respects the role of the public advocate has given legitimacy to the notion of patient representatives (usually family members or friends) assuming some or all of the burden of decision-making in hard cases, rather than this task falling solely into the hands of doctors or the health care team or some other bureaucratic mechanism such as the court. In cases where there is no one to assume the burden of decision-making, clearly the need exists for a facility, such as an interdisciplinary institutional ethics committee, to help to decide the most morally appropriate course of action to take.

Moral decision-making by institutional ethics committees[4]

The question of how an institutional ethics committee should approach moral decision-making when dealing with the matters brought before it has received surprisingly little attention over the years. While attention has been given to the nature and processes of *ethics consultation* (see, for example, La Puma and Schiedermayer 1994) — something which ethics committees can and do offer — and to the *accountability* of institutional ethics committees *apropos* the decisions they make (see, in particular, Fry-Revere 1992), little has been written on the actual decision-making processes that committee members might use to decide issues and cases brought before them. (A notable exception to this oversight is Jonathan Moreno's (1995) relatively recent work *Deciding together: bioethics and moral consensus* in which a consensus approach to bioethical decision-making is articulated and advocated.) Thus an important question to be raised here is: How might institutional ethics committees best approach moral thinking and moral decision-making on the issues brought before them — particularly when these issues involve 'hard cases'?

There is of course a variety of ways in which members of an institutional ethics committee could approach the task of moral decision-making (not least, by using traditional meeting procedures and deciding issues by 'negotiation and agreement' and/or where that fails, deciding by majority vote). For the purposes of this discussion, however, attention will focus on just one approach, and that is, an approach that is informed by the new moral perspective called 'quantum morality' (Zohar 1991; Zohar and Marshall 1993). This approach has been chosen because of the great promise it offers for dealing effectively with 'hard cases' about which members of a given institutional ethics committee (or, indeed, a health care team) might radically disagree.

Quantum morality uses a model of thinking and reasoning associated with the 'new physics' or quantum physics (see also Heisenberg 1990). Unlike the

---

4. An earlier version of the discussion on quantum morality (included under the subheading 'Moral decision-making by institutional ethics committees') first appeared in Johnstone, M-J. (1995). *Inaugural Bennett Lecture: Moral controversy and the search for solutions: some critical reflections for the nursing profession*. Faculty of Nursing, RMIT University, Melbourne, pp. 5–6.

either/or dichotomous, mechanistic and divisionary scientific way of thinking commonly associated with the classical physics of Isaac Newton (and from which Western moral philosophy has borrowed heavily), this new perspective rests on a *both/and* approach to moral thinking and decision-making. Whereas the classical model of Western moral thinking advocates an adversarial approach to interrogating ideas and discovering 'the moral truth', quantum morality advocates a cooperative approach that accepts many different moral viewpoints as having the potential to be right, rather than assuming there is only one single correct view.

Underpinning a 'quantum morality' approach is the recognition that without difference, there is no real choice — no real opportunity to develop, to grow, to evolve — no opportunity to sharpen and refine our moral thinking, and no opportunity to learn to understand another's point of view and to discover the 'creative unity in our differences' (Zohar and Marshall 1993, p. 273). Here, quantum morality takes as its starting point the view that being open to different viewpoints expands the potential of a situation, allows for more questions to be asked and more to be learnt, and ultimately allows for common ground to be found.

Moral decision-making, by this view, is seen as involving a shared and cooperative venture, where people have time and *can take time* to dialogue, to *really listen* to other people's points of view (and thereby give recognition to others by listening), and to negotiate choices that strike 'a creative balance between more fixed attitudes of control at the one extreme or total receptiveness at the other' (Zohar and Marshall 1993, p. 102). For this approach to work, however, participants must come to the moral deliberating process with a willingness to: (1) 'let go' their own point of view as the *only* point of view, and (2) to put their own views alongside others 'as one of many to be compared, contrasted and considered' (Zohar and Marshall 1993, p. 235). Through cooperative and creative dialogue, the differing viewpoints of all participants can evolve into a new 'synthesised' complex whole. In so far as evaluating whether the 'correct' choices have been made, the following applies: if the values and meanings of the choices break down 'and the moral equivalent of physical chaos sets in', the participants may conclude that 'everything has fallen apart' and that a morally good outcome has not been achieved (Zohar 1991, p. 182). Conversely, if the values and meanings of the choices made do not break down, and the moral equivalent of physical order and unity sets in, the participants may conclude that everything has stayed together as a harmonious whole evolving toward a viable futurity, and that a morally good outcome has been achieved.

Access to institutional ethics committees

The question of who should have access to institutional ethics committees has not been as widely addressed as the other more complex questions have been. Nevertheless, this in no way implies that the question of accessibility is any less important. Interestingly, again, the general view is fairly unanimous, with arguments tending to favour committees being accessible to virtually anyone (patients, staff, families) who requires assistance in working through a moral problem and making moral decisions. Since this is a relatively uncontroversial matter, I do not propose to say anything more about it here.

Can institutional ethics committees help?

There is evidence that institutional ethics committees and related consultation have achieved very positive results. La Puma et al. (1988), for example, cite a one-year study involving physicians at a university teaching hospital who used the hospital's ethics consultation service between 1 July 1986 and 30 June 1987. Of those interviewed, 71 per cent of requesting physicians stated that the ethics consultation they had was 'very important' in patient management, 'in clarifying ethical issues, or in learning about medical ethics' (p. 809). Of those physicians who used the ethics consultation service, 96 per cent indicated that they intended 'to request an ethics consultation in the future' (p. 809). Significantly, there is a paucity of research on the subject of whether nurses have access to and use ethics consultation services, and, if so, whether they have found them beneficial.

A number of other benefits have also been postulated in the bioethics literature. Brodeur (1984), for example, suggests that institutional ethics committees help to ensure good decision-making, which in turn will help to limit the risk of legal liability. More importantly, from a moral perspective, the committees help to re-emphasise *patient care* as *the* central goal of health care practice. Cranford and Doudera (1984), like Brodeur, see institutional ethics committees as ensuring better and more systematic moral decision-making. They also see the committees as helping to identify previously unrecognised moral issues on which there is no general consensus, thus paving the way for moral negotiation and the realisation of just moral outcomes. Caplan (1982), on the other hand, sees the benefit of allowing moral expertise to have a place in technical domains as, quite simply, that of improving moral understanding (see also Moreno 1991).

Institutional ethics committees are not without their problems, however. They are obviously unable to *guarantee* the quality and appropriateness of their moral analyses and decision-making, and are at risk of merely replacing, rather than changing and improving, the traditional loci of decision-making. They are also vulnerable to breeding what McCormick (1984, p. 154) calls 'inhouse protectionism' (i.e. where committee members 'operate protectively for the institution and its practitioners'), 'legal accommodationism' (i.e. where the committee becomes too narrowly focused on the law to the point that ethical considerations become diluted and even lost), and 'oversensitivity' (i.e. where committees become 'oversensitive to the felt need of consensus' to the point where they lose all the moral ingredients which otherwise distinguish them as ethically imperative). McCormick identifies the further concern that institutional ethics committees, by their very nature, may also provide the ultimate breeding ground for 'whistleblowers', particularly if the committee keeps minutes of its activities and findings or documents them in some other way. Just why this should be any more of a problem for institutional ethics committees than it is for any other kind of committee whose proceedings are confidential is not clear; it may even be, as one colleague has suggested, a *benefit*. Another problem is that institutional ethics committees can be rather cumbersome and clumsy — particularly in situations demanding 'a quick response, without prior notice, at any hour of the day or night' (Kuhse and Singer 1985, p. 183). Such problems are not insurmountable, however, and with careful forethought and planning can be prevented and/or overcome. (A particularly helpful resource on this matter is Ross et al.'s [1986] *Handbook for Hospital ethics committees: practical suggestions for ethics committee members to plan, develop, and evaluate their roles and responsibilities*.)

Implications of institutional ethics committees for the nursing profession

The last question to be addressed here is: What are the implications of institutional ethics committees for members of the nursing profession?

Possible answers to this question will depend very much on the function, power, composition and accessibility of any given ethics committee. If committees take on a multi-purpose role, as outlined earlier, it is likely that the implications for nurses will be positive. Nurses will have somewhere to go to air their concerns and will gain the opportunity of resolving moral disagreement formally. They will also gain the opportunity of developing a deeper awareness and understanding of moral issues arising from clinical practice and developing their moral problem-solving skills. And they will have the unique opportunity of gaining insights into and understanding of the kinds of moral problems and personal difficulties that other members of the health care team also experience, which will pave the way for more harmonious and interdependent working relationships. If ethics committees adopt only a narrow mono-dimensional role, however, the implication for nurses might not be so positive; indeed, the position of nurses will probably be just as frustrating as it was before any thought was given to the establishment of institutional ethics committees in the first place.

A committee's power and authority perhaps stand to have the most serious implications of all for the nursing profession — particularly in cases involving mandatory review and mandatory compliance. Where mandatory decisions stand to impinge on and infringe standards of nursing care (for example, in cases involving the withholding of food and fluids), the nursing profession could be faced with some serious problems. At the time of writing it was not known whether nurses had in fact encountered any problems associated with institutional ethics committees making decisions which required mandatory compliance.

Related to this concern is the question of composition. While it is generally accepted in the philosophical literature that nurses should be represented on ethics committees, in practice such a view is not always received sympathetically. Nurses are having to play the usual 'games' to gain representation on these committees — something which is quite unacceptable. The point — as is made evident throughout this text — is that nurses are just as vulnerable to moral problems and controversies as are doctors and others. As well as this, nurses have very real moral as well as legal responsibilities towards those who require nursing care. It is then right and proper that a 'grass roots' clinical nursing perspective be represented on ethics committees. To exclude a substantive clinical nursing perspective would be to allow the committee to have less integrity than it perhaps should have if it is to function appropriately and effectively as a mechanism for guiding and assisting the resolution of moral conflict in health care domains.

The degree of accessibility also has the potential to affect nurse practitioners. If accessibility means that the committee is literally open to all who need it, nurse practitioners need not fear suffering any undue burdens or disadvantages. If access is restricted, however, this would pose a different situation altogether. In the unlikely event of access being restricted, nurses might well suffer disproportionate burdens and disadvantages through not having the opportunity to experience the kinds of benefits that a multi-purpose ethics committee could offer.

If nurses are finding that they are not achieving fair representation on established ethics committees, or are being denied access commensurate with their needs, one solution is for nurses to establish their own working ethics committees. Indeed, many nurses have already established — or are in the process of establishing — their own nursing ethics committees. There are sound justifications for doing this. As I have discussed elsewhere (Johnstone 1998, pp. 97–107), unlike the broader institutional or hospital ethics committees, which have as their focus more general concerns relating to patient care and institutional activities, nursing ethics committees focus specifically on the moral concerns and experiences of *nurses*, and on the kinds of moral problems that nurses encounter when planning and delivering nursing care to patients. One of the major advantages of establishing nursing ethics committees is that these can provide nurses with a unique opportunity to identify and examine bioethical issues from a *nursing* point of view, and not from the point of view of those whose dominant interests tend to dictate which ethical issues will be addressed by a broader institutional ethics committee, and how, when, and by whom. This means that nurses can have the 'space', for want of a better word, to identify what *they* consider to be important ethical issues, and to determine how, when and by whom they consider these issues should be addressed. Another major advantage of nursing ethics committees is that these can provide an opportunity for nurses to identify what their (educational, support, policy reform and other) needs are and how these needs can best be met. With broader-based institutional ethics committees, these kinds of opportunities to nurses might not always be available.

Nursing ethics committees are not without disadvantages, however. Indeed, they can fall prey to exactly the same kinds of problems that more general institutional ethics committees can experience. For example, a nursing ethics committee may be lacking in institutional authority, may be lacking in direction, may have a membership which serves the interests more of the institution than of nurses and patients, may be dominated by a particular faction of nurses (for example, nursing administrators), may lack the expertise necessary for dealing with the kinds of ethical problems nurses face in their day-to-day practice, may be plagued by radical moral disagreement among committee members, may be unable or powerless to implement its decisions, may be reluctant to 'rock the boat', and so on. Despite these and like problems, however, the establishment of nursing ethics committees is a welcome and long overdue initiative in Australia. What is also needed, though, is a nursing ethics committee network through which nurses can share their knowledge and experiences; keep each other informed of the activities and achievements of their respective committees; and contribute generally to the achievement of moral practices in the health care institutions and facilities in which they work (Johnstone 1997).

Institutional ethics committee — some further considerations

Institutional ethics committees are a relatively recent phenomena in Australia and to date appear to be playing an influential role in assisting health care institutions or, more accurately, the health professionals working within them, to address a range of ethical issues (including 'morally hard cases') encountered during the course of their work (see also Johnstone 1998). The rise of institutional ethics committees has, however, had a paradoxical cost: they have become thoroughly implicated in the bureaucratisation and institutionalisation of moral decision-making (Jennings 1991, pp. 451–2; see also Bauman 1993, p. 125). As Jennings explains, this is evident by the lived reality that:

> ethical choice and agency are now embedded as never before in a network of explicit rules and formal procedures and processes for making decisions. These rules stipulate (within certain limits) what types of decisions may be made, how they may be made, by whom, and with the assistance of what resources.
>
> Equally important, these rules are increasingly becoming institutionalised: they are embedded in the organisational form of statutes, court opinions, administrative mandates, and institutional protocols; in decisions regarding terminal care, these rules inform counselling and educational mechanisms encouraging individual patients and their families to choose surrogate decision-makers and to give prior statements about wanted and unwanted treatment. As a necessary adjunct to this bureaucratisation and institutionalisation of moral decision-making, hospitals are being strongly encouraged ... to establish ethics committees to support and provide technical assistance to this process.
>
> (Jennings 1991, p. 452)

Conclusion

Conscientious objection, strike action, and institutional ethics committees are all important processes which nurses can use to 'take a stand' on important ethical issues affecting their practice. Being able to use these processes in a just and effective way, however, requires knowledge and understanding of ethics and its application to and in nursing care contexts. It also requires political savvy, astuteness, and a willingness to take 'moral risks' in the interests of questioning and calling into question 'things as they are'.

Chapter 16

Promoting ethical nursing practice[1]

Introduction

Nurses both in Australia and overseas are confronted every day with having to make morally relevant choices and to take action on the basis of these choices during the course of their work. This 'everyday' occurrence should not be taken to mean, however, that deciding and acting morally in nursing care contexts is simply a matter of habit or 'daily routine' and therefore as something 'trivial' requiring little knowledge, skill or attention. To the contrary. As both this text and our own experience reminds us, dealing with everyday ethical problems requires of decision-makers an exquisite moral sensibility, 'moral knowing', moral imagination, life experience, virtue (e.g. compassion, empathy, integrity, care, 'decency'), being generally informed (e.g. about law, social and cultural processes, human nature, politics), and a deep personal moral commitment to 'doing what is right'. In some instances, 'being moral' also requires political savvy and an ability (personal and otherwise) to transcend the many obstacles that threaten to obstruct the realisation of morally just outcomes in given contexts. At times, although it should be otherwise, deciding and acting morally can require enormous moral courage and even 'moral heroism' on the part of those choosing to take a moral course of action. This is especially so in the case of nurses who, despite an apparent increase in professional status over the past two decades, continue to lack sovereignty in their own realm of practice, continue to be burdened with enormous responsibilities without the legitimated authority to fulfil these, and continue to be coerced into silence when what they have to say on important ethical issues threatens the status quo in which others have powerful vested interests (Johnstone 1994).

All aspects of nursing (e.g. education, practice, management and research) have a profound ethical dimension. As considered elsewhere in this text, the ethical dimension is distinguished from other dimensions of nursing (for example, the legal and clinical dimensions) by the inherent moral demands to:

---

1. This chapter has drawn extensively from and has used substantial excerpts from the following two previously published works: Johnstone, M-J (1998), *Determining and responding effectively to ethical professional misconduct in nursing: a report to the Nurses Board of Victoria*, Melbourne; and Johnstone (1997), A reappraisal of everyday nursing ethics: new directions for the 1990s and beyond, *INEN Bulletin* (published by International Nursing Ethics [and Midwifery] Network, The Netherlands).

- promote human wellbeing and welfare;
- balance the needs and significant moral interests of different people; and
- make reliable judgments on what constitutes morally 'right' and 'wrong' conduct, and provide sound justifications for the decisions and actions taken on the basis of these judgments.

Members of the nursing profession cannot escape these demands or the stringent responsibilities they impose. One reason for this is that no nursing decision or action (no matter how small or trivial) occurs in a moral vacuum, or is free of moral risk or consequence. To put this another way, even the most 'ordinary' of nursing actions can affect significantly the wellbeing, welfare and moral interests of others. This is so whether in a nursing education, practice, management or research setting.

Nursing codes of ethics around the world have made explicit that nurses have a stringent moral responsibility to promote and safeguard the wellbeing, welfare and moral interests of people needing and/or receiving nursing care. These codes also variously recognise the responsibility of nurses to balance the needs and interests of different people equally in health care contexts. What is often not stated, however, is *how* nurses ought to fulfil their moral responsibilities and to deal effectively with the many ethical issues they encounter on a day-to-day basis. 'Dealing effectively' with ethical issues, in this instance, is taken as including being able to:

- identify correctly the most pertinent ethical issues facing nurses (locally and globally) at any given time;
- recognising both the short- and long-term implications of these issues for the nursing profession generally; and
- developing strategies for responding effectively to these issues once identified.

It has been a central aim of this text to assist nurses to achieve the above requirements.

A key question remains, however, and that is: How can the nursing profession best promote and maintain ethical nursing practice? It remains the task of this final chapter to briefly address this important question. Specifically, attention will focus on addressing the importance of the following:

- formulating and enacting meaningful standards of ethical nursing conduct;
- nursing ethics education;
- ethical nursing management and improving the moral culture of the organisations in which nurses work;
- nursing ethics research and scholarship;
- political action.

Formulating and enacting meaningful standards of ethical nursing conduct

Crucial to the promotion and maintenance of ethical professional conduct in nursing is the formulation and enactment of meaningful ethical standards of conduct (Johnstone 1998). In order for ethical standards to be 'meaningful', a number of conditions must be met.

- The standards in question must be part of a larger moral schema that has for its community of users (in this instance, nurses): (1) *significance* (viz. is relevant and will make a material difference to the realisation of morally desirable outcomes in the world); (2) *purpose* (viz. offers reasons why moral conduct is imperative); (3) *intention* (viz. articulates clearly its moral ends or *telos*); and (4) *value* (viz. demonstrates a worthy relation between its significance, purpose and intention) (adapted from Bohm 1989).
- The standards in question must have *emerged from within and be reflective of the lived moral reality experienced by the community of users* (in this instance, members of the nursing profession), as opposed to being imposed from outside of it (for example, by non-nurse moral philosophers). (As a point of clarification, and as discussed in the opening chapters of this text, ethical standards emerging from a group's lived reality are an essential part of the fabric of that group's lived moral experience; among other things, they serve the vital function of providing a set of common moral perceptions that can be drawn upon to 'reality test' [objectify] and validate group members' day-to-day moral judgments and interventions.)
- The community of users (here, nurses) must feel they have *a place in the larger moral scheme of things*: that is, they must feel connected with (as opposed to isolated from) other members in the community of users, have a *coherent and harmonious relationship with other members* in the community of users, and, importantly, feel they have *something to offer* (even if this something is 'small') to and in this larger moral scheme of things (adapted from Pylkkanen 1989b).

Once formulated, it is essential that ethical professional standards of conduct are 'kept before' the community of users, internalised as a way of life, and, more importantly, enacted. As is exemplified in the case of codes of ethical conduct, it is all too easy for the documented ethical standards of a profession or organisation to sit 'gathering dust on shelves' (Derry 1991). In addition, a community of users (for example, nurses) might fall into the trap of erroneously thinking that just because they have personally endorsed a formally stated code of ethics or have 'done ethics' as a subject in a nursing education course, they have discharged their moral responsibilities as ethical professionals and do not need to *do* anything more. This kind of moral hypocrisy is described comprehensively by Hoff (1982), who writes:

> It is now possible to consider ourselves morally exemplary simply because we adhere to an enlightened set of social principles. We may vote in accordance with these principles, but they require nothing of us personally; we need never lift a finger to help anyone and we need take no active part in social reform movements. We can even permit ourselves to be ruthless in relations with other people. Because morality has been sublimated into ideology, great numbers of people, the young, the educated especially, feel they have an adequate moral identity merely because they hold the 'right' views on such matters as ecology, feminism, socialism, and nuclear energy. They may lead narrow, self-indulgent lives, obsessed with their physical health, material comforts, and personal growth, yet still feel a moral advantage over those who actively work to help the needy but who are, in their eyes, ideologically unsound.
>
> (Hoff 1982, p. 13)

The application of Hoff's (1982) views to the domain of nursing is self-evident, and underscores the need for the agreed ethical standards of nursing to be distilled into action. It is crucial that these standards are seen to be more than just a list of statements which members can and have endorsed. Rather, they must be seen as a means for accomplishing shared ethical goals — as *a way of life*, and not merely as *a set of ideas* about a way of life. One way of achieving this is through the effective communication of agreed ethical standards of conduct. To be effective, the communication of ethical standards must happen repeatedly and more frequently through *actions* than through the mere distribution of documents (codes of ethics), such as through the mail or by displaying wall posters (Derry 1991). Another way of achieving the enactment of agreed standards of ethical professional conduct is through education, as will now be considered

Nursing ethics education

Another strategy crucial to the promotion and maintenance of ethical professional conduct in nursing is an effective 'preventative' nursing ethics education program. A preventative nursing ethics education program has as its principal aim the teaching of knowledge and skills that enables nurses to anticipate and identify moral problems, to engage in reflective and critical thinking about the problems anticipated and/or identified, and to take the necessary action to prevent them (adapted from McCullough 1995). To be effective, however, such a program requires a multifarious approach. Regrettably, it is beyond the scope of this present chapter to examine the topic of ethics education for nurses in the depth that is warranted. Nevertheless, there is room to make a number of key points.

Contents

To be effective, a preventative ethics education program for nurses must be *meaningful* and *substantive*. If an ethics education program is not meaningful or substantive, there is a risk that nurses could become disinterested, confused, dispirited and lacking in motivation to learn and to 'be moral'. The question remains: How might 'meaningfulness' and 'substantiveness' be determined?

As in the case of ethical standards (discussed above), to be 'meaningful' an ethics education program must have *significance*, *purpose*, *intention* and *value* for nurses. In this instance, a nursing ethics education program could be said to have these qualities when it meets the guidelines detailed below.

- *Significance* — where it is relevant to and will make a material difference to the realisation of morally desirable outcomes in nursing domains. In its approach, it draws extensively (although, not exclusively) on the lived moral experience of nurses — and, more specifically, on the empirical data of this experience — and demonstrates:
  - key ethical issues faced by nurses at any given time or place;
  - the range of moral possibilities, probabilities and 'realities' for nurses associated with these issues;
  - the profound role that experience can and does play in shaping and refining core moral values that are conducive to guiding nursing conduct that is fair and sympathetic, and which, in turn, is conducive

to fostering harmonious human relationships, and ultimately human wellbeing and survival in nursing domains (adapted from Moreno 1995, Chapter 7 'Naturalising moral consensus'; Damasio 1994, Chapter 6 'Biological regulation and survival'); and

- the role of experience in enabling nurses to develop a vast repertoire of possible moral actions which can be effectively deployed to prevent or remedy moral problems in work-related contexts.

- *Purpose* — where it articulates clearly:
  - the reasons why ethical professional conduct in nursing is imperative; and
  - the practical advantages of engaging in such conduct.
- *Intention* — where it articulates clearly the moral ends of nursing, the ultimate goals of ethical professional conduct in nursing, and is keyed to the agreed ethical standards of nursing conduct.
- *Value* — where it demonstrates the relation between the significance, purpose and intention of ethical professional conduct and the broader moral scheme of things in nursing, and the worth of this relationship.

To be *substantive*, a preventative ethic education program must focus not only on teaching the 'moral competencies' of *knowing that*, but of practical *knowing how*. It must not only teach descriptive ethics, metaethics and normative ethics as relevant to the profession and practice of nursing, but also *characterological ethics* and what it means to be — and how to be — a decent (virtuous) human being (nurse) in a world that is becoming increasingly (and destructively) morally dissociative and annihilistic (see Kruschwitz and Roberts 1987; Blum 1994; Damasio 1994; Johnstone 1995; Tester 1997). This includes teaching nurses how to deal with moral pluralism and moral disagreement in a critically reflective and creative, rather than an arbitrary and destructive, manner (Kane 1994; Johnstone 1995; see also Pylkkanen 1989a), and the importance of individual personal action aimed at preventing or alleviating moral harms (see Hoff 1982).

Location

Most ethics education for nurses occurs in a formal classroom setting. It also occurs in workshop, seminar and conference venues. And it is not denied that these are all extremely important locations of ethics education. To be effective, however, preventative ethics education must not only take place in the classroom, or in workshop, seminar and conference venues. It must also take place in the workplace, that is, in the *actual 'hands-on' contexts in which nurses work* (for example, a hospital ward, a community health care setting, an education or research unit). By 'localising' nursing ethics education within the actual lived-in moral domain of nursing work (whether this be a clinical, educational, administrative, or research setting), a number of important outcomes can be achieved.

- It enables experiential learning of preventative and professional ethics. By being taught within a workplace setting, the contents of ethics can be related directly to 'what is going on' in the lived-in domain. Ethics can be 'brought to life' (become 'in action', as it were), rather than just left standing as a set of meaningless and sterile principles and theories which only moral philosophers and teachers can understand.
- It provides nurses with an opportunity to collectively:

– identify the commonalities (commonsense moral knowledge) and differences in their moral viewpoints;
– learn about and develop alternative points of view;
– identify 'knowledge gaps' requiring attention;
– relate the micro-level of their moral experience to the macro-level;
– engage in cathartic moral talking;
– engage in critical discussion and achieve enlightenment;
– achieve a moral synthesis of differing viewpoints;
– realise the power of collective knowledge and of the nursing collective to challenge and change the status quo.

- It provides nurses with an opportunity to learn directly the art of moral problem solving; individuals can become fully engaged in the collective moral project of:
  – assessing a morally problematic situation;
  – identifying the key moral problems affecting stakeholders;
  – planning effective responses to the problems identified;
  – 'reality test' the plausibility of implementing planned responses;
  – evaluating the outcomes of moral responses initiated;
  – being morally accountable and responsible for their actions.

Duration

Today, the subject of ethics is taught in most undergraduate nursing courses and in some post-graduate nursing courses. However, the amount of time devoted to contact teaching of the subject varies across courses. The question of how much to teach, when and for how long is a matter of some controversy. Nevertheless, anecdotal evidence strongly suggests that a minimum of 26-hours contact teaching time (a full unit) is required to teach the subject effectively at undergraduate level. Furthermore, experience suggests that the subject ought to be taught as a discrete unit in its own right, and not as an integrated unit (for example, on law and ethics) as some perhaps favour. A less focused approach would, in my view, make it extremely difficult to prepare beginning practitioners to achieve the moral competencies otherwise required and prescribed by the Australian Nursing Council Inc (1994, 1997). As has been readily demonstrated in this text, (bio)ethics (and its sub-branch of nursing ethics) is a discrete field of inquiry in its own right, with its own rich history, theoretical underpinnings and practical applications. Achieving the requisite competency in moral knowledge and practice (*knowing that* and *knowing how*) — and being positioned as a beginning practitioner to engage in preventative (and remedial) ethics — students of nursing must be given an opportunity to engage in sustained and focused learning of the subject, such as would be provided by a discrete (minimum) 26-hour unit on the topic of ethics in nursing. This would enable an in-depth examination of the 'specifics' of ethical nursing practice, and a subsequent application and integration of the moral knowledge gained in other nursing subjects, both theoretical and practical in content.

In the case of postgraduate nursing education, so long as students have completed an undergraduate foundational unit on the subject of ethical issues in nursing, the number of contact teaching hours required to teach the subject can be more flexible and, to a larger extent, determined by students' interests and practice needs. It should be noted, however, that the ethical issues associated with clinical specialty areas (for example, critical care, cancer care nursing, aged care, mental health nursing, and the like) are complex and many. Effective preventative ethics education in these and similar areas would, as in the case of undergraduate courses, require discrete units in their own right taught over a (minimum) 26-hour contact teaching time period. It should not be assumed that, upon completing a unit in ethics as part of a formal nurse education program, a graduate's ethics education has been completed. To be effective, preventative ethics education must be continuous. It is important that nurses do not fall prey to the idea that once they have completed a unit in ethics as part of a formal education program, they have 'done ethics' (as it is sometime claimed), and that they would not benefit from any further education on the subject. Just as nurses need to continually update their clinical knowledge and skills, so too do nurses need to continually update their moral knowledge and skills both as *knowing that* and *knowing how*. It is important, therefore, that the subject of ethics in nursing features fully and comprehensively in all continuing (nurse) education programs (Johnstone 1998).

Remedial ethics education

In addition to preventive nursing ethics education, remedial nursing ethics education may also be required (for instance, where moral problems in practice have arisen [see Johnstone 1998]). Remedial ethics education is similar in nature to preventative ethics education but with the notable difference that its content and teaching method is 'special' insofar as it is focused specifically on a particular moral problem or problems experienced by a given individual or group. Unlike preventative ethics education where the aim is to *prevent* moral problems from occurring, remedial ethics education aims to 'cure' or remedy an extant moral problem. To be effective, not only must a remedial ethics education program be meaningful, but it must be clearly focused on addressing the moral problem(s) at hand and offer some relief through emancipatory (critical) moral thinking. Remedial ethics education can be provided over as little as a one-hour session, or over an entire 26-hour short course, depending on the seriousness of the problem and the degree to which remedial education is required in the persons involved. Remedial ethics education may sometimes be prescribed by nurse registering authorities as a disciplinary measure against nurses who have breached the agreed ethical standards of nursing (Johnstone 1998).

Who should teach nursing ethics?

In some respects, the question of 'who should teach nursing ethics?' is a trivial one, and some might wonder why I have raised it at all. The answer to this is very simple: the nursing profession is faced with the problem of not having many nurses who are appropriately qualified (by which I mean dually qualified in both nursing *and* philosophy/ethics) to teach bioethics to nurses. One unfortunate consequence of this has been that nursing students have sometimes received only a very limited moral education, or a misguided moral education, or, in cases where no lecturer was available, no moral education at all.

Some nursing education programs have overcome the problem of 'who should teach' by having moral philosophers from other departments on campus to teach the ethics component of the nursing curriculum. While there are advantages in having moral philosophers involved in teaching nurses (see, for example,

Beauchamp 1982; Singer 1982), there are also disadvantages. For instance, moral philosophers (like most people in the community) tend to have a very poor understanding of the nature of nursing practice and of the special kinds of moral problems that nurse practitioners all too frequently encounter when providing nursing care.

I would further suggest that philosophers who do not have a good understanding of the kinds of moral issues and problems nurses face will find it difficult to make their material meaningful and relevant to nursing students. This might, in turn, have the unfortunate consequence of the students simply 'switching off' — as did happen to one moral philosopher teaching ethics in the first-year program of an undergraduate nursing course.

Another disadvantage is that philosophers may attempt to educate nursing students in the classical rationalistic tradition at the expense of other moral viewpoints — such as those considered in Chapters 4, 5 and 6 of this text.

Ideally, nursing ethics should be taught by experienced nurses who also have academic credentials in bioethics/moral philosophy. Where this is not possible, bioethicists who are sympathetic to — and who have some understanding of — nursing can be a reliable and defensible alternative to nurse teachers of the subject.

Ethical nursing management and improving the moral culture of the organisations in which nurses work

The culture of the organisations and institutions in which nurses work can make it extremely difficult for nurses to function as morally accountable and responsible practitioners. As I have discussed elsewhere (Johnstone 1998), some organisations and institutions are 'morally impaired' and can be outright hostile to moral excellence. Throughout this text examples have been given to demonstrate that nurses can lose their jobs and be publicly vilified for taking a moral stand and/or upholding the agreed ethical standards of the profession. Ironically, these difficulties are compounded by nurses being educationally prepared to function as morally accountable and responsible practitioners. One reason for this is that other health care professionals with whom nurses work may not have achieved the same level of moral competency that nurses have, and thus lack the requisite knowledge and skills for discerning and responding effectively to morally problematic situations. Another reason is that while the organised nursing profession has 'institutionalised' ethical motivation, many organisations in which nurses work have not.

While nurses can probably have little influence on the ethics education of other health professionals, they can nevertheless exert some influence on improving the moral culture of the organisations in which they work. This, in turn, could have a profound influence on realising the ultimate goals of preventative ethics. Here two key questions can be raised: How can organisation support ethical behaviour? and What can nurses do to gain this support?

Organisations can support ethical behaviour in at least two ways: (1) by removing the disincentives to behaving ethically, and (2) by providing positive incentives for behaving ethically (Derry 1991). One of the greatest disincentives facing nurses is a reasonably founded fear of being punished for questioning and challenging the moral status quo (see, for example, Johnstone 1994). This disincentive is serious from a moral point of view. Among other things, if nurses fear being punished, then they may not come forward when the need arises. This, in turn, could risk otherwise avoidable and preventable moral harms occurring. Were such harms do occur, this would be an undesirable, unsatisfactory and indefensible moral outcome for all concerned. The 'unfortunate experiment' at the National Women's Hospital in New Zealand (discussed in Chapter 2 of this text) is an example of this (Coney 1988). Had nurses been less fearful in coming forward in this case, it is possible that a number of significant moral harms could have been avoided.

In contrast, positive incentives for moral conduct could encourage nurses to 'come forward'. Borrowing from Derry, incentives for moral conduct can include:

> listening, responding on the basis of others' needs rather than on the basis of one's own needs, building strong relationships, decisions on the basis of responsibility to others, giving feedback, nurturing, building cooperation rather than confrontation.
>
> (Derry 1991, pp. 121–36)

These characteristics can be expressed in the following actions:

- organisations formulating and articulating, through democratic processes, their own ethical standards of conduct (for example, in the form of an organisational code of ethics, position statements and policies);
- organisations facilitating repeated, regular and effective communication of ethical standards and policies through printed information, stakeholder access to resource people, and role modelling of ethical conduct (for example, managers need to not only *manage ethical problems well* but to *manage ethically* the problems they have to deal with as managers [Johnstone 1996]);
- organisations supporting the establishment of institutional ethics committees and other forums (for example, nursing ethics forums/ committees) for the purposes of enabling the discussion of ethical issues in a 'safe place' outside of the usual hierarchy of power and authority characteristic of institutions (see discussion on institutional ethics committees in the previous chapter);
- organisations supporting 'moral quality assurance' programs and the monitoring of 'moral performance indicators' (as Scofield [1992, p. 31] points out, 'impairment need not be fatal to anyone's personal or professional life. The *failure to monitor impairment*, however, is fatal to maintaining a real accountability and integrity' [emphasis added]);
- organisations rewarding moral conduct; this can include: 'praise, recognition, action on suggestions, responsiveness, setting examples, making positive examples of people for desired ethical actions' (adapted from Derry 1991, pp. 121–36).

Organisations, like individuals, are morally accountable and responsible entities. This accountability and responsibility includes an organisation's quality assurance of moral standards, policies and practices. Organisations, like individuals, must also behave ethically and be made to account when they fail to do so. Nurses are part of the organisations in which they work. Thus, when nurses are made to account for their moral actions and/or inactions, so too must the organisations in which they work. This is an important consideration in the effective prevention of moral problems in work-related contexts. Unless there is 'dual carriageway', morally speaking, between nurses and their employing organisations *apropos* moral accountability and responsibility, nurses will remain vulnerable to being 'scapegoated' by those who are higher up on the institutional hierarchy and thus more powerful than themselves (Johnstone 1994). Equally serious, it could obstruct ethical practice altogether, resulting in otherwise avoidable moral harms. It is therefore imperative that work-related environments are supportive of ethical nursing practice (see also Corley and Raines 1993), and that organisations actively create what Curtin (1993) calls 'moral space' for nurses to practise ethically.

Nursing ethics research and scholarship

Up until recently, there has been a questionable lack of Australasian nursing research and scholarship on ethical issues in nursing practice. At times, this lack of research and scholarship has made it extremely difficult for nurses to speak authoritatively on the many ethical issues they have had to face in health care contexts. Just why this lack of attention to nursing ethics research and scholarship has occurred is a matter for speculation. One reason may be that nurses have not been sufficiently knowledgeable about the area of ethics to undertake substantive inquiries on the subject. Another possible reason can be linked to the common though mistaken view that scholarly research is not 'proper' research — unlike 'hands on' (empirical) research, which is seen to conform more fully with traditional notions of 'research' (Jameton and Fowler 1989). Finally, there is some room to suggest that the dearth of nursing ethics research could be linked, paradoxically, to the dominance of the analytical method of philosophic inquiry and the mistaken view that 'ethics' can and should only be explored by 'pure' scholarly inquiry, rather than by other qualitative (for example, descriptive and interpretative) types of inquiries.

There is, however, mounting evidence that the status of nursing ethics research and scholarship is changing. There is now a substantially improved recognition of philosophic inquiry (of which ethics inquiry is a form) as a legitimate and important form of research within nursing; and more and more 'hands-on' studies are being done investigating topics relevant to the advancement of nursing ethics and ethical nursing practice. Two notable examples of the latter can be found in the following masters theses (both completed in 1997): *Creating equilibrium: moral decision-making of nurses working with children in New Zealand hospitals* (by Jennifer Conder, held Otago University, Dunedin, New Zealand), and *Maintaining a nursing ethic: a grounded theory of the moral practice of experienced nurses* (by Martin Woods, held Massey University, Palmerston North, New Zealand). Both these studies herald a welcome new era in nursing ethics research in Australasia. It is known anecdotally that over the next few years numerous other nursing ethics studies will also be completed.

Political action

The nursing profession has not been very successful in getting its voice heard and in getting the public to understand what nursing ethics is about. We have seen examples in this text of how the nursing perspective on bioethical issues has been conspicuously absent from history, the media, interdisciplinary conferences, and other influential domains of public activity. There can be little doubt that it is time for the nursing profession to develop a well organised action lobby, just as other professional groups have done, to remedy this situation. There is nothing unprofessional or dishonourable about engaging in lobbying activities, and there is no reason for suggesting that the nursing profession should not 'pick up the gauntlet', so to speak. Furthermore, as the National Women's Consultative Council (1988) points out:

> Action can be fun. Even when you know that it's mainly symbolic it's still more gratifying to act collectively than to fume privately. Action means getting together with other people to talk things over, finding out that other people have the same concerns that you have, and then taking those concerns to the people in power and publicly demanding that they do something about it.
>
> (National Women's Consultative Council 1988, p. 4)

As there are already several publications available on how to lobby, including, in particular, the National Women's Consultative Council's *Women into Action* (1988), I do not propose to say anything more about it here. What does warrant mention, however, is that the nursing profession would be well advised to be much better organised than it presently is if it is to make an impact. Among other things, the nursing profession would benefit from having a core group of informed, active, articulate and committed people who can scrutinise and respond to policy-making initiatives, political debate, and media activities (i.e. conduct a media watch). This group could be formally charged with the responsibilities of ensuring that a substantive nursing perspective is sought and fully represented in policy and law reforms. It could also play a fundamental role in coordinating media releases aimed at publicly declaring the nursing profession's position on matters which stand to significantly affect both its own and the public's interests. Unless the nursing profession assumes a much higher public and political profile than it has until now, it may, in the final analysis, find that it is in no position to fulfil its broader moral as well as professional responsibilities towards the community at large.

Another area which has been sorely neglected by the nursing profession is that of policy and law reform — an area which I consider to be a primary target for action lobbying by nurses. However we look at it, the fact is that nurses have suffered intolerable burdens on account of inadequate or inappropriate legal laws and institutional policies (see in particular Johnstone 1994, *Nursing and the injustices of the law*). In light of the examples given in this text and elsewhere, I would suggest that the nursing profession has a significant moral interest in researching the inadequacies and deficiencies of existing legal laws, institutional policies and similar areas, and in actively lobbying for those inadequate and deficient laws and policies to be reformed — or, in cases where laws or policies are intolerable to accountable and responsible nursing practice, even abandoned altogether. The nursing profession would also benefit from identifying areas where policy guidelines are seriously lacking — such as those pertaining to conscientious objection, Not For Resuscitation directives, informed consent, and the withholding of food and fluids. Until policy and law reforms are achieved in these and similar areas, nurses will never be free to practise nursing as they have been taught to practise it, as nursing research suggests it should be practised, and as the public is entitled to have it practised; nor will they be 'free to be moral' — that is, free to practise as morally accountable and responsible professionals (Yarling and McElmurry 1986).

The recent establishment by the Royal College of Nursing, Australia of the *Ethics Society* and the *Legal Issues Society* (open to all interested members of the Royal College of Nursing, Australia) is an important step towards achieving the level of political organisation and action lobbying needed to challenge and change existing public policies and laws that are not conducive to the ethical practice of nursing.

Conclusion

I want to conclude this text by paying tribute to two very special nurses. These nurses have been chosen not because of any great startling deeds they have performed, but because of their enormous integrity as professional caregivers, and because they have set a powerful example for other nurses to follow.

The first of these nurses is unknown. She is, however, a real person, and is recorded as once having made an important difference to a patient's wellbeing and survival. The patient in this instance was none other than the internationally reputed medical sociologist, Ann Oakley. Upon being greatly moved by the action and care of her 'invisible nurse', Oakley (1986) devoted a full chapter to the importance of nurses in her celebrated book, *Telling the truth about Jerusalem* (1986). Oakley had been admitted to hospital for treatment of a tumour on her tongue. She writes:

> I remember silently crying in front of the consultant the day the tumour was diagnosed. All he said was, 'What are you crying about? The treatment won't affect your appearance'. My appearance was not what I was worried about.

> (Oakley 1986, p. 182)

It was after this that, for the first time, despite her fifteen-year career as a medical sociologist studying health services, Oakley became aware of, and began to respect, the contributions nurses make to health care. Like so many others, Oakley had simply taken the presence of nurses 'for granted'.

Oakley's awareness changed when one day, lying in bed with a radioactive implant stitched to her tongue, she realised that her disease might be fatal — an insight which caused her to become acutely distressed. A young nurse entering the room at that moment to collect a lunch tray saw that Oakley was upset and, instead of continuing the task of removing the tray, immediately sat down to comfort and to talk to her. Oakley discussed her fears and worries — most of which derived from a lack of information about the nature of her tumour and likely prognosis. Upon learning of this, the young nurse went immediately to read Oakley's medical history and came back and informed her that, in her 'limited medical opinion' she 'would probably be all right' (Oakley 1986, p. 182).

Discussing the nurse's actions that day, Oakley writes:

> ... she stayed with me for nearly an hour, which she should not have done. I was radioactive and no one was meant to spend any longer than 10 minutes at a time with me. She was also, presumably, not supposed to tell me what was in my case-notes, so she was breaking at least two sets of rules. I never saw this nurse again after I left hospital, but I would like her to know that she was important to my survival.

> (Oakley 1986, p. 182)

The personal and professional apology offered by Ann Oakley to the 'invisible nurses' of this world is welcome. It is, however, difficult to comprehend how any researcher can spend fifteen years observing health care contexts and not notice nurses. To Oakley's credit, she admits to a 'certain blindness with respect to the contributions nurses make to health care' (p. 181), and offers a public apology — an action which is by no means insignificant.

The truly morally praiseworthy person in this case, however, is not Oakley, but the 'invisible nurse' who broke 'at least two sets of rules' in order to enhance the wellbeing of a stranger in the grip of unnecessary and avoidable suffering. The moral outcomes of this nurse's simple actions show that one does not always have to be heroic to be moral, but merely *aware of* and *sensitive to* the vulnerability of human beings, and sufficiently committed to patient wellbeing to take the actions that may be necessary in order to prevent patients from suffering unnecessarily.

The second nurse to whom tribute is owed is widely known, despite some rather extraordinary attempts by the Australian medical profession to have her achievements denied formal recognition. The nurse being referred to here is Elizabeth Kenny, a controversial figure who gained notoriety for her marvellous care and rehabilitation of polio victims during the 1930s (Willis 1979). Predictably, Kenny's methods of care and treatment were not favourably received by members of the Australian medical profession, who clearly felt threatened by what they considered an invasion of their own territory.

Kenny's work, however, had enormous public support, and her methods were widely acclaimed both in the United States and the United Kingdom (Willis 1979, p. 34). Thus, despite fierce opposition from the Australian medical profession, and despite the negative and frankly biased findings of a number of public inquiries (all of which, incidentally, were carried out entirely by doctors) into her methods, various state governments around Australia went ahead and established Kenny clinics.

Gradually the most successful of Kenny's methods were taken over and incorporated into orthodox medical treatments, thus lessening the differences between her own success rates and those of the doctors. Significantly, as Willis (1979, p. 34) points out, the medical profession took Kenny's methods 'without any acknowledgment being given to [her]'.

Like the 'invisible nurse' discussed above, Elizabeth Kenny deserves ultimate moral praise. She defied the rules of convention, and in doing so promoted the health and wellbeing (moral ends) of thousands of polio sufferers around the world. The moral outcomes of this nurse's somewhat complex actions show, again, that nurses do not necessarily have to be heroic to be moral; they do, however, need to be committed, shrewd and determined. The Kenny experience also shows the importance of nurses having public support (something which Florence Nightingale recognised long ago).

Where to from here? The answer is: to *doing*. To *doing* whatever needs to be done to make health care contexts morally tolerable — whether in a patient's own home, in the community or in an isolated unit of some major university teaching hospital. To *doing* whatever needs to be done to protect people, and to prevent them from suffering unnecessary moral harms. And to *doing* whatever needs to be done to achieve peaceable solutions to the radical moral disagreements which may arise among patients, patients' families, friends, lay carers and health professionals.

441

Nurses may not be able to change the world. They can, however, make a difference to the way a person experiences it. Whether this experience is hostile or friendly, traumatic or peaceable, painful or pleasurable, may depend, in the end, not on science, or even on reason, but on an appropriate moral attitude and on the virtues of human care, compassion, empathy, kindness, friendship, generosity, altruism, love and understanding.

Appendix I

Code for Nurses
Ethical concepts applied to nursing, 1973*
International Council of Nurses

The fundamental responsibility of the nurse is fourfold: to promote health, to prevent illness, to restore health and to alleviate suffering.

The need for nursing is universal. Inherent in nursing is respect for life, dignity and rights of man. It is unrestricted by considerations of nationality, race, creed, colour, age, sex, politics or social status.

Nurses render health services to the individual, the family and the community and coordinate their services with those of related groups.

Nurses and people

The nurse's primary responsibility is to those people who require nursing care.

The nurse, in providing care, promotes an environment in which the values, customs and spiritual beliefs of the individual are respected.

The nurse holds in confidence personal information and uses judgment in sharing this information.

Nurses and practice

The nurse carries personal responsibility for nursing practice and for maintaining competence by continual learning.

The nurse maintains the highest standards of nursing care possible within the reality of a specific situation.

The nurse uses judgment in relation to individual competence when accepting and delegating responsibilities.

The nurse when acting in a professional capacity should at all times maintain standards of personal conduct which reflect credit upon the profession.

Nurses and society

The nurse shares with other citizens the responsibility for initiating and supporting action to meet the health and social needs of the public.

Nurses and co-workers

The nurse sustains a cooperative relationship with co-workers in nursing and other fields.

The nurse takes appropriate action to safeguard the individual when his [sic] care is endangered by a co-worker or any other person.

Nurses and the profession

The nurse plays the major role in determining and implementing desirable standards of nursing practice and nursing education.

The nurse is active in developing a core of professional knowledge.

The nurse, acting through the professional organisation, participates in establishing and maintaining equitable social and economic working conditions in nursing.

---

* This code was adopted by the ICN Council of National Representatives, Mexico City, in May 1973. Reprinted by permission of the International Council of Nurses, Geneva.

Appendix II

Consumer health rights*

The Consumers' Health Forum of Australia promotes the following set of principles, rights and responsibilities to enhance the health rights of consumers individually and collectively within Australia.

Principles

A. We are entitled to a healthy and safe environment in which to live and work. That is:
    - our basic needs are met;
    - the physical environment enhances our quality of life;
    - we are protected from health hazards.

B. We are entitled to adequate, accurate information and education enabling us to make informed decisions which promote health and prevent ill health and disability.

C. We are entitled to participate in the development, monitoring and implementation of social and economic policies and programs.

D. We are entitled to equal access to health services which:
    - promote health;
    - prevent and alleviate ill health and disability; and
    - provide health care.

E. We are entitled to determine whether or not to seek assistance from health workers.

Rights

The Consumers' Health Forum of Australia supports the rights outlined below for all consumers. These rights are not all currently enforceable by law in Australia. The Forum recognises that, in exceptional circumstances, individuals may be unable to exercise their rights. In some cases a person independent of the caregiver and institution may be required to act on an individual's behalf.

1. I have a right to appropriate, quality health care, when I need it.

2. I have the right to determine what happens to me, including:
    - to choose to leave my condition untreated;
    - to give my explicit consent before any procedure can be carried out;
    - to withdraw my consent to a procedure;
    - to refuse to allow a procedure to be carried out;
    - to refuse health care from a particular health worker (including medical practitioners, allied health professionals and alternative health practitioners);
    - to refuse health care from students;
    - to refuse to participate in research and experiments.

3. I have the right to an adequate explanation, in terms and language I can understand, of:
    - the nature of my ill health and the likelihood of my return to good health;
    - the details of any proposed procedures and therapies (e.g. consultations, tests, examinations, treatment), as well as possible alternatives, including:
      — expected outcome,
      — adverse and after effects,
      — chances of success,

---

* Reprinted by permission of the Consumers' Health Forum of Australia Inc., Curtin, ACT.

- — risks,
- — costs and availability,
- — whether the procedure is experimental or to be used in research;
- • the results of any procedures which have been carried out and the implication of those results;
- • the possible consequences of not taking the advice of the health worker;
- • the name, position, qualifications and experience of health workers who are carrying out the procedures.

4. I have the right to receive health care in privacy and to be treated with respect and dignity.

5. I have the right to decide who will be present when I receive health care.
   - • I can require the presence of other people, including a friend, family member, advocate, interpreter, etc.
   - • I can refuse the presence of:
     - — health workers not directly involved in my care,
     - — students,
     - — researchers, and
     - — others, including family members.

6. I have the right to seek information and advice from other sources.

7. I have the right to seek treatment from other health workers of my choice.

8. I have the right to have all identifying personal information kept confidential. Thus no identifying information about me, my condition or treatment will be made available to anyone else without my consent.

9. I have the right of access, and to seek amendment or additions, to all information relating to my health care and condition, either personally or through another person I nominate.

10. I have the right to comment on, or complain about, my health care.

11. I have the right to receive compensation for injuries or illness caused, or aggravated by, health care or health care advice provided by a health care worker.

12. I have the right to refuse admission to, and to leave, a health care facility, regardless of my physical condition or against medical advice, and regardless of whether I have paid the bill.

Responsibilities

Exercising responsibilities in the health system can be as important as exercising rights.

However, there are many areas of life in which people find it difficult to exert control. In many instances consumers find it difficult to make an informed choice.

Nevertheless, it is in our best interests to assume as much responsibility for our health as possible.

After all, it is *our* health at stake!

In order to promote partnership between the consumer and health workers, the Consumers' Health Forum of Australia recommends that consumers:

- • provide information that enables the health care worker to provide adequate advice and care;
- • actively seek health care information;
- • treat seriously any agreement to action chosen in partnership with a health worker;
- • acknowledge responsibility for the consequences of their decision to accept or reject advice;
- • recognise that choices concerning their lifestyle affect their health;
- • advise the appropriate authority of any complaint they may have concerning their health care so that corrective action can be taken.

Appendix III

ANCI Code of Ethics for Nurses in Australia

Introduction

Nursing practice is undertaken in a variety of settings. Any particular setting will be affected to some degree by factors which are not within a nurse's control or influence. These include resource constraints, institutional policies, management decisions, and the practice of other health care providers. Nurses also recognise the potential for conflict between one person's needs and those of another, or of a group or community. Such factors may affect the degree to which nurses are able to fulfil their moral obligations and/or the number and type of ethical dilemmas they may face.

The Code contains six broad value statements. Nurses may use these statements as a guide in reflecting on the degree to which their practice demonstrates the stated value. As a means of assisting in interpretation of the six expressed values, a number of explanatory statements are provided. These are not intended to cover all the aspects a nurse should consider, but can be used as an aid in further exploration and consideration of ethical concerns in nursing practice.

A Code of Ethics is not intended to provide direction for the resolution of specific ethical dilemmas, nor can this document adequately address the definitions and exploration of terms and concepts which are part of the study of ethics. Nurses are encouraged to undertake discussion and educational opportunities in order to clarify for themselves issues related to the fulfilment of their moral obligations.

Nurses are independent moral agents and sometimes may have a personal moral stance which conflicts with participation in certain procedures. Nurses are morally entitled to refuse to participate in procedures which would violate personal moral beliefs (conscientious objection). However, nurses should not refuse involvement if there is any possibility of danger to the life or welfare of any person. Nurses accepting employment positions where they foresee they may be called on to be involved in situations at variance with their beliefs, have a responsibility to acquaint their employer or prospective employer with this fact. Employers and colleagues have a responsibility to ensure that such nurses are not discriminated against in their workplace.

The Code of Ethics is enhanced by the Code of Professional Conduct. While the Code of Ethics focuses on the morals and ideals of the profession, the Code of Professional Conduct identifies the minimum requirements for practice in the profession and focuses on the clarification of professional misconduct and unprofessional conduct. These two Codes, together with Australian nursing's published practice standards, provide a working framework for nursing practice.

Both the Code of Ethics and the Code of Professional Conduct need to be responsive to the needs and changes within the profession and, in time, these Codes will need to change in relation to changes in nursing and in society. This Code of Ethics will be reviewed within five years, or earlier if necessary.

Preamble

Nurses support and enable individuals, families and groups to maintain, restore or improve their health status, or to be cared for and comforted when deterioration of health has become irreversible. A traditional ideal of nursing is the concern for the care and nurture of human beings regardless of race, religion, status, age, gender, diagnosis or any other ground.

Nursing care is based on the development of a helping relationship and the implementation and evaluation of therapeutic processes. Therapeutic processes include health promotion and education, counselling, nursing interventions and empowerment of individuals, families or groups to exercise maximum choice in relation to their health care.

Nurses provide care and support before and during birth and throughout life, and alleviate pain and suffering during the dying process.

The Code of Ethics has been developed for nursing in the Australian context and is relevant to all nurses working in Australia. The Code of Ethics outlines nursing's intentions in practice and is supported by policies and position statements from organisations representing nurses and nursing. The Code of Ethics is complementary to the International Council of Nurses (ICN) Code for Nurses (1973).

Thus, the purpose of this Code of Ethics is to:

- identify the fundamental moral commitments of the profession;
- provide nurses with a basis for professional and self reflection and a guide to ethical practice; and
- indicate to the community the values which nurses hold.

Code of Ethics

Value statement 1

Nurses respect persons' individual needs, values and culture in the provision of nursing care.

Explanatory statements

1. Nursing care for any individual or group should not be compromised because of ethnicity, gender, spiritual values, disability, age, economic, social or health status, or any other ground.
2. Respect for a person's needs includes recognition of the individual's place in a family and community. Nurses should, therefore, facilitate the participation of significant others in the care of the individual if, and as, the person and the significant others wish.
3. Respect for individual needs, beliefs and values includes culturally sensitive care, and the provision of as much comfort, dignity, privacy and alleviation of pain and anxiety as possible.

Value statement 2

Nurses respect the rights of persons to make informed choices in relation to their care.

Explanatory statements

1. Individuals are entitled to make decisions related to their own welfare, based on accurate information given by health care providers. If persons are not present or able to speak for themselves, nurses have a role in ensuring that someone is present to accurately represent the person's perspective.
2. Nurses have a responsibility to inform people about the nursing care that is available to them, and people have free choice to accept or reject such care. Nurses respect the decisions made by each person.
3. Illness and/or other factors may compromise a person's capacity for self-determination. Where able, nurses need to provide such persons with the opportunities for choice to enable them to maintain some degree of self-direction and self-determination.

Value statement 3

Nurses promote and uphold provision of quality nursing care for all people.

Explanatory statements

1. Quality nursing care includes competent care provided by appropriately qualified individuals.
2. Promotion of quality nursing care includes valuing continuing education as a means of maintaining and increasing knowledge and skills. Continuing education refers to all formal and informal opportunities for education.

3. Standards of care are one measure of quality. Nurses implement procedures to evaluate nursing practice in order to raise standards of care, and to ensure that such standards are ethically defensible.
4. Research is necessary to the development of the profession of nursing. Research should be conducted in a manner that is ethically defensible.

Value statement 4

Nurses hold in confidence any information obtained in a professional capacity, and use professional judgment in sharing such information.

Explanatory statements

1. The nurse respects persons' rights to determine who will be provided with their personal information and in what detail. Exceptions may be necessary in circumstances where the life of the person or of other persons may be placed in danger if information is not disclosed.
2. When personal information is required for teaching, research or quality assurance procedures, care must be taken to protect the person's anonymity and privacy. Consent must always be obtained.
3. Nurses protect persons in their care against inadvertent breaches of privacy by confining their verbal communications to appropriate personnel and settings, and to professional purposes.
4. Nurses have a moral obligation to adhere to practices which limit access to personal records (whether written or computerised) to appropriate personnel.

Value statement 5

Nurses respect the accountability and responsibility inherent in their roles.

Explanatory statements

1. As morally independent agents, nurses have moral obligations in the provision of nursing care.
2. Nurses participate with other health care providers in the provision of comprehensive health care, recognising the perspective and expertise of each team member.
3. Nurses may have personal values which may cause them to experience moral distress in relation to participating in certain procedures. Nurses have a moral right to refuse to participate in procedures which would violate their reasoned moral conscience (that is, they are entitled to conscientious objection).

Value statement 6

Nurses value the promotion of an ecological, social and economic environment which supports and sustains health and wellbeing.

Explanatory statements

1. Nursing includes involvement in the detection of ill effects of the environment on the health of persons, the ill effects of human activities on the natural environment, and assisting communities in their actions on environmental health problems aimed at minimising these effects.
2. Nurses value participation in the development, implementation and monitoring of policies and procedures which promote safe and efficient use of resources.
3. Nurses acknowledge that the social environment in which persons reside has an impact on their health, and in collaboration with other health professionals and consumers, initiate and support action to meet the health and social needs of the public.

Bibliography

American Nurses' Association. 1985. *Code for Nurses*. American Nurses' Association, Kansas City.

Australian Nursing Federation. 1992. *Draft policy on conscientious objection*. Australian Nursing Federation, Melbourne.

Bandman, E. & Bandman, B. 1985. *Nursing Ethics Through the Life Span*. Prentice Hall, New York.

Beauchamp, T. & Childress, J. (1989). *Principles of Biomedical Ethics*. Oxford University Press, New York.

Canadian Nurses' Association. 1989. *Code of Ethics for Nursing*. Canadian Nurses' Association, Ottawa.

Consumers' Health Forum of Australia. 1989. *Consumer Health Rights*. Consumers' Health Forum of Australia, Canberra.

Husted, G. & Husted, J. 1981. *Ethical Decision Making in Nursing*. Mosby, St. Louis.

International Council of Nurses. 1973. *Code for Nurses: Ethical Concepts Applied to Nursing*. ICN, Geneva.

Johnstone, M-J. 1989. *Bioethics: A Nursing Perspective*. W.B. Saunders, Sydney.

The New Zealand Nurses' Association. 1988. *Code of Ethics*. The New Zealand Nurses' Association, Wellington.

Woodruff, A. 1991. Discussion paper: Code of Ethics and Code of Conduct. ANRAC Competencies Steering Committee, Adelaide.

Feedback from the Code of Ethics Think Tank. 1992.

July 1993
Reprinted October 1997

Appendix IV

Patients' Bill of Rights*
Australian Nursing Federation
(Western Australian Branch)
Position Paper

The ANF (WA Branch) believes that patients/clients, as the consumers of health care, are responsible for making decisions about their own health care.

This Patients' Bill of Rights is presented as a guide for nurses to enable them to assist patients/clients whether in the hospital or community setting, to be aware of their rights and responsibilities.

1. The legal rights of patients/clients in any health care setting are:

1.1 Right to a clear, understandable explanation in lay persons' terms of their condition, problems or disease.

1.2 Right to a clear, understandable explanation of all proposed procedures and possible alternatives. The explanation should include the nature of the condition; the proposed treatment; other alternative forms of treatment; the nature of the risks involved in the different types of treatment; and the chances of success or failure of the different types of treatment.

1.3 Right to seek 'alternative health care' and to receive such care from any person competent to provide it. 'Alternative health care' includes acupuncture, chiropractice, herbalism, homeopathy, hypnotherapy, naturopathy, osteopathy and the like.

1.4 Right to obtain a professional opinion of anyone of their choice at any stage of the health care programme. (Subject to the patients/clients or insurer paying for same.) Patients/clients also have the right to know the identity, professional status and qualifications of those providing health services.

1.5 Right to refuse any specific treatment, drug, examination or other health care procedure.

1.6 Right to change their mind and refuse treatment to which they have previously agreed.

1.7 Right to decline admission to hospital or any other health care facility.

1.8 Right to leave the health care facility regardless of their physical condition or financial status (exceptions to the right to discharge may occur if an infectious disease has been diagnosed or if the patient has been certified as mentally ill).

1.9 Right to be informed of any research and/or experimental procedures which may involve them and be given the option to agree or refuse to participate.

1.10 Right to have their case history kept confidential, except when they consent to have such information divulged or where it is required by law to be divulged.

1.11 Right to seek compensation for injuries or illness resulting from health care.

1.12 Right to refuse examination, treatment or observation by, or in the presence of, students.

1.13 Right to specify in writing any treatments that they would not wish to have carried out should they lose consciousness or the ability to communicate.

1.14 Right to be consulted before decisions are made to transfer them to any other health facility.

---

* Reprinted by permission of the Australian Nursing Federation (WA), formerly the Royal Australian Nursing Federation (WA).

The above rights are entitlements of all legally competent health care consumers (that is, sane persons over the age of eighteen). In the case of children or wards of the State, parents or guardians may exercise any of the above rights on behalf of their children or wards, provided that in exercising these rights the best interests of the patients are paramount.

2. The ANF (WA Branch) also believes that patients/clients should be entitled to:

2.1   A high standard of health care, regardless of social status, age, sex, race, religion, political beliefs or source of payments.

2.2   Prompt and appropriate treatment, according to health needs, provided in a humane manner with considerate and respectful care.

2.3   Receive information on the contents of their health record. (Legally patients/clients can appoint an agent, such as a solicitor, to obtain this information should such an action be required.)

2.4   Right of access to people outside the health care facility (parents should be able to stay with their children and nominated support persons should be able to stay with terminally ill patients twenty-four hours a day. In the case of midwifery patients, they should be able to have their partner or nominated support person with them throughout labour, delivery and the immediate post-partum period).

2.5   Be informed, by means of an information booklet or other method, of the layout of the facilities available in the health care agency.

2.6   The services of a qualified interpreter should they be required.

2.7   Nominate an advocate or representative to join the patient/client and their health therapist in making decisions.

2.8   Expect adequate instruction in self-care and for an appropriate lifestyle before being discharged from hospital; and that relatives or friends who will be caring for them receive such instruction and that arrangements be made for necessary support services.

3. The ANF (WA Branch) also believes that patients/clients have certain responsibilities. If a person is in need of health care they should, in their own interests:

3.1   Seek information as to their rights and see that their rights are satisfactorily applied.

3.2   Ensure that they have understood the purpose of all tests, treatments or other procedures, the reason for them and possible alternatives before agreeing to them.

3.3   Take responsibility for postponing, terminating or continuing part or all of the proposed health care programme, including operations. They should insist upon explanations until they feel suitably informed and should consult with all relevant persons before reaching a decision.

3.4   Know their own and their family's health history.

3.5   Keep appointments or inform those concerned of their intention not to do so.

3.6   Comply with treatment or inform the therapist of their intention not to do so.

3.7   Accept the consequences of their own informed decision.

3.8   Inform their health practitioner if they are currently in consultation with or under treatment from another practitioner in connection with the same complaint.

Acknowledgments

Medical Consumer Association of NSW: *Patients' rights*
American Hospitals Association: *A Patient's Bill of Rights*
Health Care Consumers Association of the ACT: *Patients' Bill of Rights and Responsibilities*
Health Care Consumers Association of WA: *Patients' Rights and Responsibilities*
ANF (Vic Branch): *Patients' Bill of Rights*

The ANF (WA Branch) advises that the legal rights as set out in Section 1 may vary according to the particular circumstances that the patient or health professional find themselves in.

February 1984

Appendix V*

Patients' Bill of Rights
Australian Nursing Federation (Victorian Branch)
Position Paper

Australian Nursing Federation (Victorian Branch) believes that nurses must have a clear understanding of the entitlement of all patients to certain 'rights' concerning the delivery of health care, both in the hospital setting and in the community. The following statement has been formulated as a guide to nurses.

Statement

Consumers of health care are becoming increasingly aware that they have a right and responsibility to take an active part in decision making regarding a healthy lifestyle, and when necessary to enlist the intervention of health professionals to make an informed choice regarding the nature of treatment and care.

Australian Nursing Federation (Victorian Branch) believes all nurses should respect the following 'rights' of patients no matter what the personal beliefs of the nurse may be.

1. **The right to health care**
   - right to the highest standards of health care, regardless of social status, age, sex, race, religion or political belief; this care to be prompt and appropriate;
   - right to nominate a medical practitioner of their own choice.

2. **The right to be informed**
   - right to be informed about the health care system and facilities available for their specific requirements;
   - right to know the identity and professional status and qualifications of those providing health services;
   - right to be able to request that their medical practitioner obtain a report regarding their care in any health agency and to ensure that they have access to this information;
   - right to obtain a second opinion from professional persons of their choice at any stage of the health care programme;
   - right to be acquainted, whether by means of an 'information booklet' or other method, with the layout of the facilities available in the hospital or health care agency for their personal assistance, safety and comfort;
   - right to be informed that students are present in any group wishing to interview or examine the patient;
   - right to ask for assistance from appropriate personnel if not satisfied with care and to make any suggestions which it is felt may improve this care;
   - right to expect adequate instructions in self-care and for an appropriate lifestyle before being discharged from hospital; that relatives and friends who will be caring for them receive such instructions and that arrangements are made for necessary support services;
   - right to receive itemised details of the total, final account for services rendered.

* Reprinted by permission of the Australian Nursing Federation (Vic), formerly the Royal Australian Nursing Federation (Vic).

3. **The right to consent to treatment**
   - right to participate in the decision regarding any treatment programme after:
     a. a clear, concise explanation in understandable terms, with the use of a qualified interpreter if necessary, of all proposed procedures, health problems, disease processes, diagnostic tests and prognosis;
     b. being informed of anything that is of an experimental nature, or for the purposes of research, in the proposed treatment;
     c. being informed of any known risks and of any possible alternative avenues of treatment;
     d. knowing who will be concerned in their treatment;
     e. being informed of any financial costs.

4. **The right to refuse treatment**
   - right to refuse any specific treatment, drug, examination or health procedure;
   - right to refuse to participate in any research and/or experimental procedures;
   - right to refuse to be attended by a particular member of the health team;
   - right to refuse to be interviewed or examined by medical or para-medical students;
   - right to reverse permission previously given regarding any treatments, to be informed of the likely consequences of such a refusal and to accept the responsibility for this action;
   - right to seek alternative health care, but to have the possible risks of such a decision clearly explained in a factual, non-judgmental manner;
   - right to leave the health care facility regardless of their physical condition or financial status, accepting that they can be requested to sign a release stating that they are leaving against the medical judgment of the doctor or hospital. Persons under compulsory treatment do not have the right to leave the health agency. This includes:
     — serving prisoners of the state;
     — the criminally insane;
     — those in quarantine;
     — those with certain specific infectious diseases.

5. **The right to confidentiality**
   - right to have their medical history kept confidential, except where the individual consents to have any information divulged or where it is required to be divulged by law.

6. **The right to access of persons of their own choice**
   - right to access of people outside the health care facility; to assistance in seeing a minister of religion, counsellor or solicitor; also to request that specified persons not be permitted to visit;
   - right of patients, e.g., children, terminally ill, to have a relative or close friend to remain with them during hospitalisation and take part in their care when appropriate;
   - right of midwifery patients to have their partner or nominated support person with them throughout labour, delivery and the immediate post-partum period, subject to certain medical restrictions and dependent on facilities available and the rights of other patients;
   - right to nominate a friend, advocate or representative to join with the patient and health professional in making decisions and to determine who should be informed of their condition.

7. **The right to compensation**
   - right to compensation for injuries or illness incurred in hospital care facilities or aggravated by the health professional.

8. **The right to maintenance of dignity**
   - right to be treated in a humane manner, with considerate and respectful care in an atmosphere of privacy;
   - right not to be subjected to any procedure or treatment without an adequate explanation of what is involved;
   - right to die with dignity.

The recognition of patients' rights implies the acceptance of responsibility on the part of the health care consumer for:
- following a lifestyle appropriate to the maintenance of health and carrying out self-help programmes which demonstrate assumption of their accountability for their own health status;
- seeking information about their rights;
- divulging any information known to them about their own or their family's medical history, which may have relevance to their own health care;
- keeping appointments and complying with treatment, or alternatively informing the health professional of their intention not to do so;
- accepting the consequences of their own informed decision;
- ensuring that they and their visitors at all times act in such a manner that others are not disturbed or inconvenienced;
- respecting the privacy of others and keeping in confidence any information they gain about them;
- notifying the appropriate authority of any complaints so that any necessary corrective action may be taken.

October 1984

Appendix VI

Nursing care of the person who is dying*

1. The Australian Nursing Federation recognises that:

   1.1 The role of the nurse within the context of this policy must remain within the boundaries of accepted nursing practice, which includes the professions' code of ethics and code of professional conduct, and guidelines and existing legislative framework.

   1.2 Nurses should have an understanding of their ethical and legal responsibilities in regard to providing care for the person who is dying.

   1.3 People have a right to know if they have a condition for which death is the expected outcome.

   1.4 People have a right to a choice, both in the care and treatment which is provided to them and in the way in which that care and treatment is provided.

   1.5 It is the right of the person who is dying to make choices about their care and treatment based on an adequate explanation.

   1.6 The person who is dying has the right to a death which is as dignified as possible, as the person themselves would define dignity.

   1.7 The person who is dying has the right to refuse treatment.

   1.8 The nursing role includes being an advocate for the person who is dying, and for their significant others.

2. It is the policy of the Australian Nursing Federation that:

   2.1 The nurses' professional role is to provide care and treatment, so that the person who is dying has maximal control over their care and treatment.

   2.2 The care and treatment of the person who is dying must be consistent with their beliefs and cultural expectations.

   2.3 The nurse has a responsibility to be aware of other conditions which may affect decision making in a person who is dying, such as depression, other mental illness, dementia, or the effects of mood altering drugs.

   2.4 Children and adolescents who are dying should be informed and consulted and their wishes considered in any decisions made regarding their care and treatment.

   2.5 The registered nurse responsible for the care of the person who is dying must be informed about the person's wishes and expectations in relation to their care and treatment.

   2.6 The registered nurse responsible for the care of the person who is dying has a right to know the outcome of discussions regarding care and treatment, between the person and their treating medical practitioner which are specific to their care and treatment. The outcome of these discussions should be appropriately documented and updated at regular intervals, and be available to other health professionals involved in the person's care.

   2.7 Discussions with the person who is dying and their family and significant others in relation to the initiation of cardio-pulmonary resuscitation should be part of the management plan and the outcome of those discussions clearly documented.

---

* Australian Nursing Federation Policy Statement. Nursing Care of the Person Who is Dying. Reviewed February 1998.
Reprinted with permission of the Australian Nursing Federation.

2.8   The provision of palliative care for any person who is dying is essential. This includes controlling pain, relieving other symptoms of disease and providing emotional and psychosocial support in preparation for death.

2.9   Early referral to palliative care services should be available to all persons who are dying.

2.10   Employers should provide the necessary resources to support nurses in dealing with the professional and emotional issues rising from caring for the person who is dying.

Appendix VII*

New Zealand Nurses Organisation
Code of Ethics

Foreword

by NZNO President, Nigel Kee

This Code of Ethics has been written for those who practice nursing in a country in which society is continually changing. It is linked with other NZNO policies and position papers such as the Social Policy which, of course, outlines the profession's contract with New Zealand society. The heart of the Code has remained constant: caring and partnership continue to be central concepts to the practice of nursing in Aotearoa-New Zealand.

The development of this edition of the Code has been a useful and constructive process with input, ideas, and comments from different ethnic, cultural, employment, and practice backgrounds. Some one hundred nurses attended forums and meetings in Auckland, Wellington, and Palmerston North and included nurses who came from many cultural backgrounds including Maori, Paheka, Samoan, Tongan, Niuean, Chinese, Korean, Philippino, and European. In addition, written submissions from groups of nurses and individuals were warmly received. The result has been to create a Code of Ethics unique to New Zealand which has been developed by New Zealand nurses, for New Zealand nurses; taking cognisance of the New Zealand context.

With the many challenges facing nurses, it is acknowledged that the Code of Ethics is not static and has implications for practice in the 21st Century.

Cultural Safety is integral to practice and is reflected in the Code. The nursing profession continues to lead other health professions in this important aspect of partnership.

Professional nursing practice is ethical in nature. I hope that this Code of Ethics will strengthen nurses' practice.

Acknowledgments

NZNO acknowledges the major contributions of the following individuals and working groups:

Professor Nan Kinross, Martin Woods, Irahapeti Ramsden, Chris Hopkins, Natalie Hope, Lyn Olsthoorn, Jan Rodgers, Bibby Plummer, Regina Peretini, Aileen Lawther, Elizabeth Niven, Catherine Logan, Jane Henwood, Marion Jones, Di Pennell, Carrol Mitchell and Diane Nicholson.

All the nurses who participated in the Working Groups at Auckland, Wellington and Palmerston North, and those who sent submissions.

Preamble

This Code of Ethics is a substantial revision of the 1988 version. It has been formulated by working parties of NZNO in response to the need for a code which closely reflects the current context of nursing practice. It has been developed with the specific purpose of guiding nurses' practice and communicating to society at large the ethical values of the nursing profession of Aotearoa-New Zealand.

The Code is congruent with the Social Policy Statement, of the New Zealand Nurses Organisation (1993). The Treaty of Waitangi is seen as the founding document of New Zealand society and underpins its economic and social development. In this policy statement the Treaty of Waitangi has been acknowledged as requiring protection and participation between nursing and the indigenous people, Maori. Ongoing development of this relationship is essential in arriving at a negotiated agreement which nursing and Maori could call partnership.

Since the European colonists arrived, people from many countries in Europe, Asia, Africa and the Pacific have also settled this island nation. Nurses in Aotearoa-New Zealand therefore, work with, support and care for people from a variety of cultural backgrounds, while acknowledging the unique relationship between Maori and Crown.

There has been input into this Code by people from a range of cultures who are concerned about expressions of cultural difference and culturally safe practice. Culture is not only seen as ethno specific, but includes the cultures of class, of rich, poor, sexual orientation, age and gender. Gender values characteristic of ethical systems derived from the European tradition have been used to develop value statements to guide practice. In addition, specific values have been identified which are important in the context of ethics and nursing practice.

At this time of change, challenge and uncertainty in the health service, it is important that all nurses in Aotearoa-New Zealand share, and are guided by an ethical code of practice. Not only will this be a support to individual nurses faced with an ethical dilemma, but the universal use of this Code will signal to other health professionals, managers and to the public that nurses are clear about their moral responsibilities.

Use of Code of Ethics

This code has been written for nurses to use both as a basis to further explore the ethical beliefs of Aotearoa-New Zealand nurses and as a guide to explore the detail of each situation, using the descriptions of each value as an indicator of its influence.

Each situation is unique and exists in its own context. The most important values will be specific to the particular situation. Any one value is not always an over-riding value; the balance of values and their inter-relationships may change not only with each situation but also within each situation.

This Code of Ethics does not seek to provide answers to situations encountered in practice. Ethical concerns and situations are resolved using an approach which incorporates exploring values applicable to the context and a logical process of thinking and action such as the flow chart contained in Appendix 1.

Glossary of terms

Cultural Safety in nursing   The effective nursing of a people from another culture by a nurse who has undertaken a process of reflection and rigorous examination of their own cultural identity. Cultural Safety in nursing happens when people feel fully able to use a service provided by people from another culture, without risk to their own.

Cultural Values   Morals, beliefs, attitudes, and standards that derive from a particular cultural group. Culture is not only seen as ethno specific, but must include groups from within cultures e.g. cultures of class, socialisation, sexual orientation, age etc.

Ethical Practice   The domain of nurses' moral behaviour, actions, decisions, and ethical decision making in response to conflicts of moral value.

Nurse   A nurse is a health professional who is either registered or enrolled by the Nursing Council under the Nurses Act 1977. The provision of a current practising certificate from the Nursing Council is considered to be recognition of the nurse's ability to work under the title of "nurse".

However, there are registered or enrolled nurses who, for various reasons, do not hold a practising certificate for employment. Nursing students, nurses in management, education or any other field are still representatives of the profession. This Code is just as relevant to these groups of nurses.

Nursing Practice   "Nursing practice consists of actions directed towards assisting an individual or groups of individuals to progress towards mutually acceptable health goals. It is a process of human interactioin." (NZNO 1993) Nurses practice in a variety of settings and modes — in clinical, community, educational, administrative, and research areas. Wherever nurses practice the requirement placed upon them to act ethically is paramount.

Client   In this document the term client is used to describe the individual person and/or their family/whanau/group/agent who is/are recipients of nurse(s)' practice. It encompasses the terms patient, customer, consumer, and resident or any other term appropriate to the recipient of the care. This may include the recipient's agent.

Underlying philosophy

Caring is the moral foundation of nursing. Caring is a moral value which goes beyond the mechanistic performance of duty. It is a professional and a society expectation that nurses' work requires caring, an involvement of self in a real concern for the wellbeing of another. Caring is experienced rather than measured; its complexity defies a neat definition. Caring as a philosophical base for practice is being developed and our understanding is growing. It encompasses the concepts of compassion, commitment, competence, congruence, confidence, conscience, culture, collaboration, communication, and consultation amongst others.

Assumptions

The exploration of ethical issues takes place in the unique context of the specific reality of each issue with the values of the context and participants determining the outcome. Contextual determinants include cultural, family, professional, religious and personal values.

This code is based on several assumptions that permeate nursing.

i) That relationships and interactions take place in a climate of respect for the other. This encompasses a respect for culture, religion, life choices, sexual orientation, ethnicity and other life-directing values held by individuals and groups. An example of enacting this value is shown in providing and working within the concept of cultural safety.

ii) That respect for the individual/group/community encompasses the notion of partnership/collaboration, where the client/group/community participates actively in the process of nursing. This stand acknowledges the contribution of client effort, knowledge and expertise to the partnership.

iii) That relationships and interactions seek to achieve a positive outcome for the client/ groups/community. The purpose of nursing is to affect positively the influence of a health/illness related event on the life of the individual/group/community.

Nursing takes place in a series of unique relationships with others: client, colleague, society and organisations.

This code describes New Zealand nurses' perceptions of the values underlying their practice. While not exhaustive it describes some examples of the implementation of the values in the context of the nursing relationship mentioned above. The framework of the code is summarised in the table below.

Framework of the Code[1]

Underlying Values \ Relationships	Nurse– Client Relationship	Nurse– Colleague Relationship	Nurse– Organisation Relationship	Nurse– Societal Relationship
Autonomy (outlined on page 12)	Described on Page 14	Described on Page 16	Described on Page 18	Described on Page 20
Beneficence (outlined on page 12)	Described on Page 14	Described on Page 16	Described on Page 18	Described on Page 20
Non Maleficence (outlined on page 12)	Described on Page 14	Described on Page 16	Described on Page 18	Described on Page 20
Justice (outlined on page 12)	Described on Page 14	Described on Page 16	Described on Page 18	Described on Page 20
Confidentiality (outlined on page 12)	Described on Page 15	Described on Page 16	Described on Page 18	Described on Page 20
Veracity (outlined on page 12)	Described on Page 15	Described on Page 16	Described on Page 18	Described on Page 20
Fidelity (outlined on page 13)	Described on Page 15	Described on Page 16	Described on Page 18	Described on Page 20
Guardianship of the Enviornment and its Resources (outlined on page 13)	Described on Page 15	Described on Page 16	Described on Page 18	Described on Page 21
Being Professional (outlined on page 13)	Described on Page 15	Described on Page 17	Described on Page 19	Described on Page 21

1. The page numbers in this table refer to the originals in the code booklet, however, the 'Relationships' and 'Underlying values' are covered in the tables that follow (pp. 462–7).

UNDERLYING VALUES	
In the ethics of New Zealand nurses' practice, the following values are fundamental:	
Autonomy (self determination)	• The right of individuals to self determination which encompasses an assumption that the individual/group/client/agent of the person has the wisdom to make the best choice for that person. • Particular attention should be paid to awareness and acceptance of cultural differences in the provision of health care to ensure cultural safety of clients and nurses (a situation is culturally safe when a client feels their cultural or spiritual needs are included in care or that they can ask and have those needs met without prejudice). • Many socio-cultural groups in this country place the importance of the collective on a par with the needs of and rights of the individual. The right of both the individual and the collective (whanau, hapu, iwi) must be respected.
Beneficence (doing good)	• Performing the action or actions leading to an outcome that now or in the future would be regarded as worthwhile; the concept of doing good. • Contextual variations on the meaning and value of good will influence exploration and outcome in the consideration of beneficence.
Non Maleficence (doing no harm)	• Avoidance of harm and the prevention of future harm. In a situation where harm is unavoidable, the harm is minimised. • Contextual variations on the meaning and value of harm will influence exploration and outcome in the consideration of maleficence.
Justice (fairness)	• The assumption that society has a responsibility to treat people fairly. Society confirms concepts of justice in its legal frameworks. There is an inter-relationship between law and justice which means that one does not automatically override the other. Laws are modified through practice and challenge to increase justice for society. Different health circumstances may require different resource allocation or entitlement to achieve equity.
Confidentiality (privacy)	• The privacy of written or spoken information acquired through privileged access. • The concept of privacy in each situation is modified by legal and contextual realities.
Veracity (truthfulness)	• Actions, speech and behaviour that ensure communications between individuals and/or groups are honest and truthful.
Fidelity (faithfulness)	• The obligation to remain faithful to ones commitments. • Clients have many commitments and the tension between competing commitments may require acknowledgment and compassionate understanding.
Guardianship of the Environment and its Resources	• The obligation to remain faithful to ones commitments. The assumption that Society has a responsibility to respect the environment and its resources. • Cultural/contextual variation in the relationship between person and environment will influence the value of guardianship.

Being Professional	• The belief that nursing is a profession with a defined purpose. It has a special relationship with society having been established by society to provide health related care for those of its members in need. • Nursing possesses a distinct body of knowledge, its own area of independent practice and is guided by the specific set of values, identified here.

NURSE–CLIENT RELATIONSHIP	
Underlying Values	In the context of the Nurse–Client relationship the underlying values are demonstrated by the nurse:
Autonomy (self determination)	• Creating a partnership within the nurse–client relationship, the outcome of which the client views as beneficial. • Supporting clients to enable freedom of choice and informed consent. Informed consent requires that enough relevant information is provided to enable a reasoned decision to be made, and that the information is understood. Cultural perception is an important component. Without understanding, no one can make a reasoned decision. Nurses should support clients in making informed decisions by giving information and assistance, thereby ensuring that they become active participants in their own health care. • Ensuring the health service responds to cultural diversity and that the nurse recognises cultural norms. • Being aware that people may act as individuals or as part of a collective social system.
Beneficence (doing good)	• Creating a partnership the outcome of which the client views as beneficial. • Respecting the right of clients to define safety factors related to the beneficence of nursing through their own subjective experience.
Non Maleficence (doing no harm)	• Promoting the safety of clients by means of competent and safe nursing practice. • Protecting and advocating for the rights of clients in order to minimise or prevent harm. Nurses should assist vulnerable persons who need help in the expression of personal needs and values. • Recognising cultural norms, e.g. especially when collecting and storing health information, body tissue or genetic material. • Ensuring cultural safety when nursing of people from another culture by undertaking a process of vigorous examination of their own cultural identity.
Justice (fairness)	• Accepting a client's perception of fairness and perception of what would be an appropriate outcome for them. • Respecting the rights of individual people, their dignity, needs and values. Nurses should be sensitive to such factors as the person's race, age, health status, religion, culture, sexual orientation and gender.
Confidentiality (privacy)	• Being mindful of the privileged nature of client information they gain. • Safeguarding the physical, emotional and social rights of clients from unwarranted intrusion.

Veracity (truthfulness)	• Communicating with the client in an open, honest and truthful manner.
Fidelity (faithfulness)	• Being faithful in all commitments to clients so promoting trust as an integral component of the nurse–client relationship. The withdrawal of services for whatever reason, creates a particular dilemma for nurses in relation to fidelity which needs careful consideration.
Guardianship of the Environment and its Resources	• Practising and teaching health practices which actively support the conservation of the environment and resources.
Being Professional	• Providing sound judgment and practising within this code. • Providing nursing practice which meets standards developed by the profession. • Advocating for appropriate health services for clients.

NURSE–COLLEAGUE RELATIONSHIP	
Underlying Values	In the context of the Nurse–Colleague relationship the underlying values are demonstrated by the nurse:
Autonomy (self determination)	• Being self aware to understand reasons for her/his own actions and those of others. If the nurse values her/his own abilities and performance, then s/he is better able to appreciate the contributions of others to the health of people.
Beneficence (doing good)	• Contributing knowledge and skill to create positive relationships with colleages. • Sharing knowledge and skills to contribute to effective care.
Non Maleficence (doing no harm)	• Participating in mutual/peer monitoring programmes to enhance the quality of care provided and prevent/minimise harm. • Providing support and guidance for peers to ensure they and clients are protected from any harm.
Justice (fairness)	• Being self aware in order to safeguard one's personal rights, moral values and beliefs and to acknowledge/accept those of colleagues. Nurses have a right to choose to live by their own values as long as those values do not compromise the care of their clients.
Confidentiality (privacy)	• Safeguarding the physical, emotional and social rights of colleagues from unwarranted intrusion. • Maintaining confidentiality of personal information.
Veracity (truthfulness)	• Relating to colleagues openly, honestly and truthfully in order to engender trustful and supportive relationships.
Fidelity (faithfulness)	• Being loyal to one's self, to the therapeutic team and to the professional group. Conflicting demands may require the nurse to balance client needs with specific loyalties.
Guardianship of the Environment and its Resources	• Developing and utilising processes in personal and collective professional practice which conserve the environment and resources.

Being Professional	• Working with colleagues; to keep informed of new trends, to have an up-to-date knowledge of legal issues and to be able to apply the results of relevant research in order to promote change and innovation in practice. • Being ready to accept a review of practice by peers and to intervene in instances of poor practice. Such intervention (whistle blowing) may be direct but informal in the workplace; or may require formal referral to an organisational or professional authority. • Respecting the rights and practice of professional colleagues is an integral part of nursing practice. It is inevitable that the nurse will encounter conflicting professional opinions which will require resolution by discussion. Collegial relationships are free of discrimination or harassment.

NURSE–ORGANISATION RELATIONSHIP	
Underlying Values	**In the context of practice within an organisation the underlying values are demonstrated by the nurse:**
Autonomy (self determination)	• Being aware that people may act as individuals or as part of a collective social system and that nurses themselves may be members of many different social groupings.
Beneficence (doing good)	• Working with others having regard for their individual rights. • Participating in and contributing to the establishment and review of systems and structures for care provision. • Protecting the rights of clients. • Designing and monitoring services provided. • Advocating to ensure that they meet the requirements of clients and are perceived as appropriate by those clients.
Non Maleficence (doing no harm)	• Participating in organisational activities which ensure that the organisational environment is physically, socially, spiritually, emotionally and culturally safe for clients and colleagues.
Justice (fairness)	• Supporting equality and equity by establishing systems, monitoring services and supporting resource allocation to ensure client and colleague needs are met.
Confidentiality (privacy)	• Ensuring organisational systems established to pass information from one person to another and/or to pass large volumes of personal information are not at risk of confidentiality being breached.
Veracity (truthfulness)	• Promoting open, honest and truthful communication amongst colleagues and with employers to foster a supportive trustful environment. Organisational culture may influence the nurse's ability to achieve veracity.
Fidelity (faithfulness)	• Being loyal and honouring the commitment to practice completely and perform the role which the nurse has agreed to perform.

Guardianship of the Environment and its Resources	• Informing and participating with management to ensure effective nursing practice through the efficient use of human, technical, financial and natural resources. • Matching resources to client need, monitoring and advocating for change in the allocation of resources when necessary to ensure the conservation of the environment and resources, whilst minimising risk to clients.
Being Professional	• Utilising standards for practice as an essential part of quality nursing systems together with regular review of competencies. Maintenance of standards requires the nurse to be accurate and efficient in the recording of events and to undertake regular reviews of present practice in order to develop new and better strategies. • Actively promoting within practice, co-operation between the various groups of health care professionals and colleagues.

NURSE–SOCIETAL RELATIONSHIP	
Underlying Values	In the context of the Nurse–Societal relationship the underlying values are demonstrated by the nurse:
Autonomy (self determination)	• Adapting practice to a variety of interpretations of the concept of autonomy.
Beneficence (doing good)	• Participating in research, education and innovation to ensure professional practice develops and moves forward to best meet the needs of society. • Ensuring standards for cultural safety, ethical practice and health information are established in collaboration/consultation with the community and maintained.
Non Maleficence (doing no harm)	• Monitoring services and practice in relation to the requirements of society, particularly in relation to cultural safety and the protection of vulnerable members.
Justice (fairness)	• Ensuring that services are relevant to client groups and that vulnerable clients are treated regardless of their ability to pay. • Ensuring all client groups, irrespective of age, ethnic background, sexual orientation, gender, location or health status, should have access to competent nursing services. (Accessibility issues often come to the attention of nurses who should be willing to advocate for appropriate and affordable health care for the communities within which they practice.)
Confidentiality (privacy)	• Being aware that protecting clients personal information may conflict with society's need knowledge in order to protect itself from harm. • Being prepared to analyse the contextual variations of each situation.
Veracity (truthfulness)	• Practising from the perspective that public accountability, transparency and openness are essential elements of a democratic society to promote the wellbeing of the community.

Fidelity (faithfulness)	• Being true to the commitment made to society when receiving the right to practice, that the nurse will fulfil society's expectations of a nurse.
Guardianship of the Environment and its Resources	• Practising and teaching health practices in a way which: — conserves the environment and resources — actively seeks to enhance society's relationship with the natural environment — reduces the use of substances harmful to people and the environment.
Being Professional	• Participating in continual negotiation between society and the profession to ensure the needs of society are met and that: — society is kept informed of progress — a therapeutic relationship is maintained — society is assisted to develop healthy beliefs, attitudes and lifestyles. • Supporting the concept that qualified nurses should be prepared in an approved nursing programme and should undertake regular continuing education during their working life.

Bibliography

Australian Nursing Council (1993). *Code of Ethics for Nurses in Australia.* Canberra: Australian Nursing Council and Associates.

Brien, A. (1993). *Implementing a Code of Ethics.* Unpublished paper. Palmerston North: Massey University.

Burgess, M. (1993). *A Guide to the Law for Nurses and Midwives.* Auckland: Longman Paul.

Canadian Nurses' Association (1991). *Code of Ethics for Nursing.* Ottawa: Canadian Nurses Association.

Christiansen, J. (1990). *Nursing Partnership: A Model for Nursing Practice.* Daphne Brasell Associates Press.

Cooper, M.C. Principle Orientated Ethics and The Ethic of Care: A creative tension. *Advanced Nursing Science 1991.* 14(2): 22–31.

Danish Nurses' Organisation (1992). *Ethical Guidelines for Nursing.*

Fry, S.T. (1994). *Ethics in Nursing Practice — a guide to Ethical Decision Making.* Geneva: ICN.

Johnstone, M. (1989). *Bioethics: A nursing perspective.* Sydney: Harcourt Brace Jovanovich.

New Zealand Nurses Organisation (1993). *Standards for Nursing Practice.* Wellington: NZNO.

Noddings, N. (1984). *Caring: a feminine approach to ethics and moral education.* Berkley: University of California Press.

Nursing Council of New Zealand (1995). *Code of Conduct for Nurses and Midwives.* Wellington: Nursing Council.

Oddie, G. and Perrett, R.W. (1992). *Justice, Ethics and New Zealand Society.* Auckland: Oxford University Press.

Ramsden, I. (1990). *Kawa whakarurubau — Cultural safety in nursing education in Aotearoa.* Wellington.

Thompson, I., Melia, K. and Boyd, K. (1994). *Nursing Ethics.* Edinburgh: Churchill Livingstone.

Treaty of Waitangi (1840).

Sawyer, L.M. (1989). Nursing Code of Ethics. *An International Comparison. International Nursing Review.* 36: 5: 145–148.

References

New Zealand Nurses Association (1988). *Code of Ethics*. Wellington: NZNA.
New Zealand Nurses Organisation (1993). *Social Policy Statement*. Wellington: NZNO.
Ramsden, I. (1993). *Cultural Safety in Nursing Education in Aotearoa (New Zealand)*. Wellington.

Appendix

Flowchart from How to Resolve difficult professional/ethical issues — compiled by the Professional Advisory Group of the NZNO.

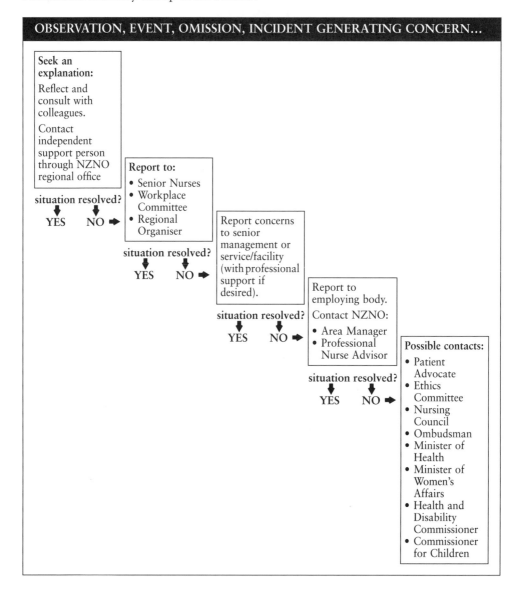

Appendix VIII

Code of Professional Conduct
United Kingdom Central Council for Nursing,
Midwifery and Health Visiting*
(June 1992)

Each registered nurse, midwife and health visitor shall act, at all times, in such a manner as to:
- safeguard and promote the interests of individual patients and clients;
- serve the interests of society;
- justify public trust and confidence; and
- uphold and enhance the good standing and reputation of the professions.

As a registered nurse, midwife or health visitor, you are personally accountable for your practice and, in the exercise of your professional accountability, must:

1. act always in such a manner as to promote and safeguard the interests and wellbeing of patients and clients;

2. ensure that no action or omission on your part, or within your sphere of responsibility, is detrimental to the interests, condition or safety of patients and clients;

3. maintain and improve your professional knowledge and competence;

4. acknowledge any limitations in your knowledge and competence and decline any duties or responsibilities unless able to perform them in a safe and skilled manner;

5. work in an open and co-operative manner with patients, clients and their families, foster their independence and recognise and respect their involvement in the planning and delivery of care;

6. work in a collaborative and co-operative manner with health care professionals and others involved in providing care, and recognise and respect their particular contributions within the care team;

7. recognise and respect the uniqueness and dignity of each patient and client, and respond to their need for care, irrespective of their ethnic origin, religious beliefs, personal attributes, the nature of their health problems or any other factor;

8. report to an appropriate person or authority, at the earliest possible time, any conscientious objection which may be relevant to your professional practice;

9. avoid any abuse of your privileged relationship with patients and clients and of the privileged access allowed to their person, property, residence or workplace;

10. protect all confidential information concerning patients and clients obtained in the course of professional practice and make disclosures only with consent, where required by the order of a court or where you can justify disclosure in the wider public interest;

11. report to an appropriate person or authority, having regard to the physical, psychological and social effects on patients and clients, any circumstances in the environment of care which could jeopardise standards of practice;

---

* Reproduced with permission of the United Kingdom Central Council for Nursing, Midwifery and Health Visiting.

12. report to an appropriate person or authority any circumstances in which safe and appropriate care for patients and clients cannot be provided;

13. report to an appropriate person or authority where it appears that the health or safety of colleagues is at risk, as such circumstances may compromise standards of practice and care;

14. assist professional colleagues, in the context of your own knowledge, experience and sphere of responsibility, to develop their professional competence, and assist others in the care team, including informal carers, to contribute safely and to a degree appropriate to their roles;

15. refuse any gift, favour or hospitality from patients or clients currently in your care which might be interpreted as seeking to exert influence to obtain preferential consideration; and

16. ensure that your registration status is not used in the promotion of commercial products or services, declare any financial or other interests in relevant organisations providing such goods or services and ensure that your professional judgment is not influenced by any commercial considerations.

Notice to all Registered Nurses, Midwives and Health Visitors

This code of Professional Conduct for the Nurse, Midwife and Health Visitor is issued to all registered nurses, midwives and health visitors by the United Kingdom Central Council for Nursing, Midwifery and Health Visiting. The Council is the regulatory body responsible for the standards of these professions and it requires members of the professions to practice and conduct themselves within the standards and framework provided by the Code.

The Council's Code is kept under review and any recommendations for change and improvement would be welcomed and should be addressed to the:

Registrar and Chief Executive
United Kingdom Central Council for Nursing, Midwifery and Health Visiting
23 Portland Place
London
W1N 3AF

Appendix IX

American Nurses' Association Code For Nurses*

Preamble

A code of ethics makes explicit the primary goals and values of the profession. When individuals become nurses, they make a moral commitment to uphold the values and special moral obligations expressed in their code. The Code for Nurses is based on a belief about the nature of individuals, nursing, health, and society. Nursing encompasses the protection, promotion, and restoration of health; the prevention of illness; and the alleviation of suffering in the care of clients; including individuals, families, groups and communities. In the context of these functions, nursing is defined as the diagnosis and treatment of human responses to actual or potential health problems.

Since clients themselves are the primary decision-makers in matters concerning their own health, treatment, and wellbeing, the goal of nursing actions is to support and enhance the client's responsibility and self-determination to the greatest extent possible. In this context, health is not necessarily an end in itself, but rather a means to a life that is meaningful from the client's perspective.

When making clinical judgments, nurses base their decisions on consideration of consequences and of universal moral principles, both of which prescribe and justify nursing actions. The most fundamental of these principles is respect for persons. Other principles stemming from this basic principle are autonomy (self-determination), beneficence (doing good), non-maleficence (avoiding harm), veracity (truth-telling), confidentiality (respecting privileged information), fidelity (keeping promises), and justice (treating people fairly).

In brief, then, the statements of the code and their interpretation provide guidance for conduct and relationships in carrying out nursing responsibilities consistent with the ethical obligations of the profession and with high quality in nursing care.

Introduction

A code of ethics indicates a profession's acceptance of the responsibility and trust with which it has been invested by society. Under the terms of the implicit contract between society and the nursing profession, society grants the profession considerable autonomy and authority to function in the conduct of its affairs. The development of a code of ethics is an essential activity of a profession and provides one means for the exercise of professional self-regulation.

Upon entering the profession, each nurse inherits a measure of both the responsibility and the trust that have accrued to nursing over the years, as well as the corresponding obligation to adhere to the profession's code of conduct and relationships for ethical practice. The *Code for Nurses with Interpretive Statements* is thus more a collective expression of nursing conscience and philosophy than a set of external rules imposed upon an individual practitioner of nursing. Personal and professional integrity can be assured only if an individual is committed to the profession's code of conduct.

A code of ethical conduct offers general principles to guide and evaluate nursing actions. It does not assure the virtues required for professional practice within the character of each nurse. In particular situations, the justification of behavior as ethical must satisfy not only the individual nurse acting as a moral agent but also the standards for professional peer review.

---

* Reproduced with the permission of the American Nurses' Association, © 1976, 1985. *The Code for Nurses with Interpretive Statements* is published by the American Nurses' Association.

The Code for Nurses was adopted by the American Nurses' Association in 1950 and has been revised periodically. It serves to inform both the nurse and society of the profession's expectations and requirements in ethical matters. The code and the interpretive statements together provide a framework within which nurses can make ethical decisions and discharge their responsibilities to the public, to other members of the health team, and to the profession.

Although a particular situation by its nature may determine the use of specific moral principles, the basic philosophical values, directives, and suggestions provided here are widely applicable to situations encountered in clinical practice. The Code for Nurses is not open to negotiation in employment settings, nor is it permissible for individuals or groups of nurses to adapt or change the language of this code.

The requirements of the code may often exceed those of the law. Violations of the law may subject the nurse to civil or criminal liability. The state nurses' associations, in fulfilling the profession's duty to society, may discipline their members for violations of the code. Loss of the respect and confidence of society and of one's colleagues is a serious sanction resulting from violation of the code. In addition, every nurse has a personal obligation to uphold and adhere to the code and to ensure that nursing colleagues do likewise.

Guidance and assistance in applying the code to local situations may be obtained from the American Nurses' Association and the constituent state nurses' associations.

Code for nurses

1. The nurse provides services with respect for human dignity and the uniqueness of the client unrestricted by considerations of social or economic status, personal attributes, or the nature of health problems.

2. The nurse safeguards the client's right to privacy by judiciously protecting information of a confidential nature.

3. The nurse acts to safeguard the client and the public when health care and safety are affected by the incompetent, unethical, or illegal practice of any person.

4. The nurse assumes responsibility and accountability for individual nursing judgments and actions.

5. The nurse maintains competence in nursing.

6. The nurse exercises informed judgment and uses individual competence and qualifications as criteria in seeking consultation, accepting responsibilities, and delegating nursing activities to others.

7. The nurse participates in activities that contribute to the ongoing development of the profession's body of knowledge.

8. The nurse participates in the profession's efforts to implement and improve standards of nursing.

9. The nurse participates in the profession's efforts to establish and maintain conditions of employment conducive to high quality nursing care.

10. The nurse participates in the profession's effort to protect the public from misinformation and misrepresentation and to maintain the integrity of nursing.

11. The nurse collaborates with members of the health professions and other citizens in promoting community and national efforts to meet the health needs of the public.

Appendix X

Code of Ethics for Nursing*
Canadian Nurses' Association

Preface

In 1955, the Canadian Nurses' Association adopted its first Code of Ethics, based on a code developed by the International Council of Nurses (ICN). This code (with minor changes) continued to guide members in their ethical decision making well into the 1970s.

Over the years, however, a growing need was expressed for an ethical code tailored to nursing in Canada. At the CNA's 1978 Annual Meeting, the development of a new national code was made a priority, and in 1979, Sister Simone Roach was appointed as project director. In February 1980, the Board approved *CNA Code of Ethics: an ethical basis for nursing in Canada*. But shortly afterwards, many members began to voice concern over certain aspects of the new Code — Section Three in particular — which appeared to violate the nurse's right to equitable working conditions. It was also felt that the code should be written in a form that could be used in everyday practice.

As a result, in February 1981, the Board decided that a completely new code would need to be written, using the 1980 document as background. Two months later, an ad hoc committee was established, consisting of nursing leaders, a consultant ethicist/writer, and a CNA staff resource person.

Throughout the drafting and revision process, the committee sought input from nurses all across Canada — to ensure the new Code would be truly national in scope. In February 1984, a draft Code was published in the CNA journals, and members were encouraged to provide feedback. Their comments, plus consultations with member associations, led to several changes that clarified and improved the Code. This process of 'sifting and sorting' through ideas — so crucial to the development of our profession — could have been extended even further. However, the Committee felt that this document represented the 'state of the art' for the profession, and that it was time to give the Code a chance to 'live'.

To avoid confusing this Code with others, it should be emphasised that ethical codes can be understood at three levels — provincial, national, and international — each expressing different values. In several provinces, the registering/licensing bodies have adopted codes of ethics or guidelines that set standards specifically for nurses working in those jurisdictions. The national guidelines, on the other hand, express the values shared by nurses across Canada, while the ICN Code reflects those values shared by nurses all over the world.

The work of arriving at a national code, acceptable to the majority of the membership, has been a long and arduous task. On behalf of the Board of Directors, I would like to thank Stephany Grasset, Jocelyn Hezekiah, Judith Lougheed, Jeanette Pick, and Anne Thorne for their dedicated work on the Ad Hoc Committee. Dr. Benjamin Freedman also provided valuable consulting services, and Marianne Lamb acted as the CNA staff resource.

The Code is now a living document — and one that we can live with for some time to come. Provision has been made for the Code to be reviewed at least every five years to keep it responsive to changing needs and values, both within our profession and within society. Change is inevitable; however, certain truths will always remain for us to identify and respond to in our work with the human condition. This Code, it is hoped, will provide an ethical framework to guide us in this process.

Lorine Besel
President

---

* Adopted in 1985. Reprinted here with permission of the Canadian Nurses' Association.

Preamble

Nursing practice can be defined generally as a 'dynamic, caring, helping relationship in which the nurse assists the client to achieve and maintain optimal health'.[1] Nurse educators, administrators and researchers, although not necessarily assisting the client directly, have too as their ultimate goal, the maintenance and improvement of nursing practice. 'Nurses direct their energies toward the promotion, maintenance and restoration of health, the prevention of illness, the alleviation of suffering and the ensuring of a peaceful death when life can no longer be sustained'.[2]

The nurse, by entering and maintaining a commitment to the profession, is committed to its professional ethics. As persons and as citizens, nurses continue to be bound by the moral and legal norms shared by all other participants in society. In addition, nurses assume a professional commitment to the health and the wellbeing of clients. Nursing as such encompasses moral activities.

The adoption of this Code represents a conscious undertaking on the part of the Canadian Nurses' Association and its members to be responsible for upholding the following statements (values, standards, and limitations). This Code expresses and seeks to clarify those ethical principles that are definitive of ethical nursing activity. For those entering the profession, this Code identifies the basic moral commitments of nursing and may serve as a source for education and reflection. For those within the profession, the Code also serves as a basis for self-evaluation and for peer review. For those outside the profession, this Code may serve to establish expectations regarding the ethical conduct of nurses.

Ethical Problems and Dilemmas

Ethical *problems* fall into two distinct categories:

(a) Ethical *violations* involve the neglect of moral obligation; for example, a nurse who neglects to provide competent care to a client because of personal inconvenience has ethically failed the client.
(b) Ethical *dilemmas*, however, arise when ethical reasons both for and against a particular course of action are present. For example, a nurse whose client is likely to refuse some appropriate form of health care presents the nurse with an ethical dilemma. In this case, substantial moral reasons may be offered on behalf of several opposed options.

This Code provides clear direction with respect to the avoidance of ethical violations. When a course of action is mandated by the Code, and there exists no opposing ethical principle, ethical conduct requires that course of action.

This Code cannot serve the same function for all ethical dilemmas. There is room within the profession of nursing for conscientious disagreement among nurses. The resolution of a dilemma often depends upon the special factual circumstances of the case in question. Resolution may also depend upon the relative weight of the opposing principles, a matter about which reasonable people may disagree.

For dilemmas, no particular resolution may be definitive of good nursing practice. However, the Code constitutes an attempt to provide *guidance* for those nurses who face ethical dilemmas. A proper consideration of the Code may rule out some suggested resolutions of the ethical dilemmas. For example, a nurse whose client is likely to refuse some form of appropriate health care, as was noted, presents the nurse with an ethical dilemma. Even so, it would be wrong for the nurse to engineer consent by deceiving the client about the nature of the care to be provided. (For example, see Value II, Standard 4.)

Elements of the Code

This Code contains different elements designed to help the nurse in its interpretation. The values and standards are presented by topic and not in order of importance. There is variation in the normative (the nurse *should* or *ought* to or is *obliged* to) terminology used in the Code. These terms have been used interchangeably and no difference in moral force of the statements is intended. A number of distinctions between ethics and morals may be found in the literature. Since no distinction has been uniformly adopted by writers on ethics, these terms are used interchangeably in this Code as well.

- *Values* express broad ideals of nursing. They establish the correct directions for nursing. In the absence of a conflict of ethics, the fact that a particular action promotes a *value* of nursing may be decisive in some specific instances. Nursing behavior can always be appraised in terms of values: how closely did it approach the value, how widely did it deviate from it. Because they are so broad however, values may not give specific guidance in difficult instances.

- *Standards* are moral obligations that have their basis in nursing values. Standards provide more specific direction for conduct than do values, however; they spell out what a value requires under particular circumstances.

- *Limitations* describe exceptional circumstances in which a value or standard cannot receive its usual application. Limitations have been included separately to emphasize that, in the ordinary run of events, the values and standards will be decisive.

It is also important to emphasize that even when a value or standard must be limited, it nonetheless carries moral weight. For example, a nurse who is compelled to testify in a court of law regarding confidential matters is still subject to the values and standards of confidentiality. While the requirement to testify is a justified limitation upon confidentiality, in other respects confidentiality must be observed. The nurse must only reveal that confidential information which is pertinent to the case at hand and such revelation must take place within the appropriate context. The general obligation to preserve the client's confidences remains despite particular limiting circumstances.

Rights and Obligations

Clients possess *rights*, both legal and moral. In general, the statements in this Code are cast in the form of the moral obligations of nurses rather than in terms of the rights of clients. Those legal and moral rights exist with or without professional acceptance. The obligations of nurses *exceed* that which would be required by the legal rights of clients and this Code tries to reflect that fact. (For example, see Value II, Standard 3.) In many instances, it is beyond the power of nurses to *secure* the right of a client. A client's right to be treated in a dignified fashion must be reflected in the nurse's own behavior towards the client and in attempts to influence the actions of other members of the health care team. The task of this Code is to state clearly the moral obligations that are incumbent upon nurses.

Nurses too possess legal and moral rights, as persons and as nurses. It is beyond the scope of this Code to address the personal rights of nurses. To the extent that conditions of employment are essential to the establishment of ethical nursing, however, this Code must deal with that issue.

The satisfaction of some ethical responsibilities requires action taken by the nursing profession as a whole. The fourth section of the Code contains values and standards concerned with those collective responsibilities of nursing and are particularly addressed to professional associations. Ethical reflection must be an ongoing affair, and its facilitation is a continuing responsibility of the Canadian Nurses' Association.

The body of the Code is divided into sections that correspond to the sources of nursing obligations:

- *Clients*
- *Health Team*
- *The Social Context of Nursing*
- *Responsibilities of the Profession*

Clients

I. A nurse is obliged to treat clients with respect for their individual needs and values.

Standards

1. Factors such as the client's race, religion, ethnic origin, social status, sex, age or health status may not be permitted to compromise the nurse's commitment to that client's care.

2. The expectations and normal life patterns of clients are acknowledged. Individualized programs of nursing care are designed to accommodate the psychological, social, cultural and spiritual needs of clients, as well as their biological needs.

3. The nurse does more than respond to the requests of clients, by accepting an affirmative obligation to aid clients in their expression of needs and values within the context of health care.

4. Recognizing the client's membership in a family and a community, the nurse, with the client's consent, attempts to facilitate the participation of significant others in the care of the client.

II. Based upon respect for clients and regard for their right to control their own care, nursing care should reflect respect for the right of choice held by clients.

Standards

1. The competent client's consent is an essential precondition to the provision of health care. Nurses bear the primary responsibility to inform clients about the nursing care that is available to them.

2. Consent may be signified in many different ways. Verbal permission or knowledgeable cooperation are the usual forms in which clients consent to nursing care. In each case, however, a valid consent represents the free choice of the competent client to undergo that care which is to be provided.

3. Consent properly understood is the process by which a client becomes an active participant in care. All clients should be aided in becoming active participants in their care to the maximum extent that circumstances permit. Professional ethics may require of the nurse actions that exceed the legal requirements of consent. For example, although a child may be legally incompetent to consent, nurses should nevertheless attempt to inform and involve the child in treatment.

4. Force, coercion and manipulative tactics must not be employed in the obtaining of consent.

5. Illness or other factors may compromise the client's capacity for self-direction. Nurses have a continuing obligation to value autonomy in such clients, for example, by creatively providing them with opportunities for choices, within their capabilities, thereby aiding them to maintain or regain some degree of autonomy.

6. Whenever information is provided to a client, this must be done in a truthful, understandable and sensitive way. It must proceed with an awareness of the individual client's needs, interests and values.

7. Nurses should respond freely to their client's requests for information and explanation when in possession of the knowledge required to respond accurately. When the questions of the client require information beyond that of the nurse, the client should be informed of that fact and referred to a more appropriate health care practitioner for a response.

III. The nurse is obliged to hold confidential all information regarding a client learned in the health care setting.

Standards

1. The rights of persons to control the amount of personal information that will be revealed applies with special force in the health care setting. It is, broadly speaking, up to clients to determine who shall be told of their condition, and in what detail.

2. In describing professional confidentiality to a client, its boundaries should be revealed:
   (a) Competent care requires that other members of a team of health personnel have access to or be provided with the relevant details of a client's condition.
   (b) In addition, discussions of the client's care may be required for the purpose of teaching, research or quality assurance. In this case, special care must be taken to protect the client's anonymity.

   Whenever possible, the client should be informed of these necessities at the onset of care.

3. An affirmative duty exists to institute and maintain practices that protect client confidentiality, for example, by limiting access to records.

Limitations

The nurse is not morally obligated to maintain confidentiality when the failure to disclose information will place the client or third parties in danger. Generally, legal requirements to disclose are morally justified by these same criteria. In facing such a situation, the first concern of the nurse must be the safety of the client or third party.

Even when the nurse is confronted with the necessity to disclose, confidentiality should be preserved to the maximum possible extent. Both the amount of information disclosed and the number of people to whom disclosure is made should be restricted to the minimum necessary to prevent the feared harm.

IV. The nurse has an obligation to be guided by consideration for the dignity of clients.

Standards

1. Nursing care should be carried out with consideration for the personal modesty of clients.

2. A nurse's conduct at all times should acknowledge the client as a person. For example, discussion of care in the presence of the client should actively involve or include that client.

3. As ways of dealing with death and the dying process change, nursing is challenged to find new ways to preserve human values, autonomy and dignity. In assisting the dying client, measures must be taken to afford as much comfort, dignity and freedom from anxiety and pain as possible. Special consideration is given to the need of the client's family to cope with their loss.

V. The nurse is obligated to provide competent care to clients

Standards

1. Nurses should engage in continuing education and in the upgrading of skills relevant to the practice setting.

2. In seeking or accepting employment, nurses should accurately state their areas of competence as well as limitations.

3. Nurses who are assigned to work outside of an area of present competence should seek to do that which, under the circumstances, is in the best interests of their clients. Supervisors or others should be informed of the situation at the earliest possible moment so that protective measures can be instituted. As a temporary measure, the safety and welfare of clients may be better served by the best efforts of the nurse under the circumstances than by no nursing care at all.

4. When called upon outside of an employment setting to provide emergency care, nurses fulfill their obligations by providing the best care that circumstances, experience and education permit.

Limitations

A nurse is not ethically obliged to provide requested care when compliance would involve a violation of her or his moral beliefs. When that request falls within recognized forms of health care, however, the client should be referred to a more appropriate health care practitioner. Nurses who have or are likely to encounter such situations are morally obligated to seek to arrange conditions of employment so that the care of clients is not jeopardized.

VI. The nurse is obliged to represent the ethics of nursing before colleagues and others.

Standards

1. Nurses serving on committees concerned with health care or research should see their role as including the vigorous representation of nursing's professional ethics.

2. Many public issues include health as a major component. Involvement in civic activities may afford the nurse the opportunity to further the objectives of nursing as well as to fulfill the duties of a citizen.

VII. The nurse is obligated to advocate the client's interest.

Standards

1. Advocating the interests of the client includes assistance in achieving access to quality health care. For example, by providing information to clients privately or publicly, the nurse enables them to satisfy their rights to health care.

2. When speaking to public issues or in court as a nurse, the public is owed the same duties of accurate and relevant information as are clients within the employment setting.

VIII. In all professional settings, including education, research and administration, the nurse retains a commitment to the welfare of clients. The nurse bears an obligation to act in such a fashion as will maintain trust in nurses and nursing.

Standards

1. Nurses accepting professional employment must ascertain that conditions will permit provision of care consistent with the values and standards of the Code. Prospective employers should be informed of the provisions of the Code so that realistic and ethical expectations may be established at the beginning of the nurse–employer relationship.

2. Accurate performance appraisal is required by a concern for present and future clients and is essential to the growth of nurses. Nurse administrators and educators are morally obligated to provide timely and accurate feedback to nurses, and their supervisors, student nurses and their teachers.

3. Administrators bear special ethical responsibilities that follow from a concern for present and future clients. The nurse administrator seeks to ensure that the competencies of personnel are used efficiently. Working within available resources, the administrator seeks to ensure the welfare of clients. When competent care is threatened due to inadequate resources or for some other reason, the administrator acts to minimize the present danger and to prevent future harm.

4. An essential element of nursing education is the student–client encounter. This encounter must be conducted in accordance with ethical nursing practices, with special attention to the dignity of the client. The nurse educator is obligated to ensure that nursing students are acquainted with and comply with the provisions of the Code.

5. Research is necessary to the development of the profession of nursing. Nurses should be acquainted with advances in research, so that established results may be incorporated into practice. The individual nurse's competencies and circumstances may also be used to engage in, or to assist and encourage research designed to enhance the health and welfare of clients.

The conduct of research must conform to ethical nursing practice. The self-direction of clients takes on added importance in this context. Further direction is provided in the Canadian Nurses' Association publication entitled, *Ethical Guidelines for Nursing Research Involving Human Subjects*.

Health Team

IX. Client care should represent a cooperative effort, drawing upon the expertise of nursing and other health professions. Acknowledging personal or professional limitations, the nurse recognizes the perspective and expertise of colleagues from other disciplines.

Standards

1. The nurse participates in the assessment, planning, implementation and evaluation of comprehensive programs of care for clients.

2. The nurse accepts a responsibility to work with others through professional nurses' associations to secure quality care for clients.

X. The nurse, as a member of the health care team, is obliged to take steps to ensure that the client receives competent and ethical care.

Standards

1. The first consideration of the nurse who suspects incompetence or unethical conduct should be the welfare of present clients or potential harm to future clients. Subject to that principle, the following should be considered:
    (a) The nurse is obliged to ascertain the facts of the situation in deciding upon the appropriate course of action.
    (b) Institutional mechanisms for reporting incidents or risks of incompetent or unethical care should be followed.
    (c) It is unethical for a nurse to participate in efforts to deceive or mislead clients regarding the cause of their injury.
    (d) Relationships in the health care team should not be disrupted unnecessarily. If a situation can be resolved without peril to present or future clients by direct discussion with the colleague suspected of providing incompetent or unethical care, that should be done.

2. The nurse who attempts to protect clients threatened by incompetent or unethical conduct may be placed in a difficult position. Colleagues and professional associations are morally obliged to support nurses who fulfill their ethical obligations under the Code.

3. Guidance concerning those activities that may be delegated by nurses to assistants and other health care workers is found in legislation and policy statements. When functions are delegated, the nurse should be satisfied regarding the competence of those who will be fulfilling these functions. The nurse has a duty to provide continuing supervision in such a case.

The Social Context of Nursing

XI. Conditions of employment should contribute to client care and to the professional satisfaction of nurses. Nurses are obliged to work towards securing and maintaining conditions of employment that satisfy these connected goals.

Standards

1. In the final analysis, the improvement of conditions of nursing employment is often to the advantage of clients. Over the short term however, there is a danger that action directed toward this goal will work to the detriment of clients. Nurses bear an ethical

responsibility to present as well as future clients and so the following principles should be noted:

(a) The safety of clients should be the first concern in planning and implementing any job action.

(b) Individuals and groups of nurses participating in job actions share this ethical commitment to the safety of clients. However, their responsibilities may lead them to express this commitment in different, but equally appropriate ways.

(c) Clients whose safety requires ongoing or emergency nursing care are entitled to have those needs satisfied throughout the duration of any job action. Members of the public are entitled to know of the steps that have been taken to ensure the safety of clients.

(d) Individuals and groups of nurses participating in job actions have a duty of coordination and communication to take steps reasonably designed to ensure the safety of clients.

Responsibility of the Profession

XII. Professional nurses' organizations recognize a responsibility to clarify, secure and sustain ethical nursing conduct. The fulfillment of these tasks requires that professional organizations remain responsive to the rights, needs and legitimate interests of clients and nurses.

Standards

1. Sustained communication and cooperation between the Canadian Nurses' Association, provincial associations and other organizations of nurses, is an essential step towards securing ethical nursing conduct.

2. Professional nurses' associations must at all times accept responsibility for assuring quality care for clients.

3. Professional nurses' associations have a role in representing nursing interests and perspectives before non-nursing bodies, including legislatures, employers, the professional organizations of other health disciplines and the public media of communication.

4. Professional nurses' associations should provide and encourage organizational structures that facilitate ethical nursing conduct.

   (a) Changing circumstances may call for reconsideration and adaptation of this Code. Supplementation of the code may be necessary in order to address special situations. Professional associations should consider the ethics of nursing on a regular and continuing basis and be prepared to provide assistance to those concerned with its implementation.

   (b) Education in the ethical aspects of nursing should be available to nurses throughout their careers. Nurses' associations should actively support or develop structures designed towards this end.

Notes

1. Canadian Nurses' Association, *A Definition of Nursing Practice, Standards for Nursing Practice*, Ottawa, Canadian Nurses' Association, 1980, p. vi.
2. Ibid, p. v.

Appendix XI

Position statement
Ethics in nursing practice[*]

Introduction

Nurses are involved with people in human situations, which are often complex and occur in dynamic environments. Ethical issues arise daily in every aspect of the practice of nursing requiring appropriate responses from individual practitioners. Ethics entails the rational and conscious reflection of what should happen in human situations and the enunciation of principles and standards to guide behaviour. The practice of ethics in the discipline of nursing is '... designed to illuminate what we ought to do by asking us to consider and reconsider our ordinary actions, judgments and justifications' (Beauchamp T. & Childress J. 1983 *Principles of biomedical ethics*. 2nd ed, Oxford University Press, New York, p. xii). Rational reflection on the ethical aspects of nursing is a continuing responsibility for the nursing profession as a whole, as well as for individual practitioners.

Royal College of Nursing, Australia believes that:

Nurses aspire to, and have a responsibility to uphold, the highest possible ethical standards in their practice.

Ethics is integral to all areas of nursing: education, research, administration and clinical practice.

The nursing profession has a significant contribution to make to public debate and policy development on ethical issues relevant to the Australian community.

Rationale

- Changing values in the health field, in other human and behavioural sciences and society, raise new and previously unthought of ethical issues to which health care providers, including nurses, must respond.
- Nurses, as health professionals, share a responsibility to inform the public and contribute to public debate on ethical issues affecting the community at large by clearly articulating ethical issues arising in contemporary nursing practice.
- Providing guidance and support to nurses to assist them in ethical decision making and to practise ethically is the responsibility of the whole of the profession.
- Royal College of Nursing, Australia subscribes to the 'Code of Ethics for Nurses in Australia' and supports the values espoused in the Code.

Royal College of Nursing, Australia recommends that:

- Governments ensure a nursing perspective is represented by formal groups dealing with ethical matters of concern to the community.
- Editors, publishers and other media entities seek consultation with nurses on ethical issues relevant to the health field.
- Institutional ethics committees, whether in health care or academic settings, include nurses as core members.

---

[*] Reproduced with permission of the Royal College of Nursing, Australia.

Royal College of Nursing, Australia resolves to:

- Support its Ethics Society to identify ethical issues for the consideration of the nursing profession and to recommend ways for the College to respond appropriately.
- Encourage its Ethics Society to consider and identify ways that the College can support education, research and scholarship activities aimed at the understanding of ethical issues by nurses.
- Encourage its Legal Issues Society to identify legal constraints to the ethical practice of nursing and to identify ways that the College might seek reforms to change the situation.
- Actively lobby the National Health and Medical Research Council and other bodies for nursing representation on all committees, groups or working parties dealing with concerns and/or policy development in areas of ethics.

Authorised by Council of Royal College of Nursing, Australia
Date of issue: April 1997
Date to be revised: April 1999

Appendix XII

Position statement
Conscientious objection[*]

Introduction

Health and nursing care contexts have become increasingly characterised by moral uncertainty, controversy and perplexity. With this predicament has come an increasing recognition that our moral standards are not absolute and that different people can hold diverse though equally valid points of view on an issue. It is inevitable, therefore, that people may find themselves in marked disagreement about the morality of certain processes and procedures in health care contexts (for example, abortion, euthanasia, organ transplantation, blood transfusion, involuntary psychiatric treatment, circumcision) and that this moral disagreement may not be resolved to everyone's satisfaction.

Nurses are not immune from the problems of moral uncertainty, controversy and disagreements that occur in the workplace. Further, nurses may sometimes even be opposed, on conscientious grounds, to participating in certain medical/nursing procedures and practices which others have judged to be morally acceptable. The *Code of Ethics for Nurses in Australia* (1993) recognises that, in non-emergency situations, nurses are morally entitled to refuse to participate in certain procedures and practices which would violate nurses' sincerely held personal moral beliefs and values. With this entitlement, however, it is also acknowledged that nurses who are conscientiously opposed to certain practices and procedures have a moral responsibility to advise their employers, or prospective employers, of their position. Employers and colleagues in turn have a responsibility to ensure that nurse and co-workers are not treated unfairly or discriminated against on account of their conscientious beliefs.

Conscientious objection refers to a statement of a particular application of adopted moral standards in a given context. The statement can also be translated as indicating that a moral disagreement has arisen between the objector and others in regard to which moral standards apply and what one's moral duty is in the situation at hand. The moral standards adopted may be either religious or secular in nature.

Criteria for conscientious objection

In order for a claim of conscientious objection to be accepted the following five criteria must be met:

- The objection is motivated by distinctly moral concerns and not by self interest, fear, convenience or prejudice.

- The claim is based on autonomous, informed and critically reflective choice.

- The conscientious objection is claimed as a last resort and only after other means of addressing the problem at hand have been exhausted.

- It is acknowledged by the conscientious objector that others might have an equal claim to conscientious objection to the matter in hand.

- The act, process or procedure at issue is of a demonstrably morally uncertain and controversial nature.

---

[*] Reproduced with permission by the Royal College of Nursing, Australia.

Royal College of Nursing, Australia believes that:

- Nurses have a stringent professional responsibility to be informed about the ethical, legal, cultural and clinical implications of claiming conscientious objection in health care contexts.

- Nurses are entitled to have their conscientious beliefs respected in non-emergency situations provided the criteria of conscientious objection are met.

- When considering new/alternative employment opportunities, nurses should ensure that they are fully conversant with the philosophy, objectives and nature of the services offered by the employing agency and the compatibility of those values and services with their own conscientious beliefs.

- Nurses have a responsibility to advise their employers, or prospective employers, of their conscientious beliefs, particularly if the expression of these beliefs would significantly interfere with the provision of services offered by the employing agency.

- When claiming conscientious objection nurses should ensure that patient care is not compromised and that the legal duty of care is maintained, for example by the timely organisation of replacement staff.

- Employers and co-workers have a responsibility to ensure that nurses and co-workers are treated fairly and not discriminated against on account of their conscientious beliefs.

Rationale

Members of the College comprise people from a variety of cultural, social, political, economic and religious backgrounds. They are employed in various health care settings where it is likely that they will encounter a diversity of moral viewpoints on certain medical, nursing and other health care practices.

Through their care of individuals, families, groups and communities, and as members of the multidisciplinary health care teams, nurses are exposed to and are often required to participate in a variety of morally controversial health care practices and procedures. It is, therefore, important that nurses are informed about the legal, ethical, cultural and clinical aspects of these practices and procedures and the possible implications of conscientiously refusing to participate in them.

The College has a responsibility to provide professional leadership in assisting its membership, as well as the broader profession, to become informed and knowledgeable about conscientious objection in health care contexts.

The College recognises that unless professional nursing organisations formulate a position on conscientious objection it may be difficult to support and advise nurses claiming conscientious objector status in the workplace.

Royal College of Nursing, Australia recommends that:

- Employing organisations develop and implement policies which recognise diversity in the moral beliefs of their employees and which accommodates conscientious objection from employees without discrimination.

- Employing organisations identify the appropriate form by which conscientious objection is made known and to whom it should be known.

- Employing organisations identify appropriate personnel to assist the nurse in the decision-making process and any required documentation.

- Employing organisations treat as confidential those situations of conscientious objection that might arise in the course of employment.

Royal College of Nursing, Australia resolves to:

- Assist in the dissemination of information on conscientious objection to help guide and advise its membership and the broader nursing profession on how to respond effectively and justly to claims of conscience in the workplace.

- Respond, as appropriate, to social and legal policy initiatives in all Australian States and Territories to ensure that provisions are made to protect nurses claiming conscientious objector status in the case of morally controversial practices (e.g. abortion, euthanasia/assisted suicide, organ transplantation, and so on).

References

Australian Nursing Council Inc. *1993 Code of Ethics for Nurses in Australia*, ANCI, Canberra.

Johnstone, M. (1994). *Bioethics: a nursing perspective*, Second edition, W.B. Saunders/ Baillière Tindall, Sydney.

Johnstone, M. (1995). *Inaugural Bennett lecture: Moral controversy and the search for solutions: some critical reflections for the nursing profession*. Faculty of Nursing, RMIT, Melbourne.

Authorised by Council of Royal College of Nursing, Australia
Date of issue: February 1998
Date to be revised: February 2000

References

Chapter 1 The changing moral world and its implications for the nursing profession

Andersen, S. (1990). Patient advocacy and whistle-blowing in nursing: help for the helpers. *Nursing Forum* 25(3), pp. 5–13.

Anderson, W. Truett. (1990). *Reality isn't what it used to be*. Harper, San Francisco.

Bauman, Z. (1993). *Postmodern ethics*. Blackwell, Oxford UK/Cambridge, Mass.

Bishop, A. and Scudder, J. (1987). Nursing ethics in an age of controversy. *Advances in Nursing Science* 9(3), pp. 34–43.

Boyle, J. (1994). Radical moral disagreement in contemporary health care: a Roman Catholic perspective. *Journal of Medicine and Philosophy* 19(2), pp. 183–200.

Courier-Mail (1995). 13 May, Queenslander supports killing doctors who perform abortion. Reprinted in *Monash Bioethics Review* 14(3), p. 11.

Engelhardt, H. Tristram (1996). *The foundations of bioethics*, 2nd edn. Oxford University Press, New York.

Fasching, D. (1993). *The ethical challenge of Auschwitz and Hiroshima: apocalypse or utopia?* State University of New York Press, Albany.

Forrow, L., Arnold, R. and Frader, J. (1991). Teaching clinical ethics in the residency years: preparing competent professionals. *Journal of Medicine and Philosophy* 16(1), pp. 93–112.

Freire, P. (1970). *Cultural action for freedom*. Penguin Books, Harmondsworth, Middlesex.

—— (1972). *Pedagogy of the oppressed*. Penguin Books, London.

Friedman, J. (1994). *Cultural identity and global process*. Sage Publications, London.

Johnstone, M-J. (1994). *Nursing and the injustices of the law*. W.B. Saunders/Baillière Tindall, Sydney.

—— (1998). *Determining and responding effectively to ethical professional misconduct: A report to the Nurses Board of Victoria*, Melbourne.

Kane, R. (1994). *Through the moral maze: searching for absolute values in a pluralistic world*. North Castle Books. Armonk, New York/London, UK.

Khushf, G. (1994). Intolerant tolerance. *Journal of Medicine and Philosophy* 19(2), pp. 161–81.

Kuhse, H. (1992). Quality of life and the death of 'Baby M'. *Bioethics* 6(3), pp. 233–50.

McCullough, L. (1995). Preventive ethics, professional integrity, and boundary setting: the clinical management of moral uncertainty. *Journal of Medicine and Philosophy* 20(1), pp. 1–11.

McCullough, L. and Jonsen, A. (1991). Bioethics education: diversity and critique. *Journal of Medicine and Philosophy* 16(1), pp. 1–4.

Macklin, R. (1993). *Enemies of patients*. Oxford University Press, New York.

Milo, R. (1986). Moral deadlock. *Philosophy* 61, pp. 453–71.

Nagel, T. (1991). *Mortal questions*. Canto edition. Cambridge University Press (1979), Cambridge, UK.

Reichlin, M. (1994). Observations on the epistemological status of bioethics. *Journal of Medicine and Philosophy* 19(1), pp. 79–102.

Rohter, L. (1993). Anti-abortion protester kills doctor. *The Age*, 12 March, p. 7.

Sharkey, A. (1994). Killing for life. *The Age, Extra*, pp. 3–4.

Singer, P. and Kuhse, H. (1994). Bioethics and the limits of tolerance. *Journal of Medicine and Philosophy* 19(2), pp. 129–45.

Smith, M. (1994). *The moral problem*. Blackwell Publishers, Oxford, UK.

Wear, S. (1991). The irreducibly clinical character of bioethics. *Journal of Medicine and Philosophy* 16(1), pp. 53–70.

Wear, S., Lagaipa, S. and Logue, G. (1994). Toleration of moral diversity and the conscientious refusal by physicians to withdraw life-sustaining treatment. *Journal of Medicine and Philosophy* 19(2), pp. 147–59.

Wildes, K. (1993). Moral authority, moral standing, and moral controversy. *Journal of Medicine and Philosophy* 18(4), pp. 347–50.

—— (1994). Toleration and moral diversity: Bosnia or Pennsylvania. *Journal of Medicine and Philosophy* 19(2), pp. 123–28.

Winslow, B. and Winslow, G. (1991). Integrity and compromise in nursing ethics. *Journal of Medicine and Philosophy* 16(3), pp. 307–23.

Zohar, D. (1991). *The quantum self*. Flamingo, London.

Zohar, D. and Marshall, I. (1993). *The quantum society*. Flamingo, London.

Chapter 2 'Be good women but do not bother with a Code of Ethics'

Aikens, C. (1943). *Studies in ethics for nurses*, W.B. Saunders, Philadelphia (first published 1916).

Aly, G. and Roth, K. (1984). The legalization of mercy killings in medical and nursing institutions in Nazi Germany from 1938 until 1941: a commented documentation, *International Journal of Law and Psychiatry* 7, pp. 145–63.

Barritt, E.R. (1973). Florence Nightingale's values and modern nursing education. *Nursing Forum* 12 (1), pp. 7–47.

Beauchamp, T.L. and Childress, J.F. (1989). *Principles of biomedical ethics*, 3rd edn. Oxford University Press, New York.

Bergman, R. (1973). Ethics — concepts and practice. *International Nursing Review* 20 (5), pp. 140–2.

Bickley, J. (1988). What the cervical cancer inquiry report means for nurses. *New Zealand Nursing Journal* 81 (9), pp. 14–15.

—— (1993). Watchdogs or wimps? Nurses' response to the Cartwright Report. In Coney, S. (ed), *Unfinished business: what happened to the Cartwright Report? Writings on the aftermath of 'the unfortunate experiment' at National Women's Hospital.* Women's Health Action, Auckland, NZ, pp. 125–36.

Birnbach, N. and Lewenson, S. (eds). (1991). *First words: selected addresses from the national League for Nursing 1894–1933*, National League for Nursing, New York.

Blum, J.D. (1984). The code of nurses and wrongful discharge. *Nursing Forum* 21, pp. 149–51.

Bock, A. (1992). Nurses in call for euthanasia inquiry. *The Age*, 3 March, p. 6.

Bridges, D.C. (1968). 'International Nursing Review' past, present — and progress? *International Nursing Review* 15 (1), pp. 9–17.

Briggs, P. and McDonald, B. (1992). 'Straw Men' in the euthanasia debate. *The Age*, 24 March, p. 12.

Caplan, A. (ed.) (1992). *When medicine went mad: bioethics and the holocaust*. Humana Press, Totowa, New Jersey.

Centre for Human Bioethics (1986). *Proceedings of the conference, 'AIDS: Social Policy, Ethics and Law'*. Centre for Human Bioethics, Monash University, Melbourne.

—— (1987a). *Proceedings of the conference, 'The role of the nurse: doctors' handmaiden, patients' advocate, or what?* Centre for Human Bioethics, Monash University, Melbourne.

—— (1987b). *Proceedings of the conference, 'IVF: the Current Debate'*. Centre for Human Bioethics, Monash University, Melbourne.

Clay, T. (1987). *Nurses: power and politics*. Heinemann Nursing, London.

Coney, S. (1988). *The unfortunate experiment*. Penguin Books, Auckland, NZ.

—— (1990). *Out of the frying pan: inflammatory writing 1972–89*. Penguin Books, Auckland, NZ.

—— (ed). (1993). *Unfinished business: what happened to the Cartwright Report? Writings on the aftermath of 'the unfortunate experiment' at National Women's Hospital.* Women's Health Action, Auckland, NZ.

Coney, S. and Bunkle, P. (1987). An 'unfortunate experiment' at National Women's. *Metro*, June, pp. 47–65.

Cotterhill, D. (1992). Views not representative. *Australian Nurses Journal* 21 (10), p. 4.

Coulter, C. (1987). Women, infertility and IVF. In *Proceedings of the conference, 'IVF: the Current Debate'*. Centre for Human Bioethics, Monash University, Melbourne, pp. 156–68.

Densford, J. and Everett, M. (1947). *Ethics for modern nurses: professional adjustments 1*. W.B. Saunders, Philadelphia.

Dock, L.L. (1900). Ethics — or a code of ethics? In L.L. Dock, *Short papers on nursing subjects*. M. Louise Longeway, New York.

Dolan, J.A., Fitzpatrick, M.L. and Herrmann, E.K. (1983). *Nursing in society: an historical perspective*, 15th edn. W.B. Saunders, Philadelphia.

Ewing, T. (1998). Abortion crusader fights for just one political cause, *The Age*, 23 March, p. 8.

Free v Holy Cross Hospital 505 NE2d 1188 (Ill App 1 Dist 1987).

Gartland, S. (1992). Nurses death aid 'no shock'. *Herald-Sun*, 3 March, p. 5.

Gladwin, M. (1930). *Ethics talks to nurses*, W.B. Saunders, Philadelphia.

Heitman, L. and Robinson, B. (1997). Developing a nursing ethics round table. *American Journal of Nursing*, 97(10), pp. 36–8.

Herald-Sun (1992). Nurses admit death role. 2 March, p. 3.

Hunt, G. (ed). (1994). *Ethical issues in nursing*. Routledge, London and New York.

In re the Alleged Unfair Dismissal of Ms K Howden by the City of Whittlesea 6/9/90 (Case No 90/3672, Decision D90/1933), IRCV (unreported).

Jameton, A. (1984). *Nursing practice: the ethical issues*, Prentice-Hall. Englewood Cliffs, New Jersey.

Johns, G. (1988). The commanding presence of George Herbert Green. *New Zealand Herald*, 6 August, p. 9.

Johnstone, M-J. (1987). Nursing and professional ethics. In *Proceedings of the conference, 'The Role of the Nurse: Doctor's Handmaiden, Patients' Advocate or What?'* Centre for Human Bioethics, Monash University, Melbourne.

—— (1988a). Law, professional ethics and the problem of conflict with personal values. *International Journal of Nursing Studies* 25 (2), pp. 147–57.

—— (1988b). A critical bioethical issue. *Australian Nurses Journal* 18 (1), p. 8.

—— (1988c). Ethical issues in neonatal nursing. Paper presented at the conference 'Storking the Future', Monash Medical Centre, 27 August, Melbourne.

—— (1989). *Bioethics: a nursing perspective*. 1st edn. W.B. Saunders/Baillière Tindall, Sydney.

—— (1993). The development of nursing ethics in Australia: an historical overview. *Papers of the First National Nursing History Conference: Australian nursing ... the story*, Royal College of Nursing, Australia, Melbourne, pp. 33–51.

—— (1994). *Nursing and the injustices of the law*. W.B. Saunders/Baillière Tindall, Sydney.

—— (1997). The role and function of nursing ethics committees. *Ethics Society Newsletter*, 2(4), December, pp. 1–4.

—— (1998). *Determining and Responding Effectively to Ethical Professional Misconduct in Nursing: A Report to the Nurses Board of Victoria*, Melbourne.

Johnstone, M-J., Kanitsaki, O., Wallace, M., and O'Connor, M. (1996). Conclusion: taking a position on the euthanasia question. In Johnstone, M-J. (ed), *The politics of euthanasia: a nursing response*. Royal College of Nursing, Canberra, Australia, pp. 117–28.

Kelly, L.Y. (1985). *Dimensions of professional nursing*, 5th edn. Macmillan Publishing, New York.

Koonz, C. (1987). *Mothers in the Fatherland: women, the family and Nazi politics*. St Martin's Press, New York.

Kuhse, H. and Singer, P. (1992). Euthanasia: a survey of nurses' attitudes and practices. *Australian Nurses Journal* 21 (9), pp. 21–2.

Lagnado, L. and Dekel, S. (1991). *Children of the flames: Dr Josef Mengele and the untold story of the twins of Auschwitz*. Sidgwick & Jackson, London.

Lifton, R.J. (1986). *The Nazi doctors: a study of the psychology of evil*. Macmillan, London.

Luckes, E. (1888). *Hospital sisters and their duties*, J. and A. Churchill, London.

Magazanik, M. (1992a). Nurses back euthanasia, survey finds. *The Age*, 2 March, p. 1.

—— (1992b). When death is part of the quality of life. *The Age*, 4 March, p. 3.

—— (1992c). Euthanasia should be legal, says clergyman. *The Age*, 5 March, p. 3.

—— (1992d). Euthanasia law is unrealistic: doctor. *The Age*, 5 June, p. 1.

—— (1992e). Law Commission supports reform on treatment of sick babies. *The Age*, 6 June, p. 5.

Mathews, S. (1988). Nurses overlooked. *The Age*, 24 March, p. 12.

McIntosh, P. (1988). Nurses must be more aggressive. *Australian Dr Weekly*, 10 June, pp. 1, 10.

Millership, R. (1992). A better way. *Australian Nurses Journal* 21 (10), p. 4.

Monkivitch, A. (1992). Euthanasia result not accurate. *The Age*, 5 March, p. 12.

Muirden, N., Jackson, K., Pisasale, M., Williams, B., Bingham, J. and Evans, B. (1992). A survey among palliative care nurses would give differing views. *The Age*, 10 March, p. 12.

Nadelson, C.C. and Notman, M.T. (1978). Women as health professionals. In Reich, W.T. (ed.), *Encyclopedia of bioethics*. The Free Press, New York, pp. 1713–20.

New Zealand Herald (1987a). Cancer cases quoted. 12 August, p. 13.

—— (1987b). 'Absolutely appalled' over tests. 12 November, p. 14.

—— (1987c). Dr Collison denies imposing staff gag. 18 November.

—— (1987d). Inquiry judge seeks more nurses' views. 3 December.

—— (1987e). Consent 'not asked' for samples. 10 December.

—— (1988a). Swabbed girls 'often Maoris and Islanders'. 20 January.

—— (1988b). Dr Green 'Did not treat all cases'. 28 January, p. 3.

Nightingale, F. (1970 edn). *Notes on nursing*. Duckworth, London. (First published 1859 by Harrison & Sons.)

Nursing Times (1990). Nurses obliged to lie to cancer patients. 86 (28), 11 July, p. 9.

O'Brien, N. (1998a). Stop abortions or face charges, nurses told. *The Australian*, 12 February, p. 3.

—— (1998b). Doctors demand abortion overhaul. *The Australian*, 17 February, p. 7.

—— (1998c). Abortion laws 'as bad as Cambodia's'. *The Australian*, 24 February, p. 4.

O'Brien, N. and Price, M. (1998a). Abortion charges create state of panic. *The Australian*, 11 February, p. 5.

—— (1998b). AMA tells doctors to refuse abortions. *The Australian*, 10 February, p. 5.

O'Connor, M. (1992). Representative sample? *Australian Nurses Journal* 21 (10) May, p. 4.

Parsons, S. (1916). *Nursing problems and obligations*, Whitcomb & Barrows, Boston (facsimile, Garland Publishing, New York, 1985).

Pirrie, M. (1987). A disabled baby's right to live. *The Age*, 28 April, p. 11.

Proctor, R. (1988). *Racial hygiene: medicine under the Nazis*. Harvard University Press, Cambridge, Mass.

—— (1992). Nazi biomedical politics. In Caplan (ed.), *When medicine went mad: bioethics and the holocaust*, pp. 23–42.

Reeves, P. (1998). WA nurses caught in abortion row. *Australian Nursing Journal*, 5(8), p. 11.

Reich, W.T. (ed.) (1978). *Encyclopedia of bioethics*. The Free Press, New York.

—— (ed). (1995). *The encyclopedia of bioethics*, revised edition. Simon & Schuster Macmillan, New York/Simon & Schuster and Prentice Hall International.

Report of the Cervical Cancer Inquiry (1988). Prepared by the Committee of Inquiry into Allegations Concerning the Treatment of Cervical Cancer at National Women's Hospital and into Other Related Matters. Government Printing Office, Auckland, NZ.

Report of the Study of Professional Issues in Nursing (1988). Health Department (Vic.), Melbourne

Robb, I. Hampton. (1903). *Nursing ethics: for hospital and private use*, J.B. Savage, Cleveland.

Roberts, J. (1987). Women not told of intimate checks. *Sunday Star* (Auckland), 26 September.

Rudd, S. (1992). Ethics committees — a forum for nurses? *Australian Medicine*, 4(12), 6 July, p. 15.

Rumbold, G. (1986). *Ethics in nursing practice*. Baillière Tindall, London.

Sanders, K. (1988). Obeying doctor's orders: professional accountability. In *Proceedings of 'Nursing Law and Ethics'. First Victorian State Conference. Theme: 'Matters of Life and Death'*, School of Nursing, Phillip Institute of Technology, Melbourne.

Sawyer, L.M. (1989). Nursing code of ethics: an international comparison. *International Nursing Review* 36 (5), pp. 145–8.

Schumpeter, P. (1988). No-resuscitation rules are unclear: lecturer. *The Age*, 1 October, p. 21.

Skene, L. (1992). Doctor ending baby's pain should not face risk of jail. *The Age*, 9 June, p. 12.

Smith, W.B. and Lew, Y.L. (1968). *Nursing care of the patient*. Dymock, Sydney.

Stanley, T. (1978). Nursing. In Reich (ed.), *Encyclopedia of bioethics*, pp. 1138–46.

Steppe, H. (1991). Nursing in the Third Reich. *History of Nursing Journal* 3 (4), pp. 21–37.

—— (1992). Nursing in Nazi Germany. *Victorian Journal of Nursing Research* 14 (6), pp. 744–53.

Sun-Herald (1990). Medically unfit. 17 June, p. 168.

Svendsen, I. (1987). Lecturer calls for code of nursing conduct, *The Age*, 17 November, p. 21.

Syme, R. (1992). A missing voice in euthanasia debate. *The Age*, 21 March, p. 10.

The Age (1992). Editorial — The law and the right to die. 5 March, p. 13.

Thompson, I., Melia, K. and Boyd, K. (1994). *Nursing ethics*, 3rd edn. First published in 1983. Churchill Livingstone, Edinburgh.

Tighe, M. (1992). Slippery slope to killing patients. *The Age*, 21 March, p. 10.

Tschudin, V. (1986). *Ethics in nursing: the caring relationship*. Heinemann Nursing, London.

Viens, D.C. (1989). A history of nursing's code of ethics. *Nursing Outlook* 37 (1), pp. 45–9.

Waikato Times (1987a). Patient recall: decision later. 1 September.

—— (1987b). Rape by medical students? 18 September.

—— (1990). Ethical guidelines underway. 15 October, p. 3.

Warthen v Toms River Community Memorial Hospital, Superior Court of New Jersey, AD, 8/1/85–14/2/85. In *Atlantic Reporter*, 2nd Series, New Jersey, pp. 229–34.

Wikler, D. and Barondess, J. (1993). Bioethics and anti-bioethics in light of Nazi medicine: what must we remember? *Kennedy Institute of Ethics Journal* 3(1), pp. 39–55.

Winslow, B. and Winslow, G. (1991). Integrity and compromise in nursing ethics. *Journal of Medicine and Philosophy*, 16(3), pp. 307–23.

Woodham-Smith, C. (1964). *Florence Nightingale 1820–1910*. Collins Fontana, London.

Yarling, R.R. and McElmurry, B.J. (1986). The moral foundation of nursing. *Advances in Nursing Science* 8(2), pp. 63–73.

Zink, M. and Titus, L. (1994). Nursing ethics committees — where are they? *Nursing Management*, 25(6), pp. 70–6.

Chapter 3 Ethics, bioethics and nursing ethics: some working definitions

Abel, E.K. and Nelson, M.K. (eds) (1990). *Circles of care: work and identity in women's lives*. State University of New York Press, Albany.

Allen, R.E. (ed.) (1966). *Greek philosophy: Thales to Aristotle*. The Free Press, MacMillan, New York, pp. 57–255.

Barnard, D. (1988). 'Ship? What ship? I thought I was going to the doctor!': patient-centred perspectives on the health care team. In N.M.P. King, L.R. Churchill and A.W. Cross, *Physician as captain of the ship*, D. Reidel, Dordrecht, pp. 89–111.

Barry, V. (1982). *Moral aspects of health care*. Wadsworth, Belmont, California.

Bayles, M.D. (1981). *Professional ethics*. Wadsworth, Belmont, California.

Beauchamp, T. and Childress, J. (1994). *Principles of biomedical ethics*, 4th edn. Oxford University Press, New York.

—— (1983). *Principles of biomedical ethics*, 2nd edn. Oxford University Press, New York.

—— (1989). *Principles of biomedical ethics*, 3rd edn. Oxford University Press, New York.

Beecher, H. (1966). Ethics and clinical research. *New England Journal of Medicine*, 274(2), June, pp. 1354–60.

Benner, P. (1991). The role of experience, narrative, and community in skilled ethical comportment. *Advances in Nursing Science*, 14(2), pp. 1–21.

—— (ed). (1994). *Interpretive phenomenology: embodiment, caring, and ethics in health and illness*. Sage, Thousand Oaks.

Bilton, M. and Sim, K. (1992). *Four hours in My Lai: a war crime and its aftermath*. Viking, London.

Bishop, A. and Scudder, J. (1990). *The practical, moral, and personal sense of nursing: a phenomenological philosophy of practice*. State University of New York Press, Albany.

Blackburn, S. (1984). *Spreading the word*. Clarendon Press, Oxford.

Boddy, J. (ed.) (1985). *Health: perspectives and practices*. The Dunmore Press, Palmerston North, New Zealand.

Brandt, R. (1959). *Ethical theory*. Prentice Hall, Englewood Cliffs, New Jersey (see in particular Chapter 4, 'The use of authority in ethics').

Carlton, W. (1978). *'In our professional opinion ...': the primacy of clinical judgment over moral choice*. University of Notre Dame Press, Notre Dame.

Chrisman, N.J. (1981). Nursing in the context of social and cultural systems. In P. Mitchell and A. Loustau, *Concepts basic to nursing*, McGraw-Hill, New York, pp. 37–52.

Churchill, L. (1989). Reviving a distinctive medical ethic. *Hastings Center Report*, May–June, 19(3), pp. 28–34.

Clouser, K. Danner (1978). Bioethics. In Reich, *Encyclopedia of bioethics*, pp. 115–27.

Coady, C. (1996). On regulating ethics. In M. Coady and S. Bloch (eds). *Codes of ethics and the professions*. Melbourne University Press, Melbourne, pp. 269–87.

Dock, L.L. (1900). Ethics — or a Code of Ethics? In L.L. Dock, *Short papers on nursing subjects*, M. Louise Longeway, New York, pp. 37–56 (p. 57 missing).

Eberst, R.M. (1984). Defining health: a multidimensional model. *JOSH* 54 (3), March, pp. 99–104.

Engelhardt, H. Tristram Jr (1986). *The foundations of bioethics*. Oxford University Press, New York.

Fagin, C.M. (1975). Nurses' rights. *American Journal of Nursing* 75 (1), pp. 82–5.

Fineman, M.A. and Thomadsen, N.S. (eds) (1991). *At the boundaries of law: feminism and legal theory*. Routledge, New York and London.

Freckelton, I. (1996). Enforcement of ethics. In M. Coady and S. Bloch (eds).

Fullinwider, R. (1996). Professional codes and moral understanding. In Coady, M. and Bloch, S. (eds), *Codes of ethics and the professions*, Melbourne University Press, Melbourne, pp. 72–87.

Gauthier, D.P. (1986). *Morals by agreement*. Clarendon Press, Oxford.

Goldman, A.H. (1980). *The moral foundations of professional ethics*. Rowman & Littlefield, Totowa, New Jersey.

Grennan, E. (1930). The Somera case. *International Nursing Review* 5, December/January, pp. 325–33.

Gross, E. (1986). Conclusions: what is feminist theory? In C. Pateman and E. Gross (eds). *Feminist challenges: social and political theory*. Allen & Unwin, Sydney, pp. 190–204.

Hare, R.M. (1964). *The language of morals*. Oxford University Press, Oxford.

—— (1981). *Moral thinking*. Clarendon Press, Oxford.

Hart, H.L.A. (1958). Positivism and the separation of law and morals. *Harvard Law Review* 71 (1–4), pp. 593–629.

—— (1961). *The concept of law*. Oxford University Press (Clarendon Law Series), Oxford.

Herman, J.L. (1992). *Trauma and recovery*. Basic Books, New York.

Hobbes, T. (1968 edn). *Leviathan* (reprinted from 1651 edn, with notes by C.B. MacPherson). Penguin Books, Harmondsworth, Middlesex.

Hodge, B. (1993). Uncovering the ethic of care. *Nursing Praxis in New Zealand*, 8(2), pp. 13–22.

Hume, D. (1888 edn). *Treatise of human nature* (edited by L.A. Selby-Bigge). Oxford University Press, London.

In re alleged unfair dismissal of Ms K. Howden by the City of Whittlesea 6/9/90 (Case No 90/3672, Decision D90/1933) IRCV (unreported)).

Johnstone, M-J. (1986). *Professional ethics and the problems of conflict with ordinary morality*. Minor thesis completed in partial fulfilment of the requirements for the Master's Preliminary (Philosophy), Monash University, Melbourne.

—— (1987a). Professional ethics in nursing: a philosophical analysis. *Australian Journal of Advanced Nursing* 4 (3), pp. 12–21.

—— (1987b). Nursing and professional ethics. *Proceedings of the conference 'The Role of the Nurse: Doctors' Handmaiden, Patients' Advocate or What?'*, Centre for Human Bioethics, Monash University, Melbourne.

—— (1988). Ethical issues in planning rehabilitation in patients with advanced cancer. Paper presented at seminar, 'Rehabilitation in patients with advanced cancer — a contradiction in terms?', College of Nursing, Australia, in conjunction with Victorian Association of Hospice Care Programs, Melbourne, 17 October.

—— (1994a). Ethical aspects. In J. Romanini and J. Daly, *Critical care nursing: Australian perspectives*, W.B. Saunders/Baillière Tindall, Sydney.

—— (1994b). *Nursing and the injustices of the law*. W.B. Saunders/Baillière Tindall, Sydney.

—— (1998). *Determining and responding effectively to ethical professional misconduct in nursing: a report to the Nurses Board of Victoria*. Melbourne.

Jonsen, A. (1993). The birth of bioethics. *Hastings Center Report, Special Supplement*, 23(6), S1–S4.

Kairys, D. (ed.) (1982). *The politics of law: a progressive critique*. Pantheon Books, New York.

Kanitsaki, O. (1988). Cancer and informed consent: a cultural perspective. Paper presented at seminar, 'Controversial Ethical Issues in Patients with Cancer', Heidelberg Repatriation General Hospital, Melbourne, 13 October.

—— (1989). Crosscultural sensitivity in palliative care. In P. Hodder and A. Turney (eds), *The creative options of palliative care*, Pandora, Sydney, pp. 13–19.

—— (1993). Transcultural human care: its challenge to and critique of professional nursing care. In D.A. Gaut, *A global agenda for caring*, National League for Nursing Press, New York, pp. 19–45.

—— (1994). Cultural and linguistic diversity. In J. Romanini and J. Daly, *Critical care nursing: Australian perspectives*, W.B. Saunders/Baillière Tindall, Sydney.

Kant, I. (1972 edn). *The moral law* (translated by H. J. Paton). Hutchinson, London.

Keireini, E. (1983). International Council of Nurses, Council of National Representatives Meeting, Brasilia, Brazil, 6–10 June 1983. *New Zealand Nursing Journal* 76 (9), pp. 3–9.

Kelly, L.Y. (1985). *Dimensions of professional nursing*, 5th edn. Macmillan, New York.

Kelman, H.C. and Hamilton, V.L. (1989). *Crimes of obedience*. Yale University Press, New Haven and London.

Kleinman, A. (1980). *Patients and healers in the context of culture*. University of California Press, Berkeley, Los Angeles.

Kuhse, H. (1987). *The sanctity-of-life doctrine in medicine: a critique*. Clarendon Press, Oxford.

Kuhse, H. and Singer, P. (1988). Doctors' practices and attitudes regarding voluntary euthanasia. *Medical Journal of Australia* 148 (June 20), pp. 623–7.

Kultgen, J. (1982). The ideological use of professional codes. *Business and Professional Ethics Journal* 1 (3), Spring, pp. 53–69.

Ladd, J. (1978). The task of ethics. In Reich, *Encyclopedia of bioethics*, pp. 400–7.

Lanham, D. (1993). *Taming death by law*. Longman Professional, Melbourne.

Leininger, M. (ed) (1991). *Ethical and moral dimensions of care*. Wayne State University Press, Detroit.

Lichtenberg, J. (1996). What are codes of ethics for? In M. Coady and S. Bloch (eds). *Codes of ethics and the professions*. Melbourne University Press, Melbourne, pp. 13–27.

Mackie, J.L. (1977). *Ethics: inventing right and wrong*. Penguin Books, Harmondsworth, Middlesex.

Makereti (1986). *The old-time Maori*. New Women's Press, Auckland, New Zealand.

May, W.F. (1983). Code and covenant or philanthropy and contract? In Gorovitz, S., Macklin, R., Jameton, A.L., O'Connor, J.M. and Sherwin, A. (eds), *Moral problems in medicine*, 2nd edn. Prentice Hall, Englewood Cliffs, New Jersey, pp. 83–99.

McNeill, P. (1993). *The ethics and politics of human experimentation*. Cambridge University Press, Cambridge, UK.

Melia, K. (1994). The task of nursing ethics. *Journal of Medical Ethics*, 20(1), pp. 7–11.

Mordacci, R. and Sobel, R. (1998). Health: a comprehensive concept. *Hastings Center Report*, 28(1), pp. 34–37.

Newman, M.A. (1986). *Health as expanding consciousness*. C. V. Mosby, St Louis, Missouri.

Nordenfelt, L. (1987). *On the nature of health*. D. Reidel, Dordrecht.

Pappworth, M. (1967). *Human guinea pigs: experimentation on man*. Penguin Books, Harmondsworth, Middlesex, UK.

Parker, R. (1990). Nurses stories: the search for a relational ethic of care. *Advances in Nursing Science*, 13(1), pp. 31–40.

Peers, Lt Gen. W.R. (1979). *The My Lai Inquiry*. W.W. Norton, New York.

Potter, V. (1971). *Bioethics: bridge to the future*. Prentice-Hall, Englewood Cliffs, New Jersey.

Pyne, R.H. (1981). *Professional discipline in nursing: theory and practice*. Blackwell Scientific Publications, Oxford.

Rawls, J. (1971). *A theory of justice*. Oxford University Press, Oxford.

Rea, K. (1987). Negligence. *Nursing. The Add-on Journal of Clinical Nursing* 3 (14), pp. 533–6.

Reich, W. (ed.) (1978). *Encyclopedia of bioethics*. The Free Press, New York.

—— (1994). The word 'bioethics': its birth and the legacies of those who shaped it. *Kennedy Institute of Ethics Journal* 4(4), pp. 319–35.

—— (1995a). *Introduction to the Encyclopedia of Bioethics*, revised edition. Simon & Schuster Macmillan, New York/Simon & Schuster and Prentice Hall International.

—— (1995b). The word 'bioethics': the struggle over its earliest meanings. *Kennedy Institute of Ethics Journal* 5(1), pp. 19–34.

Romanin, S. (1988). TV telephone poll was unsatisfactory. *The Age*, 11 February, p. 12.

Ross, S.D. (1972). *Moral decision: an introduction to ethics*. Freeman, Cooper & Company, San Francisco, California.

Rowland, R. (1988). *Woman herself: a transdisciplinary perspective on women's identity*. Oxford University Press, Melbourne.

Sax, S. (1984). *A strife of interests: politics and policies in Australian health services*. George Allen & Unwin, Sydney.

Seedhouse, D. (1988), *Ethics: the heart of health care*. John Wiley & Sons, Chichester.

Singer, P. (1994). *Rethinking life & death: the collapse of our traditional ethics*. The Text Publishing Company, Melbourne.

Skene, L. (1996). A legal perspective on codes of ethics. In M. Coady and S. Bloch (eds). *Codes of ethics and the professions*. Melbourne University Press, Melbourne, pp. 111–29.

Stephens, P. (1987). Tolerance of abortion is much wider now. *The Age*, 7 December, p. 5.

Thompson, I., Melia, K. and Boyd, K. (1994). *Nursing ethics, third edition*. Churchill Livingstone, Edinburgh.

Thornton, M. (1990). *The liberal promise: anti-discrimination legislation in Australia*. Oxford University Press, Melbourne.

Toy, M. (1998). Heavy burden on women. *The Age*, 4 February, p. 2.

United Kingdom Central Council for Nursing, Midwifery and Health Visiting [UKCC] (1984). *Code of Professional Conduct for the Nurse, Midwife and Health Visitor*, 2nd edn. UKCC, London.

Veatch, R.M. (1985). Nursing ethics, physician ethics and medical ethics. *Bioethics Reporter* 6 (7), pp. 381–3.

Veatch, R.M. and Fry, S.T. (1987). *Case studies in nursing ethics*. J.B. Lippincott Company, Philadelphia.

Waikato Times (1984a). Waikato Hospital chief says: morphine off limits to trainee. 16 February, p. 3.

—— (1984b). Police to lay no charges. 11 July, p. 1.

Wainer, J. (1989). Report on the pro-abortion march in Washington. *Alive and WEL* (Women's Electoral Lobby) (May), pp. 4–5.

Walton D.N. (1980). The ethical force of definitions. *Journal of Medical Ethics* 6, pp. 16–18.

Waring, M. (1988). *Counting for nothing: what men value and what women are worth*. Allen & Unwin, Port Nicholson Press, Wellington (NZ).

Warnock G.J. (1967). *Contemporary moral philosophy*. Macmillan Education, Basingstoke, UK.

Warthen v Toms River Community Memorial Hospital 488 A 2d 229 (NJ Super AD 1985).

Winslow, G.R. (1984). From loyalty to advocacy: a new metaphor for nursing. *Hastings Center Report* 14 (3), June, pp. 32–40.

With AAP. (1998). Most nurses in NSW support voluntary euthanasia. *Australian Nursing Journal*, 5(8), p. 9.

Chapter 4 Theoretical perspectives informing ethical conduct

Allen, R.E. (ed.) (1966). *Greek philosophy: Thales to Aristotle*. The Free Press, New York.

Anderson, W. Truett. (1990). *Reality isn't what it used to be: Theatrical politics, ready-to-wear religion, global myths, primitive chic, and other wonders of the postmodern world*. Harper San Francisco, New York.

Australian Nurses Journal (1988). A costly misjudgment. Anonymous. *Australian Nurses Journal* 17 (6), December/January, p. 3.

Baier, K. (1978a). Deontological theories. In Reich, W.T. (ed.) (1978). *Encyclopedia of bioethics*. The Free Press, New York, pp. 413–17.

—— (1978b). Teleological theories. In Reich, W.T. (ed.) (1978). *Encyclopedia of bioethics*. The Free Press, New York, pp. 417–21.

Bauman, Z. (1993). *Postmodern ethics*. Blackwell, Oxford UK & Cambridge, Mass.

Beauchamp, T. and Childress, J. (1989). *Principles of biomedical ethics*, 3rd edn. Oxford University Press, New York.

—— (1994). *Principles of biomedical ethics*, 4th edn. Oxford University Press, New York.

Beauchamp, T.L. and Walters, L. (eds) (1982). *Contemporary issues in bioethics*, 2nd edn. Wadsworth, Belmont, California.

Benhabib, S. and Dallmayr, F. (eds)(1990). *The communicative ethics controversy*. The MIT Press, Cambridge, Mass.

Benn, S.I. (1971). Privacy, freedom, and respect for persons. *Nomos* 13 (J.R. Pennock and J.W. Chapman (eds) American Society for Political and Legal Philosophy: Privacy, Artherton Press, New York), pp. 1–21.

Benner, P. (1984). From novice to expert: excellence and power in clinical nursing practice. Addison-Wesley, Nursing Division, Menlo Park, California.

Bentham, J. (1962). An introduction to the principles of morals and legislation (reprinted from 1789 edition). In Warnock, M. (ed.) (1962). *Utilitarianism*. Fontana Library/Collins, London, pp. 33–77.

Blum, L. (1980). *Friendship, altruism and morality*. Routledge & Kegan Paul, London, UK.

—— (1988). Moral exemplars: reflections on Schindler, the Trocmes, and others. *Midwest Studies in Philosophy*, 13, pp. 196–221.

—— (1994). *Moral perception and particularity*. Cambridge University Press, New York.

Blustein, J. (1991). *Care and commitment: taking the personal point of view*. Oxford University Press, New York.

Bohm, D. (1989). Meaning and information. In Pylkkanen, P. (ed), *The search for meaning: the new spirit in science and philosophy*. Crucible (an imprint of The Aquarian Press), Wellingborough, Northamptonshire, pp. 43–85.

Burdekin, B., Guilfoyle, M., and Hall, D. (1993). *Human rights & mental illness: Report of the National Inquiry into the Human Rights of People with Mental Illness*. Australian Government Publishing Service, Canberra.

Clouser, K. Danner. (1995). Common morality as an alternative to principlism. *Kennedy Institute of Ethics Journal*, 5(3), pp. 219–36.

Cortese, A. (1990). *Ethnic ethics: the restructuring of moral theory*. State University of New York Press, Albany.

Curtin, L.L. (1986). The nurse as advocate: a philosophical foundation for nursing. In P. Chinn (ed.), *Ethical issues in nursing*, Aspen System, Rockville, Maryland, pp. 11–20.

Dancy, J. (1993). *Moral reasons*. Blackwell, Oxford, UK.

Davis-Floyd, R. and Arvidson P. Sven (eds). (1997). *Intuition: the inside story. Interdisciplinary perspectives*. Routledge, New York.

Dworkin, R. (1977). *Taking rights seriously*. Duckworth, London.

Elliott, C. (1992). Where ethics comes from and what to do about it. *Hastings Center Report*, 22 (4), pp. 28–35.

Engelhardt, H. Tristram Jr (1986). *The foundations of bioethics*. Oxford University Press, New York.

Engelhardt, H. Tristram. (1996). *The Foundations of bioethics*, 2nd edn. Oxford University Press, New York.

Feinberg, J. (1978). Rights. In Reich, W.T. (ed.) (1978). *Encyclopedia of bioethics*. The Free Press, New York, pp. 1507–11.

—— (1979). The rights of animals and unborn generations. In R.A. Wasserstrom (ed.), *Today's moral problems*, Macmillan, New York, pp. 581–601.

—— (1984). *Harm to others: the moral limits of the criminal law*. Oxford University Press, New York.

Fletcher, J. (1966). *Situation ethics*. SCM Press, Bloomsbury Street, London.

Flew, A. (ed.) (1979). A *dictionary of philosophy*. Pan Books, London.

Frankena, W.K. (1973). *Ethics*, 2nd edn. Prentice Hall, Englewood Cliffs, New Jersey.

Gert, B. (1984). Moral theory and applied ethics. *The Monist* 67 (4), October, pp. 532–48.

Gillam, L. (ed.) (1989). *Proceedings of the conference 'The Fetus as Tissue Donor: Use or Abuse?'*, Centre for Human Bioethics, Monash university, Melbourne.

Goldberg, P. (1983). *The intuitive edge*. Jeremy Tarcher, Los Angeles.

Grennan, E. (1930). The Somera case. *International Nursing Review* 5 (December/January), pp. 325–33.

Habermas, J. (1990). *Moral consciousness and communicative action*. The MIT Press, Cambridge, Mass.

Hare, R.M. (1981). *Moral thinking: its levels, method and point*. Clarendon Press, Oxford.

Harmon, G. (1977). *The nature of morality*. Oxford University Press, New York.

Harrison, J. (1954). When is a principle a moral principle? *Aristotelian Society*, supplementary vol. 28, July 9–11, pp. 111–34.

Hinman, L. (1994). *Ethics: a pluralistic approach to moral theory*. Harcourt Brace Jovanovich, Fort Worth, Texas.

Hobbes, T. (1968). *Leviathan* (reprinted from 1651 edition with notes by C.B. Macpherson). Pelican Books, Harmondsworth, Middlesex.

Hughes, J. (1995). Ultimate justification: Wittgenstein and medical ethics. *Journal of Medical Ethics*, 21, pp. 25–30.

Hume, D. (1888). *A treatise of human nature*. Clarendon Press, Oxford.

—— (1947). Of the original contract (reprinted from 1748 edition). In Sir Ernest Barker, *Social contract*, Oxford University Press, London, pp. 209–36.

International Council of Nurses. (1973). *Code for Nurses*. International Council of Nurses, Geneva.

Johnston, P. (1989). *Wittgenstein and moral philosophy*. Routledge, London, UK.

Johnstone, M-J. (1987). Ethics in focus. *Australian Nurses Journal* 17 (3), September, pp. 41–2.

—— (1990). *Ethics and nursing: Module 601E — An external course for registered nurses*. Royal College of Nursing, Australia, Melbourne.

—— (1993). The development of nursing ethics in Australia: an historical overview. *Papers of the First National Nursing History Conference: Australian nursing ... the story*, Royal College of Nursing, Australia, Melbourne, pp. 33–51.

—— (1994). *Nursing and the injustices of the law*. W.B. Saunders/Baillière Tindall, Sydney.

—— (1998). *Determining and responding effectively to ethical professional misconduct in nursing: a report to the Nurses Board of Victoria*, Melbourne.

Jonsen, A. (1995). Casuistry: an alternative or complement to principles? *Kennedy Institute of Ethics Journal*, 5(3), pp. 237–51.

Jonsen, A. and Toulmin, S. (1988). *The abuse of casuistry: a history pf moral reasoning*. University of California Press, Berkeley and Los Angeles, California.

Kant, I. (1972). The moral law (translated by H.J. Paton). Hutchinson University Library, London.

Klostermaier, K. (1998). The truth & the goodness of nature. *The Quest*, 86(2), Spring, pp. 34–41, 52–3.

Kopelman, L. (1995). Conceptual and moral disputes about futile and useful treatments. *Journal of Medicine and Philosophy*, 20(2), pp. 109–21.

Kruschwitz, R. and Roberts, R. (eds) (1987). *The virtues: contemporary essays on moral character*. Wadsworth Publishing Co, Belmont, California.

Leininger, M. (1990). Culture: the conspicuous missing link to understand ethical and moral dimensions of human care. In M. Leininger (ed.), *Ethical and moral dimensions of care*, Wayne State University Press, Detroit, pp. 49–66.

Locke, J. (1947). An essay concerning the true, original extent and end of civil government (reprinted from 1690 edition). In Sir Ernest Barker, *Social contract*, Oxford University Press, London. pp. 3–206.

MacIntyre, A. (1966). *A short history of ethics*. Routledge & Kegan Paul, London.

—— (1985). *After virtue: a study in moral theory*, 2nd edn. Duckworth, London.

—— (1988). Whose justice? Which rationality? Duckworth, London.

Mackie, J.L. (1962). Omnipotence. *Sophia* 1 (2), July, pp. 14–25.

Martin, R. and Nickel, J.W. (1980). Recent work on the concepts of rights. *American Philosophical Quarterly* 17 (3), July, pp. 165–80.

McNaughton, D. (1988). *Moral vision: an introduction to ethics*. Basil Blackwell, Oxford.

Meinke, S.A. (1989). *Anencephalic infants as potential organ sources: ethical and legal issues: Scope Notes 12*. Kennedy Institute of Ethics, Georgetown University, Washington DC.

Mill, J.S. (1962a). On liberty (reprinted from 1859 edn). In Warnock, M. (ed.) (1962). *Utilitarianism*. Fontana Library/Collins, London. pp. 126–250.

—— (1962b). Utilitarianism (reprinted from 1861 edn). In Warnock, M. (ed.) (1962). *Utilitarianism*. Fontana Library/Collins, London. pp. 251–342.

Moody, H. (1992). *Ethics in an aging society*. The John Hopkins University Press, Baltimore.

Moreno, J. (1995). *Deciding together: bioethics and moral consensus*. Oxford University Press, New York.

Musgrave, C.F. (1987). The ethical and legal implications of hospice care. *Cancer Nursing* 10 (4), pp. 183–9.

Newton, L. (1981). Lawgiving for professional life: reflections on the place of the professional code. *Business and Professional Ethics Journal* 1 (1), pp. 41–53.

Nielsen, K. (1989). *Why be moral?* Prometheus Books, Buffalo, New York.

Outka, G. (1972). *Agape: an ethical analysis.* Yale University Press, New Haven and London.

Pellegrino, E. (1995). Toward a virtue-based normative ethics for the health professions. *Kennedy Institute of Ethics Journal*, 5(3), pp. 253–77.

Pence, G. (1984). Recent work on virtues. *American Philosophical Quarterly*, 21(4), pp. 281–97.

—— (1991). Virtue theory. In Singer, P. (ed), *A companion to ethics.* Basil Blackwell, Oxford, UK, pp. 249–58.

Plato (1966). Euthyphro. In Allen, R.E. (ed), *Greek philosophy: Thales to Aristotle.* The Free Press, New York. pp. 59–74.

Pylkkanen, P. (ed). (1989). *The search for meaning: the new spirit in science and philosophy.* Crucible (an imprint of The Aquarian Press), Wellingborough, Northamptonshire.

Rasmussen, D. (ed.) (1990). *Universalism vs communitarianism: contemporary debates in ethics.* The MIT Press, Cambridge, Mass.

Rawls, J. (1971). *A theory of justice.* Oxford University Press, Oxford.

Reich, W.T. (ed.) (1978). *Encyclopedia of bioethics.* The Free Press, New York.

Ross, W.D. (1930). *The right and the good.* Clarendon Press, Oxford.

Rousseau, J.-J. (1947). The social contract (reprinted from 1762 edition). In Sir Ernest Barker, *Social contract*, Oxford University Press, London, pp. 239–440.

Sanders, K. and Moore, B. (eds) (1991). *Anencephalics, infants and brain death treatment options and the issue of organ donation. Proceedings of Consensus Development Conference.* Law Reform Commission of Victoria, Royal Children's Hospital, Melbourne, and Australian Association of Paediatric Teaching Centres, Melbourne.

Senate Legal and Constitutional Committee. 1997. *Consideration of Legislation Referred to the Committee: Euthanasia Laws Bill 1996.* Commonwealth of Australia, Canberra.

Singer, p. (1979a). Famine, affluence, and morality. In R.A. Wasserstrom (ed.), *Today's moral problems*, Macmillan, New York, pp. 561–72.

—— (1979b). *Practical ethics.* Cambridge University Press, Cambridge.

—— (ed.) (1991). *A companion to ethics.* Basil Blackwell, Oxford.

Smart, J.J.C. and Williams, B. (1973). *Utilitarianism: for and against.* Cambridge University Press, Cambridge.

Solomon, R.C. and Murphy, M.C. (eds) (1990). *What is justice? Classic and contemporary readings.* Oxford University Press, New York.

Solomon, W.D. (1978). Rules and principles. In Reich, W.T. (ed.) (1978). *Encyclopedia of bioethics.* The Free Press, New York, pp. 407–12.

Stevenson, C.L. (1944). Ethics and language. Yale University Press, New Haven.

Stout, J. (1988). *Ethics after Babel: the languages of morals and their discontents.* Beacon Press, Boston.

Swanton, C. (1987). The rationality of ethical intuitionism. *Australasian Journal of Philosophy* 65 (2), June, pp. 172–81.

United Nations (1959). *Declaration of the Rights of the Child.* United Nations, New York.

—— (1978). *The International Bill of Human Rights.* United Nations, New York.

Urmson, J.O. (1958). Saints and heroes. First published in Melden, A.I. (ed.), *Essays in moral philosophy*, University of Washington Press, pp. 198–216; reprinted in J. Feinberg (1969), *Moral concepts*, Oxford University Press, Oxford, pp. 60–73.

—— (1975). A defence of intuitionism. *Proceedings of the Aristotelian Society* 65, pp. 111–19.

Vardey, L. (1995). *Mother Teresa: a simple path.* Rider, London.

Vaughan, F.E. (1979). *Awakening intuition.* Anchor Books/Doubleday, New York.

Waithe, M.E. (ed.) (1987). *A history of women philosophers. Volume 1: 600 BC–500 AD.* Martinus Nijhoff, Dordrecht.

Walton, D. (1986), *Courage: a philosophical investigation.* University of California Press, Berkeley and Los Angeles, California.

Walzer, M. (1987). *Interpretation and social criticism.* Harvard University Press, Cambridge, Mass.

Warnock, G.J. (1967). *Contemporary moral philosophy.* Macmillan Education, Houndmills, Basingstoke, Hampshire.

Warnock, M. (ed.) (1962). *Utilitarianism.* Fontana Library/Collins, London.

Williams, B. (1985). *Ethics and the limits of philosophy.* Fontana and Collins, London.

Chapter 5 A feminist perspective on ethics and bioethics

Alec, M. (1986). *Hypatia's heritage.* The Women's Press, London.

Allmark, P. (1995). Can there be an ethics of care? *Journal of Medical Ethics,* 21(1), pp. 19–24.

Andolsen, B. Hilkert, Gudorf, C.E. and Pellauer, M.D. (eds) (1987). *Women's consciousness, women's conscience.* Harper & Row, San Francisco (first published by Winston Press, 1985).

Aristotle (1957 edn). *The politics.* Penguin Books, Harmondsworth, Middlesex.

—— (1976 edn). *Ethics.* Penguin Books, Harmondsworth, Middlesex.

Baier, A. (1985). *Postures of the mind: essays on mind and morals.* Methuen, London. Chapter 6: Caring about caring: a reply to Frankfurt.

Benner, P. (1984). *From novice to expert.* Addison-Wesley, Menlo Park, California.

Benner, P. and Wrubel, J. (1989). *The primacy of caring.* Addison-Wesley, Menlo Park, California.

Berkowitz, M. (1982). The role of discussion in ethics training. *Topics in Clinical Nursing* 4 (1), April, pp. 33–48.

Bishop, A.H. and Scudder, J.R. (1991). *Nursing: the practice of caring.* National League for Nursing Press, New York.

Blum, L. (1980). *Friendship, altruism and morality.* Routledge & Kegan Paul, London.

—— (1994). *Moral perception and particularity.* Cambridge University Press, New York.

Bok, S. (1980). *Lying: moral choice in public and private life.* Quartet Books, London.

Bowden, P. (1994). The ethics of nursing care and 'the ethic of care'. *Nursing Inquiry,* 2, pp. 10–21.

Brabeck, M.M. (ed.) (1989). *Who cares? Theory, research, and educational implications of the ethic of care.* Praeger, New York.

Braidotti, R. (1986). Ethics revisited: Women and/in philosophy. In C. Pateman and E. Gross (eds) (1986), *Feminist challenges,* Allen & Unwin, Sydney.

Bridston, E. (1982). An educational strategy for enhancement of moral–ethical decision making. *Topics in Clinical Nursing* 4 (1), April, pp. 57–65.

Broughton, J.M. (1983). Women's rationality and men's virtues: a critique of gender dualism in Gilligan's theory of moral development. *Social Research* 50 (3), Autumn, pp. 597–642.

Brown, J.M., Kitson, A.L. and McKnight, T.J. (1992). *Challenges in caring: explorations in nursing and ethics.* Chapman & Hall, London.

Card, C. (ed.) (1991). *Feminist ethics.* University of Kansas Press, Lawrence, Kansas.

Carper, B. (1986). The ethics of caring. In P. Chinn (ed.), *Ethical issues in nursing,* Aspen Systems, Rockville, Maryland.

Ching, M. (1993). The use of touch in nursing practice. *Australian Journal of Advanced Nursing,* 10(4), pp. 4–9.

Chinn, P.L. (ed.) (1991). *Anthology on caring.* National League for Nursing Press, New York.

Code, L. (1991). *What can she know? Feminist theory and the construction of knowledge.* Cornell University Press, Ithaca and London.

Code, L., Mullett, S. and Overall, C. (eds) (1988). *Feminist perspectives: philosophical essays on methods and morals.* University of Toronto Press, Toronto.

Cole, E.B. and Coultrap-McQuin, S. (eds) (1992). *Explorations in feminist ethics: theory and practice.* Indiana University Press, Bloomington and Indianapolis.

Connelly, R. (1991). Nursing responsibility for the placebo effect. *Journal of Medicine and Philosophy,* 16(3), pp. 325–41.

Cooper, M.C. (1991). Principle-orientated ethics and the ethic of care: a creative tension. *Advances in Nursing Science* 14 (2), pp. 22–31.

Cortese, A. (1990). *Ethnic ethics: the restructuring of moral theory.* State University of New York Press, Albany.

Crittenden, B. (1979). The limitations of morality as justice in Kohlberg's theory. In D.B. Cochrane, C.M. Hamm and A.C. Kazepides (eds), *The domain of moral education,* Paulist Press, New York, pp. 251–66.

Curzer, H. (1993). Is care a virtue for health care professionals. *Journal of Medicine and Philosophy,* 18(1), pp. 51–69.

Damasio, A. (1994). *Descartes error: emotion, reason, and the human brain.* Avon Books, New York.

Daniels, N. (1984). Understanding physician power: a review of the social transformation of American medicine. *Philosophy and Public Affairs* 13 (4), Fall, pp. 347–57.

de Bono, E. (1990). I *am right — you are wrong.* Penguin, London.

Dossey, L. (1991). *Meaning & medicine.* Bantam Books, New York.

—— (1993). *Healing words: the power of prayer and the practice of medicine.* Harper San Francisco, New York.

Drengson, A.R. (1985). Critical notice. *Canadian Journal of Philosophy* 15 (1), March, pp. 111–31.

Edwards, J.C. (1982). *Ethics without philosophy: Wittgenstein and the moral life.* University Presses of Florida, Tampa.

Elliott, C. (1992). Where ethics comes from and what to do about it. *Hastings Center Report* 22 (4), pp. 28–35.

Engelhardt, H. Tristram Jr (1986). *The foundations of bioethics.* Oxford University Press, New York.

Fisher, B. and Tronto, J. (1990). Toward a feminist theory of caring. In E.K. Abel and M.K. Nelson (eds), *Circles of care, work and identity in women's lives.* State University of New York Press, Albany, pp. 35–62.

Flanagan, O. and Jackson, K. (1987). Justice, care, and gender: the Kohlberg–Gilligan debate revisited. *Ethics* 97, April, pp. 622–37.

Frazer, E., Hornsby, J. and Lovibond, S. (eds) (1992). *Ethics: a feminist reader.* Blackwell, Oxford.

Fry, S. (1988a). The ethic of caring: can it survive in nursing? *Nursing Outlook* 36 (1), p. 48.

—— (1988b). Response to 'Virtue, ethics, caring and nursing'. *Scholarly Inquiry for Nursing Practice: An International Journal* 2 (2), pp. 97–101.

—— (1989a). Toward a theory of nursing ethics. *Advances in Nursing Science* 11 (4), pp. 9–22.

—— (1989b). The role of caring in a theory of nursing ethics. *Hypatia* 4 (2). Reprinted in Holmes, H.B. and Purdy, L.M. (eds) (1992). *Feminist perspectives in medical ethics.* Indiana University Press, Bloomington and Indianapolis, pp. 93–106.

Gastmans, C., Dierckx de Casterle, B., and Schotsmans, P. (1998). Nursing considered as moral practice: a philosophical-ethical interpretation of nursing. *Kennedy Institute of Ethics Journal,* 8(1), pp. 43–69.

Gatens, M. (1986). Feminism, philosophy and riddles without answers. In C.O. Pateman and E. Gross (eds), *Feminist challenges,* Allen & Unwin, Sydney, pp. 13–29.

Gaut, D.A. (ed.) (1992). *The presence of caring in nursing.* National League for Nursing Press, New York.

Gaut, D.A. and Leininger, M.M. (eds) (1991). *Caring: the compassionate healer.* National League for Nursing Press, New York.

Gauthier, D. (1986). *Morals by agreement.* Clarendon Press, Oxford.

Geary, P. and Hawkins, J. (1991). To cure, to care, or to heal. *Nursing Forum,* 26(3), pp. 5–13.

Gibson, M. (1976). Rationality. *Philosophy and Public Affairs* 6 (3), pp. 193–225.

Gilligan, C. (1982). *In a different voice: psychological theory and women's development.* Harvard University Press, Cambridge, Mass. (See in particular Chapter 3, 'Concepts of self and morality'.)

—— (1987). Moral orientation and moral development. In Kittay, E.F. and Meyers, D.T. (eds) (1987). *Women and moral theory*. Rowman & Littlefleld, Totowa, New Jersey, pp. 19–33.

Grimshaw, J. (1986). *Feminist philosophers*. Wheatsheaf Books, Brighton, Sussex.

Harding, S. (ed.) (1987). *Feminism and methodology: social science issues*. Indiana University Press, Bloomington and Indianapolis, and Open University Press, Milton Keynes.

—— (ed.) (1991). *Whose Science? Whose knowledge? Thinking from women's lives*. Open University Press, Milton Keynes.

Harding, S. and Hintikka, M.B. (eds) (1983). *Discovering reality*. D. Reidel, Dordrecht.

Hare, R.M. (1981). *Moral thinking*. Clarendon Press, Oxford.

Hekman, S. (1995). *Moral voices, moral selves: Carol Gilligan and feminist moral theory*. Polity Press, Cambridge, UK.

Held, V. (1987). Feminism and moral theory. In Kittay, E.F. and Meyers, D.T. (eds) (1987). *Women and moral theory*. Rowman & Littlefleld, Totowa, New Jersey, pp. 111–28.

Hoagland, S.L. (1988). *Lesbian ethics: toward new value*. Institute of Lesbian Studies, Palo Alto, California.

Hodge, B. (1993a). Practising within an ethic of care. *Newsletter, Bioethics Research Centre*, 2(3), September, pp. 6–8 (Otago University, Dunedin, Wellington NZ).

—— (1993b). Uncovering the ethic of care. *Nursing Praxis in New Zealand*, 8(2), pp. 13–22.

Holmes, H.B. and Purdy, L.M. (eds) (1992). *Feminist perspectives in medical ethics*. Indiana University Press, Bloomington and Indianapolis.

Hutton, B. (1987). The oft-forgotten grandmothers of Western philosophy. *The Age*, 23 September, p. 20.

Jaggar, A.M. (1983). *Feminist politics and human nature*. Rowman & Allanheld, Totowa, New Jersey.

Johnstone, M.-J. (1994). *Nursing and the injustices of the law*. W.B. Saunders/Baillière Tindall, Sydney.

Kanitsaki, O. (1996). Care and caring in a multicultural society: a critical examination. Paper presented at *Patterns of Caring: Universal Connections. 18th International Association of Human Caring Research Conference*. April. Mayo Medical Center, Rochester, Minnesota, USA.

Katzenstein, M.F. and Laitin, D.D. (1987). Politics, feminism, and the ethics of caring. In Kittay, E.F. and Meyers, D.T. (eds) (1987). *Women and moral theory*. Rowman & Littlefleld, Totowa, New Jersey, pp. 261–81.

Kittay, E.F. and Meyers, D.T. (eds) (1987). *Women and moral theory*. Rowman & Littlefleld, Totowa, New Jersey.

Klimek, M. (1990). Virtue, ethics, and care: developing the personal dimension of caring in nursing education. In Leininger, M.M. and Watson, J. (eds) (1990). *The caring imperative in education*. National League for Nursing Press, New York, pp. 177–87.

Kohlberg, L. (1981). *The philosophy of moral development: moral stages and the idea of justice*. Harper & Row, San Francisco.

Larson, P. and Ferketich, S. (1993). Patients' satisfaction with nurses' caring during hospitalisation. *Western Journal of Nursing Research*, 15(6), pp. 690–707.

Leftwich, R. (1993). Care and cure as healing processes in nursing. *Nursing Forum*, 28(3), pp. 13–17.

Leininger, M.M. (ed.) (1988). *Care: the essence of nursing and health*. Wayne State University Press, Detroit.

—— (ed.) (1990a). *Ethical and moral dimensions of care*. Wayne State University Press, Detroit.

—— (1990b). Culture: the conspicuous missing link to understand ethical and moral dimensions of human care. In Leininger 1990a, pp. 49–66.

—— (ed.) (1991). *Culture care diversity and universality: a theory of nursing*. National League for Nursing Press, New York.

Leininger, M.M. and Watson, J. (eds) (1990). *The caring imperative in education*. National League for Nursing Press, New York.

Little, M. (1996). Why a feminist approach to bioethics? *Kennedy Institute of Ethics Journal*, 6(1), pp. 1–18.

Lloyd, G. (1984). *The man of reason: 'male' and 'female' in Western philosophy*. Methuen, London.

MacIntyre, A. (1985). *After virtue: a study in moral theory*. Duckworth, London.

Malcolm, N. (1958). *Ludwig Wittgenstein: a memoir*. Oxford University Press, London.

Marshall, P.A. (1992). Anthropology and bioethics. *Medical Anthropology Quarterly* 6 (1), pp. 49–73.

Matthews, C. (1991). *Sophia goddess of wisdom: the divine feminine from black goddess to world-soul*. Mandala (an imprint of HarperCollins), London, UK.

McAlister, L. Lopez (ed.) (1989). *Hypatia*. Special issue 4 (1), Spring, *The history of women in philosophy*.

McMillan, C. (1982). *Women, reason and nature: some philosophical problems with feminism*. Princeton University Press, Princeton, New Jersey.

Midgley, M. (1980). *Beast and man*. Methuen, London.

Midgley, M. and Hughes, J. (1983). *Women's choices*. Weidenfeld & Nicolson, London.

Mill, J.S. (1929 edn). The subjection of women. In M. Wollstonecraft, *A vindication of the rights of woman*, and J.S. Mill, *The subjection of women*, Everyman's Library, London, pp. 219–317.

—— (1962). Utilitarianism (reprinted from 1861 edn). In Warnock, M. (ed.) (1962). *Utilitarianism*. Fontana Library/Collins, London.

Moore, G.E. (1903). *Principia ethica*. Cambridge University Press, London.

Moore, N. and Komras, H. (1993). *Patient-focused healing: integrating caring and curing in health care*. Jossey-Bass Publishers, San Francisco.

Morgan, K.P. (1988). Women and moral madness. In Code, L., Mullett, S. and Overall, C. (eds) (1988). *Feminist perspectives: philosophical essays on methods and morals*. University of Toronto Press, Toronto, pp. 146–67.

Moulton, J. (1983). A paradigm of philosophy: the adversary method. In Harding, S. and Hintikka, M.B. (eds) (1983). *Discovering reality*. D. Reidel, Dordrecht, pp. 149–64.

Mullett, S. (1988). Shifting perspectives: a new approach to ethics. In Code, L., Mullett, S. and Overall, C. (eds) (1988). *Feminist perspectives: philosophical essays on methods and morals*. University of Toronto Press, Toronto, pp. 109–26.

Nicolayev, J. and Phillips, D.C. (1979). On assessing Kohlberg's stage theory of moral development. In Cochrane, D.B., Hamm, C.M. and Kazepides A.C. (eds), *The domain of moral education*. Paulist Press, New York, pp. 231–50.

Nietzsche, F. (1972 edn). *Beyond good and evil*. Penguin Books, Harmondsworth, Middlesex.

Noddings, N. (1984). *Caring: a feminine approach to ethics and moral education*. University of California Press, Berkeley.

O'Brien, M. (1981). *The politics of reproduction*. Routledge & Kegan Paul, London, UK.

Oliver, N. (1990). Nurse, are you a healer? *Nursing Forum*, 25(2), pp. 11–14.

Parsons, S. (1986). Feminism and moral reasoning. *Australasian Journal of Philosophy*. Supplement to vol. 64, June, pp. 75–90.

Pateman, C. (1989). *The disorder of woman*. Polity Press, Cambridge.

Pellegrino, E. (1995). Toward a virtue-based normative ethics for the health professions. *Kennedy Institute of Ethics Journal*, 5(3), pp. 253–77.

Peterson, C. and Bossio, L. (1991). *Health and optimism*. The Free Press, New York.

Plato (1955 edn). *The Republic*. Penguin Classics, Harmondsworth, Middlesex.

Porter, E. (1991). *Women and moral identity*. Allen & Unwin, Sydney, pp. 19–44.

Puka, B. (1989). The liberation of caring: a different voice for Gilligan's 'different voice'. In Brabeck, M. (ed), *Who cares? Theory, research, and educational implications of the ethic of care*. Praeger, New York.

Rachels, J. (1988). Can ethics provide answers? In D. Rosenthal and F. Shehadi (eds). *Applied ethics and ethical theory*. University of Utah Press, Salt Lake City, pp. 3–24.

Rawls, J. (1971). *A theory of justice*. Oxford University Press, Oxford.

Rich, A. (1979). *On lies, secrets and silence: selected prose 1966–1978*. Virago Press, London.

Roach, Sister M. Simone (1987). *The human act of caring: a blueprint for the health professions*. Canadian Hospital Association, Ottawa, Ontario.

Robb, C.S. (1985). A framework for feminist ethics. In Andolsen, B. Hilkert, Gudorf, C.E. and Pellauer, M.D. (eds) (1987). *Women's consciousness, women's conscience*. Harper & Row, San Francisco, pp. 211–33.

Rousseau, J.-J. (1911 edn). *Emile*. Everyman's Library, London.

Segal, L. (1987). *Is the future female? Troubled thoughts on contemporary feminism*. Virago Press, London.

Sherwin, S. (1992). *No longer patient: feminist ethics & health care*. Temple University Press, Philadelphia.

—— (1996). Feminism and bioethics. In Wolf, S. (ed.) *Feminism & bioethics: beyond reproduction*. Oxford University Press, New York, pp. 47–66.

Singer, P. (ed.) (1991). *A companion to ethics*. Basil Blackwell, Oxford.

Spender, D. (1988). *Women of ideas, and what men have done to them*. Pandora Press, London (first published by Routledge & Kegan Paul, 1982). (See in particular essay on Harriet Taylor [1807–58], pp. 184–96.)

Starck, P. and McGovern, J. (eds) (1992). *The hidden dimension of illness: human suffering*. National League for Nursing Press, New York.

Stout, J. (1988). *Ethics after Babel: the languages of morals and their discontents*. Beacon Press, Boston.

Swanson, K. (1993). Nursing as informed caring for the wellbeing of others. *IMAGE: Journal of Nursing Scholarship*, 25(4), pp. 352–57.

Taylor, B. (1995). Nursing as healing work. *Contemporary Nurse*, 4(3), pp. 100–106.

Taylor, C. (1998). Reflections on 'nursing considered as moral practice'. *Kennedy Institute of Ethics Journal*, 8(1), pp. 71–82.

Tronto, J.C. (1993). *Moral boundaries: a political argument for an ethic of care*. Routledge, New York/London.

Twomey, J.G. (1989). Analysis of the claim to distinct nursing ethics: normative and non-normative approaches. *Advances in Nursing Science*, 11 (3), pp. 25–32.

Von Wright, G.H. (1958). Biographical sketch. In Malcolm, N. *Ludwig Wittgenstein: a memoir*. Oxford University Press, London.

Waithe, M. (ed)(1995). *A history of women philosophers. Volume 4: 1900-today*. Kluwer Academic Publishers, Dordrecht.

Waithe, M.E. (ed.) (1987). *A history of women philosophers*. Volume I: *Ancient women philosophers, 600 BC–500 AD*, Martinus Nijhoff, Dordrecht.

—— (ed.) (1989a). *A history of women philosophers*. Volume II: *Medieval, Renaissance and Enlightenment women philosophers, AD 500–1600*. Kluwer Academic Publishers, Dordrecht.

—— (1989b). Twenty-three hundred years of women philosophers: toward a gender indifferentiated moral theory. In Brabeck, M.M. (ed.), *Who cares? Theory, research, and educational implications of the ethic of care*. Praeger, New York, pp. 3–18.

—— (ed.) (1991). *A history of women philosophers*. Volume III: *Modern women philosophers, 1600–1900*. Kluwer Academic Publishers, Dordrecht.

Walker, M.U. (1992). Moral understanding: alternative 'epistemology' for a feminist ethics. In Cole, E.B. and Coultrap-McQuin, S. (eds). *Explorations in feminist ethics: theory and practice*. Indiana University Press, Bloomington and Indianapolis, pp. 165–75.

Walzer, M. (1987). *Interpretation and social criticism*. Harvard University Press, Cambridge, Mass.

Watson, J. (1985a). *Nursing: the philosophy and science of caring*. Colorado Associated University Press, Boulder, Colorado.

—— (1985b). *Nursing: human science and human care: a theory of nursing*. Appleton-Century-Crofts, Norwalk, Connecticut.

Webb, S. (1988). Is the hospital system sick? *Sunday Examiner*, Tasmania, 19 June, p. 6.

Wertheimer, M. (1990). Separate roles for doctors and nurses need to be recognised. *Medicine* 2 (7), 16 April, p. 11.

Williams, B. (1972). *Morality: an introduction to ethics*. Cambridge University Press, Cambridge.

—— (1981). *Moral luck*. Cambridge University Press, Cambridge.

—— (1985). *Ethics and the limits of philosophy*. Fontana/Collins, London.

Wittgenstein, L. (1965 edn). A lecture on ethics. *Philosophical Review* 74, January, pp. 3–12.

Wolf, S. (1996a). Gender and feminism in ethics. In Wolf, S. (ed), *Feminism & bioethics: beyond reproduction*. Oxford University Press, New York, pp. 3–43.

—— (ed). (1996b). *Feminism & bioethics: beyond reproduction*. Oxford University Press, New York.

Wollstonecraft, M. (1929 edn). A vindication of the rights of woman. In Wollstonecraft, M., *A vindication of the rights of woman*, and J.S. Mill, *The subjection of women*, Everyman's Library, London, pp. 3–215.

Chapter 6   A transcultural perspective on ethics and bioethics

Bauman, Z. (1993). *Postmodern ethics*. Blackwell, Cambridge, Mass.

Beals, A.R. (1979). *Culture in process*. Holt, Rinehart & Winston, New York.

Beauchamp, T.L. and Childress, J.F. (1989). *Principles of biomedical ethics*, 3rd edn. Oxford University Press, New York.

—— (1994). *Principles of biomedical ethics*, 4th edn. Oxford University Press, New York.

Benhabib, S. and Dallmayr, F. (eds) (1990). *The communicative ethics controversy*. MIT Press, Cambridge, Mass.

Boulware-Miller, K. (1985). Female circumcision: challenges to the practice as a human rights violation. *Harvard Women's Law Journal*, 8, pp. 155–77.

Brink, D.O. (1989). *Moral realism and the foundations of ethics*. Cambridge University Press, Cambridge.

Bullivant, B.M. (1981). *Race, ethnicity and curriculum*. Macmillan, Melbourne.

—— (1984). *Pluralism, cultural maintenance and evolution*. Bank House, Clevedon, Avon.

Chopra, D. (1989). *Quantum healing*. Bantam Books, New York.

Cohen, Y.A. (1968). *Man in adaptation: the cultural present*. Aldine, Chicago.

Cortese, A. (1990). *Ethnic ethics: the restructuring of moral theory*. State University of New York Press, Albany.

Dalla-Vorgia, P., Katsouyanni, K., Garanis, T.N., Touloumi, G., Drogari, P. and Koutselinis, A. (1992). Attitudes of a Mediterranean population to the truth-telling issue. *Journal of Medical Ethics* 18 (2), pp. 67–74.

Dancy, J. (1993). *Moral reasons*. Blackwell, Oxford, UK and Cambridge, USA.

Dossey, L. (1982). *Space, time and medicine*. New Science Library, Boston, Mass.

—— (1991). *Meaning and medicine*. Bantam Books, New York.

Elliott, C. (1992). Where ethics comes from and what to do about it. *Hastings Center Report* 22 (4), pp. 28–35.

Fasching, D. (1993). *The ethical challenge of Auschwitz and Hiroshima: apocalypse or utopia?* State University of New York Press, Albany.

Fieldhouse, P. (1986). *Food and nutrition: customs and culture*. Croom Helm, London.

Gergen, K. (1994). *Realities and relationships: soundings in social constructions*. Harvard University Press, Cambridge, Mass.

Gilmore, K. (nd). Proforma letter from the National Director of Amnesty International Australia, addressed to 'Friends' (distributed with an attached information leaflet on female genital mutilation via membership list, April, 1998).

Helman, C. (1990). *Culture, health and illness*. Wright, London.

James, S. (1994). Reconciling international human rights and cultural relativism: the case of female circumcision. *Bioethics*, 8(1), pp. 1–26.

Johnstone, M.-J. and Kanitsaki, O. (1991). Some moral implications of cultural and linguistic diversity in health care. *Bioethics News* 10 (2), pp. 22–32.

Kanitsaki, O. (1989a). Health–illness–suffering experiences of a sample of Greek-born members of 12 Greek–Australian families living in Melbourne. Minor thesis completed in partial fulfilment of the requirements for the Degree of Master of Educational Studies, Faculty of Education, Monash University, Melbourne.

—— (1989b). Cross-cultural sensitivity in palliative care. In P. Hodder and A. Turley (eds), *The creative option of palliative care: a manual for health professionals*, Melbourne City Mission, Melbourne, pp. 68–71.

—— (1992). Meeting the challenge of patients' rights: a transcultural perspective. *Proceedings of Fourth Victorian State Conference on Nursing Law and Ethics: 'Meeting the challenge of patients rights — issues for the 1990s'*, held Dallas Brooks Hall, 20 November. Faculty of Nursing, RMIT, Bundoora, Melbourne.

—— (1993). Transcultural human care: its challenge and critique of professional nursing care. In Gaut, D. (ed.), *A global agenda for caring*. National League for Nursing Press, New York, pp. 19–45.

—— (1994). Cultural and linguistic diversity. In Romanini, J. and Daly, J. (eds), *Critical care nursing: Australian perspectives*, W.B. Saunders/Baillière Tindall, Sydney.

—— (1996). Care and caring in a multicultural society: a critical examination. Paper presented at *Patterns of Caring: Universal Connections. 18th International Association of Human Caring Research Conference*. April. Mayo Medical Center, Rochester, Minnesota, USA.

Kluckhohn, C. (1962). *Culture and behavior*. The Free Press, New York.

Kuczewski, M. (1996). Reconceiving the family: the process of consent in medical decision making. *Hastings Center Report*, 26(2), pp. 30–7.

Leininger, M. (1990). Culture: the conspicuous missing link to understanding ethical and moral dimensions of human care. In M. Leininger (ed.), *Ethical and moral dimensions of care*, Wayne State University Press, Detroit, pp. 49–66.

—— (ed.) (1991). *Culture care diversity and universality: a theory of nursing*. National League for Nursing Press, New York.

Macklin, R. (1998). Ethical relativism in a multicultural society. *Kennedy Institute of Ethics Journal*, 8(1), pp. 1–22.

Marshall, P. A. (1992). Anthropology and bioethics. *Medical Anthropology Quarterly* 6 (1), pp. 49–73.

McNaughton, D. (1988). *Moral vision: an introduction to ethics*. Basil Blackwell, Oxford.

Mead, M. (1955). *Cultural patterns and technical change*. Mentor Books, New York.

Midgley, M. (1991a). *Can't we make moral judgements?* The Bristol Press, Bristol.

—— (1991b). *The origins of ethics*. In Singer 1991, pp. 3–13.

Moyers, B. (1993). *Healing and the mind*. Doubleday, New York.

Robson, A. (1994). Female circumcision. *Amnesty International Australian Newsletter*, 12(2), March, p. 15.

Saunders, D. (1994). Health officials to supervise circumcised girls, court rules. *The Age*, 1 March, p. 2.

Sherwin, S. (1992). *No longer patient: feminist ethics & health care*. Temple University Press, Philadelphia.

Silberbauer, G. (1991). Ethics in small-scale societies. In Singer, P. (ed), (1991). *A companion to ethics*. Basil Blackwell, Cambridge, Mass., pp. 14–28.

Singer, P. (ed). (1991). *A companion to ethics*. Basil Blackwell, Cambridge, Mass.

Sorokin, P. (1957). *Social and cultural dynamics*. Extending Horizons. Books–Porter Sargent, Boston.

Spindler, G.D. (1974). *Education and cultural process: towards an anthropology of education*. Holt, Rinehart & Winston, New York.

Stout, J. (1988). *Ethics after Babel: the languages of morals and their discontents*. Beacon Press, Boston.

Surbone, A. (1992). Truth telling to the patient. *JAMA* 268(13), pp. 1661–62.

Walker, A. and Parmar, P. (1993). *Warrior marks: female genital mutilation and the sexual blinding of women*. Jonathan Cape, London, UK.

Weil, A. (1983). *Health and healing: understanding conventional and alternative medicine*. Houghton Mifflin, Boston.

Williams, R. (1989). *Resources of hope: culture, democracy, socialism*. Verso, London.

Wolff, R.P., Moore, B. and Marcuse, H. (1969). *A critique of pure tolerance*. Beacon Press, Boston.

Wuthnow, R., Hunter, J.D., Bergesen, A. and Kurzweil, E. (1984). *Cultural analysis*. Routledge & Kegan Paul, London.

Chapter 7 Moral problems and moral decision-making in nursing

Amato, J.A. (1990). *Victims and values: a history and theory of suffering*. Praeger, New York.

Andersen, S. (1990). Patient advocacy and whistleblowing in nursing: help for the helpers. *Nursing Forum*. 25(3), pp. 5–13

Andrews, M. and Fargotstein, B. (1986). International nursing consultation: a perspective on ethical issues. *Journal of Professional Nursing*. 2(5), pp. 302–8.

Aroskar, M.A. (1986). Are nurses' mind sets compatible with ethical practice? In P.L. Chinn (ed.), *Ethical issues in nursing*, Aspen Systems, Rockville, Maryland, pp. 69–79.

Atkinson, R.L., Atkinson, R.C. and Hilgard, E.R. (1983). *Introduction to psychology*, 8th edn. Harcourt Brace Jovanovich, New York.

Beauchamp, T. and Childress, J. (1994). *Principles of biomedical ethics*, 4th edn. Oxford University Press, New York/Oxford.

Beauchamp, T.L. and Walters L. (eds) (1982). *Contemporary issues in bioethics*, 2nd edn. Wadsworth, Belmont, California.

Benner, P. (1984). *From novice to expert: excellence and power in clinical nursing practice*. Addison-Wesley, Nursing Division, Menlo Park, California.

—— (1991). The role of experience, narrative, and community in skilled ethical comportment. *Advances in Nursing Science* 14 (2), pp. 1–21.

Bergman, R. (1973). Ethics, concepts and practice. *International Nursing Review* 20 (5), p. 140.

Bishop, A.H. and Scudder, J.R. (1990). *The practical, moral and personal sense of nursing: a phenomenological philosophy of practice*. State University of New York Press, Albany.

Blum, L. (1980). *Friendship, altruism and morality*. Routledge & Kegan Paul, London/ Boston.

—— (1994). *Moral perception and particularity*. Cambridge University Press, Cambridge, UK/New York.

Bond, E. (1996). *Ethics and human wellbeing*. Blackwell, Cambridge, Massachusetts/ Oxford, UK.

Bowden, P. (1994). The ethics of nursing care and 'the ethic of care'. *Nursing Inquiry*, 2, pp. 10–21.

Bromberger, B. and Fife-Yeomans, J. (1991). *Deep Sleep: Harry Bailey and the scandal of Chelmsford*. Simon & Schuster, Sydney.

Cahn, M. (1989). *The nurse as moral hero: a case for required dissent*. Thesis component of the Doctor of Nursing Sciences degree in the School of Nursing, Indiana University. UMI Dissertation Services, Ann Arbor, Michigan (no. 8822134).

Carlton, W. (1978). *'In our professional opinion ...': the primacy of clinical judgment over moral choice*. University of Notre Dame Press, Notre Dame.

Chapell, A. (1994). Protecting the public. *Nursing New Zealand*, August, pp. 28–9.

Coney, S. (1988). *The unfortunate experiment*. Penguin Books, Auckland.

Cooper, M. (1988). Covenantal relationships: grounding for the nursing ethic. *Advances in Nursing Science* 10 (4), pp. 48–59.

—— (1990). Reconceptualizing nursing ethics. *Scholarly Inquiry for Nursing Practice: An International Journal* 4 (3), pp. 209–18.

—— (1991). Principle-orientated ethics and the ethic of care: a creative tension. *Advances in Nursing Science* 14 (2), pp. 22–31.

Corley, M. and Raines, D. (1993). Environments that support ethical nursing practice. *AWHONN'S Clinical Issues.* 4(4), pp. 611–19.

Craig, O. (1989). Life or death? How doctors decide which patient gets a 'black dot'. *Sun-Herald* (Sydney), 12 March.

Curtin, L. and Flaherty, M.J. (1982). *Nursing ethics: theories and pragmatics.* Prentice Hall, Bowie, Maryland, p. 61.

Damasio, A. (1994). *Descartes error: emotion, reason, and the human brain.* Avon Books, New York.

Davis, A. (1982). Helping your staff address ethical dilemmas, *Journal of Nursing Administration* 12 (2), February, pp. 9–13.

de Bono, E. (1985). *Conflicts: a better way to resolve them.* Penguin Books, London.

—— (1990). *I am right — you are wrong.* Penguin Books, London.

Dreyfus, H. and Dreyfus, S. (1991). Towards a phenomenology of ethical expertise. *Human Studies,* 14, pp. 229–50.

Frankena, W. (1973). *Ethics,* 2nd edn. Prentice-Hall, Englewood Cliffs, New Jersey.

Freckelton, I. (1996). Enforcement of ethics. In Coady, M. and Bloch, S. (eds). *Codes of ethics and the professions.* Melbourne University Press, Melbourne, pp. 130–65.

Free v Holy Cross Hospital 505 NE 2d 1199 (III App 1 Dist 1987).

Gastmans, C., Dierckx de Casterle, B., and Schotsmans, P. (1998). Nursing considered as moral practice: a philosophical-ethical interpretation of nursing. *Kennedy Institute of Ethics Journal,* 8(1), pp. 43–69.

Gaut, D. and Leininger, M.M. (eds) (1991). *Caring: the compassionate healer.* National League for Nursing Press, New York.

Gergen, K. (1994). *Realities and relationships: soundings in social construction.* Harvard University Press, Cambridge, Mass.

Gilligan, C. (1982). *In a different voice.* Harvard University Press, Cambridge, Mass. (See in particular Chapter 3, 'Concepts of self and morality'.)

Gilligan, C. (1987). Moral orientations and moral development. In E.F. Kittay and D.T. Meyers (eds) (1987). *Women and moral theory.* Rowman & Littlefield, Totowa, New Jersey, pp. 19–33.

Hare, R.M. (1963). *Freedom and reason.* Oxford University Press, London. (See in particular chapter 9, 'Toleration and fanaticism'.)

—— (1981). *Moral thinking.* Clarendon Press, Oxford. (See in particular Chapter 10, 'Fanaticism and amoralism'.)

Jameton, A. (1984). *Nursing practice: the ethical issues.* Prentice-Hall, Englewood Cliffs, New Jersey.

Johnstone, M.-J. (1987). Nursing and professional ethics. In *Proceedings of the conference, 'The Role of the Nurse: Doctors' Handmaiden, Patients' Advocate or What?'* Centre for Human Bioethics, Monash University, Melbourne, pp. 18–44.

—— (1994). *Nursing and the injustices of the law.* W.B. Saunders/Baillière Tindall, Sydney.

—— (1998). *Determining and responding effectively to ethical professional misconduct in nursing: a report to the Nurses Board of Victoria,* Melbourne.

Johnstone, M. and Kanitsaki, O. (1991). Some moral implications of cultural and linguistic diversity in health care. *Bioethics News,* 10(2), pp. 22–32.

Kanitsaki, O. (1988). Cancer and informed consent: a cultural perspective. Paper presented at seminar, Controversial Ethical Issues in Patients with Cancer. Heidelberg Repatriation General Hospital Melbourne, 13 October.

—— (1989). Health–illness–suffering experiences of a sample of Greek-born members of 12 Greek–Australian families living in Melbourne. Minor thesis completed in partial fulfilment of the requirements for the Degree of Master of Educational Studies, Faculty of Education, Monash University, Melbourne.

—— (1993). Transcultural human care: its challenge to and critique of professional nursing care. In Gaut, D. (ed.), *A global agenda for caring,* National League for Nursing Press, New York, pp. 19–45.

—— (1994). Cultural and linguistic diversity. In Romanini, J. and Daly, J. (eds), *Critical care nursing: Australian perspectives*, W.B. Saunders/Baillière Tindall, Sydney.

Kent, A. (1990). Protecting the public? *Nursing Times*, 86(37), p. 20.

King, P.A. (1985). Unprofessional conduct and the nursing profession: the *Tuma case*. *Bioethics Reporter* 6 (7), pp. 159–62.

Lemmon, E.J. (1987). Moral dilemmas. In C.W. Gowans (ed.), *Moral dilemmas*, Oxford University Press, New York, pp. 101–14.

Lynn, J. (ed.) (1989). *By no extraordinary means: the choice to forgo life-sustaining food and water*. Indiana University Press, Bloomington and Indianapolis.

MacKinnon, C.A. (1987). *Feminism unmodified: discourses on life and law*. Harvard University Press, Cambridge, Mass.

McNaughton, D. (1988). *Moral vision: an introduction to ethics*. Basil Blackwell, Oxford.

Miller, C. (1988). Nurses told, let sick die. *Herald* (Melbourne), 30 September, p. 3.

—— (1989). NFR system is 'dangerous'. *Australian Dr Weekly*, 20 January.

Milo, R.D. (1986). Moral deadlock. *Philosophy* 61, pp. 453–71.

Nexus (1996). Hearings. October Issue, 2(2), pp. 6–7. (Official newsletter of the Nurses Board of Victoria.)

Nielsen, K. (1989). *Why be moral?* Prometheus Books, Buffalo, New York.

O'Hanlan, K., Cabaj, R., Schatz, B., Lock, J. and Nemrow, P. (1997). A review of the medical consequences of homophobia with suggestion for resolutions. *Journal of Gay and Lesbian Medical Association*, 1(1), pp. 25–39.

Packard, J.S. and Ferrara, M. (1988). In search of the moral foundation of nursing. *Advances in Nursing Science* 10 (4), pp. 60–71.

Report of the Royal Commission into Deep Sleep Therapy (1990). Government Printer, Sydney.

Rice, S. (1988). *Some doctors make you sick: the scandal of medical incompetence*. Angus & Robertson, Sydney.

Roach, M.S. (1987). *The human act of caring: a blueprint for the health professions*. Canadian Hospital Association, Ottawa, Ontario.

Ross, W.D. (1930). *The right and the good*. Oxford University Press, London.

Schumpeter, P. (1988). No-resuscitation rules are unclear: lecturer. *The Age*, 1 October, p. 21.

Seary v State Bar of Texas (1980), 604 SW2d 256 at 258.

Singer, P. (1993). *Practical ethics*, 2nd edn. Cambridge University Press, New York.

Stevens, J. and Herbert, J. (1997). Ageism and nursing practice in Australia. *Nursing Review*. September issue, special section, pp. 17–24.

Stout, J. (1988). *Ethics after Babel: the languages of morals and their discontents*. Beacon Press, Boston.

Tuma v Board of Nursing of the State of Idaho 593 P 2d 711 (1979).

Twomey, J.G. (1989). Analysis of the claim to distinct nursing ethics: normative and non-normative approaches. *Advances in Nursing Science* 11 (3), pp. 25–32.

Unwin, N. (1985). Relativism and moral complacency. *Philosophy* 60, pp. 205–14.

Upfront (1988). 'Not for Resuscitation' orders leave nurses in a moral, legal and professional dilemma. 7 (4), December, pp. 6, 13.

Van Hooft, S. (1987). Caring and professional commitment. *Australian Journal of Advanced Nursing* 4 (4), pp. 29–38.

Vessey, J. (1994). The ghost of Tuskegee. *Nursing Research*, 43(2), p. 67.

Warthen v Toms River Community Memorial Hospital 488 A 2d 299 (NJ Super AD 1985).

Watson, J. (1985). *Nursing: human science and human care*. Appleton-Century-Crofts, Norwalk, Connecticut.

Wilkinson, J. (1987/1988). Moral distress in nursing practice: experience and affects. *Nursing Forum*. 23(1), pp. 16–29.

Williams, B. (1973). Ethical consistency. In C. W. Gowans (ed.) (1987), *Moral dilemmas*, Oxford University Press, New York, pp. 115–37.

Wilson-Barnett, J. (1986). Ethical dilemmas in nursing. *Journal of Medical Ethics* 12, pp. 123–6, 135.

Yarling, R.R. and McElmurry, B.J. (1986). The moral foundation of nursing. *Advances in Nursing Science* 8 (2), pp. 63–73.

Chapter 8 Patients' rights to and in health care

Andrews, K. (1985). Informed consent: adrift on a trans-Atlantic crossing. *Lawyer* 3 (6), August, pp. 12–16 (published by Victorian Young Lawyers).

Australian Consumers' Association (1988). *Your health rights.* Australasian Publishing Company and Australian Consumers' Association, Sydney.

Australian Nursing Council Inc. (1993). *Code of ethics for nurses in Australia.* Australian Nursing Council, Inc., Canberra.

Bates, E. and Linder-Pelz, S. (1987). *Health care issues.* Allen & Unwin, Sydney.

Beauchamp, T.L. and Childress, J.F. (1989). *Principles of biomedical ethics,* 3rd edn. Oxford University Press, New York.

Beauchamp, T, and Childress, J. (1994). *Principles of biomedical ethics,* 4th edn. Oxford University Press, New York.

Beauchamp, T. (1978). Paternalism. In Reich, W. (ed), *Encyclopedia of bioethics.* The Free Press, New York/Collier Macmillan, London, UK, pp. 1194–201.

—— (1980). Suicide. In Regan, T. (ed), *Matters of life and death: new introductory essays in moral philosophy.* Random House, New York, pp. 67–108.

—— (1995). Paternalism. In Reich, W. (ed), *Encyclopedia of Bioethics,* revised edition. Simon & Schuster Macmillan, New York/Simon & Schuster and Prentice Hall International, pp. 1914–920.

Bioethics News (1985). Request to die. *Bioethics News* 5 (1), October.

Bok, S. (1980). *Lying: moral choice in public and private life.* Quartet Books, London.

Bone, P. (1987). Pelvic check 'by patient's consent' only. *The Age,* 18 September, p. 5.

Brody, B. (1986). Should there be a distinctively Jewish medical ethics? *Isaac Frank Memorial Lecture,* Kennedy Institute of Ethics, Georgetown University, Washington DC, ICC Auditorium, 2 June.

Bromberger, B. and Fife-Yeomans, J. (1991). *Deep Sleep: Harry Bailey and the scandal of Chelmsford.* Simon & Schuster, Sydney.

Buchanan, A. (1978). Medical paternalism. *Philosophy and Public Affairs,* 7(4), pp. 371–90.

—— (1984). The right to a decent minimum of health care. *Philosophy and Public Affairs* 13 (1), Winter, pp. 55–78.

Buchanan, A.E. and Brock, D.W. (1989). *Deciding for others: the ethics of surrogate decision making.* Cambridge University Press, Cambridge.

Campbell, E.J., Baker, M.D. and Crites-Silver, P. (1988). Subjective effects of humidification of oxygen for delivery by nasal cannula: a prospective study. *Chest* 93 (2), February, pp. 289–93.

Capron, A. (1974). Informed consent in catastrophic disease and treatment. *University of Pennsylvania Law Review* 123, December, pp. 364–76 (cited in T.L. Beauchamp and J.F. Childress [1983], *Principles of biomedical ethics,* 2nd edn, Oxford University Press, New York, pp. 67, 102).

Childress, J. (1982). *Who should decide? Paternalism in health care.* Oxford University Press, New York.

Chopra, D. (1989). *Quantum healing: exploring the frontiers of mind/body medicine.* Bantam Books, New York.

Conley, J. (1987). AMA will consider secret AIDS tests. *The Age,* 4 July, p. 1.

Consumers' Health Forum (1990). *Legal recognition and protection of the rights of health consumers.* Consumers' Health Forum of Australia, Curtin, ACT.

Council for Science and Society (1982). *Expensive medical techniques.* Calvert's Press, London.

Daley, D.W. (1983). Tarasoff and the psychotherapist's duty to warn. In Gorovitz, S., Macklin, R., Jameton, A.L., O'Connor, J.M. and Sherwin, A. (eds), *Moral problems in medicine*, 2nd edn, Prentice Hall, Englewood Cliffs, New Jersey, pp. 234–46.

Dossey, L. (1991). *Meaning and medicine: a doctor's tales of breakthrough and healing.* Bantam Books, New York.

Dworkin, G. (1972). Paternalism. *Monist*, 56(1), pp. 64–84.

—— (1988). *The theory and practice of autonomy.* Cambridge University Press, New York.

Engelhardt, H.T. (1986). *The foundations of bioethics.* Oxford University Press, New York.

Engstrom, B. (1986). Communication and decision-making in a study of multidisciplinary team conference with the registered nurse as conference chairman. *International Journal of Nursing Studies* 23 (4), pp. 299–314.

Faden, R.R. and Beauchamp, T.L. (1986). *A history and theory of informed consent.* Oxford University Press, New York.

Feather, R.B. (1985). The institutionalised mental health patient's right to refuse psychotropic medication. *Perspectives in Psychiatric Care* 23 (2), pp. 45–68.

Feinberg, J. (1971). Legal paternalism. *Canadian Journal of Philosophy*, 1, pp. 105–24.

Field, M. (1997). NZ health uproar after life fight fails. *The Age*, 13 October, p. 10.

Fordham, J. (1988). *Doctors' orders or patient choice?* Leo Cussen Institute, Melbourne.

Freedman, B. (1978). A meta-ethics for professional morality. *Ethics* 89, pp. 1–19.

Fried, C. (1982). Equality and rights in medical care. In Beauchamp, T.L. and Walters L. (eds) (1982). *Contemporary issues in bioethics*, 2nd edn. Wadsworth, Belmont, California, pp. 395–401.

Fuchs, V.R. (1983). *Who shall live? Health, economics and social choice.* Basic Books, New York.

Gert, B. and Culver, C. (1976). Paternalistic behaviour. *Philosophy and Public Affairs*, 6(1). pp. 45–57.

Gilbert, S. (1997). *Wrongful death: a memoir.* WW Norton & Co., New York.

Gilmour, J. (1992). *Michael: a mother's battle for the rights of her child.* Little Hills Press, Sydney.

Goffman, E. (1963). *Stigma: notes on the management of spoiled identity.* Penguin Books, London, UK.

Gross, P.F. (1985). Nursing care in the 1980s and beyond: the challenge to be relevant, ethical and accepted. *Australian Nurses Journal*, 15 (1) July, pp. 46–8.

Hart, H. (1963). *Law, liberty, and morality.* Stanford University Press, Stanford, Cal.

Health Call (1987). *Health complaints advisory link line annual report, 1 May, 1986–30 April, 1987.* Health Call, Melbourne.

—— (1988). *Health Call annual report 1988.* Health Issues Centre, Melbourne.

Health Issues Centre (1991). *Our better health: getting it together.* Health Issues Centre, Melbourne.

—— (1992). *Casemix: quality and consumers.* Health Issues Centre, Melbourne.

Hobbes, T. (1968 edn). *Leviathan* (reprinted from 1651 edition with notes by C.B. Macpherson). Penguin Books, Harmondsworth, Middlesex.

Inlander, C.B., Levin, L.S. and Weiner, E. (1988). *Medicine on trial: the appalling story of ineptitude, malfeasance, neglect, and arrogance.* Prentice Hall, New York.

International Code of Medical Ethics (1983). In Amnesty International, *Ethical codes and declarations relevant to the health professions*, Amnesty International, London, 1985.

International Council of Nurses, Code for Nurses (1973). International Council of Nurses, Geneva, Switzerland.

Johnstone, M-J. (1998). *Determining and responding effectively to ethical professional misconduct in nursing: a report to the Nurses Board of Victoria.* Melbourne.

—— (1990). Bioethics and the health care economics debate: a nursing perspective. Paper presented at the NSW Nurses' Association's 45th Annual Conference/Professional Seminar Day, Bioethical Considerations and Opportunity Cost, Sydney. Reprinted in full in M.-J. Johnstone (1992), *Module 601E. Ethics and Nursing — Book of Readings.* Distance Education Division of Royal College of Nursing Australia, Melbourne, Reading 2.1.

—— (1991). Government's rationalisation of language services spells disaster for NESB patients. *Transcultural Health Care Council Newsletter*, March–April, pp. 1–4.

—— (1994). *Nursing and the injustices of the law.* W.B. Saunders/Baillière Tindall, Sydney.

Kanitsaki, O. (1983). Acculturation — a new dimension in nursing. *Australian Nurses Journal* 13 (5), November, pp. 42–5, 53.

—— (1988a). Transcultural nursing: challenge to change. *Australian Journal of Advanced Nursing* 5 (3), March–May, pp. 4–11.

—— (1988b). Cancer and informed consent: a cultural perspective. Paper presented at seminar, Controversial Ethical Issues in Patients with Cancer, Heidelberg Repatriation General Hospital, Melbourne, 13 October.

—— (1992). Meeting the challenge of patients' rights: a transcultural perspective. *Proceedings of the conference 'Meeting the Challenge of Patient's Rights — Issues for the 1990s', RMIT Faculty of Nursing, Nursing Law and Ethics, 4th Victorian State Conference*, held 20 November, Dallas Brooks Hall, Melbourne Institute of Technology, Faculty of Nursing, Melbourne.

Kant, I. (1959edn). *Fundamental principles of the metaphysics of ethics.* (translated by T. Kingmill Abbott), Longmans, London, UK.

—— (1972 edn). *The moral law* (translated by H.J. Paton). Hutchinson University Press, London.

Kerr, J. Fairbanks (1987). *Don't call a doctor.* Veritas, Bullsbrook, Western Australia.

King, N.M., Churchill, L.R. and Cross, A.W. (1988). *The physician as captain of the ship.* D. Reidel, Dordrecht.

Kirby, M. (1995). Patients' rights — why the Australian courts have rejected 'Bolam'. *Journal of Medical Ethics*, 21(1), pp. 5–8.

Kirkman, M. and Bell, S. (1989). AIDS and confidentiality. *Nursing Forum*, 24(3/4), pp. 47–51.

Kuczewski, M. (1996). Reconceiving the family: the process of consent in medical decision making. *Hastings Center Report*, 26(2), pp. 30–7.

Law Reform Commission of Victoria, Australian Law Reform Commission, and New South Wales Law Reform Commission (1987). *Informed consent to medical treatment*, discussion paper no 7. Law Reform Commission of Victoria, Melbourne.

Lindorff, D. (1992). *Marketplace medicine: the rise of the for-profit hospital chains.* Bantam Books, New York.

McCloskey, H.J. (1980). Privacy and the right to privacy. *Philosophy* 55, pp. 17–38.

McCullough, L.B. (1983). The right to health care. In Gorovitz, S., Macklin, R., Jameton, A.L., O'Connor, J.M. and A. Sherwin (eds), *Moral problems in medicine*, 2nd edn. Prentice Hall, Englewood Cliffs, New Jersey, pp. 536–44.

Mendelsohn, R.S. (1982). *Male practice: how doctors manipulate women.* Contemporary Books, Chicago.

Miller, C. (1988). 1500 Aboriginals tested for AIDS — 5 positive. *The Herald* (Melbourne), 31 August, pp. 1, 2.

Moyers, B. (1993). *Healing and the mind.* Doubleday, New York.

Mulley, A.G. (1984). The triage decision. In S. J. Reiser and M. Anbar (eds), *The machine at the bedside.* Cambridge University Press, Cambridge, pp. 221–6.

Muyskens, J. L. (1982). *Moral problems in nursing: a philosophical investigation.* Rowman & Littlefield, Totowa, New Jersey.

New Zealand Nurses' Association. (1988). *Code of Ethics.* New Zealand Nurses' Association, Wellington, NZ.

Ooi, C. (1988) 'Paediatrics — a new version', unpublished paper.

Parker, R. (1974). A definition of privacy. *Rutgers Law Review* 27 (2), pp. 275–96.

Reed, C. (1996). Man sues physician who made him live. *The Age*, 20 June, p. 14.

Rice, S. (1988). *Some doctors make you sick.* Angus & Robertson, Sydney.

Rivers, F. (1996). *The way of the owl: succeeding with integrity in a conflicted world.* HarperSanFrancisco, New York.

Roberts, M. (1987). The nurse as an advocate between patient and family. *Proceedings of the conference, 'The Role of the Nurse: Doctors' Handmaiden, Patients' Advocate or What?* Centre for Human Bioethics, Monash University, 16 November, pp. 98–111.

Robertson, G. (1981). Informed consent to medical treatment. *The Law Quarterly Review* 97, January, pp. 102–26.

Robinson, G. and Merav, A. (1983). Informed consent: recall by patients tested postoperatively. In Gorovitz, S., Macklin, R., Jameton, A.L., O'Connor, J.M. and Sherwin, A. (eds), *Moral problems in medicine*, 2nd edn. Prentice Hall, Englewood Cliffs, New Jersey, pp. 182–6.

Roth, L.H., Meisel, A. and Lidz, C.W. (1983). Tests of competency to consent to treatment. In Gorovitz, S., Macklin, R., Jameton, A.L., O'Connor, J.M. and Sherwin, A. (eds), *Moral problems in medicine*, 2nd edn. Prentice Hall, Englewood Cliffs, New Jersey, pp. 172–9 (reprinted from *American Journal of Psychiatry* 134 (4), pp. 279–84).

Royal Australian Nursing Federation (Vic) (1987). Position paper: patients' bill of rights. In Royal Australian Nursing Federation, *Ethics in perspective*, vol. 1, RANF, Melbourne, pp. 123–6.

Royal Australian Nursing Federation (WA) (1987). Position paper: patients' bill of rights. In Royal Australian Nursing Federation, *Ethics in perspective*, vol. 1, RANF, Melbourne, pp. 119–22.

Russell, H. (1987). What you don't know can hurt. *Health Issues*, 11 September, pp. 17–19.

Sade, R.M. (1983). From 'Medical care as a right: a refutation'. In Gorovitz, S., Macklin, R., Jameton, A.L., O'Connor, J.M. and Sherwin, A. (eds), *Moral problems in medicine*, 2nd edn. Prentice Hall, Englewood Cliffs, New Jersey, pp. 532–5.

Schauble, J. and Willox, I. (1987). Government reviews law on consent to medical treatment. *The Age*, 21 August, p. 19.

Sheehan, M. and Wells, D. (1985). The allocation of medical resources. In Buchanan, C.L. and Prior, E.W. (eds), *Medical care and markets: conflicts between efficiency and justice*, George Allen & Unwin, Sydney, pp. 55–69.

Skinner, B.F. (1973). *Beyond freedom and dignity*. Penguin Books, Harmondsworth, Middlesex, England.

Social Development Committee (Vic) (1986). *First report on inquiry into options for dying with dignity*. March, Government Printer, Melbourne.

—— (1987). *Inquiry into options for dying with dignity: second and final report*. April, Government Printer, Melbourne.

Somerville, M. (1986). Rights to, in and against medical treatment. *Bioethics News* 5 (3), April, pp. 5–17.

Spitzer, R.B. (1988). Meeting consumer expectations. *Nursing Administration Quarterly* 12 (3), pp. 31–9.

Staunton, P. and Whyburn, B. (1997). *Nursing and the law*, 4th edn. W.B. Saunders/ Baillière Tindall, Sydney.

Stone, D. (1991). Hospitals forced to use cleaners as interpreters. *The Sunday Age*, 10 February, p. 4.

Sugirtharjah, S. (1994). The notion of respect in Asian traditions. *British Journal of Nursing*, 3(14), pp. 739–41.

Swenson, D.F. (1981). The dignity of human life. In Klemke, E.D. (ed.), *The meaning of life*, Oxford University Press, New York, pp. 20–30.

Tadd, G. (1998). *Ethics and values for care workers*. Blackwell Science, Oxford, UK.

Thomasma, D. (1990). Establishing the moral basis of medicine: Edmund D. Pellegrino's philosophy of medicine. *Journal of Medicine and Philosophy*, 15(3), pp. 245–67.

Thomson, J.J. (1975). The right to privacy. *Philosophy and Public Affairs* 4 (4), Summer, pp. 295–314.

United Nations (1978). *The International Bill of Human Rights*, United Nations, New York.

Uyer, G. (1986). Effect of nursing approach in understanding of physicians' directions, by mothers of sick children in an out-patient clinic. *International Journal of Nursing Studies* 23 (1), pp. 79–85.

Vandeveer, D. (1980). The contractual argument for withholding medical information. *Philosophy and Public Affairs* 9 (2), pp. 198–205.

Victorian Health Services Commissioner Annual Report 1991. Flash Print, Melbourne.

Walker, Q.J. and Langlands, A.O. (1986). The misuse of mammography in the management of breast cancer. *Medical Journal of Australia* 145, 1 September, pp. 185–7.

Wallace, M. (1991). *Health care and the law: a guide for nurses*. The Law Book Company, North Ryde.

Wallace, M. (1992). Meeting the challenge of patients' rights: a legal perspective. *Proceedings of the conference 'Meeting the Challenge of Patients' Rights — Issues for the 1990s', RMIT Faculty of Nursing, Nursing Law and Ethics, 4th Victorian State Conference*, held 20 November, Dallas Brooks Hall, Melbourne, Royal Melbourne Institute of Technology, Faculty of Nursing, Melbourne.

Winslade, W. (1995). Confidentiality. In Reich, W. (ed), *The encyclopedia of bioethics*, revised edition. Simon & Schuster Macmillan, New York/Simon & Schuster and Prentice Hall International, pp. 451–59.

Chapter 9   Human rights and the mentally ill

Australian Health Ministers. (1995). *National Mental Health Policy*, Australian Government Publishing Service, Canberra.

Australian Nursing Council, Inc. (1993). *Code of Ethics for Nurses in Australia*. Australian Nursing Council, Inc., Canberra.

Beauchamp, T.L. and Childress, J.F. (1994). *Principles of Biomedical Ethics*, 4th edn. Oxford University Press, New York.

Bloch, S. and Chodoff, P. (eds) (1991). *Psychiatric Ethics*, 2nd edn. Oxford University Press, New York.

Bromberger, B. and Fife-Yeomans, J. (1991). *Deep Sleep: Harry Bailey and the Scandal of Chelmsford*, Simon & Schuster, Sydney.

Buchanan, A.E. and Brock, D.W. (1989). *Deciding for Others: The Ethics of Surrogate Decision Making*. Cambridge University Press, New York.

Burdekin, B., Guilfoyle, M., and Hall, D. (1993). *Human Rights and Mental Illness: Report of the National Inquiry into the Human Rights of People with Mental Illness* (2 volumes). Australian Government Publishing Service, Canberra.

Carter, W.J. (1991). *Report of the Commission of Inquiry into the Care and Treatment of Patients in the Psychiatric Unit of the Townsville General Hospital between 2nd March, 1975 and 20th February, 1988*, (2 volumes). Government Printing Services, Brisbane.

Daley, D.W. (1983). Tarasoff and the psychotherapist's duty to warn. In Gorovitz, S., Macklin, R., Jameton, A., O'Connor, J., and Sherwin, S. (eds) *Moral Problems in Medicine*, 2nd edn. Prentice-Hall, Englewoods Cliffs, New Jersey.

Engelhardt, H.T. (1995). *The Foundations of Bioethics*, 2nd edn. Oxford University Press, New York.

Gorovitz, S., Macklin, R., Jameton, A., O'Connor, J., and Sherwin, S. (eds) (1983). *Moral Problems in Medicine*, 2nd edn. Prentice-Hall, Englewoods Cliffs, New Jersey.

Health Care Committee Expert Panel on Mental Health. (1991). *Homelessness and Severe Mental Disorders*. Australian Government Publishing Service, Canberra.

Hekman, S.J. (1995). *Moral Voices, Moral Selves: Carol Gilligan and Feminist Moral Theory*. Polity Press, Cambridge, UK.

Johnstone, M-J. (1994). *Nursing and the Injustices of the Law*, W.B. Saunders/Baillière Tindall, Sydney.

—— (1995). Guest Editorial: The scandalous neglect of mental health care ethics. *Contemporary Nurse*, 4, 142–4.

—— (1998). *Determining and responding effectively to ethical professional misconduct in nursing: a report to the Nurses Board of Victoria*. Melbourne.

Mental Health Consumers Outcomes Task Force. (1995). *Mental Health Statement of Rights and Responsibilities*. Australian Government Publishing Service, Canberra.

Raphael, B. (1995). Foreword, in Mental Health Consumers Outcomes Task Force, *Mental Health Statement of Rights and Responsibilities.* Australian Government Publishing Service, Canberra.

Rave, E.J. and Larsen, C.C. (eds) (1995). *Ethical Decision Making in Therapy: Feminist Perspectives.* The Guilford Press, New York.

Senate Community Affairs References Committee. (1995). *Psychotherapeutic Medication in Australia: Report of the Senate Community Affairs References Committee.* Commonwealth of Australia, Senate Printing Unit, Parliament House, Canberra.

South East Centre Against Sexual Assault. (1994). *Certified Truths: Women Who Have Been Sexually Assaulted — Their Experiences of Psychiatric Services.* South East Centre Against Sexual Assault, Monash Medical Centre, Melbourne.

Tarasoff v Regents of the University of California 13 Cal. 3d 177, 529 P.2d 553, 118 Cal. Rptr. 129 (1974).

Tippett, V., Elvy, G., Hardy, J., and Raphael, B. (1994). *Mental Health in Australia: A Review of Current Activities and Future Directions.* Australian Government Publishing Service, Canberra.

Tomison, A. (1996) Child maltreatment and mental disorder. *Child Abuse Prevention,* discussion paper no. 3. Australian Institute of Family Studies, Melbourne.

Torrey, E.F. (1988). *Nowhere to Go: The Tragic Odyssey of the Homeless Mentally Ill,* Harper and Row, New York.

Weinstein, H.M. (1990). *Psychiatry and the CIA: Victims of Mind Control.* American Psychiatric Press, Washington DC.

Chapter 10   Ethical issues associated with the reporting of child abuse

Amato, J. (1990). *Victims and values: a history and a theory of suffering.* Praeger, New York.

Archard, D. (1993). *Children: rights and childhood.* Routledge, London/New York.

Australian Institute of Health and Welfare (AIHW) (1998). *Child protection, Australia 1996–97.* AIHW cat. no. CWS 4, Canberra (Child Welfare Series no. 20).

Beauchamp, T. and Childress, J. (1994). *Principles of biomedical ethics,* 4th edn. Oxford University Press, New York/Oxford.

Birrell, R and Birrell, J. (1966). The 'maltreatment syndrome' in children. *Medical Journal of Australia,* 2, pp. 1134–138.

—— (1968). The 'maltreatment syndrome' in children: a hospital survey. *Medical Journal of Australia,* 2, pp. 1023–29.

Blum, L. (1980). *Friendship, altruism and morality.* Routledge & Kegan Paul, London/Boston.

—— (1994). *Moral perception and particularity.* Cambridge University Press, Cambridge, UK/New York.

Bok, S. (1978). *Lying: moral choice in public and private life.* Vintage Books, New York.

—— (1983). *Secrets: on the ethics of concealment and revelation.* Vintage Books, New York.

Bond, E. (1996). *Ethics and human wellbeing.* Blackwell, Cambridge, Massachusetts/Oxford, UK.

Bowman, J. (1995). Genetics and racial minorities. In W.T. Reich (ed), *Encyclopedia of Bioethics,* revised edition. Simon & Schuster Macmillan, New York, p. 982.

Briere, J. (1992). *Child abuse trauma: theory and treatment of the lasting effects.* Sage, Newbury Park, Ca.

Callahan, J. (ed). (1995). *Reproduction, ethics and the law: feminist perspectives.* Indiana University Press, Bloomington and Indianapolis.

Chandler, J. (1993). Doctors might relent on abuse reporting. *The Age,* 27 March, p. 28.

Child Protection Victoria. (1993). *Reporting Child Abuse.* Health and Community Services, Melbourne.

Coffey, M. (1996). 100 children die in care. *Herald Sun,* 31 October, pp. 1, 4.

Coyler, V. (1986). Why not get tough about child abuse? *The Age,* 15 October.

Daly, M., Farouque, F. and Adams, D. (1996). Children left in danger by care workers: report. *The Age,* 26 October, p. 1.

Daniels, N. (1996). *Justice and justification: reflective equilibrium in theory and practice*. Cambridge University Press, Cambridge, UK/New York.

Drane, J. (1995). Alternative therapies: ethical and legal issues. In Reich, W.T. (ed), *The encyclopedia of bioethics*, revised edition. Simon & Schuster Macmillan, New York, pp. 135–43.

Elliott, M. (ed). (1993). *Female sexual abuse of children: the ultimate taboo*. Longman, Harlow, Essex.

Engelhardt, H. (1986). *The foundations of bioethics*. Oxford University Press, New York.

—— (1996). *The foundations of bioethics*, 2nd edn. Oxford University Press, New York.

Farouque, F. (1993a). Inquest told of boy's bruises. *The Age*, 11 November, p. 3.

—— (1993b). Doctor left Valerio's mother to get advice. *The Age*, 12 November, p. 3.

Feinberg, J. (1984). *Harm to others: the moral limits of the criminal law*. Oxford University Press, New York/Oxford.

Fletcher, J. (1973). Ethics and euthanasia. *American Journal of Nursing*, 73(4), pp. 670–5.

Fogarty, J. (1993). *Protective services for children in Victoria: a report* (July). Melbourne.

Fogarty, J. and Sargeant, D. (1989). *Protective services for children in Victoria – an interim report* (February). Melbourne.

Folks, H. (1902). *Care of the destitute, neglected, and delinquent children*. Macmillan, New York.

Frankena, W. (1973). *Ethics, second edition*. Prentice-Hall, Englewood Cliffs, New Jersey.

Gallagher, J. (1995). Collective bad faith: 'Protecting' the fetus. In Callahan, J. (ed), *Reproduction, ethics and the law: feminist perspectives*. Indiana University Press, Bloomington and Indianopolis, pp. 343–79.

Gandevia, B. (1978). *Tears often shed: child health and welfare in Australia from 1788*, Charter, Gordon.

Garner, H. How we lost Daniel's life. *Time* magazine, 8 March (10), pp. 23–25.

Giovannoni, J. (1982). Mistreated children. In Yelaja, S. (ed), *Ethical issues in social work*. Charles C. Thomas, Springfield, Illinois, pp. 105–20.

Goddard, C. (1996). *Child abuse and child protection: a guide for health, education and welfare workers*. Churchill Livingstone, Melbourne.

Gorovitz, S., Macklin, R., Jameton, A., O'Connor, J., and Sherwin, S. (eds) (1983). *Moral problems in medicine*, 2nd edn, Prentice Hall, Englewood Cliffs, New Jersey.

Grodin, M. and Glantz, L. (1994). *Children as research subjects: science, ethics & law*. Oxford University Press, New York/Oxford.

Hawes, R. and Honeysett, S. (1996). State accused over child abuse deaths. *The Australian*, 31 October, p. 3.

Herman, J. (1992). *Trauma and recovery: the aftermath of violence — from domestic abuse to political terror*. Basic Books, a Division of HarperCollins, New York.

Higgins, G. O'Connell. (1994). *Resilient adults: overcoming a cruel past*. Jossey-Bass Publishing, San Franciso.

Hiskey, E. (1980). Child protection in Victoria, Part 1. *Australian Child and Family Welfare*, 5(3).

Hoff, C. (1982). When public policy replaces private ethics. *Hastings Center Report*, 12(4), pp. 13–14.

Holmes, H. and Purdy, L (eds). (1992). *Feminist perspectives in medical ethics*. Indiana University Press, Bloomington and Indianopolis.

Jecker, N., Jonsen, A. and Pearlman, R. (1997). *Bioethics: an introduction to the history, methods, and practice*. Jones and Bartlett, Sudbury, Massachusetts.

Johnson v State, 21 Tenn. 291, 292 (1840).

Johnstone, M-J (in press). Reporting child abuse: ethical issues for nurse registering authorities. A report to the Nurses' Board of Victoria, Melbourne (due for publication September 1999).

Kissane, K. (1993). No place like home. *Time magazine*, 8 March (10), pp. 24–5.

—— (1995). Falling through a larger net. *The Age*, 4 July, p. 13.

LaFollette, H (ed). (1997). *Ethics in practice: an anthology*. Blackwell, Cambridge, Massachusetts/Oxford, UK.

Lantos, J. (1995). Child abuse. In Reich, W.T. (ed), *The encyclopedia of bioethics*, revised edition. Simon & Schuster Macmillan, New York, pp. 42–6.

Levine, C. (ed). (1995). *Taking sides: clashing views on controversial bioethical issues*, 6th edn. The Dushkin Publishing Group, Guilford, Connecticut.

Lewin, L. (1994). Child abuse: ethical and legal concerns. *Journal of Psychosocial Nursing*, 32(12), pp. 15–18.

Longdon, C. (1993). A survivor's and therapist's viewpoint. In Elliott, M. (ed), *Female sexual abuse of children: the ultimate taboo*. Longman, Harlow, Essex, pp. 50–60.

Lord, G. (1997). Untitled. In L. Mullinar and C. Hunt (eds). *Breaking the silence: survivors of child abuse speak out*. Hodder & Stoughton, Sydney, p. i.

Loring, M. (1994). *Emotional abuse*. Lexington Books (an imprint of Macmillan), New York.

Macklin, R. (1993). *Enemies of patients*. Oxford University Press, New York/Oxford.

MacNair, R. (1992). Ethical dilemmas of child abuse reporting: implications for mental health counsellors. *Journal of Mental Health Counselling* 14(2), pp. 127–36.

Magazanik, M. (1993). Protecting our children. *The Age*, 27 February, p. 18.

McNaughton, D. (1988). *Moral vision: an introduction to ethics*. Basil Blackwell, Oxford, UK/New York.

Mendes, P. (1996). The historical and political context of mandatory reporting and its impact on child protection practice in Victoria. *Australian Social Work*, 49(4), pp. 25–32.

Milburn, C. (1996). Call for national probe on children. *The Age*, 7 November, p. 3.

Miller, R. and Weinstock, R. (1987). Conflict of interest between therapist-patient confidentiality and the duty to report sexual abuse of children. *Behavioral Sciences and the Law*, 5(2), pp. 161–74.

Minow, M. (1990). *Making all the difference: inclusion, exclusion, and American law*. Cornell University Press, Ithaca/London.

Monash Review. (1986). Australia gets serious about battered children. October, 5(86), p. 11.

Mono. (1997). The myth of false memory. In L. Mullinar and C. Hunt (eds). *Breaking the silence: survivors of child abuse speak out*. Hodder & Stoughton, Sydney, p. 40–2.

Mullinar, L. and Hunt, C. (eds). (1997). *Breaking the silence: survivors of child abuse speak out*. Hodder & Stoughton, Sydney.

Myers, J. (ed) (1994). *The backlash: child protection under fire*. Sage, Thousand Oaks, California.

O'Hagan, K. (1993). *Emotional and psychological abuse of children*. Open University Press, Buckingham, UK.

Oliver, K. (1989). Marxism and surrogacy. In H. Holmes and L Purdy (eds). (1992). *Feminist perspectives in medical ethics*. Indiana University Press, Bloomington and Indianopolis, pp. 266–83.

Pegler, T. (1996). Life of crime for one in five wards. *The Age*, 21 June, p. 4.

Pegler, T. and Farouque, F. (1996). State fails children: auditor. *The Age*, 21 June, p. 1.

Phillips, M. and Frederick, C. (1995). *Healing the divided self: clinical and Ericksonian hypnotherapy for post-traumatic and dissociative conditions*. WW Norton, New York/London.

Porterfield, K. (1993). *Blind faith: recognizing and recovering from dysfunctional religious groups*. CompCare, Minneapolis.

Quinn, C. (1992). Protection and prevention: an integral approach to child sexual assault. In J. Breckenridge and M. Carmody (eds). *Crimes of violence: Australian responses to rape and child sexual assault*. Allen & Unwin, Sydney, pp. 86–96.

Radi, H. (1979). Whose child? Custody of children in NSW 1854-1934. In J. MacKinolty and H. Radi (eds). *In pursuit of justice: Australian women and the law 1788–1979*. Hale & Iremonger, Sydney, pp. 119–13.

Reich, W. (ed) (1995). *The encyclopedia of bioethics*, revised edition. Simon & Schuster Macmillan, New York.

Renvoize, J. (1993). *Innocence destroyed: a study of child sexual abuse*. Routledge, London/New York.

Sanford, L. (1990). *Strong at the broken places: overcoming the trauma of childhood abuse*. Random House, New York.

Schrag, F. (1995). Rights of children. In Reich, W.T. (ed), *Encyclopedia of Bioethics*, revised edition. Simon & Schuster Macmillan, New York, pp. 355–57.

Scott, D. and O'Neil, D. (1996). *Beyond child rescue: developing family-centred Practice at St Luke's*. Allen & Unwin in association with Institute of Public Affairs, Sydney.

Sherwin, S. (1992). *No longer patient: feminist ethics & health care*. Temple University Press, Philadelphia.

Singer, P. (1993). *Practical ethics*, 2nd edn. Cambridge University Press, New York.

Strang, H. (1996). Children as victims of homicide. *Trends and issues in crime and criminal justice*, no. 53, Australian Institute of Criminology, Canberra.

Tanne, J. (1991). Jail for pregnant cocaine users in US. *British Medical Journal* 303 (6807), p. 873.

Terr, L. (1994). *Unchained memories: true stories of traumatic memories, lost and found*. Basic Books, New York.

Thomas, M. (1972). Child abuse and neglect: Part 1. Historical overview, legal matrix, and social perspectives. *North Carolina Law Review*, 50, pp. 293–349.

Tilden, V., Schmidt, T., Limandri, B., Chiodo, G., Garland, M., and Loveless, P. (1994). Factors that influence clinicians' assessment and management of family violence. *American Journal of Public Health*, 84(4), pp. 628–33.

Valent, P. (1993). *Child survivors: adults living with childhood trauma*. William Heinemann Australia, Melbourne.

van der Kolk, B. (1996). The complexity of adaptation to trauma: self-regulation, stimulus, discrimination, and characterological development. In van der Kolk, B., McFarlane, A., and Weisaeth, L. (eds). *Traumatic stress: the effects of overwhelming experience on mind, body, and society*. The Guilford Press, New York/London, pp. 182–213.

van der Kolk, B., McFarlane, A and Weisaeth, L. (eds). *Traumatic stress: the effects of overwhelming experience on mind, body, and society*. The Guilford Press, New York/London.

Vicki, J. (1995). *Sex and the sect*. Essien, Melbourne.

Watkins, S. (1990). The Mary Ellen Myth: correcting child welfare history. *Social Work*, 35(6), pp. 500–503.

Wilson, J. and Raphael, B. (1993). *International handbook of traumatic stress syndromes*. Plenum Press, New York/London.

Winslade, W. (1995). Confidentiality. In Reich, W.T. (ed), *Encyclopedia of Bioethics*, revised edition. Simon & Schuster Macmillan, New York, pp. 451–59.

Chapter 11   Abortion and the nursing profession

AFP (1989). Toronto Court has rethink to allow women's abortion. *Australian*, 13 July, p. 8.

Ansell, K. (1988). Nile's abortion bill would jail doctors. *The Age*, 28 June, p. 21.

Badham, P. (1987). Christian belief and the ethics of in vitro fertilization and abortion. *Bioethics News* 6.(2), January, pp. 7–18.

Baltimore Sun (1993). US abortion clinics lose civil rights protection. *The Age*, 15 January, p. 6.

Bandman, E.L. and Bandman B. (1985). *Nursing ethics in the life span*. Appleton-Century-Crofts, Norwalk, Connecticut.

Barrett, G. (1992a). Ireland abortion law poll likely. *The Age*, 20 February, p. 9.

—— (1992b). Abortion ruling is threat to EC treaty. *The Age*, 21 February, p. 8.

—— (1992c). Parents of girl in abortion row to appeal against ban. *The Age*, 22 February, p. 7.

—— (1992d). Pressure for change in Irish abortion ban. *The Age*, 24 February, p. 8.

—— (1992e). Court rules against Ireland on abortion. *The Age*, 31 October, p. 8.

—— (1992f). Election, abortion vote in Ireland. *The Age*, 26 November, p. 7.

Barrett, L.I. (1992). Abortion: the issue Bush hopes will go away. *Time* magazine, 13 July, pp. 54–5.

Benner, P. and Wrubel, J. (1989). *The primacy of caring.* Addison-Wesley, Menlo Park, California.

Beyer, L. (1989). The globalization of the abortion debate. *Time* magazine, 21 August, pp. 60–1.

Bioethics News (1993). Pope: rape victims should not have abortions. 12.(3), April, p. 3.

Bolton, M. Brandt (1983). Responsible women and abortion decisions. In Gorovitz, S., Macklin, R., Jameton, A.L., O'Connor, J.M. and Sherwin, A. (eds), *Moral problems in medicine*, 2nd edn. Prentice Hall, Englewood Cliffs, New Jersey, pp. 330–8.

Brody, B. (1982). The morality of abortion. In T.L. Beauchamp and L. Walters, *Contemporary issues in bioethics*, 2nd edn. Wadsworth, Belmont, California, pp. 240–50.

Broekhuijse, P. (1988). Nurse loses job over abortion. *Sunday Telegraph*, 21 February, p. 13.

Buckle, S. and Dawson, K. (1988). Individuals and syngamy. *Bioethics News* 7.(3), April, pp. 15–30.

Canadian Press (1988). Abortion ruling: What does it mean? *Leader Post*, 29 January, p. 1.

Cannold, L. (1994). Consequences for patients of health care professional's conscientious actions: the ban on abortion in South Australia. *Journal of Medical Ethics*, 20(2), pp. 80–6.

—— (1998). *The abortion myth: feminism, morality and the hard choices women make.* Allen & Unwin, Sydney.

Char, W.F. and McDermott, J.F. (1972). Abortions and acute identity crisis in nurses. *American Journal of Psychiatry* 128.(8), pp. 952–7.

Chesler, P. (1987). *Mothers on trial: the battle for children and custody.* Harcourt Brace Jovanovich, New York.

Corlett, D. (1993). Former Yugoslavia. *Victorian Foundation for Survivors of Torture Newsletter*, Spring, p. 4.

Cornwell, R. (1993). US plans to reverse abortion, labor laws. *The Age*, 2 April, p. 8.

Davis, A. and Aroskar, M. (1983). *Ethical dilemmas and nursing practice*, 2nd edn. Appleton-Century-Crofts, Norwalk, Connecticut.

Debelle, P. (1991). Ethics in embryo. *Good Weekend, The Age magazine*, 9 January, pp. 18–24.

Doder, D. (1993). Balkans rape babies face life of shame, rejection. *The Age*, 5 July, p. 8.

Dworkin, R. (1993). *Life's dominion: an argument about abortion and euthanasia.* HarperCollins*Publishers*, London, UK.

Ehrenreich, B. (1985). After two abortions, a clear choice and few regrets. *The Age* 'Saturday Extra', 23 March, p. 7.

Eisenstein, Z.R. (1988). *The female body and the law.* University of California Press, Berkeley.

Engelhardt, H. Tristram Jr (1986). *The foundations of bioethics.* Oxford University Press, Oxford.

—— (ed.) (1989). *Journal of Medicine and Philosophy* 14.(1). Special edition: *Harvesting cells, tisssues, and organs from fetuses and anencephalic newborns.*

Ewing, T. (1998). Abortion crusader fights for just one political cause. *The Age*, 23 March, p. 3.

Fisher, A. and Buckingham, J. (1985). *Abortion in Australia.* Dove Communications, Melbourne.

Gallagher, J. (1995). Collective bad faith: 'Protecting' the fetus. In Callahan, J. (ed.) *Reproduction, ethics, and the law: feminist perspectives.* Indiana University Press, Bloomington and Indianapolis, pp. 343–79.

Gibbs, N. (1990). The gift of life — or else. *Time Magazine*, 10 September, p. 49.

Gillam, L. (ed.) (1989). *Proceedings of the Conference: The Fetus as Tissue Donor: Use or Abuse?* Centre for Human Bioethics, Monash University, Melbourne.

Glover, J. (1977). *Causing deaths and saving lives.* Penguin Books, Harmondsworth, Middlesex.

Graycar, R. and Morgan, J. (1990). *The hidden gender of law.* Federation Press, Sydney.

Griffiths, L. (1988). Fetal transplants spark controversy. *Australian Dr Weekly*, 20 May.

Harper, P. (1983). Lost, but still alive — the natural parents' need to know. In *Proceedings of the Conference: Adoption and AID: Access to Information?* Centre for Human Bioethics, Monash University, Melbourne, 2 November, pp. 29–38.

Health and Community Services (1992). *Adoption: myth and reality. The Adoption Information Service in Victoria*. Health and Community Services Promotions and Media Unit, Melbourne.

Henderson, B. (1975). *Abortion: the Bobigney affair*. Wild & Woolley, Sydney.

Holden, W. (1994). *Unlawful carnal knowledge: the true story of the Irish 'X' case*. HarperCollins *Publishers*, London, UK.

Holmes, P. (1988). Over the limit? *Nursing Times* 20.(84), p. 19.

Howe, D., Sawbridge, P. and Hinings, D. (1992). *Half a million women: mothers who lose their children by adoption*. Penguin, London.

Independent (1992). Jubilation in Ireland as abortion ban lifted. *The Age*, 28 February, p. 6.

Independent, New York Times (1992). Abortion trip ban on rape victim, 14. *The Age*, 19 February, p. 9.

International Council of Nurses (1977). *The nurse's dilemma*. International Council of Nurses, Florence Nightingale International Foundation, Geneva, Switzerland.

Joyce, J. (1997). Gay gene abortion slammed. *BrotherSister*, 126 (20 February), p. 3.

Keown, J. (1988). *Abortion, doctors and the law*. Cambridge University Press, Cambridge.

Lancaster, K. (1983). Secrecy in adoption: a historical perspective'. In *Proceedings of the Conference: Adoption and AID: Access to Information?* Centre for Human Bioethics, Monash University, Melbourne, 2 November, pp. 21–8.

Le Grand, C. (1998). Doctors still risk fines for abortion. *Weekend Australian* 23–24 May, p. 11.

Leo, J. (1983). Sharing the pain of abortion. *Time* Magazine, 26 September, p. 59.

Lifton, B. (1994). *Journey of the adopted self*. Basic Books, New York.

Lifton, R.J. (1986). *The Nazi doctors: a study of the psychology of evil*. Macmillan, London.

Loudon, B. and Wilson, K. (1997). Doctor in gay gene abort call. *Herald-Sun*, 17 February, p. 3.

Lowther, W. (1988). Father seeks right to stop wife's abortion. *The Age*, 26 August, p. 8.

Luker, K. (1984). *Abortion and the politics of motherhood*. University of California Press, Berkeley.

Macklin, R. (1993). *Enemies of patients*. Oxford University Press, New York.

Mandel, T.E. (1985). The use of immature pancreas as a source of tissue for transplantation in diabetes. *Bioethics News* 5.(1), October, pp. 14–22.

McCorvey, N. (1994). *I am Roe: My life, Roe v Wade, and the freedom of choice*. HarperCollins*Publishers*, New York.

Messer, E. and May, K.E. (1988). *Back rooms: voices from the illegal abortion era*. Simon & Schuster, New York.

Morrow, L. (1991). When one body can save another. *Time Magazine*, 17 June, pp. 46–50.

Muyskens, J.L. (1982). *Moral problems in nursing: a philosophical investigation*. Rowman & Littlefield, Totowa, New Jersey.

Noonan, J.T. (1983). From 'An almost absolute value in history'. In Gorovitz, S., Macklin, R., Jameton, A.L., O'Connor, J.M. and Sherwin, A. (eds), *Moral problems in medicine*, 2nd edn. Prentice Hall, Englewood Cliffs, New Jersey, pp. 303–8.

Nursing Times (1985). Midwives demand 24-week time limit for abortions. 81.(30), 24 July, p. 5.

Nursing Times (1988). Nurses in abortion row. 84.(7), 17 February, p. 8.

O'Brien, N. and Price, M. (1998). Abortion charges create state of panic. *The Australian*, 11 February, p. 5.

PA (1987). Law Lords reject father's plea to stop abortion. *The Age*, 26 February, p. 8.

Petchesky, R.P. (1986). *Abortion and women's choice: the state. sexuality, and reproductive freedom*. Verso (imprint of New Left Books), London.

Pojman, L. and Beckwith, F. (eds) (1994). *The abortion controversy: a reader*. Jones and Bartlett, Boston.

Purdy, L. (1996). *Reproducing persons: issues in feminist bioethics*. Cornell University Press, Ithaca, New York.

Rea, K. (1981). Legal semantics. *Nursing Times* 77.(9), p. 351.

Reardon, D. (1998). Pro-life grief over abortion laws. *The Age*, 3 April, p. 7.

Reeves, P. (1998). Stakes raised in WA pay campaign. *Australian Nursing Journal*, 5(8), p. 11.

Reuter (1990a). Belgian king steps down over legalising abortion. *The Age*, 5 April, p. 7.

Reuter (1990b). Abortion issue threatens German treaty. *The Age*, 31 August, p. 7.

Rhode, D. L. (1989). *Justice and gender: sex discrimination and the law*. Harvard University Press, Cambridge, Mass.

Rogers, J. (1992). Rights for rapists. *The Age*, 'Access Age', 19 February, p. 12.

Rohter, L. (1993). Anti-abortion protester kills doctor. *The Age*, 12 March, p. 7.

Rothenberg, L.S. (1987). An ethicist urges offering all options in disability cases. *Kennedy Institute of Ethics Newsletter* 1.(8), February/March, pp. 1–2.

Rowland, R. (1992). *Living laboratories: women and reproductive technologies*. Pan Macmillan, Sydney.

Royal College of Nursing v DHSS (CA) [1981] AC.800.

Rumbold, G. (1986). *Ethics in nursing practice*. Baillière Tindall, London.

Schnookal, R. (1990). Re-introduction of the Bill to abolish Medicare funding of abortion announced. *Alive and WEL* (official newsletter of the Women's Electoral Lobby), October, p. 2.

Senate Select Committee on the Human Embryo Experimentation Bill 1985. (1986). *Human embryo experimentation in Australia*. Australian Government Publishing Service, Canberra.

Shanley, M. (1995). Father's rights, mother's wrongs? Reflections on unwed fathers' rights, patriarchy, and sex equality. In Callahan, J. (ed.), *Reproduction, ethics, and the law: feminist perspectives*. Indiana University Press, Bloomington and Indianapolis, pp. 219–48.

Smart, C. (ed.) (1992). *Regulating womanhood: historical essays on marriage, motherhood and sexuality*. Routledge, London and New York.

Stephens, P. (1987). Tolerance of abortion is much wider now. *The Age*, 7 December, p. 5.

Teo, W. (1975). Abortion: the husband's constitutional rights. *Ethics*, 85(4), pp. 337–42.

The fetal brain cell debate (1988). *Bioethics News* 7.(4), July, pp. 10–11.

Thomas, S. (1986). *Genetic risk*. Penguin Books, Harmondsworth, Middlesex.

Thompson, J.B. and Thompson, H.O. (1981). *Ethics in nursing*. Macmillan, New York.

Thomson, J.J. (1971). A defense of abortion. *Philosophy and Public Affairs* 1.(1), pp. 47–66.

Toner, R. (1993). President in move to reverse policy on abortion. *The Age*, 25 January, p. 6.

Tooley, M. (1972). Abortion and infanticide. *Philosophy and Public Affairs* 2.(1), Fall, pp. 37–65.

Tribe, L. (1985). *Constitutional choices*. Harvard University Press, Cambridge, Mass.

Tschudin, V. (1986). *Ethics in nursing: the caring relationship*. William Heinemann Medical Books, London.

Wainer, J. (1990). Abortion funding abolition Bill. *Alive and WEL* (official newsletter of the Women's Electoral Lobby), February, p. 8.

Wallace, M. (1998). Misrepresentation = confusion on abortion in WA. *Newsletter of the Legal Issues Society, Royal College of Nursing Australia*, 2(1), p. 2–3.

Warren, M. (1997). On the moral and legal status of abortion. In LaFollette, H. (ed.), *Ethics in practice: an anthology*. Blackwell Publishers, Cambridge, Mass, pp. 79–90.

Warren, M.A. (1973). On the moral and legal status of abortion. *The Monist* 57.(1), January, pp. 43–61.

—— (1977). Do potential people have moral rights? *Canadian Journal of Philosophy* 7.(2), June, pp. 275–89.

—— (1985). *Gendercide: the implications of sex selection*. Rowman & Allanheld, Totowa, New Jersey.

—— (1988). The moral significance of birth. *Bioethics News* 7.(2), January, pp. 32–44.

Watson, J. (1985). *Nursing: human science and human care*. Appleton-Century-Crofts, Norwalk, Connecticut.

Werner, R. (1979). Abortion: the ontological and moral status of the unborn. In Wasserstrom, R.A. (ed.), *Today's moral problems*, 2nd edn. Macmillan, New York, pp. 51–74.

Wikler, D. and Barondess, J. (1993). Bioethics and anti-bioethics in light of Nazi medicine: what must we remember? *Kennedy Institute of Ethics Journal* 3.(1), pp. 39–55.

Williams, C. (1993). Children of rape in Bosnia trapped by new policy. *The Age*, 26 July, p. 8.

Winkler, R. and van Keppel, M. (1983). The long term adjustment of the relinquishing mothers in adoption: a research summary. Reprinted as an appendix in *Proceedings of the Conference: Adoption and AID: Access to Information?* Centre for Human Bioethics, Monash University, Melbourne, 2 November, pp. 39–40.

Chapter 12   Euthanasia and assisted suicide

Admiraal, P.V. (1991). Is there a place for euthanasia? *Bioethics News* 10.(4), pp. 10–23.

Amato, J.A. (1990). *Victims and values: a history and a theory of suffering*. Praeger, New York.

Athersmith, F. (1986). Euthanasia could be abused by selfish relatives, says doctor. *The Age*, 3 July, p. 10.

Australasian Nurses Journal (1912). The right to die. 19.(9), 16 September, pp. 304–8.

Australian Dr Weekly (1990). Mercy killing survey, 10 August, p. 10.

Battin, M. Pabst (1983). The least worst death. *Hastings Center Report* 13(2), April, pp. 13–16.

Baume, P. (1996). Voluntary euthanasia and law reform. *Australian Quarterly*, 68(3), pp. 17–25.

Beauchamp, T.L. and Davidson, A.I. (1979). The definition of euthanasia. *Journal of Medicine and Philosophy* 4(3), pp. 294–312.

Beauchamp, T.L. and Perlin, S. (1978). *Ethical issues in death and dying*. Prentice Hall, Englewood Cliffs, New Jersey.

Beloff, J. (1992). Do we have a duty to die? In *Voluntary Euthanasia Society* (1992), pp. 52–6.

Bindels, P., Krol, A., van Ameijden, E., Mulder-Folkerts, D., van den Hoek, J., van Griensven, G., and Coutinho, R. (1996). Euthanasia and physician-assisted suicide in homosexual men with AIDS. *The Lancet*, 347 (24 February), pp. 499–504.

British Medical Association (1986). *News Review* 11.(1), pp. 22–3.

Brock, D. (1993). *Life and death: philosophical essays in biomedical ethics*. Cambridge University Press, New York.

Brovins, J. and Oehmke, T. (1993). *Dr Death: Dr Jack Kevorkian's Rx: Death*. Lifetime Books, Hollywood.

Browne, A. (1990). Assisted suicide and active voluntary euthanasia. *Bioethics News* 9.(4), pp. 9–38.

Campbell, C.S. (1992). Religious ethics and active euthanasia in a pluralistic society. *Kennedy Institute of Ethics Journal* 2.(3), pp. 253–77.

Carrick, P. (1985). *Medical ethics in antiquity*. D. Reidel, Dordrecht.

Cassell, E. (1991). *The nature of suffering and the goals of medicine*. Oxford University Press, New York.

Cassell, E.J. (1982). The nature of suffering and the goals of medicine. *New England Journal of Medicine* 306, pp. 639–45.

Cattanach, J.F. (1985). The distinction between membership of the human species and characteristics of the human being. *Bioethics News* 5.(1), October, pp. 28–30.

Chopra, D. (1989). *Quantum healing: exploring the frontiers of mind/body medicine*. Bantam Books, New York.

Coutinho, R. (1996). Euthanasia and physician-assisted suicide in homosexual men with AIDS. *The Lancet*, 347, 24 February, pp. 499–504.

de Beauvoir, S. (1964 [1987 edn]). *A very easy death*. Penguin, Harmondsworth, Middlesex.

de Wachter, M.A.M. (1992). Euthanasia in the Netherlands. *Hastings Center Report* 22.(2), pp. 23–30.

Dix, A., Errington, M., Nicholson, K., and Powe, R. (1996). *Law for the medical profession in Australia*, 2nd edn. Butterworth-Heinemann, Melbourne.

Donovan, M., Dillon, P. and McGuire, L. (1987). Incidence and characteristics of pain in a sample of medical–surgical inpatients. *Pain* 30, pp. 68–78.

Dossey, L. (1991). *Meaning & medicine*. Bantam Books, New York.

Ewing, T. (1994). Spinal damage: scientists cross the frontier. *The Age*, 13 January, p. 1.

Fletcher, J. (1973). Ethics and euthanasia. *American Journal of Nursing* 73.(4), April, pp. 670–5.

Gibbs, N. (1990). Dr Death's suicide machine. *Time Magazine*, 18 June, pp. 70–1.

—— (1993). Death giving. *Time Magazine*, 31 May, pp. 49–53.

Glaser, R.J. (1975). A time to live and a time to die: the implications of negative euthanasia. In J.A. Behnke and S. Bok (eds). *The dilemmas of euthanasia*. Anchor Books, Anchor Press/Doubleday, Garden City, New York, pp. 133–50.

Glick, H. (1992). *The right to die: public policy innovation and its consequences*. Columbia University Press, New York.

Glover, J. (1977). *Causing death and saving lives*. Penguin Books, Harmondsworth, Middlesex.

Gordon, M. and Singer, P. (1995). Decisions and care at the end of life. *The Lancet*, 346(8968), 15 July, pp. 163–6.

Green, O.H. (1980). Killing and letting die. *American Philosophical Quarterly* 17.(3), July, pp. 195–204.

Greipp, M. (1992). Undermedication for pain: an ethical model. *Advances in Nursing Science*, 15(1), pp. 44–53.

Gruzalski, B. (1981). Killing by letting die. *Mind* 90, pp. 91–8.

Gunn, M.J. and Smith, J.C. (1985). *Arthur*'s Case and the right to life of a Down's Syndrome child. *Criminal Law Review*, November, pp. 693–756.

Hamilton, H. (1995). *Euthanasia: an issue for nurses*. Royal College of Nursing, Australia, Canberra.

Harari, F. (1987). Death can't be legislated, euthanasia committee finds. *The Age*, 1 May, p. 1.

Harari, F. and Clarke, S. (1987). Criticism for bill on rights of dying. *The Age*, 14 October, p. 3.

Hart, R. and Snell, J. (1992). Dr Cox: the nurse's story. *Nursing Times*, 7(88), p. 19.

Hill, C. Stratton (1992). Suffering as contrasted to pain, loss, grief, despair, and loneliness. In Starck, P. and McGovern, J. (1992). *The hidden dimension of illness: human suffering*. National League for Nursing Press, New York, pp. 69–80.

Hirschler, B. (1993). Dying with dignity in Holland. *The Age*, 11 February, p. 7.

Horan, D.J. (1982). Infanticide: when doctor's orders read 'murder'. *Registered Nurse* 45.(1), pp. 75–82.

Humphries, D. (1983). Poll shows most favour voluntary euthanasia. *The Age*, 26 November, reprinted in *The Age reprint booklet, no. 44: Euthanasia*, The Age Education Unit, Melbourne, p. 14.

Johnstone, M.-J. (1988). Quality versus quantity of life: who should decide? *Australian Journal of Advanced Nursing* 6.(1), September–November, pp. 30–7.

—— (ed.) (1996a). *The politics of euthanasia: a nursing response*. Royal College of Nursing, Australia, Canberra.

—— (1996b). The politics of euthanasia: an introduction. In Johnstone, M-J. (ed.), *The politics of euthanasia: a nursing response*. Royal College of Nursing, Australia, Canberra, pp. 13–19.

—— (1996c). The political and ethical dimensions of euthanasia. In Johnstone, M-J. (ed.), *The politics of euthanasia: a nursing response*. Royal College of Nursing, Australia, Canberra, pp. 21–47.

Kamisar, Y. (1978). Euthanasia legislation: some non-religious objections. In Beauchamp, T.L. and Perlin, S. (1978). *Ethical issues in death and dying*. Prentice Hall, Englewood Cliffs, New Jersey, pp. 220–31.

Kanitsaki, O. (1993). Transcultural human care: its challenge to and critique of professional nursing care. In D. A. Gaut (ed.), *A global agenda for caring*, National League for Nursing Press, New York, pp. 19–45.

—— (1994). Cultural and linguistic diversity. In Romanini, J. and Daly, J., *Critical care nursing: Australian perspectives*, W.B. Saunders/Baillière Tindall, Sydney, pp. 94–125.

Kass, L. (1993). Is there a right to die? *Hastings Center Report* 23.(1), pp. 34–43.

Keown, J. (1992). On regulating death. *Hastings Center Report* 22.(2), pp. 39–43.

Kevorkian, J. (1991). *Prescription: medicide. The goodness of planned death*. Prometheus Books, Buffalo, New York.

Kilner, J.F. (1990). *Who lives? Who dies? Ethical criteria in patient selection*. Yale University Press, New Haven and London.

Klemke, E.D. (ed.) (1981). *The meaning of life*. Oxford University Press, New York.

Klotzko, A. (1995). CQ Interview: Arlene Judith Klotzko and Dr. Boudewijn Chabot discuss assisted suicide in the absence of somatic illness. *Cambridge Quarterly of Health Care Ethics Journal*, 4(2), pp. 239–49.

Kuhse, H. (1982). Commenting on David B. Allbrook's paper, 'Medicine and the prolongation of life: does "can" imply "ought"?' *Issues in ethics. Proceedings of the Conference on Medical Science and the Preservation of Life: Ethical and Legal Dilemmas*, November 1981, Centre for Human Bioethics, Monash University, Melbourne, pp. 35–44.

—— (1984). A modern myth. That letting die is not the intentional causation of death: some reflections on the trial and acquittal of Dr Leonard Arthur. *Journal of Applied Philosophy* 1.(1), pp. 21–38.

—— (1987). *The sanctity-of-life doctrine in medicine: a critique*. Clarendon Press, Oxford.

—— (1991). Introduction to the Australian edition. In Humphry, D. (1991). *Final exit: the practicalities of self-deliverance and assisted suicide for the dying*. Penguin Books, Ringwood, Victoria, pp. xi–xv.

—— (1995). Editorial: Oregon — medically assisted suicide becomes law. *Monash Bioethics Review* 14(1), pp. 1–3.

Kuhse, H. and Singer, P. (1985). *Should the baby live?* Oxford University Press, Oxford.

—— (1988). Doctors' practices and attitudes regarding voluntary euthanasia. *Medical Journal of Australia* 148.(20), pp. 623–7.

Lewins, F. (1996). *Bioethics for health professionals: an introduction and critical approach*. Macmillan Education Australia, Melbourne.

Maslen, G. (1986). Should the baby die? *The Age*, 28 June, Saturday Extra, p. 7.

McGuire, C. (1987). Euthanasia without consent. *The Age*, Letter to the Editor, 19 October, p. 12.

Moody, H. (1992). *Ethics in an aging society*. John Hopkins University Press, Baltimore and London.

Muirden, N. (1993). Palliative care and the terminally ill. *St Vincent's Bioethics Centre Newsletter* 11.(1), pp. 13–19.

Nurses' Board of the Northern Territory. (1996). *Position Statement on the Nurse's Role in Euthanasia*. Nurses' Board of the Northern Territory, Darwin.

Nursing Times (1987). Dutch nurses in euthanasia drama. 83.(12), 25 March, p. 8.

Ogilvie, A. and Potts, S. (1994). Assisted Suicide for depression: the slippery slope in action? *British Medical Journal*, 309, 20–27 August, pp. 492–3.

Parker, M. (1994). Active voluntary euthanasia and physician assisted suicide. *Monash Bioethics Review* 13(4), pp. 34–42.

Rachels, J. (1975). Active and passive euthanasia. *New England Journal of Medicine* 292, pp. 490–7.

Radic, L. (1982). Most support the right to die. *The Age*, 23 August, reprinted in *The Age Reprint Booklet, no. 44: Euthanasia*, The Age Education Unit, Melbourne, p. 3.

Reiser, S.J. (1975). The dilemma of euthanasia in modern medical history: the English and American experience. In Behnke, J.A. and Bok, S. (eds). *The dilemmas of euthanasia*. Anchor Books, Anchor Press/Doubleday, Garden City, New York, pp. 27–49.

Rights of the Terminally Ill Act 1995 (NT).

Riley, M. (1998). Mercy death doctor to stand trial for murder, *The Age*, 11 December, p. 11.

Robertson, J.A. (1981). Dilemma in Danville. *Hastings Center Report* 11.(5), October, pp. 5–8.

Royal College of Nursing, Australia. (1996). *Position Statement on Voluntary Euthanasia/ Assisted Suicide*. Royal College of Nursing, Australia, Canberra.

Royal College of Nursing. (1994). Living Wills: Guidance for Nurses, in *Issues in nursing and health*, Royal College of Nursing, London.

Schwartz, R.L. (1993). Autonomy, futility and the limits of medicine. *Bioethics News* 12.(3), pp. 31–6.

Senate Legal and Constitutional Committee. 1997. *Consideration of Legislation Referred to the Committee: Euthanasia Laws Bill 1996*. Commonwealth of Australia, Canberra.

Somerville, M. 1996. Legalising euthanasia: why now? *Australian Quarterly*, 68(3), pp. 1–14.

Staal, H. (1995). Verpleegkundige veroordeeld voor plegen euthanasie. *NRC Handelsblad*: 7 (translated by W Chenhall).

Starck, P. and McGovern, J. (1992). *The hidden dimension of illness: human suffering*. National League for Nursing Press, New York.

Steinbock, B. (1983). The intentional termination of life. In Gorovitz, S., Macklin, R., Jameton, A.L., O'Connor, J.M. and Sherwin, A. (eds). *Moral problems in medicine*, 2nd edn. Prentice Hall, Englewood Cliffs, New Jersey, pp. 290–5.

ten Have, H.A.M. and Welie, J.V.M. (1992). Euthanasia: normal medical practice? *Hastings Center Report* 22.(2), pp. 34–8.

The Age (1986a). AMA chief opposes active euthanasia. 4 August.

—— (1986b). Euthanasia. 1 July, 31 December.

Tooley, M. (1980). An irrelevant consideration: killing versus letting die. In B. Steinbock. *Killing and letting die*. Prentice Hall, Englewood Cliffs, New Jersey, pp. 56–62.

Trammell, R.L. (1978). The presumption against taking life. *Journal of Medicine and Philosophy* 3.(1), pp. 53–67.

Trollope, S. (1995). Legislating a right to die: the Rights of the Terminally Ill Act 1995 (NT). *Journal of Law & Medicine* 3(1), pp. 19–29.

Turton, P. (1987). Last rights. *Nursing Times* 83.(17), 29 April, pp. 18–19.

—— (1992). Euthanasia and the nurses: last rights. In Voluntary Euthanasia Society (ed.) (1992). *Your ultimate choice: the right to die with dignity*. Souvenir Press, London, pp. 92–4.

Twycross, R.G. and Lack, S.A. (1984). *Therapeutics in terminal cancer*. Churchill Livingstone, Edinburgh.

van de Pasch, T. (1995). Letter from the Netherlands. *International Nursing Review* 42(4), p. 108.

van der Arend, A. (1995). President, International Nursing Ethics (& Midwifery) Network (INEN). Letter-to-Megan-Jane Johnstone, dated 15 August.

van der Maas, P., van der Wal, G., Haverkate, I., de Graaff, C., Kester, J., Onwuteaka-Philipsen, B., van der Heide, A., Bosma, J., and Willems, D. (1996). Euthanasia, physician-assisted suicide, and other medical practices involving the end of life in the Netherlands, 1900–1995. *New England Journal of Medicine*, 335(22), pp. 1699–1705.

van der Wal, G. and Dillmann, R. (1994). Euthanasia in the Netherlands. *British Medical Journal*, 308, 21 May, pp. 1346–49.

van der Wal, G., van der Maas, P., Bosma, J., Onwuteaka-Philipsen, B., Willems, D., Haverkate, I. and Kostense, P. (1996). Evaluation of the notification procedure for physician-assisted death in the Netherlands. *New England Journal of Medicine*, 335(22), pp. 1706–11.

Vatican (1980). *Declaration on euthanasia*. Vatican Polygot Press, Vatican City, Rome.

Veatch, R.M. and Fry, S. (1987). *Case studies in nursing ethics*. J.B. Lippincott, Philadelphia.

Vervoorn, A. (1987). Voluntary euthanasia in the Netherlands: recent developments. *Bioethics News* 6.(2), pp. 19–26.

Voluntary Euthanasia Society (ed.) (1992). *Your ultimate choice: the right to die with dignity*. Souvenir Press, London.

Wallace, M. (1991). *Health care and the law: a guide for nurses*. The Law Book Company, North Ryde, Sydney.

Weinryb, E. (1980). Omissions and responsibility. *Philosophical Quarterly* 30.(118), January, pp. 1–18.

Zerwekh, J.V. (1983). The hydration question. *Nursing 83* 13.(1), January, pp. 47–51.

Chapter 13   Suicide and parasuicide

Alvarez, A. (1980). The background. In Battin, M. Pabst and Mayo, D. *Suicide: the philosophical issues*. Peter Owen, London, pp. 7–32.

Amundsen, D. (1989). Suicide and early Christian values. In Brody, B. (ed.), *Suicide and euthanasia: historical and contemporary themes*. Kluwer Academic Publishers, Dordrecht, pp. 77–153.

Aquinas, St Thomas (1978). Whether it is lawful to kill oneself. Reprinted from *Summa Theologica* in Beauchamp, T. and Perlin, S. (eds). *Ethical issues in death and dying*. Prentice Hall, Englewood Cliffs, New Jersey, pp. 102–5.

Aristotle (1976 edn). *Nicomachean ethics* (translated by J.A.K. Thomson). Penguin, Harmondsworth, Middlesex.

Bailey, S. (1994). Critical care nurses' and doctors' attitudes to parasuicide patients. *Australian Journal of Advanced Nursing* 11.(3), pp. 11–17.

—— (1998). An exploration of critical care nurses' and doctors' attitudes towards psychiatric patients. *Australian Journal of Advanced Nursing*, 15(3), pp. 8–14.

Barrington, M. (1983). Apologia for suicide. In Gorovitz, S., Macklin, R., Jameton, A.L., O'Connor, J.M. and Sherwin, A. (eds). *Moral problems in medicine*, Prentice Hall, Englewood Cliffs, New Jersey, pp. 472–6.

Battin, M. Pabst (1982). *Ethical issues in suicide*. Prentice Hall, Englewood Cliffs, New Jersey.

Battin, M. Pabst and Mayo, D. (1980). *Suicide: the philosophical issues*. Peter Owen, London.

Baume, P. (1988). Perspectives on youth suicide. *Australian Journal of Advanced Nursing* 5.(3), pp. 40–8.

Beauchamp, T. (1978a). What is suicide? In Beauchamp, T. and Perlin, S. (eds). *Ethical issues in death and dying*. Prentice Hall, Englewood Cliffs, New Jersey, pp. 97–102.

—— (1978b). An analysis of Hume and Aquinas on suicide. In Beauchamp, T. and Perlin, S. (eds). *Ethical issues in death and dying*. Prentice Hall, Englewood Cliffs, New Jersey, pp. 111–22.

—— (1980). Suicide. In Regan, T. (ed.), *Matters of life and death: new introductory essays in moral philosophy*, Random House, New York, pp. 67–108.

—— (1989). Suicide in the age of reason. In Brody, B. (ed.), *Suicide and euthanasia: historical and contemporary themes*. Kluwer Academic Publishers, Dordrecht, pp. 183–219.

Beauchamp, T. and Childress, J. (1989). *Principles of biomedical ethics*, 3rd edn. Oxford University Press, New York.

Beauchamp, T. and Perlin, S. (eds) (1978). *Ethical issues in death and dying*. Prentice Hall, Englewood Cliffs, New Jersey.

Boyle, J. (1989). Sanctity of life and suicide: tensions and developments within common morality. In Brody, B. (ed.), *Suicide and euthanasia: historical and contemporary themes*. Kluwer Academic Publishers, Dordrecht, pp. 221–50.

Brandt, R. (1978). The morality and rationality of suicide. In Beauchamp, T. and Perli, S. (eds). *Ethical issues in death and dying*. Prentice Hall, Englewood Cliffs, New Jersey, pp. 122–33.

—— (1980). The rationality of suicide. In Pabst Battin, M. and Mayo, D., *Suicide: the philosophical issues*. Peter Owen, London, pp. 117–32.

Brody, B. (ed.) (1989a). *Suicide and euthanasia: historical and contemporary themes*. Kluwer Academic Publishers, Dordrecht.

—— (1989b). A historical introduction to Jewish casuistry on suicide and euthanasia. In Brody (1989a), pp. 39–75.

Browne, A. (1990). Assisted suicide and active voluntary euthanasia. *Bioethics News* 9.(4), pp. 9–38.

Carr, E.H. (1961). *The romantic exiles: a nineteenth-century portrait gallery*. Beacon Press, Boston.

Christian, M. (1997). No suicide dollars. Letter to the Editor. *BrotherSister*, 25 December (no. 148), p. 9.

Clemons, J. (ed.) (1990). *Perspectives on suicide*. Westminster/John Knox Press, Louisville, Kentucky.

Colt, G. Howe (1991). *The enigma of suicide*. Simon & Schuster, New York.

Cooper, J. (1989). Greek philosophers on euthanasia and suicide. In Brody, B. (ed.), *Suicide and euthanasia: historical and contemporary themes*. Kluwer Academic Publishers, Dordrecht, pp. 9–38.

Daly, M. (1978). *Gyn/ecology: the metaethics of radical feminism*. The Women's Press, London.

Davis, A. (1992). Suicidal behaviour among adolescents: its nature and prevention. In Kosky, R., Eshkevari, H. and Kneebone, G. (eds).*Breaking out: challenges in adolescent mental health in Australia*. Australian Government Publishing Service, Canberra.

Deane, J. (1992). Teen suicide. *Sunday Herald-Sun* (Melbourne), 2 February, p. 81.

Demopolous, H. (1968). Suicide and Church canon law. Unpublished doctoral dissertation, Claremont School of Theology, California.

Donnelly, J. (ed.) (1990). *Suicide: right or wrong?* Prometheus Books, Buffalo, New York.

Durkheim, E. (1952). *Suicide*. Routledge & Kegan Paul, London.

Farber, M. (1975). Psychological variables in Italian suicide. In Farberow, N. (ed.), *Suicide in different cultures*. University Park Press, Baltimore, pp. 179–84.

Farberow, N. (ed.) (1975a). *Suicide in different cultures*. University Park Press, Baltimore.

—— (1975b). Cultural history of suicide. In Farberow (1975a), pp. 1–15.

Ferngren, G. (1989). The ethics of suicide in the Renaissance and Reformation. In Brody, B. (ed.), *Suicide and euthanasia: historical and contemporary themes*. Kluwer Academic Publishers, Dordrecht, pp. 155–81.

Foucault, M. (1973). *The birth of the clinic*. Tavistock Publications, London.

—— (1977). *Discipline and punish: the birth of the prison*. Penguin, London.

French, M. (1985). *Beyond power: on women, men and morals*. Abacus, London.

Gibson, P. (1994). Gay male and lesbian youth suicide. In Remafedi, G. (ed), *Death by denial: studies of suicide in gay and lesbian teenagers*. Alyson Pubs, Boston, pp. 15–68.

Glover, J. (1977). *Causing death and saving lives*. Penguin, Harmondsworth, Middlesex.

Hauerwas, S. (1986). *Suffering presence*. University of Notre Dame Press, South Bend, Indiana.

Heckler, R. (1994). *Waking up alive: the descent to suicide and return to life*. Piatkus, London.

Heyd, D. and Bloch, S. (1981). The ethics of suicide. In Bloch, S. and Chodoff, P. (eds). *Psychiatric ethics*, Oxford University Press, Oxford, pp. 185–202.

Holy Bible (new King James version). Thomas Nelson, Nashville, Tennessee.

Hume, D. (1983). Essay on suicide. In Gorovitz, S., Macklin, R., Jameton, A.L., O'Connor, J.M. and Sherwin, A. (eds). *Moral problems in medicine*, Prentice Hall, Englewood Cliffs, New Jersey, pp. 437–42.

Kant, I. (1983 edn). Suicide. In Gorovitz, S., Macklin, R., Jameton, A.L., O'Connor, J.M. and Sherwin, A. (eds). *Moral problems in medicine*, Prentice Hall, Englewood Cliffs, New Jersey, pp. 434–7.

Kaplan, K. and Schwartz, M. (1993). *A psychology of hope: an antidote to the suicidal pathology of Western civilization*. Praeger, Westport, Connecticut.

Kennedy, H. (1992). Why do the kids suicide? Kyneton stunned by youth suicides. *Sunday Herald-Sun*, Melbourne, 16 August, pp. 4–5.

Knight, J. (1992). The suffering of suicide: the victim and family considered. In Starck, P. and McGovern, J. (eds). *The hidden dimension of illness: human suffering*, National League for Nursing Press, New York, pp. 245–68.

Kreitman, N. (1969). Parasuicide. *British Journal of Psychiatry*, 115, p. 746.

Leenaars, A. (ed). (1993). *Suicidology: essays in honor or Edwin Shneidman*. Jason Aronson, Northvale, New Jersey.

Lester, D. and Tallmer, M. (1994). *Now I lay me down: suicide in the elderly*. The Charles Press, Philadelphia.

Lifton, R. (1979). *The broken connection*. Simon & Schuster, New York.

Lindars, J. (1991). Holistic care in parasuicide. *Nursing Times* 87.(15), pp. 30–1.

Margolis, J. (1975). Suicide. Reprinted in Beauchamp and Perlin (1978), pp. 92–7.

Middleton, K. (1994). Act on suicide's tragic toll: expert. *The Age*, 1 March, p. 3.

Motto, J. (1983). The right to suicide: a psychiatrist's view. In Gorovitz, S., Macklin, R., Jameton, A.L., O'Connor, J.M. and Sherwin, A. (eds). *Moral problems in medicine*, Prentice Hall, Englewood Cliffs, New Jersey, pp. 443–6.

Murphy, G. (1983). Suicide and the right to die. In Gorovitz, S., Macklin, R., Jameton, A.L., O'Connor, J.M. and Sherwin, A. (eds). *Moral problems in medicine*, Prentice Hall, Englewood Cliffs, New Jersey, p. 442.

Pegler, T. (1993). Coroner urges tight surveillance of psychiatric patients. *The Age*, 19 June, p. 26.

Plato (1903 edn). *The trial and death of Socrates, being The Euthyphron, Apology, Crito, and Phaedo of Plato* (translated by F. J. Church). Macmillan, London.

—— (1969 edn). *The last days of Socrates* (translated by H. Tredennick). Penguin, Harmondsworth, Middlesex.

Power, T. (1993). Mother's illness drove six-year-old to commit suicide. *The Age*, 17 June, p. 9.

Rauscher, W. (1981). *The case against suicide*. St Martin's Press, New York.

Remafedi, G. (ed). (1994a). *Death by denial: studies of suicide in gay and lesbian teenagers*. Alyson Pubs, Boston.

—— (1994b). Introduction: The state of knowledge on gay, lesbian, and bisexual youth suicide. In Remafedi, G. (ed), *Death by denial: studies of suicide in gay and lesbian teenagers*. Alyson Pubs, Boston, pp. 7–14.

Ryle, G. (1993). Suicide deaths outstrip state's road fatalities. *The Age*, 8 January, p. 3.

Shneidman, E (1985). *Definition of suicide*. Wiley, New York.

—— (1993). *Suicide as psychache: a clinical approach to self-destructive behaviour*. Jason Aronson, Northvale, New Jersey.

Slater, E. (1980). Choosing the time to die. In Pabst Battin, M. and Mayo, D., *Suicide: the philosophical issues*. Peter Owen, London, pp. 199–204.

Smith, D. and Perlin, S. (1978). Suicide. In Reich, W.T. (ed.), *Encyclopedia of bioethics*, The Free Press, New York, pp. 1618–27.

Sophocles (1911 edn). *Oedipus King of Thebes* (translated by G. Murray), George Allen & Unwin, London.

Soubrier, J-P. (1993). Definitions of suicide. In Leenaars, A. (ed), *Suicidology: essays in honor or Edwin Shneidman*. Jason Aronson, Northvale, New Jersey, pp. 35–41.

Stengel, E. (1970). *Suicide and attempted suicide*. Penguin Books, Harmondsworth, Middlesex.

Stubbs, D. (1994). Foreword, to R. Heckler. *Waking up alive: the descent to suicide and return to life*. Piatkus, London, pp. xixiv.

Suicide Prevention Victorian Task Force (1997). *Suicide Prevention Victorian* Task Force Report. Melbourne (available from Information Victoria, 1/356 Collins Street, Melbourne).

Szasz, T. (1988). The ethics of suicide. In T. Szasz. *The theology of medicine*. Syracuse University Press, New York, pp. 68–85.

The Leader (1992). Save young lives. 19 August, p. 8.

Wennberg, R. (1989). *Terminal choices: euthanasia, suicide, and the right to die*. William B. Eerdmans Publishing Company, Grand Rapids, Michigan, and The Paternoster Press, Exeter, UK.

Williams, M. (1997). *Cry of pain: understanding suicide and self-harm*. Penguin Books, London.

Windt, P. (1980). The concept of suicide. In Pabst Battin, M. and Mayo, D., *Suicide: the philosophical issues*. Peter Owen, London, pp. 39–47.

Chapter 14 Quality of life, 'Not For Treatment' and 'Not For Resuscitation' directives

Adams, M. (1984). On life.......and death.......and dots. *Nursing 84* 14.(6), June, pp. 53–8.

Annas, G. (1982a). CPR: the beat goes on. *Hastings Center Report* 12.(4), August, pp. 24–5.

Annas, G. (1982b). CPR: when the beat should stop. *Hastings Center Report* 12.(5), October, pp. 30–1.

Bandman, E. and Bandman, B. (1985). *Nursing ethics in the life span*. Appleton-Century-Crofts, Norwalk, Connecticut.

Bioethics News (1992). 'Not for resuscitation' orders — Britain. 12.(1), October, p. 4.

Brody, B. and Halevy, A. (1995). Is futility a futile concept? *Journal of Medicine and Philosophy*, 20(2), pp. 123–44.

Buchanan, F. (1983). Resuscitation procedures. Letter to the Editor, *Nursing Times* 79.(34), p. 7.

Carson, R. (1982). Commentary. *Hastings Center Report* 12.(5), October, p. 28.

Clinical Ethics Committee, Council of Physicians and Dentists (1984). *Use of life support systems: ethical guidelines relating to use of life support systems*. Royal Victoria Hospital, Montreal, Quebec.

Council on Ethical and Judicial Affairs, American Medical Association (1991). Guidelines for the appropriate use of Do-Not-Resuscitate orders. *Journal of the American Medical Association* 265.(14), pp. 1868–71.

Cowles, K. (1984). Definitions of life and death continue to elude us. *Nursing Outlook* 32.(3), May/June, pp. 169–72.

Curtin, L. (1979). CPR policies: the art of the possible — optimal care vs maximal treatment. *Supervisor Nurse* 10, August, pp. 16–18.

Cushing, M. (1981). No code orders: current developments and the nursing director's role. *Journal of Nursing Administration* 11.(26), April, pp. 22–9.

Dolan, M.B. (1988). Coding abuses hurt nurses, too. *Nursing 88* 18.(12), December, p. 47.

Downie, R.S. and Calman, K.C. (1987). *Healthy respect: ethics in health care*. Faber & Faber, London.

Dunnum, L. (1990). Life satisfaction and spinal cord injury: the patient perspective. *Journal of Neuroscience Nursing*, 22, pp. 43–7.

Fader, A.M., Gambert, S.R., Nash, M., Gupta, K.L. and Escher, J. (1989). Implementing a 'Do-Not-Resuscitate' (DNR) policy in a nursing home. *Journal of the American Geriatrics Society* 37.(6), pp. 544–6.

Foltz, A.T. (1987). The influence of cancer on self-concept and life quality. *Seminars in Oncology Nursing* 3.(4), November, pp. 303–12.

Fredette, S. LaFortune and Beattie, H.M. (1986). Living with cancer: a patient education program. *Cancer Nursing* 9.(6), pp. 308–16.

Freeman, J. and McDonnell, K. (1987). *Tough decisions: a casebook in medical ethics*. Oxford University Press, New York.

Gerhart, K., Koziol-McLain, J., Lowenstein, S., and Whiteneck, G. (1994). Quality of life following spinal cord injury: knowledge and attitude of emergency care providers. *Annals of Emergency Medicine*, 23(4), pp. 807–12.

Germino, B.B. (1987). Symptom distress and quality of life. *Seminars in Oncology Nursing* 3.(4), November, pp. 299–302.

Gert, B., Culver, C., and Clouser, K. Danner. (1997). *Bioethics: a return to fundamentals*. Oxford University Press, New York.

Graham, K.Y. and Longman, A.J. (1987). Quality of life and persons with melanoma. *Cancer Nursing* 10.(6), December, pp. 338–46.

Haines, I.E., Zalcberg, J. and Buchanan, J.D. (1990). Not-for-resuscitation orders in cancer patients — principles of decision-making. *Medical Journal of Australia* 153.(4), pp. 225–9.

Hastings Center (1982). Does 'doing everything' include CPR? *Hastings Center Report* 12.(5), October, pp. 27–8.

Hickie, J.B. (1990). Guidelines for the decision making process for treatment with cardiopulmonary resuscitation. *Reflections* (an occasional publication of the Bioethics Committee of St Vincent's Hospital, University Campus, Sydney), November, p. 1.

Honan, S., Helseth, C., Bakke, J., Karpiuk, K., Krsnak, G. and Torkelson, R. (1991). Perception of 'No Code' and the role of the nurse. *Journal of Continuing Education in Nursing* 22.(2), pp. 54–61.

Humphry, D. and Wickett, A. (1986). *The right to die: understanding euthanasia*. Collins/Harper & Row, Sydney.

Jecker, N. (1993). Saying 'no' to futile treatment. *8th National Bioethics Conference 1993 Presentation Papers*. Christian Centre for Bioethics at Sydney Adventist Hospital, Sydney, pp. 29–41.

Jecker, N. and Schneiderman, L. (1995). When families request that 'everything possible' be done. *Journal of Medicine and Philosophy*, 20(2), pp. 146–63.

Johnstone, M.-J. (1988). A critical bioethical issue. *Australian Nurses Journal* 8.(1), July, p. 8.

—— (1994a). Death and dying in aged care: some ethical considerations. *Proceedings of the Conference Nursing Home Nursing, June 1994*. Ausmed Publications, Melbourne.

—— (1994b). *Nursing and the injustices of the law*. W.B. Saunders/Baillière Tindall, Sydney.

Kanitsaki, O. (1988). Cancer and informed consent: a cultural perspective. Paper presented at Seminar on Controversial Ethical Issues in Patients with Cancer, Heidelberg Repatriation General Hospital, 13 October 1988, Melbourne.

Kellmer, D. (1986). No code orders: guidelines for policy. *Nursing Outlook* 34.(4), July/August, pp. 179–83.

Kopelman, L. (1995). Conceptual and moral disputes about futile and useful treatments. *Journal of Medicine and Philosophy*, 20(2), pp. 109–21.

Kroeger Mappes, E. (1985). Ethical dilemmas for nurses: physicians' orders versus patients' rights. *Bioethics Reporter* 6/7, pp. 408–13.

Kuhse, H. (1987). *The sanctity-of-life doctrine in medicine: a critique*. Clarendon Press, Oxford.

Lipton, H.L. (1989). Physicians' Do-Not-Resuscitate decisions and documentation in a community hospital. *Quarterly Review Bulletin*, April, pp. 108–13.

Lo, B. (1991). Unanswered questions about DNR orders. *Journal of the American Medical Association* 265.(14), pp. 1874–5.

Lo, B., McLeod, G.A. and Saika, G. (1986). Patient attitudes to discussing life-sustaining treatment. *Archives of Internal Medicine* 146, pp. 1613–15.

Loewy, E.H. (1991). Involving patients in Do Not Resuscitate (DNR) decisions: an old issue raising its ugly head. *Journal of Medical Ethics* 17.(1), pp. 156–60.

Macklin, R. (1993). *Enemies of patients*. Oxford University Press, New York.

Mead, G. and Turnbull, C. (1995). Cardiopulmonary resuscitation in the elderly: patients' and relatives views. *Journal of Medical Ethics*, 21, pp. 39–44.

Mitchel, K., Kerridge, I. and Lovat, T. (1993). Medical futility, treatment withdrawal and the persistent vegetative state. *Journal of Medical Ethics*, 19(2), pp. 71–5.

Murphy, D., Burrows, D., Santilli, S., Kemp, A., Tenner, S., Kreling, B. and Teno, J. (1994). The influence of the probability of survival on patients' preferences. *The New England Journal of Medicine*, 330(8), pp. 545–49.

New South Wales Health Department (1993). *Dying with dignity: interim guidelines on management*. NSW Health Department, Sydney.

Nursing Times (1983). RCN slams 'life and death' choice. 79.(24), p. 20.

Parliament of Victoria, Legislative Council, 50th Parliament, 2nd Session (1988). *Parliamentary Debates (Hansards)* 6 (3, 4, 5 & 6), May. See in particular the debate on the Medical Treatment Bill (no. 2), 3 May 1988, pp. 1012–44.

Pellegrino, E. (1985). Moral choice, the good of the patient, and the patient's good. In J. Moskop and L. Kopelman (eds). *Ethics and critical care medicine*. D. Reidel, Dordrecht, pp. 117–38.

Perry, S.W., Schwart, H.I. and Amchin, J. (1986). Determining resuscitation status: a survey of medical professionals. *General Hospital Psychiatry* 8, pp. 198–202.

Rabkin, M.T., Gillerman, G. and Rice, N.R. (1979). CPR policies: the art of the possible — orders not to resuscitate. *Supervisor Nurse* 10, August, pp. 26, 29–30.

Rachels, J. (1986). *The end of life: euthanasia and morality*. Oxford University Press, Oxford.

Regan, K.M. (1983). Life at all costs? Letter to the Editor, *Nursing Times* 79.(26), p. 6.

Reich, W.T. (1978). Quality of life. In Reich, W.T. (ed.), *Encyclopedia of bioethics*. The Free Press, New York, pp. 829–39.

Sage, W.M., Hurst, C. R., Silverman, J.F. and Bortz, W.M. (1987). Intensive care for the elderly: outcome of elective and nonelective admissions. *Journal of the American Geriatrics Society* 35.(4), April, pp. 312–18.

Saunders, J.M. and Valente, S.M. (1986). The question that won't go away. *Nursing 86* 16.(3), pp. 61–4.

Schade, S.G. and Muslin, H. (1989). Do not resuscitate decisions: discussions with patients. *Journal of Medical Ethics* 15.(4), pp. 186–90.

Scofield, G. R. (1991). Is consent useful when resuscitation isn't? *Hastings Center Report* 21.(6), pp. 28–36.

Siegler, M. (1982). Commentary. *Hastings Center Report* 12.(5), October, pp. 28–9.

Social Development Committee, Parliament of Victoria (1987). *Inquiry into options for dying with dignity: second and final report*, April. Government Printer, Melbourne.

Stanley, D.P. and Reid, D.P. (1989). Withholding cardiopulmonary resuscitation: one hospital's policy. *Medical Journal of Australia* 151, 4 September, pp. 257–62.

Stewart, K. and Rai, G. (1989). A matter of life and death. *Nursing Times* 85.(35), pp. 27–9.

The Regan Report on Hospital Law (1985). Institution — 'no CPR policy': Constitutional Issue 25.(12) May, p. 1.

Thom, A. (1988). Who decides? *Nursing Times* 85.(2), pp. 35–7.

Tomlinson, R. and Brody, H. (1990). Futility and the ethics of resuscitation. *Journal of the American Medical Association* 264.(10), 12 September, pp. 1276–80.

Tong, R. (1995). Towards a just, courageous, and honest resolution of the futility debate. *Journal of Medicine and Philosophy*, 20(2), pp. 165–89.

Veatch, R. (1977). *Death, dying, and the boiological revolution*. Yale University Press, New Haven.

Victorian Hospital Association Report (1988). 'Stickers recommended', 42, August–September, p. 3.

Victorian Nursing Council (1988). Resuscitation by the nurse. *Position Statements*, Victorian Nursing Council, Melbourne.

Welch-McCaffrey, D. (1985). Cancer, anxiety, and quality of life. *Cancer Nursing* 8.(3), June, pp. 151–8.

Yarling, R. and McElmurry, B. (1986). Rethinking the nurse's role in 'Do Not Resuscitate' orders: a clinical policy proposal in nursing ethics. In Chinn, P. (ed.), *Ethical issues in nursing*. Aspen Systems, Rockville, Maryland, pp. 123–34.

Chapter 15 Taking a stand: conscientious objection, strike action and institutional ethics committees

Allender, J. and Robinson, P. (1989). Hospital AIDS ban to be outlawed. *The Australian*, 8 March, p. 1.

Almond, B. (ed.) (1990). *AIDS — a moral issue: the ethical, legal and social aspects*. Macmillan, Houndmills, Basingstoke, Hampshire.

anonymous (1983). AMA judicial chairman sees emergence of hospital ethics panels as an inevitability. *Federation of American Hospitals Review* 16, November/December, pp. 30–2.

Athersmith, F. (1989a). Hospital's ban on AIDS to be made illegal. *The Age*, 8 March, p. 3.

—— (1989b). Four per cent of nurses hurt by needles, survey finds. *The Age*, 5 May, p. 3.

Baly, M. (1984). *Professional responsibility*, 2nd edn. H.M. & M. Nursing Publications, Division of John Wiley & Sons, Chichester, UK.

Bauman, Z. (1993). *Postmodern ethics*. Blackwell, Cambridge, Mass.

Beard, B., Lester, L., Ivy, S. and Prince, N. (1988). Obstetrical nurses' attitudes about AIDS: an international study. *4th International Conference on AIDS. Book 1: Final program. Abstracts, Monday June 13, Tuesday June 14*. Stockholm International Fairs, Stockholm, Sweden, p. 505 (no. 9116).

Beardshaw, V. (1982). A question of conscience. *Nursing Times* 78.(9), pp. 349–51.

Beauchamp, T.L. and Childress, J.F. (1989). *Principles of biomedical ethics*, 3rd edn. Oxford University Press, New York.

Benjamin, M. and Curtis, J. (1986). *Ethics in nursing*, 2nd edn. Oxford University Press, New York.

Benn, S.I. and Peters, R.S. (1959). *Social principles and the democratic state*. George Allen & Unwin, London.

Bickley, J. (1988). Why NZNA supports direct action. *New Zealand Nursing Journal* 81.(3), March, p. 6.

Bioethics News (1991). National Bioethics Consultative Committee disbanded. 10.(4), July, p. 1.

Birnbauer, B. (1986). Government wants to hire 500 UK nurses to ease waiting lists. *The Age*, 30 January, p. 3.

Blake, D.C. (1992). The hospital ethics committee: health care's moral conscience or white elephant? *Hastings Center Report* 22.(1), pp. 6–11.

Brennan, L. and the editors of *Nursing 88* (1988). The battle against AIDS: areport from the nursing front. *Nursing 88*, (18)4, pp. 60–4.

Brennan, T.A. (1988). Ethics committees and decisions to limit care. *Journal of the American Medical Association* 260.(6), 12 August, pp. 803–7.

Broad, C.D. (1940). Conscience and conscientious action. First published in *Philosophy*, volume 15; reprinted in J. Feinberg, *Moral concepts*, Oxford University Press, Oxford, 1969, pp. 74–9.

Brodeur, Rev. D. (1984). Towards a clear definition of ethics committees. *Linacre Quarterly* 51.(3), August, pp. 233–47.

Caplan, A.L. (1982). Mechanics on duty: the limitations of a technical definition of moral expertise for work in applied ethics. *Canadian Journal of Philosophy*, supplementary vol. 8, pp. 1–17.

Childress, J.F. (1979). Appeals to conscience. *Ethics* 89, pp. 315–35.

Cole-Adams, P. (1986). As public support fades, the nurses reach a turning point. *The Age*, 12 December, p. 1.

Consumers' Health Forum of Australia (1990). *Legal recognition and protection of the rights of health consumers*. Consumers' Health Forum of Australia, Curtin, ACT.

Cossar, L. (1988). Hospital helps woman to die. *The Herald*, 22 March, p. 1.

Cossar, L. and Evans, J. (1986). Nurses: wider role closer for 'aides'. *The Herald*, 12 December, p. 1.

Coster, P. (1986). After 39 days in a crisis the doctors battle for patients — the nurses to keep their patience. *The Herald*, 8 December, p. 1.

Crabbe, G. (1988). The lonely dilemma. *Nursing Times* 84.(9), p. 18.

Cranford, R.E. and Doudera, J.D. (1984). The emergence of institutional ethics committees. *Law, Medicine and Health Care* 12.(1), February, pp. 13–20.

Curtis, M. (1989). Nurse AIDS anger. *The Sun*, 10 March, p. 3.

Davis, M. (1986a). Use nursing aides, AMA urges. *The Age*, 11 December, p. 10.

—— (1986b). Unions plan strike to support nurses. *The Age*, 26 November, p. 5.

—— (1986c). Casualty nurses to walk out today. *The Age*, 8 December, p. 1.

Davis, M. and Menagh, C. (1986a). Bans threat as unions back nurses' strike. *The Age*, 19 November, p. 1.

—— (1986b). Nurses angered by aides plan. *The Age*, 13 December, p. 1.

Davis M. and Noble, T. (1986). Threats to nurses upset police. *The Age*, 5 November, p. l.

Fitzpatrick, F.J. (1988). *Ethics in nursing practice: basic principles and their application*. The Linacre Centre, London.

Fletcher, J. (1966). *Situation ethics*. SCM Press, Bloomsbury Street, London.

Forrell, C. (1986). Concerned nurses should walk out on their leadership. *The Age*, 10 December, p. 13.

Freedman, B. (1978). A meta-ethics for professional morality. *Ethics* 89, pp. 1–19.

—— (1981). One philosopher's experience on an ethics committee. *Hastings Center Report* 11.(2), April, pp. 20–2.

Fry-Revere, S. (1992). *The accountability of bioethics committees and consultants*. University Publishing Group Inc., Frederick, Maryland.

Gardner, H. and McCoppin, B. (1986). Vocation, career or both? Politicization of Australian nurses, Victoria 1984–1986. *Australian Journal of Advanced Nursing* 4.(1), September–November, pp. 25–35.

Garnett, A.C. (1965). Conscience and conscientiousness. First published in *Rice University Studies*, volume 51; reprinted in K. Kolenda (ed.), *Insight and vision*, Trinity University Press, 1966, pp. 71–83; subsequently reprinted in J. Feinberg, *Moral concepts*, Oxford University Press, Oxford, 1969, pp. 80–92.

Gonsalves, M. A. (1985). *Right and reason: ethics in theory and practice*, 8th edn. Times Mirror/Mosby College, St Louis.

Hart, H.L.A. (1957). Positivism and the separation of law and morals. *Harvard Law Review* 71, pp. 593–629.

—— (1961). *The concept of law*. Oxford University Press, Oxford.

Heisenberg, W. (1990). *Physics and philosophy*. Penguin Books, London.

Hicks, C. (1982). Why I am opposing the doctors. *Nursing Times* 76.(36), pp. 1579–80.

Himsworth, Sir Harold (1953). Change and permanence in education for medicine. *The Lancet* 6790, 17 October, pp. 789–91.

Huerta, S.R. and Oddi, L.F. (1992). Refusal to care for patients with human immunodeficiency virus/acquired immunodeficiency syndrome: issues and responses. *Journal of Professional Nursing* 8.(4), pp. 221–30.

Hughes, Judge C.J. (1978). In the matter of Karen Quinlan. In T.L. Beauchamp and S. Perlin (eds). *Ethical issues in death and dying*. Prentice Hall, Englewood Cliffs, New Jersey, pp. 290–8.

Hume, D. (1888 edn). A *treatise of human nature*. Oxford University Press, London.

International Council of Nurses (1973). *Code for Nurses*. International Council of Nurses, Geneva, Switzerland.

Jennings, B. (1991). Possibilities of consensus: toward democratic moral discourse. *Journal of Medicine and Philosophy*, 16(4), pp. 447–63.

Johnstone, M.-J. (1988). Law, professional ethics and the problem of conflict with personal values. *International Journal of Nursing Studies* 25.(2), pp. 147–57.

—— (1989). *Bioethics: a nursing perspective*, 1st edn. W.B. Saunders/Baillière Tindall, Sydney.

—— (1994). *Nursing and the injustices of the law.* W.B. Saunders/Baillière Tindall, Sydney.

—— (1997). The role and function of nursing ethics committees. *Ethics Society Newsletter* 2(4), pp. 1–4 (published by the Royal College of Nursing, Australia).

—— (1998). *Determining and responding effectively to ethical professional misconduct: a report to the Nurses Board of Victoria*, Melbourne.

Kant, I. (1930 edn). *Lectures on ethics* (translated by L. Infield and J. MacMurray). Methuen, London. See in particular 'Conscience', pp. 129–35.

Kelly, L. (1985). *Dimensions of professional nursing*, 5th edn. Macmillan, New York.

Kordig, C.R. (1976). Pseudo-appeals to conscience. *Journal of Value Inquiry* 10, pp. 7–17.

Kuhse, H. (ed.) (1988). Ethics Committees. *Bioethics News* 7.(4), July, special supplement.

Kuhse, H. and Singer, P. (1985). *Should the baby live?* Oxford University Press, Oxford.

La Puma, J. and Schiedermayer, D. (1994). *Ethics consultation: a practical guide.* Jones and Bartlett, Boston.

La Puma, J., Stocking, C.B., Silverstein, M.D., DiMartini, A. and Siegler, M. (1988). An ethics consultation service in a teaching hospital. *Journal of the American Medical Association* 260.(6), 12 August, pp. 808–11.

Lester, L. and Beard, B. (1988). Student nurses' fear of AIDS. *4th International Conference on AIDS. Book 1: Final program. Abstracts, Monday June 13, Tuesday June 14*. Stockholm International Fairs, Stockholm, Sweden, p. 504 (no. 9113).

Levine, C. (1977). Institutional ethics committees: a guarded prognosis. *Hastings Center Report* 7.(3), June, pp. 25–8.

—— (1984). Questions and (some very tentative) answers about institutional ethics committees. *Hastings Center Report* 14.(3), June, pp. 9–12.

Lewy, G. (1970). Superior orders, nuclear warfare, and the dictates of conscience. In R.A. Wasserstrom. *War and morality.* Wadsworth, Belmont, California, pp. 115–34.

Machan, T. (1983). Individualism and the problem of political authority. *The Monist* 66.(4), October, pp. 500–16.

McCormick, R.A. (1984). Ethics committees: promise or peril? *Law, Medicine and Health Care* 12.(4), September, pp. 150–5.

McKenzie, N.F. (ed.) (1991). *The AIDS reader: social, political, ethical issues.* Meridian, New York.

McNeill, P.M., Berglund, C.A. and Webster, I.W. (1990). Reviewing the reviewers: a survey of institutional ethics committees in Australia. *Medical Journal of Australia* 152 (March), pp. 289–96.

Mill, J.S. (1962 edn). Utilitarianism (reprinted from 1861 edn). In Warnock, M. (ed.), *Utilitarianism.* Fontana Library/Collins, London, pp. 251–87.

Miller, C. (1989). Outrage as hospital bans AIDS. *The Herald* (Melbourne), 7 March, p. 1.

Moreno, J. (1995). *Deciding together: bioethics and moral consensus.* Oxford University Press, New York.

—— (1991). Ethics consultation as moral engagement. *Bioethics News* 10.(2), January, *Ethics committees: a special supplement*, pp. 3–13.

Muir, Judge R. (1978). Opinion in the matter of Karen Quinlan. In T.L. Beauchamp and S. Perlin (eds). *Ethical issues in death and dying.* Prentice Hall, Englewood Cliffs, New Jersey, pp. 285–90.

Muyskens, J.L. (1982a). Collective responsibility and the nursing profession. In Barry, V. (ed.), *Moral aspects of health care.* Wadsworth, Belmont, California, pp. 120–7.

—— (1982b). *Moral problems in nursing: a philosophical investigation.* Rowman & Littlefield, Totowa, New Jersey.

—— (1982c). Nurses' collective responsibility and the strike weapon. *Journal of Medicine and Philosophy* 7.(1), February, pp. 101–12.

National Health and Medical Research Council (1988). *Discussion paper on the ethics of limiting life sustaining treatment.* NH & MRC, Woden, ACT.

New Zealand Nursing Journal (1988). Prostitutes support nurses. 81.(4), April, p. 5.

Newton, L. (1981). Lawgiving for professional life: reflections on the place of the professional code. *Business and Professional Ethics Journal* 1.(1), Fall, pp. 41–53.

Noble, C.N. (1982). Ethics and experts. *Hastings Center Report* 12.(3), June, pp. 7–9.

Nowell-Smith, P.H. (1954). *Ethics.* Penguin Books, Harmondsworth, Middlesex.

Nursing Mirror (1984). ECT nurse loses appeal. 158.(24), 20 June, p. 2.

Nursing Times (1982a). MP calls for conscience clause in Bill. 78.(42), 20 October, p. 1738.

—— (1982b). Secret Wexham report slams Walsh. 78.(38), 22 September, p. 1573.

—— (1983a). Sacked ECT student presses for new hearing. 79.(32), 10 August, p. 18.

—— (1983b). Third nurse sacked over ECT issue. 79.(14), 6 April, p. 17.

—— (1986a). Health staff avoid nurses tending AIDS patients. 82.(44), 29 October, p. 10.

—— (1986b). Nurse loses appeal over refusing to give ECT. 82.(52), 31 December, p. 7.

—— (1988). Nurses urged to strike worldwide. 84.(14), 6 April, p. 5.

Parsons, L. (1982). Why ECT is an ethical issue. *Nursing Times* 78.(9), 3 March, p. 352.

Pirrie, M. (1988). Woman's request to stop respirator had legal basis: hospital. *The Age*, 23 March, p. 3.

Price, T. (1989). New fears on AIDS: hospital ban may spread. *The Sun*, 8 March, p. 3.

Randal, J. (1983). Are ethics committees alive and well? *Hastings Center Report* 13.(6), December, pp. 10–12.

Rawls, J. (1971). *A theory of justice.* Oxford University Press, Oxford.

Ross, J., Wilson, Bayley C., Michel, V. and Pugh, D. (1986). *Handbook for hospital ethics committees: practical suggestions for ethics committee members to plan, develop, and evaluate their roles and responsibilities.* American Hospital Publishing, Chicago.

Royal Australian Nursing Federation (RANF) (Vic) (1986a). *Newsflash.* 10 November, Melbourne.

—— (1986b). *Nurses Action.* September, RANF, Melbourne.

—— (1986c). *Nurses Action.* October, RANF, Melbourne.

—— (1986d). *Nurses Action.* November, RANF, Melbourne.

—— (1986e). *Nurses Action.* December, RANF, Melbourne.

—— (1987). *Nurses Action.* February, RANF, Melbourne.

Rudd, S. (1992). Ethics committees — a forum for nurses? *Australian Medicine* 4 (12), July 6, p. 15.

Rumbold, G. (1986). *Ethics in nursing practice.* Baillière Tindall, London.

Seeskin, K.R. (1978). Genuine appeals to conscience. *Journal of Value Inquiry* 12, pp. 296–300.

Singer, P. (1979). Famine, affluence, and morality. In Wasserstrom, R.A. (ed.), *Today's moral problems*, 2nd edn. Macmillan, New York, pp. 561–72.

Staff of the National Health Law Program (1991). Health benefits: how the system is responding to AIDS. In McKenzie, N.F. (ed.), *The AIDS reader: social, political, ethical issues.* Meridian, New York, pp. 247–72.

Stephens, P. (1986). Should essential workers lose their right to strike? *The Age*, 12 December, p. 13.

The Herald (1986). The achievement of Irene Bolger. Editorial comment, 2 December, p. 6.

Timms, N. (1983). *Social work values: an enquiry.* Routledge & Kegan Paul, London. (See in particular Chapter 3, 'Conscience in social work: towards the practice of moral judgment', pp. 33–44.)

Tschudin, V. (1986). Ethics in nursing: the caring relationship. Heinemann (Nursing), London.

Urmson, J. O. (1958). Saints and heroes. First published in A. I. Melden (ed.), *Essays in moral philosophy*, University of Washington Press, pp. 198–216; reprinted in J. Feinberg, *Moral concepts*, Oxford University Press, Oxford, 1969, pp. 60–73.

Veatch, R. (1972). Medical ethics: professional or universal? *Harvard Theological Review* 65, pp. 531–9.

—— (1977). Institutional ethics committees: is there a role? *Hastings Center Report* 7.(3), June, pp. 22–5.

Viele, C., Dodd. M. and Morrison, C. (1984). Caring for acquired immune deficiency syndrome patients. *Oncology Nursing Forum* 11, pp. 56–60.

Voumard, S. (1988). Ethics committees out of kilter with public opinion, says doctor. *The Age*, 18 May, p. 17.

Vousden, M. (1985). Swallow your pride, or lose your job? *Nursing Mirror* 160.(1), 2 January, p. 23.

Williams, G. (1988). Industrial Report. *New Zealand Nursing Journal* 81.(3), pp. 6–14.

Wilmoth, P. and Pirrie, M. (1988). Whose life is it anyway? *The Age* (Saturday Extra), 23 April.

Women's Electoral Lobby (1987). Comment reported in *Victorian Diary Newsletter* (February), Melbourne.

Young, A. (1994). *Law and professional conduct in nursing*, 2nd edn. Scutari Press, London.

Young, E.W. (1988). Nurses' attitudes toward homosexuality: analysis of change in AIDS workshops. *Journal of Continuing Education in Nursing* 19.(1), pp. 9–12.

Youngner, S., Coulton, C., Juknialis, B.W. and Jackson, D.L. (1984). Patients' attitudes toward institutional ethics committees. *Law, Medicine and Health Care* 12.(1), February, pp. 21–5.

Zohar, D. (1991). *The quantum self*. Flamingo, London.

Zohar, D. and Marshall, I (1993). *The quantum society*. Flamingo, London.

Chapter 16 Promoting ethical nursing practice

Australian Nursing Council Inc. (1997). *National Competency Standards for the Registered and Enrolled Nurse*. ANCI, Canberra.

—— (1994). *National Competencies for the Registered and Enrolled Nurse in Recommended Domains*. ANCI, Canberra.

Beauchamp, T.L. (1982). What philosophers can offer. *Hastings Center Report* 12.(3), June, pp. 13–14.

Blum, L. (1994). *Moral perception and particularity*. Cambridge University Press, New York.

Bohm, D. (1989). Meaning and information. In Pylkkanen, P. (ed), *The search for meaning: the new spirit in science and philosophy*. Crucible, an imprint of The Acquarian Press. Wellingborough, Northamptonshire, UK, pp. 43–85.

Coney, S. (1988). *The unfortunate experiment*. Penguin Books, Auckland.

Corley, M and Raines, D. (1993). Environments that support ethical nursing practice. *AWHONN's Clinial Issues*, 4(4), pp. 611–19.

Curtin, L. (1993). Creating moral space for nurses. *Nursing Management* 24(3), pp. 18–19.

Damasio, A. (1994). *Descartes error: emotion, reason, and the human brain*. Avon Books, New York.

Derry, R. (1991). How can an organisation support and encourage ethical behaviour? In Freeman, R. (ed), *Business ethics: the state of the art*. Oxford University Press, New York, pp. 121–36.

Hoff, C. (1982). When public policy replaces private ethics. *Hastings Center Report* 12(4), pp. 13–14.

Jameton, A. and Fowler, M.D.M. (1989). Ethical inquiry and the concept of research. *Advances in Nursing Science* 11.(3), pp. 11–24.

Johnstone, M-J. (1994). *Nursing and the injustices of the law*. W.B. Saunders/Baillière Tindall, Sydney.

—— (1995). *Inaugural Bennett Lecture. Moral controversy and the search for solutions: some critical reflections for the nursing profession*. Faculty of Nursing, RMIT University, Melbourne.

—— (1996). Ethical decision making in nursing management. In Anderson, J. (ed), *Thinking management: focusing on people*. Ausmed Publications, Melbourne, pp. 214–31.

—— (1998). *Determining and responding effectively to ethical professional misconduct in nursing: a report to the Nurses Board of Victoria*. Melbourne.

Kane, R. (1994). *Through the moral maze: searching for absolute values in a pluralistic world*. North Castle Books, Armonk, New York.

Kruschwitz, R. and Roberts, R. (1987). *The virtues: contemporary essays on moral character*. Wadsworth, Belmont, California.

McCullough, L. (1995). Preventive ethics, professional integrity, and boundary setting: the clinical management of moral uncertainty. *Journal of Medicine and Philosophy*, 20(1), pp. 1–11.

Moreno, J. (1995). *Deciding together: bioethics and moral consensus*. Oxford University Press, New York.

National Women's Consultative Council (1988). *Women into action*. CPN Publications, Canberra.

Oakley, A. (1986). *Telling the truth about Jerusalem*. Basil Blackwell, Oxford.

Pylkkanen, P. (ed). (1989a). *The search for meaning: the new spirit in science and philosophy*. Crucible, an imprint of The Acquarian Press, Wellingborough, Northamptonshire, UK.

—— (1989b). Introduction. In Pylkkanen, P. (ed), *The search for meaning: the new spirit in science and philosophy*. Crucible, an imprint of The Acquarian Press. Wellingborough, Northamptonshire, UK, pp. 13–39.

Scofield, G. (1992). The problem of the impaired clinical ethicist. *Quarterly Review Bulletin*, 18(1), pp. 26–32.

Singer, P. (1982). How do we decide? *Hastings Center Report* 12.(3), June, pp. 9–11.

Solomon, M., Jennings B., Guilfoy, V., Jackson, R., O'Donnell, L., Wolf, S., Nolan, K., Koch-Weser, D. and Donnelley, S. (1991). Toward an expanded vision of clinical ethics education: from the individual to the institution. *Kennedy Institute of Ethics Journal* 1.(3), pp. 225–45.

Tester, K. (1997). *Moral culture*. Sage, London.

Waithe, M.E. and Ozar, D.T. (1990). The ethics of teaching ethics. *Hastings Center Report* 20.(4), pp. 17–21.

Willis, E. (1979). Sister Elizabeth Kenny and the evolution of the occupational division of labour in health care. *Australian and New Zealand Journal of Sociology* 15.(3), November, pp. 30–8.

Yarling, R.R. and McElmurry, B.J. (1986). The moral foundation of nursing. *Advances in Nursing Science* 8.(2), pp. 63–73.

Index

TO THE OWNER OF THIS BOOK

We are interested in your reaction to *Bioethics: a nursing perspective*, 3rd edition, by Megan-Jane Johnstone.

1. What was your reason for using this book?

    _____ university course _____ continuing education course
    _____ college course   _____ personal interest
    _____ TAFE course   _____ other (specify)

2. In which tertiary institution are you enrolled? _____

3. Approximately how much of the book did you use?
    _____ 1/4   _____ 1/2   _____ 3/4   _____ all

4. What is the best aspect of the book?

5. Have you any suggestions for improvement?

6. Would more diagrams / illustrations help?

7. Is there any topic that should be added?

Fold here

(Tape shut)

No postage stamp required
if posted in Australia

Reply Paid 5
The Product Manager
Elsevier (Australia) Pty Limited
Locked Bag 16
ST PETERS 2044